DATE DUE

AUG 0 8 2005		
NOV – 6 2005		
SEP 1 2 2006		
OCT 3 0 2012		
GAYLORD		PRINTED IN U.S.A.

Adult Perioperative Anesthesia THE REQUISITES IN ANESTHESIOLOGY

SERIES EDITOR

Roberta L. Hines, M.D.

Chair and Professor
Department of Anesthesiology
Yale University School of Medicine
New Haven, Connecticut

OTHER VOLUMES IN THE REQUISITES IN
ANESTHESIOLOGY SERIES

Pediatric Anesthesia

Cardiac and Vascular Anesthesia

Regional Anesthesia

Critical Care

Obstetric and Gynecologic Anesthesia

Pain Medicine

Ambulatory Anesthesia

Adult Perioperative Anesthesia

THE REQUISITES IN ANESTHESIOLOGY

Daniel J. Cole, M.D.
Professor of Anesthesiology
Mayo Clinic College of Medicine
Chair, Department of Anesthesiology
Mayo Clinic Scottsdale
Arizona

Michelle Schlunt, M.D.
Assistant Professor of Anesthesiology
Loma Linda University School of Medicine
Loma Linda, California

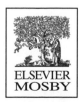

ELSEVIER
MOSBY

ELSEVIER
MOSBY

The Curtis Center
170 S Independence Mall W 300 E
Philadelphia, Pennsylvania 19106

ADULT PERIOPERATIVE ANESTHESIA: THE REQUISITES IN ANESTHESIOLOGY   ISBN: 0-323-02044-5

NOTICE

Anesthesiology is an ever-changing field. Standard safety precautions must be followed, but as new
research and clinical experience broaden our knowledge, changes in treatment and drug therapy may
become necessary or appropriate. Readers are advised to check the most current product information
provided by the manufacturer of each drug to be administered to verify the recommended dose, the
method and duration of administration, and contraindications. It is the responsibility of the treating
physician, relying on experience and knowledge of the patient, to determine dosages and the best
treatment for each individual patient. Neither the Publisher nor the editor assumes any liability for any
injury and/or damage to persons or property arising from this publication.

Library of Congress Cataloging-in-Publication Data

Cole, Daniel J. (Daniel John), 1956-
  Adult perioperative anesthesia: the requisites in anesthesiology/Daniel J. Cole, Michelle
Schlunt.—1st ed.
    p.   ; cm.
  ISBN 0-323-02044-5
  1. Anesthesia.   2. Postoperative care.   3. Surgery, Operative.   4. Anesthesiology.   I.
Schlunt, Michelle.   II. Title.
  [DNLM: 1. Anesthesia—Adult.   2. Surgical Procedures, Operative.   3. Anesthetics.   4.
Perioperative Care. WO 200 C689a 2004]
RD81.C596 2004
617.9'6—dc22

                                                    2004042591

Acquisitions Editor: Natasha Andjelkovic
Developmental Editor: Anne Snyder
Project Manager: Daniel Clipner

Printed in the United States of America

Last digit is the print number: 9   8   7   6   5   4   3   2   1

Contributors

Richard L. Applegate II, MD
Professor
Department of Anesthesiology
Loma Linda University School of Medicine
Loma Linda, California

Sara Arnold, MD
Resident
Department of Anesthesiology
   and Peri-Operative Medicine
Oregon Health and Science University
Portland, Oregon

M.S. Batra, MD
Senior Staff Anesthesiologist
Department of Anesthesiology
Virginia Mason Medical Center
Seattle, Washington

Lauren C. Berkow, MD
Assistant Professor
Department of Anesthesia and Critical Care Medicine
Johns Hopkins Medical Institution
Baltimore, Maryland

Edwin A. Bowe, MD
Professor and Chair
Department of Anesthesiology
University of Kentucky
Lexington, Kentucky

Daniel J. Cole, MD
Professor of Anesthesiology
Mayo Clinic College of Medicine
Department of Anesthesiology
Mayo Clinic Scottsdale
Arizona

Aisling M. Conran, MD
Assistant Professor of Anesthesia and
   Critical Care
Department of Anesthesia and
   Critical Care
University of Chicago
Chicago, Illinois

Annie Côté, MD, FRCPC
Associate-Professor
Department of Anesthesia
McGill University
Montreal
Quebec, Canada

Yulia Demidovich, MD
Resident
Department of Anesthesia and
   Critical Care
University of Chicago
Chicago, Illinois

Thomas P. Engel, MD
Associate Professor of Clinical
   Anesthesiology
Department of Anesthesiology
UC Davis Medical Center
Sacramento, California

Joanne D. Fortier, MD, FRCPC
Associate-Professor
Department of Anesthesia
University of Montreal
Montreal
Quebec, Canada

James S. Hicks, MD
Associate Professor of Anesthesiology
   and Peri-Operative Medicine
Department of Anesthesiology and Peri-Operative
   Medicine
Oregon Health and Science University
Portland, Oregon

Kianusch Kiai, MD, MS
Assistant Clinical Professor
Department of Anesthesiology
David Geffen School of Medicine
University of California, Los Angeles
Los Angeles, California

Michelle S. Kim, MD
Assistant Professor
Department of Anesthesiology
Children's Memorial Hospital
Chicago, Illinois

Jeffrey R. Kirsch, MD
Professor & Chairman
Department of Anesthesiology
   and Peri-Operative Medicine
Oregon Health and Science University
Portland, Oregon

Kenneth Kuchta, MD
Assistant Clinical Professor
Department of Anesthesiology
David Geffen School of Medicine
University of California, Los Angeles
Los Angeles, California

Charles Lee, MD
Staff Anesthesiologist
Department of Anesthesiology
Santa Barbara Cottage Hospital
Santa Barbara, California

Linda J. Mason, MD
Professor of Anesthesiology and Pediatrics
Department of Anesthesiology
Loma Linda University School of Medicine
Loma Linda, California

Rima Matevosian, MD
Associate Clinical Professor
David Geffen School of Medicine
University of California, Los Angeles
Los Angeles, California

Pedro Alejandro Mendez-Tellez, MD
Assistant Professor
Department of Anesthesiology and Critical Care
   Medicine
Johns Hopkins Hospital
Baltimore, Maryland

Michael F. Mulroy, MD
Staff Anesthesiologist, Medical Director of the
   Ambulatory Surgery Unit
Virginia Mason Medical Center
Seattle, Washington

Hamid Nourmand, MD
Assistant Clinical Professor of Anesthesiology
Department of Anesthesiology
David Geffen School of Medicine
University of California, Los Angeles
Los Angeles, California

Parwane S. Parsa, MD
Assistant Professor of Clinical Anesthesia
Department of Anesthesia and Critical Care
University of Chicago
Chicago, Illinois

Piyush M. Patel, MD, FRCPC
Professor of Anesthesiology
Department of Anesthesia
University of California, San Diego
San Diego, California

Ronald W. Pauldine, MD
Assistant Professor
Department of Anesthesiology
Johns Hopkins Bayview Medical Center
Baltimore, Maryland

John Penner, MD, MS
Assistant Professor
Department of Anesthesia and
   Critical Care
University of Chicago
Chicago, Illinois

Michel-Antoine Perreault, MD, FRCPC
Associate-Professor
Department of Anesthesia
University of Montreal
Montreal
Quebec, Canada

Annie Pharand, MD, FRCPC
Staff Anesthesiologist
Department of Anesthesia
University of Montreal
Montreal
Quebec, Canada

José M. Rodríguez-Paz, MD
Assistant Professor
Department of Anesthesiology and
    Critical Care
Johns Hopkins School of Medicine
Baltimore, Maryland

David M. Rosenfeld, MD
Instructor of Anesthesiology
Mayo Clinic College of Medicine
Department of Anesthesiology
Mayo Clinic Scottsdale
Arizona

Melissa R. Rosenfeld, MD
Valley Anesthesiology Consultants
Phoenix, Arizona

Randall M. Schell, MD
Professor
Department of Anesthesiology
University of Kentucky
Lexington, Kentucky

David P. Seamans, MD
Instructor of Anesthesiology
Mayo Clinic College of Medicine
Department of Anesthesiology
Mayo Clinic Scottsdale
Arizona

David M. Sibell, MD, DABA, SCPM
Assistant Professor
Department of Anesthesiology and
    Peri-Operative Medicine
Oregon Health and Science University
Portland, Oregon

Gary R. Stier, MD
Associate Professor
Department of Anesthesiology
Loma Linda University School of Medicine
Loma Linda, California

Lila A. Sueda, MD
Staff Anesthesiologist
Department of Anesthesiology
Virginia Mason Medical Center
Seattle, Washington

Brandon Lucas Villarreal, MD
Assistant Professor
Department of Anesthesiology
David Geffen School of Medicine
University of California, Los Angeles
Los Angeles, California

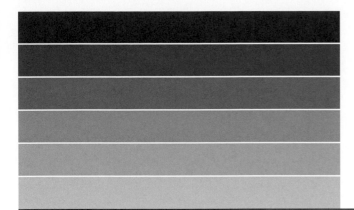

Preface

ADULT PERIOPERATIVE ANESTHESIA should serve as a concise but thorough presentation to the clinical aspects of anesthesia not covered in the other seven volumes of the "Requisites in Anesthesiology" series.

This book is intended for residents rotating through the subspecialties, for practitioners who are preparing for board examinations or recertification, and for the practicing anesthesiologist who desires a quick review for a particular clinical case.

Adult Perioperative Anesthesia is divided into three distinct sections. The first section delineates basics concepts of anesthesia for the perioperative physician. By intent, this section has more detail than the other two sections. The second section focuses on fundamental concepts and the "how to" for specialty specific anesthesia. And finally, a third section addresses special considerations that the practicing anesthesiologist must be familiar with.

Where appropriate, an effort has been made to include educational visual aids which include synoptic boxes that summarize current controversies, clinical caveats, and drug interactions; figures and tables; and in many chapters a relevant case study.

We wish to acknowledge the support and assistance of Allan Ross and Anne Snyder for their invaluable role in the conclusion of this project. Finally, we wish to dedicate this work to the many "teachers" whom we all interact with who extend that extra effort to ensure that we understand the concepts and acquire the skills that are necessary to deliver the highest quality of care to our patients.

Contents

GENERAL
CONSIDERATIONS

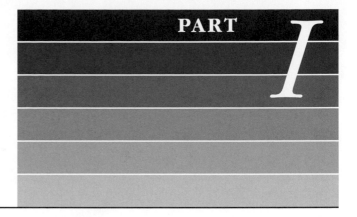

CHAPTER 1

Preoperative Evaluation and Testing

GARY R. STIER

3

INTRODUCTION

The preanesthesia evaluation is a vital component of the anesthesiologist's perioperative responsibilities and practice. The preanesthesia evaluation is defined as the process of clinical assessment that precedes the delivery of care for surgery and nonsurgical procedures and its associated sedative/anesthetic administration; and involves the review of information from multiple sources including the patient's medical records, history, physical examination, and the results from medical tests and evaluations (Box 1-1).

The preoperative anesthesia evaluation involves the following five steps:

1. Identification of disease: this is accomplished by obtaining an accurate medical history, either from the patient, the patient's private physician, or through available medical records, and performing a pertinent physical examination and reviewing available laboratory or diagnostic tests.

2. Assessment of the severity of the underlying disease: this is based upon the assimilation of information obtained from step 1, and modified by further laboratory or diagnostic testing (e.g., stress testing, spirometry) as deemed necessary.

3. Medical optimization or treatment of identified disease; this may include the addition of more aggressive preoperative therapy (e.g., beta-blockers, steroids, antibiotics, anti-hypertensive medications, hemodynamic monitoring, etc.) or surgical delay to allow more time for medical therapy (e.g., treatment of poorly controlled hypertension).

4. An assessment of the preoperative anesthetic risk that is based upon underlying medical diseases, results of the preanesthesia evaluation, and the surgical procedure planned.

5. A discussion of available anesthetic techniques and options including a discussion of postoperative pain control measures.

The preanesthesia history and physical examination should be completed before ordering specific preanesthesia tests. Preoperative tests may be indicated:

• in order to diagnose or identify a disease or disorder that may affect perioperative anesthetic care

• to assess known disease or medical therapy that may impact upon perioperative anesthetic care

• as an aid in the development of a perioperative anesthetic plan.

The timing of the initial preanesthesia evaluation is influenced by such factors as the patient's underlying medical diseases and the particular type of surgical procedure planned (Table 1-1). In general, the preanesthesia evaluation should be performed prior to the day of surgery for the majority of patients, as this allows

Box 1-1   American Society of Anesthesiologists Basic Standards for Preanesthesia Care

These standards apply to all patients who receive anesthesia or monitored anesthesia care. Under unusual circumstances, e.g., extreme emergencies, these standards may be modified. When this is the case, the circumstances shall be documented in the patient's record.

Standard I: An anesthesiologist shall be responsible for determining the medical status of the patient, developing a plan of anesthesia care and acquainting the patient or the responsible adult with the proposed plan.

The development of an appropriate plan of anesthesia care is based upon:

1. Reviewing the medical record
2. Interviewing and examining the patient to:
    a. Discuss the medical history, previous anesthetic experiences and drug therapy.
    b. Assess those aspects of the physical condition that might effect decisions regarding perioperative risk and management.
3. Obtaining and/or reviewing tests and consultations necessary to the conduct of anesthesia.
4. Determining the appropriate prescription of preoperative medications as necessary to the conduct of anesthesia.

The responsible anesthesiologist shall verify that the above has been properly performed and documented in the patient's record.

Approved by the House of Delegates, American Society of Anesthesiologists October 14, 1987.

From the website of: American Society of Anesthesiologists, 520 N. Northwest Highway, Park Ridge, Illinois 60068–2573.

adequate time for preoperative testing and consultations to be completed. For selected patients with low severity of disease and medium- or low-risk surgical procedures, the preanesthesia assessment may be done on the day of surgery. A preoperative patient assessment questionnaire is particularly useful in making the determination of which patients to see before surgery. In those preoperative clinics where the questionnaire is reviewed by appropriate preoperative medical staff prior to scheduling the preoperative visit, nearly one-third of patients may be eligible to have their preoperative medical assessment performed on the day of surgery. This process reduces the number of patients requiring a preoperative visit prior to the day of surgery, and can be utilized to limit the number of tests ordered.

Table 1-1 Recommended Timing of the Preanesthetic Interview and Physical Examination

	Surgical Invasiveness		
	High	Medium	Low
High Severity of Disease			
Prior to the day of surgery	Yes	Yes	Yes
On or before the day of surgery	No	±	±
Only on the day of surgery	No	No	No
Low severity of disease			
Prior to the day of surgery	Yes	±	No
On or before the day of surgery	±	Yes	No
Only on the day of surgery	No	±	Yes

±, evaluation may be acceptable depending upon individual circumstances. Modified from American Society of Anesthesiologists. Practice advisory for pre-anesthesia evaluation: a report by the American Society of Anesthesiologists. *Anesthesiology* 2002;96:485–496.

HISTORY

Obtaining an adequate patient history is the most important part of the preoperative assessment process. This includes a review of a series of pertinent organ-specific questions (Table 1-2), identifying medical diseases (medical records, previous hospitalizations and surgical procedures), noting current treatments, and reviewing the results of recent tests. These questions can be included in a preprinted questionnaire that is completed by the patient. The answers can then be reviewed by a qualified preoperative staff member (i.e., nurse, nurse practitioner, physician) and a decision made regarding whether the patient should be seen a day or more before the scheduled surgery or on the day of surgery (this decision also depends upon the type of surgery planned).

PHYSICAL EXAMINATION

The physical examination is a very important part of the preoperative assessment and should initially focus upon a general examination of the patient (e.g., obesity, cachexia, breathing pattern), followed by an examination of specific organ systems, particularly the airway, cardiac, and pulmonary systems (Table 1-3). In patients with a history of significant disease in other organ systems (e.g., liver disease), the examination should also focus on a general assessment of these organ systems (e.g., peripheral edema, ecchymoses, petechiae).

Airway assessment is the most important part of the physical examination. The initial airway assessment is made by a general survey of the patient's head and neck. Obvious problems such as morbid obesity, short neck, cervical collars, and any breathing difficulties should be noted. The presence of any craniofacial abnormalities may suggest a potentially difficult airway. The presence of a full beard may make mask ventilation more difficult. Mouth opening should be assessed, as it is often related to the ease of laryngoscopy. Adults should be able to open their mouths about two large fingerbreadths between the upper and lower incisors. Limited mouth opening can make visualization of any laryngeal structures challenging. Edentulous patients are typically easy to intubate, while patients with a significant overbite can be more challenging. The presence of loose teeth should be noted and documented on the record. It is important to discuss with the patient the possibility of damage to any loose teeth and a note of this discussion should be recorded in the patient record. Next, the oral pharynx is examined with special notation made of the size of the tongue in relation to mouth opening. The Mallampati classification is commonly utilized in estimating the difficulty of laryngoscopy (Table 1-4). The Mallampati classification uses a simple grading system that is based upon the preoperative ability to visualize the faucial pillars, soft palate, and base of the uvula with the tongue protruded maximally (Fig. 1-1). The degree of difficulty in visualizing these three structures has been shown to be an accurate predictor of difficulty with direct laryngoscopy.

A simple scoring system based upon multivariate predictors of airway difficulty was recently used in preoperative airway assessment. The independent predictors found to correlate with difficult laryngoscopic visualization were: mouth opening, thyromental distance, oropharyngeal (Mallampati) classification, neck movement, ability to prognath, body weight, and history of difficult tracheal intubation. This multivariate airway risk index was determined to be more accurate as compared to only the Mallampati classification at both low- and high-risk levels.

Another measure of potentially difficult laryngoscopic visualization is the thyromental space, estimated by measuring the distance from the inner surface of the mandible to the thyroid cartilage. In adults, this distance should be at least three large fingerbreadths. The size of this area is important as glottic exposure may be difficult if the space is narrowed. A receding chin is associated with an "anterior larynx", which is often a warning that laryngoscopy may be difficult. Finally, the neck should be examined for obvious masses as well as for the degree of extension. A patient with a short, thick neck may result in difficulty with mask ventilation as well as make laryngoscopy difficult. Consequently, the patient should be asked to flex and extend the neck maximally, provided there are no contraindications to this maneuver.

Table 1-2   Preoperative History and Representative Questions (by Organ System)

Organ System	Important Questions
Airway	Do you wear dentures or other dental hardware?
	Do you have loose, cracked, or chipped teeth?
	Do you have difficult opening your mouth fully?
	Do you snore, or do others say you snore?
	Do you have daytime sleepiness or trouble concentrating?
	Do you have neck stiffness or pain on moving your head?
	Have you ever had anesthesia? If yes, did anyone ever say it was hard to place the breathing tube?
	Have you ever been treated for problems with the joints of the head (e.g., temporomandibular joint or "TMJ" problems)?
Cardiac	Have you ever had a heart attack
	Have you ever had chest pain, chest tightness, or angina? If so, does it come with activity or at rest?
	Have you had a complete heart evaluation in the last two years?
	Have you ever had heart surgery?
	Have you ever had fainting spells?
	Do you frequently feel your heart skip beats?
	Have you ever had heart failure?
	Do you take water pills (diuretics)?
	Could you climb one flight of stairs carrying two bags of groceries? If not, why not?
	Do you exercise regularly?
	Do you get short of breath or fatigued when walking briskly?
	Do you have high blood pressure? If so, for how long?
	Do you have high cholesterol? If so, for how long?
Pulmonary	Do you cough regularly? If so, is it a productive cough?
	Do you have emphysema or bronchitis?
	Do you have asthma? If so, do you feel that your wheezing is well controlled?
	Have you ever had to go to the emergency department because you had difficulty breathing?
	Have you ever been on a mechanical ventilator to help you breathe?
	Have you ever taken steroids to help your breathing?
	Do you take inhalers regularly?
	Have you had an upper respiratory tract infection during the last two weeks?
	Have you ever smoked? If so, do you still smoke?
	Have you ever smoked more than a half a pack or more of cigarettes per day?
Gastrointestinal/Hepatic	Do you have frequent heartburn?
	Have you ever been told you have a hiatal hernia?
	Have you ever had hepatitis?
	Have you ever had jaundice?
	Do you have, or been told you have, liver cirrhosis?
	Do you drink more than 6 beers (or equivalent) per day?
Hematologic	Have you ever had a blood transfusion? If so, when?
	Have you ever had prolonged or unusual bleeding from cuts, nosebleeds, minor bruises, tooth extractions, or surgery?
	Has a family member or blood relative ever had a serious bleeding problem?
Endocrine	Have you ever been told that you have high blood sugars?
	Do you have diabetes mellitus? If so, for how long?
	Have you ever taken insulin for your diabetes? If so, how long?
	Have you ever taken pills to control your blood sugar levels?
	Do you take, or have you taken, steroids or cortisone in the last year?
	Do you have thyroid gland problems?
	Have you ever taken thyroid medicine or had radioactive iodine for thyroid disease?
Renal	Have you ever had any kidney problems (infections, stones)?
	Do you have burning with urination?
	Do you have an increased frequency of urination?
	Have you ever had kidney failure?
	Have you ever been on kidney dialysis?
Neurologic	Have you ever had a seizure?
	Have you ever had a stroke?

Table 1-2 Preoperative History and Representative Questions (by Organ System)—cont'd

Organ System	Important Questions
Miscellaneous	Have you ever had numbness, or a tingling feeling in your arm or leg that has lasted more than a few hours? Have you ever been diagnosed as having a tremor? Have you ever had multiple sclerosis, or any other disorder of the nervous system? Have you taken antidepressant, sedative, tranquilizing, or anti-seizure medications in the last year? Within the last 2 years, have you used recreational drugs such as amphetamines, cocaine, crack, heroin, or other narcotics? Have you ever been exposed to someone with HIV (body fluids)? Has any close family relative ever had a high fever requiring hospitalization or died after an anesthetic? Have you ever had any problems with a previous anesthetic? If so, what was the problem?

Extension of the head should be assessed, with normal extension being about 80°; lesser degrees of extension represent limitation and may be associated with difficult laryngoscopy.

After the airway examination, the pulmonary examination begins with an overall view of the breathing pattern of the patient. A labored or tachypneic breathing pattern may indicate poorly controlled or end-stage pulmonary disease. Auscultation of the lungs should focus on breath sounds. The presence of rales should suggest interstitial pulmonary edema from congestive heart failure (CHF), while wheezing is indicative of reactive airway disease that is poorly controlled. Wheezing occurring in the expiratory phase is more indicative of reactive airway disease (e.g., asthma), while inspiratory wheezing may indicate partial airway obstruction (glottic or tracheal stenosis).

The cardiac examination includes a determination of blood pressure and auscultation of the heart. Particular attention should be focused upon the rate and rhythm, as well as the presence of heart murmurs. If a murmur is present, the location and radiation of the murmur as well as the phase of the cardiac cycle in which the murmur is heard should be noted. (e.g., systole, diastole). A loud coarse murmur heard best in systole along the right parasternal border at the level of the second interspace that radiates to the neck may indicate aortic stenosis. The presence of additional heart sounds such as a third or fourth heart sound should be noted.

PREOPERATIVE TESTING

Patients scheduled for elective surgery typically undergo a battery of routine preoperative tests. The purpose of preoperative testing accomplishes a number of goals:

- to detect abnormalities that may change anesthetic management and reduce perioperative morbidity and mortality

- to reduce overall cost through a decrease in utilization of hospital resources (e.g., length of hospitalization)
- to improve outcome.

Unfortunately, the very process of routine preoperative testing is costly and often leads to further testing if results are abnormal. This, in turn, may delay surgery while the patient undergoes further medical investigation. Consequently, the need for routine preoperative tests in healthy patients scheduled for elective surgery must be clearly beneficial for this process to be supported. Unfortunately, routine preoperative testing is not supported by the literature. Multiple studies on routine preoperative screening have found only 1–2% of tests to be significantly abnormal. In addition, there is little evidence to show that these abnormalities have any effect on overall perioperative management. The data supports a conclusion that, if the history and physical examination disclose no preoperative indications for laboratory testing, then anesthesia and surgery may proceed without further testing with virtually no increased perioperative risk. Even in elderly patients, the data do not support a correlation between abnormal preoperative laboratory values and postoperative outcome. Accordingly, preoperative testing for hemoglobin, creatinine, glucose, and electrolytes on the basis of age alone does not appear to be indicated. Preoperative testing should, therefore, be based primarily upon indications specific to a patient in whom either clinical findings or risk factors for particular diseases that may impact perioperative outcome (Table 1-5) are present. If preoperative testing is based on this rationale, nearly 60% of preoperative tests may be eliminated.

SPECIFIC PREOPERATIVE TESTS

Electrocardiogram

Although preoperative screening electrocardiograms (ECG) are of benefit in certain patient groups (Table 1-6), little benefit is seen in healthy patients <50 years of age

Table 1-3 Keypoints in the Physical Examination by Organ System

Organ system	Areas of focus
Airway	Mouth opening
	Thyromental distance
	Oropharyngeal (Mallampati) classification
	Neck movement
	Ability to prognath (move jaws forward)
	Body weight
	History of difficult tracheal intubation
Cardiac	Rate
	Rhythm
	Murmurs (systolic or diastolic, quality location, grade)
	Presence of a S_3 or S_4
	Carotid pulsation (rate of upstroke, bruit)
Pulmonary	Breathing pattern (tachypnea, retractions)
	Breath sounds (present, locally absent, wheezing, rhonchi, rales)
	Scoliosis
	Kyphosis
	Barrel chest
Hepatic	Ascites
	Cachexia
	Bruising
	Jaundice
Hematologic	Skin color (pale)
	Petechiae
	Ecchymoses
Renal	Signs of debilitation
	Peripheral edema
	Bruising
	Neurologic irritability (e.g., asterixis in uremia)
Neurologic	Mental status
	Focal neurologic deficits
	Movement disorders (e.g., Parkinsonism)
Musculoskeletal	Muscle strength
	Deformities (spinal, joint)
	Arthritis

Table 1-4 Mallampati Airway Classification

Class	Visualization of Oral Structures	Laryngoscopic View
I	Soft palate, fauces, uvula, pillars	Excellent
II	Soft palate, fauces, uvula	Good
III	Soft palate, tip of uvula only	Poor
IV	Hard palate only	Difficult to absent

Modified from Dierdorf SF. Anesthesia and informed consent. *Curr Opin Anaesthesiol* 2002;15:349–350.

Hemoglobin

The preoperative determination of hemoglobin has generally been routine. Although the traditional goal has historically been to keep the hemoglobin above 10 g/dL, no data have ever been presented to substantiate any improvement in perioperative outcome by obtaining set hemoglobin targets. Of more clinical relevance is the practice of correlating the level of hemoglobin with the patient's underlying medical condition. For example, a patient with acute anemia and extensive underlying cardiopulmonary disease scheduled for moderate-major surgery (intrathoracic, major vascular, upper abdominal, intracranial operations) would most probably benefit from a preoperative increase in hemoglobin, while a dialysis patient with well-compensated chronic anemia of renal disease and absent cardiopulmonary disease might be expected to better tolerate a given level of anemia. In otherwise healthy patients, the incidence of undiagnosed anemia ranges from 0.5% to

with no cardiovascular risk factors. Indeed, the finding of significant ECG abnormalities (e.g., Q waves, ST-segment abnormalities, or T-wave inversions) has little prognostic significance in terms of perioperative outcome and long-term survival. Moreover, the physical examination and history should detect any significant dysrhythmias that might occur in an asymptomatic healthy patient younger than 50 years. Conversely, a screening preoperative ECG should be obtained in patients with known cardiovascular disease, or significant risk factors for cardiovascular disease.

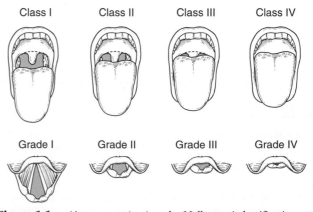

Figure 1-1 Airway examination: the Mallampati classification and laryngeal grade.

Table 1-5 Preoperative Indications for Specific Tests

Preoperative Test	Indications
Electrocardiogram	Age >50 years
	Cardiac disease (present or past)
	Hypertension
	Vascular disease (present or past)
	Diabetes mellitus (age >40 years)
	Respiratory disease
	Type and invasiveness of surgery
Chest radiograph	Active cardiac disease or history of myocardial infarction/congestive heart failure
	Recent upper respiratory tract infection with symptoms
	Chronic obstructive pulmonary disease with symptoms or acute episode within 6 months
	Significant smoking history with symptoms
	Cardiothoracic, major vascular, major upper abdominal procedures
Hemoglobin/Hematocrit	Extremes of age (neonates, elderly)
	History of anemia
	Bleeding disorders
	Neoplasia
	Hematologic diseases
	Chemotherapy
Complete blood count	Hematologic disorder
	Vascular procedure
	Chemotherapy
Coagulation studies	Bleeding disorders
	Renal dysfunction
	Liver dysfunction
	Anticoagulant therapy
	Vascular procedure
	Major blood loss surgery
Serum electrolytes	Renal dysfunction
	Diuretics
	Diabetes
	Endocrine disorders
	History of serious dysrhythmias
	Digoxin
	Major vascular surgery (with aortic cross-clamp)
Blood glucose	Diabetes mellitus
	Elderly (>60 years) undergoing moderate–major surgery
	Steroids
	Obesity
	Intracranial procedures or cardiac surgery (with bypass)
Pulmonary function tests (spirometry)	Severe reactive airway disease
	Severe chronic obstructive pulmonary disease
	Scoliosis
	Type and invasiveness of surgery
Pregnancy test	Uncertain pregnancy history
	History suggestive of current pregnancy
Urinalysis	Urinary symptoms
	Prosthesis implantation
	Urologic surgery

5%, the highest incidence of anemia being in infants less than 1 year old, in young women, and in older men (>65 years). It would therefore be reasonable for these higher-risk patients to undergo routine preoperative hemoglobin determination. The clinical indications for preoperative hemoglobin determination are listed in Box 1-2.

Chest Radiography

Chest radiographs are routinely ordered as part of the preoperative clearance process. Unfortunately, little evidence has been obtained that a preoperative chest radiograph, even in high-risk patients, changes perioperative management, improves perioperative outcome, or

Table 1-6   Indications for Preoperative Screening Electrocardiography (ECG) in Selected Patient Groups

Patient Group	Screening ECG	Comments
Healthy, ≤50 years old, no cardiac risk factors*	No	Annual incidence of coronary artery disease in this patient population is low Incidence of significant dysrhythmias usually detected by history and physical examination Incidence of significant ST-segment abnormalities low Incidence of ECG abnormalities in asymptomatic patient without risk factors has little effect on perioperative outcome or long-term survival
Healthy >50 years old	Yes	Increased incidence of occult cardiac disease
Healthy >50 years old for major surgery† (e.g., vascular)	Yes	Incidence of perioperative ECG changes and myocardial ischemia is increased
Cardiovascular risk factors	Yes	Prevalence of coronary artery disease is increased Increased incidence of intra- and postoperative abnormalities Baseline ECG may avoid postoperative cardiac workup
Previous ECG		
Patient <50 years; previous ECG normal; no change in clinical symptoms	No	Little benefit found in this patient group
Increased risk of coronary artery disease	Yes	Patients with diabetes and/or cardiovascular disease should have a repeat ECG within 2 months of surgery because of a higher likelihood of significant changes
Previously abnormal ECG	Yes	Increased likelihood of significant changes

* Significant risk factors include: known atherosclerotic heart disease (previous myocardial infarction, angina), peripheral vascular disease, long-standing hypertension, diabetes mellitus, left ventricular hypertrophy, congestive heart failure, hypercholesterolemia, or diseases with high probability of cardiac involvement (end-stage renal disease, collagen vascular diseases, bacteremia, metastatic neoplasms).
† Major surgery is defined as intrathoracic, major vascular, upper abdominal, or intracranial operations.

predicts postoperative cardiopulmonary complications. A preoperative chest radiograph should, therefore, be limited to clinical situations where there is an increased risk of abnormalities or when the history or physical examination suggests active pulmonary disease (Box 1-3).

Box 1-2   Indications for Preoperative Hemoglobin Determination

All female patients
Males >65 years
Neonates (<60 weeks postconceptual age)
Patients who have a >20 pack-year history of smoking
Operations where there is a high likelihood of major blood loss
Chronic renal failure
Known anemia
Bleeding disorders (including patients taking anticoagulant medications)
Hemorrhage
Malignancy (especially hematologic malignancy)
Radiation/chemotherapy
Other potentially relevant diseases (e.g. some infections, liver diseases, or malnutrition)

Prothrombin and Partial Thromboplastin Times

Preoperative coagulation testing is indicated only in selected clinical situations (Box 1-4). A routine screening preoperative prothrombin time (PT) and partial thromboplastin time (PTT) are of no value in asymptomatic patients without risk factors for bleeding abnormalities. Moreover, bleeding times are inaccurate in predicting intraoperative bleeding tendencies and are no longer used in the preoperative setting. In patients scheduled for a major surgical procedure with the potential for significant blood loss, a screening preoperative PT and PTT may be of value as a baseline for comparison with postoperative coagulation studies should clinical coagulopathy appear in the postoperative period.

Electrolytes, Glucose, Blood Urea Nitrogen, Creatinine

Preoperative serum electrolyte determinations are not routinely indicated. Rather, such testing should be based upon the presence of risk factors suggesting abnormalities, as determined by history and physical examination,

Box 1-3   Indications for Preoperative Chest Radiographs

Cardiovascular disease
- Congestive heart failure or suspected cardiomegaly (long-standing hypertension)*
- Ischemic cardiac disease
- Known or suspected valvular heart disease
- Symptoms of active cardiovascular disease (dyspnea)

Pulmonary disease
- Chronic pulmonary disease (asthma, obstructive pulmonary disease) with symptoms
- Recent upper respiratory tract infection with symptoms
- Long history of smoking (>20 years) for major surgery

Oncologic process (where chance of pulmonary metastasis is present)

Major thoracic, vascular, or upper abdominal surgery

These recommendations apply to patients undergoing moderate to major surgical procedures. Chest radiographs in patients scheduled for minor surgery are not routinely ordered for any patient unless physical and history indicate the result may change anesthetic management.

* If cardiomegaly is present on chest radiograph, an echocardiographic examination should be considered to assess left ventricular function.

underlying medical diseases, or previous abnormalities. Specific indications for electrolyte testing are listed in Box 1-5.

Patients with hypokalemia (<3.0 mEq/L) present a common problem. Of most importance is whether the abnormality is acute or chronic. Rapid correction of chronic hypokalemia is probably more dangerous than no treatment. Although no definite level of hypokalemia

Box 1-4   Indications for Preoperative Coagulation Testing

ABSOLUTE INDICATIONS FOR TESTING

Positive risk factors
- Anticoagulant therapy
- Liver disease
- Alcoholism
- Malnourishment
- Malabsorption syndromes
- Family history of bleeding disorders with prior operations or dental work

RELATIVE INDICATIONS FOR TESTING

Major surgical procedures where large blood loss is anticipated (e.g., major vascular)

Box 1-5   Indications for Preoperative Testing of Serum Electrolytes

Cardiac disease
- Congestive heart failure
- Dysrhythmias
- Ischemic heart disease

Pulmonary disease

Renal disease

Hepatic disease

Diabetes mellitus

Pharmacologic
- Diuretics
- Corticosteroids
- Chemotherapy (e.g., *cis*-platinum)
- Amphotericin B

Bowel preparation

Patients older than 60 years undergoing prolonged surgery with major blood loss

contraindicates surgery, few perioperative problems have been documented in healthy patients with chronic hypokalemia as low as 2.5 mEq/L; however, elective cases are typically postponed for values less than 3.0 mEq/L unless adequate documentation is present to note that the hypokalemia has been chronically present. Preoperative testing of blood glucose levels, blood urea nitrogen (BUN), and serum creatinine (Cr) should be performed in those patients where the known incidence of significant abnormalities is elevated (Boxes 1-6 and 1-7)

Liver Function Tests

The likelihood of finding elevated liver enzymes in the asymptomatic patient is very low (1 in 700); therefore, preoperative testing of liver function should be limited to selected patients with risk factors or clinical findings as listed in Box 1-8. In patients with an aspartate aminotransferase (AST) level greater than twice normal, further

Box 1-6   Indications for Preoperative Glucose Testing

Known diabetes mellitus (type 1 or 2)

Patients >60 years undergoing moderate to major surgery

Patients on systemic steroids undergoing moderate-major surgery

Obese patients undergoing moderate–major surgery

Surgery for ongoing soft tissue infection

Surgery involving cardiac bypass

Craniotomies

Box 1-7 Indications for Preoperative Blood Urea Nitrogen and Serum Creatinine Testing

Diseases with increased incidence of renal dysfunction
- Diabetes mellitus
- Moderate–severe hypertension
- Severe liver dysfunction
- Severe atherosclerotic vascular disease

Recent use of nephrotoxic drugs
- Intravenous contrast dye
- Aminoglycosides
- Recent initiation of angiotensin-converting-enzyme inhibitors without previous creatinine determination

Operations at risk of perioperative renal ischemia
- Aortic cross-clamping
- Cardiac bypass surgery

clinical evaluation should include repeat AST testing, and if still elevated, a full liver enzyme panel, along with a serum bilirubin, hepatitis panel, and possibly preoperative consultation.

Urinalysis

A preoperative screening urinalysis is not indicated in asymptomatic patients scheduled for surgery. If, however, the patient has signs or symptoms suggesting a urinary tract infection (UTI), then a urinalysis should be performed preoperatively. If evidence exists for a UTI, preoperative treatment is generally indicated. Diabetic patients might reasonably have a preoperative screening urinalysis to search specifically for proteinuria, an indication of early diabetic nephropathy. In patients scheduled for surgical procedures involving the genitourinary tract, a preoperative urinalysis is often desired by the surgical team as the risk of infection may be increased with manipulation of the urinary

Box 1-8 Indications for Preoperative AST Liver Enzyme Testing

History of excessive alcohol intake
History of or known exposure to hepatitis
Patients undergoing major upper abdominal surgery in which surgical traction can cause hepatic ischemia
Drugs associated with liver damage (hydralazine, methotrexate, other known liver toxins)
Morbid obesity
Malignancy

tract. Patients undergoing other procedures such as hip or knee arthroplasty typically have a preoperative screening urinalysis performed; however, the evidence to support such a practice is lacking. No other types of surgical procedure are impacted upon by the results of a preoperative screening urinalysis (Table 1-7).

Repeat Laboratory Testing Before Surgery

Although the time between testing and the scheduled surgery is still debated, in general, for healthy patients or patients with specific risk factors whose previous testing disclosed no abnormalities and there has been no change in clinical status, test results within 1–6 months prior to surgery is generally acceptable. Repeat testing may be indicated when the medical condition has changed, or when test results may be required to make choices regarding anesthetic techniques (e.g., regional anesthesia in the setting of anticoagulation therapy).

AMERICAN SOCIETY OF ANESTHESIOLOGISTS PHYSICAL CLASSIFICATION

After obtaining the patient history, performing the physical examination, reviewing laboratory and diagnostic testing, and taking into consideration the type and length of the surgical procedure, an American Society of Anesthesiologists (ASA) Physical Classification assignment should be applied (Table 1-8). This classification serves as a general categorization of patient sickness rather than an accurate predictor of perioperative risk. In short, the results of the preanesthesia evaluation will enable the anesthesiologist to determine whether the patient is in the best possible shape for surgery given the underlying medical condition. An appropriate anesthetic plan can then be formulated, taking into consideration the postoperative period.

INFORMED CONSENT

Informed consent is a necessary part of the preoperative assessment. The inability to obtain an informed consent may place the anesthesiologist at an increased medicolegal risk should an adverse event occur. Informed consent is obtained when a competent adult agrees to a therapeutic or diagnostic procedure after the risks of the procedure and any alternatives have been explained. The side effects, risks, and complications of the procedure should be presented in the context of the patient's underlying medical diseases. The role of the person obtaining the consent, therefore, is to present patients with the

Table 1-7   Summary of Selected Preoperative Testing

Patient Type	ECG	Hb (M)	Hb (F)	CBC	Electrolytes/ Glucose	BUN/Cr	PT/PTT	UA	LFTs	CXR
Healthy 50										
Age <50 years			X							
Age ≥50 years	X		X							
Neonate		X	X							
Medical Disease										
Cardiac disease	X	X	X		X	X				X
Pulmonary disease	X	X	X							X
Smoking (>20 pack-years)	X	X	X							X
Renal disease	X	X	X		X	X				
Hepatic disease		X	X	X	X	X	X		X	
Hypertension	X	X	X		X	X				
Diabetes	X	X	X		X	X		X		
Vascular disease	X	X	X		X	X				
Neurologic disease	X	X	X		X	X				
Cancer		X	X	X	X					X
Symptoms of UTI								X		
Chemotherapy		X	X	X	X	X				
Diuretics	X				X	X				
Corticosteroids				X						
Anticoagulants		X	X	X			X			
Major surgery	X	X	X	X	X	X	X			
Urologic surgery							X			
Cardiac surgery	X	X	X	X	X	X	X		X	

BUN, blood urea nitrogen; CBC, complete blood count; Cr, creatinine; CXR, chest radiograph; ECG, electrocardiogram; F, female; Hb, hemoglobin; LFTs, liver function tests; M, male; PT, prothrombin time; PTT, partial thromboplastin time; UA, urinalysis; UTI, urinary tract infection.

Table 1-8   American Society of Anesthesiologists (ASA) Physical Status Classification

Status	Disease State
ASA Class I	No organic, physiologic, biochemical, or psychiatric disturbance
ASA Class II	Mild to moderate systemic disturbance that may not be related to the reason for surgery
ASA Class III	Severe systemic disturbance that may or may not be related to the reason for surgery
ASA Class IV	Severe systemic disturbance that is life-threatening with or without surgery
ASA Class V	Moribund patient who has little chance of survival but is submitted to surgery as a last resort (resuscitative effort)
Emergency Operation (E)	Any patient in whom an emergency operation is required

information required to permit them to make a rational choice. The information discussed should be that which a reasonable patient would consider necessary, and should be discussed with the patient's perspective kept in mind. The informed consent is thus a shared decision-making process with the patient. The time spent explaining the plan for anesthesia and the potential complications is important in establishing rapport between patient and physician and may avert future complaints. A preprinted anesthesia-specific consent form can be helpful as the starting point for the informed consent discussion and the patient's signature at least verifies that the discussion took place (see Appendix). Careful consideration of what information the patient would like to receive and preparation of a carefully crafted consent document can improve the effectiveness and efficiency of obtaining informed consent.

Anesthesia Risk

Risk is the degree of likelihood that an adverse event will occur. Estimating perioperative risk is difficult and inaccurate because of differences in the terminology used (anesthesia-related versus anesthesia alone) and

Table 1-9 Risk Factors and Perioperative Mortality	
Risk Factor	**Mortality in Hospital (%)**
Age >80	5.8
Ischemic heart disease	2.9
Myocardial infarction	
>1 year	4.0
<1 year	7.7
Congestive heart failure	9.0
Chronic obstructive pulmonary disease	5.0
Renal failure	5.9
Diabetes mellitus	2.1
Emergency surgery	2.8
Surgery >300 minutes	4.9
Major surgery	3.1

Modified from Mangano DT, Layug EL, Wallace A, Tateo I. Effect of atenolol on mortality and cardiovascular morbidity after noncardiac surgery. *N Engl J Med* 1996;335:1713-1720.

the presence of confounding variables such as the existence and severity of coexisting disease, the age of the patient, the type and length of surgery, and the skill of the anesthesiologist and surgeon. Attempts at estimating perioperative risk are illustrated by the ASA physical classification system (see Table 1-8), Goldman's cardiac risk index, and Shapiro's pulmonary index to name just a few. Each of these risk prediction models accurately estimates risk in certain risk groups (Table 1-9), however, these models become less accurate when applied to consecutive patients. Common clinical causes of death in the perioperative period are: pneumonia, CHF, myocardial infarction, pulmonary embolism, and respiratory failure. In those studies that have estimated the risk of death due solely to anesthesia, two periods of time have emerged with distinct characteristics – prior to 1980 and after 1980. Prior to 1980, the risk of death due to anesthesia was estimated to range from 1 in 536 to 1 in 6,158 anesthetics; after 1980, the risk was substantially less, ranging from 1 in 13,207 to 1 in 188,076 anesthetics. A recent estimate of anesthetic risk that included 184,472 patients (ASA classification I–V) across two hospitals revealed an anesthesia-related mortality rate of 1 per 13,000 anesthetics. An older study which included 1,001,000 ASA classification I and II patients examined outcome data supplied by a malpractice insurance carrier and noted a death rate of 1 per 200,200. Ultimately, risk is minimized by a thorough preanesthesia assessment and optimization of medical status, meticulous intraoperative care, and effective postoperative therapy. No particular anesthetic technique has been shown to be the safest; rather, the skill and judgment of the anesthesia care provider is of most importance.

PREMEDICATION

Introduction

A knowledge of the indications for the use of preoperative medication is an essential component of the preanesthesia evaluation process. In choosing premedicants, a number of factors should be considered (Box 1-9). No single agent or combination of agents satisfies all premedicant requirements for all clinical situations. Of most importance is choosing the premedicant(s) that accomplishes the desired preoperative clinical goals (Table 1-10).

It is important to note that particular patient groups clearly benefit from sedative premedications while for other patient groups premedication is contraindicated (Table 1-11).

When using premedication, the appropriate timing of administration is crucial for the greatest patient benefit. In general, drugs given orally are administered 60–90 minutes before surgery, those given intramuscularly are

---

Box 1-9   Factors to Consider in Choosing Adult Premedication

Type of surgery scheduled (e.g. cancer or heart surgery)

PATIENT-SPECIFIC FACTORS

Degree of apprehension and fear
Patient age and weight
Physical health status
Usual daily medications
Allergies to medications
Previous adverse experiences with drugs used for preoperative medication
Endocarditis prophylaxis
Steroid dependency
History of postoperative nausea and vomiting (PONV) or motion sickness
Risk of aspiration
Tolerance for depressant drugs
Elective or emergency surgery
Inpatient or outpatient surgery
Indications and contraindications to sedative premedicants

CLINICAL ENDPOINTS DESIRED

Anxiolysis
Pain relief
Both anxiolysis and pain relief
Antisialagogue effects
Medical therapy
• Aspiration prophylaxis
• Endocarditis prophylaxis
• Corticosteroid supplementation

Table 1-10   Adult Premedication, by Drug Category, and Usual Dosages

Category	Medication	Dosage
Anxiolysis	Midazolam	1–2 mg IV; 2–5 mg IM
	Lorazepam	1–4 mg PO/IV
	Diazepam	5–20 mg PO
Analgesia	Morphine	0.05–0.1 mg/kg IM
	Meperidine	0.5–1.5 mg/kg IM
	Fentanyl	25–50 µg IV
Aspiration prophylaxis	Cimetidine	400 mg PO hs & am
	Ranitidine	150 mg PO hs & am
	Famotidine	40 mg PO hs & am
	Metoclopramide	10 mg PO/IV
	Nonparticulate antacid	30 mL PO
Antisialagogue	Glycopyrrolate	0.2–0.3 mg IM/IV
	Atropine	0.3–0.6 mg IM/IV
	Scopolamine	0.3–0.6 mg IM/IV
Antiemetic	Droperidol	0.625–1.25 mg IV
	Metoclopramide	10 mg IV
	Ondansetron	4 mg IV; 8 mg PO
	Dolasetron	12.5–25 mg IV

am, in the morning; hs, at night; IM, intramuscularly; IV, intravenously; PO, by mouth.

administered 30–60 minutes before surgery, and drugs administered intravenously (except lorazepam) are given 1–5 minutes before surgery.

Drugs and Dosages Typically Used for Adult Premedication

Typically, adult premedication involves a single drug or a combination of drugs chosen from among five basic categories (Table 1-12). The particular drug(s) chosen are selected based upon a desired clinical endpoint (anxioly-

Table 1-11   Indications and Contraindications for CNS-depressant Premedication

Contraindications	Indications
Very young (<1 yr)	Cardiac surgery
Elderly	Cancer surgery
Debilitated	Co-existing pain
Decreased level of consciousness	Regional anesthesia
Intracranial pathology	Pediatric (>4 yrs)
Severe pulmonary disease	Anxious healthy adults
Hypovolemia	
Non anxious adults	

sis, pain relief, anticholinergic effects, antiemetic properties, aspiration prophylaxis). Table 1-12 outlines the most common drugs used for adult premedication and a discussion of each category follows.

Benzodiazepines

Surgery is a psychologically stressful event. Preoperative anxiety is typically treated with benzodiazepines alone or in combination with other premedicants (e.g., opioids). Benzodiazepines are used because they produce relief of anxiety, sedation, and amnesia. They do not have pain-relieving properties. Benzodiazepines interact with specific "benzodiazepine receptors" in the central nervous system that, when stimulated, facilitate transmission of the inhibitory neurotransmitter gamma-aminobutyric acid (GABA), which produces sedation (see Table 1-12). Anxiolysis is produced by the glycine-mediated inhibition of neuronal pathways in the brain and brainstem, whereas amnesia is produced by a poorly understood mechanism. The benzodiazepines used most commonly as premedicants are midazolam, lorazepam, and diazepam. The administration of intravenous benzodiazepines depresses respiration with a resulting increase in P_aCO_2 by 1.5–6.0 mm Hg. Rapid administration of intravenous midazolam may produce apnea. Synergistic central nervous system depressant effects occur when benzodiazepines are combined with other sedative agents (Table 1-13).

Narcotic Premedicants

Opioids (see Table 1-12) are best used in patients who are experiencing pain preoperatively. Opioids are not ideal agents for relieving anxiety, producing sedation, or preventing recall of perioperative events and should not, therefore, be used alone if these effects are desired. Morphine and meperidine are the opioids most frequently used for premedication. Fentanyl is not the best choice because of its potency and short clinical effects. No matter which opioid is used, the dose should be reduced in elderly or debilitated patients. Premedication with opioids has several side effects: orthostatic hypotension (via interference with compensatory vasoconstriction), histamine release (morphine), blunting of the carbon dioxide response at the medullary respiratory center, decreased responsiveness to hypoxemia related to inhibition of the carotid body, nausea and vomiting via stimulation of the chemoreceptor trigger zone, biliary sphincter spasm, flushing, dizziness, and miosis. When used for premedication, opioids are usually combined (in reduced doses) with benzodiazepines or scopolamine (in reduced doses) for enhanced sedative and/or amnestic properties (Table 1-14).

Anticholinergic Premedicants

Anticholinergic premedicants (see Table 1-12) are primarily used for specific clinical indications such as: an

Table 1-12 Category of Premedicant and Mechanism of Action

Category	Drug	Mechanism of Action
Antianxiety	Midazolam Lorazepam Diazepam	The clinical effects of the benzodiazepines occur by an interaction with specific receptors in the central nervous system. Sedation occurs by the facilitation and enhancement of inhibitory transmission mediated by gamma-aminobutyric acid (GABA). Anxiolysis occurs via glycine-mediated inhibition of neuronal pathways in the brain and brainstem. The pathway producing amnesia is unknown.
Opioids	Morphine Demerol Fentanyl	The clinical effects of these agents occur by stimulation of the opioid receptors in the central nervous system
H_2-blocking agents	Cimetidine Ranitidine Famotidine	Competitive inhibition of histamine at the H_2-receptor of the gastric parietal cells resulting in reduced gastric acid secretion, gastric volume, and hydrogen ion concentration.
Gastric motility	Cisapride	Enhances the release of acetylcholine at the myenteric plexus. Has serotonin-4 receptor ($5\text{-}HT_4$) agonistic properties that may increase gastrointestinal motility and cardiac rate. Has no dopamine receptor blocking activity, hence no extrapyramidal side effects or central antiemetic activity. Increases lower esophageal peristalsis and accelerates gastric emptying.
Anticholinergic	Scopolamine	Antagonizes the action of acetylcholine at cholinergic postganglionic nerve endings. Has greater antisialagogue and ocular effects than atropine and lesser effects on the heart (tachycardia), bronchial smooth muscle (bronchodilatation), and gastrointestinal tract. It is a tertiary amine and therefore readily crosses the blood–brain barrier in the central nervous system. Produces a more marked and longer-lasting sedative effect than atropine, and therapeutic doses may cause amnesia, drowsiness, and fatigue (especially when used in combination with an opioid such as morphine).
Antiemetic	Ondansetron Dolasetron	Selective $5\text{-}HT_3$ receptor antagonists, blocking serotonin both peripherally on vagal nerve terminals and centrally in the chemoreceptor trigger zone.
	Metoclopramide	Blocks dopamine receptors in the chemoreceptor trigger zone; enhances the response to acetyl gastric choline of tissue in upper gastrointestinal tract increasing gastrointestinal motility and accelerating emptying without stimulating gastric, biliary, or pancreatic secretions.
	Droperidol	Butyrophenone derivative, chemically related to haloperidol; interferes with central nervous system transmission at dopamine, norepinephrine, serotonin, and GABA synaptic sites. Produces marked tranquilization and sedation, inducing a state of mental detachment and indifference while maintaining a state of reflex alertness. Antiemetic effects due to receptor blockade in the chemoreceptor trigger zone. Has alpha-1 adrenergic antagonist action, which may lower systemic vascular resistance and blood pressure.

awake fiberoptic intubation (to reduce secretions), the anticholinergic (heart-rate-supporting) effect in a pediatric patient, or scopolamine's amnestic and sedative effect when combined with an opioid (e.g., morphine). Tables 1-15 and 1-16 compare the general clinical effects of the commonly used anticholinergic medications – atropine, glycopyrrolate, and scopolamine.

Antiemetic Prophylaxis (see Table 1-12)

Postoperative nausea and vomiting (PONV) occurs in 18%–96% of cases. PONV is extremely distressing to patients, many of whom consider it to be as incapacitating as the pain of surgery itself. Well-known factors that increase the incidence of PONV include gender (higher in females), age, obesity, type of surgical procedure (especially laparoscopic abdominal procedures), length of the surgery, anxiety, previous history of motion sickness or PONV, and type of anesthetic agent used. Agents available to treat PONV are listed in Box 1-10 and Table 1-17.

Of the antiemetics available for the management of PONV, the most commonly used agents have been droperidol, ondansetron, and metoclopramide. Droperidol and metoclopramide are both central dopaminergic antagonists, while the serotonin (5-HT) antagonists (ondansetron, dolasetron) induce their antiemetic effects by blocking $5\text{-}HT_3$ receptors in the medullary chemoreceptor trigger zone of the area postrema, and in the nerve terminals of the vagus nerve in the periphery (gastrointestinal tract). Administration of an antiemetic medication is most useful just before emergence from anesthesia or in the postoperative care unit if the signs/symptoms of nausea emerge (especially with 5-HT antiemetics)

Agents Used as Prophylaxis Against Aspiration Pneumonitis

Patients at risk for regurgitation and aspiration of gastric contents should be identified and appropriate prophylactic medications administered before surgery. Box 1-11 outlines the major risk factors for pulmonary aspiration, while

Table 1-13 Anxiolytic/Sedation Premedicants

Drug	Trade Name	Route of Administration	Adult Dosage	Time to Clinical Effect	Clinical Effects	Elimination Half-life	Metabolism	Active Metabolites?	Notes
Benzodiazepines									
Midazolam	Versed	IV, IM, PO, rectal	IV: 0.05–0.1 mg/kg (adults: 1–5 mg) IM: 0.05–0.2 mg/kg; PO: 0.5–0.75 mg/kg Rectal: 0.3–0.35 mg/kg) Dilute in 5 mL saline	IV: 1–3 min IM: onset, 5–10 min with peak effect 15–30 min, PO: 20 min	Anxiolysis, amnesia, sedation	1–4 h (prolonged in the elderly)	Hepatic microsomal enzymes	No	Amnesia lasts 20–32 min; may be extended by IM administration or potentiated by scopolamine
Lorazepam	Ativan	IV, IM, PO, SL	IV: 1–4 mg PO: 25–50 μg/kg (≤4 mg)	IV: max effects 30–40 min; PO: max effect 2–6 h	Anxiolysis, amnesia, sedation	10–20 h	Hepatic conjugation	No (less affected by age or liver disease)	More potent amnestic than midazolam
Diazepam	Valium	IV, IM, PO, rectal	IV: 2.5–10 mg IM: 0.1–0.2 mg PO: 5–20 mg Rectal: 0.5 mg/kg	IV: 5 min PO: adult, 30–60 min; children, 15–30 min	Anxiolysis, amnesia, sedation	21–37 h in healthy adults; prolonged in the elderly	Hepatic microsomal enzymes	Yes	Insoluble in water, pain on injection, phlebitis
Oxazepam	Serax	PO	PO: 10–15 mg	2–4 h	Anxiolysis, amnesia, sedation	5–15 h	Hepatic conjugation	No	
Barbiturates									
Pentobarbital	Nembutal	IM, PO, IV	IM: 150–200 mg PO: 50–200 mg IV: 100 mg	IM: 10–15 min PO: 15–60 min IV: 1–2 min	Preoperative sedation, hypnosis	22–50 h	Hepatic microsomes	No	Caution in liver disease, cardiac disease, elderly, hypovolemic
Secobarbital	Seconal	IM, PO, IV, rectal	IM: 4–5 mg/kg PO: 100–200 mg IV: 50–100 mg	IM: 15–30 min PO: 10–30 min IV: <2 min	Sedation, hypnosis	15–40 hours	Hepatic microsomes	No	May produce disorientation, anti-analgesic effect

Table 1-13 Anxiolytic/Sedation Premedicants—cont'd

Drug	Trade Name	Route of Administration	Adult Dosage	Time to Clinical Effect	Clinical Effects	Elimination Half-life	Metabolism	Active Metabolites?	Notes
Butyrophenones									
Droperidol	Inapsine	IV, IM	2.5–7.5 mg	3–10 min	Sedation, antiemetic	2 h	Liver	No	Dysphoria, restlessness, extrapyramidal signs
Haloperidol	Haldol	IV, IM, PO	PO: 0.5–2 mg IM: 2–5 mg IV: 2–5 mg	PO: 3–5 h IM: 20 min IV: <5 min	Sedation, tranquilization	12–38 h	Liver	Pro-antiemetic	
Phenothiazines									
Promethazine	Phenergan	IV, IM, PO	PO: 25–50 mg IV/IM: 25–50 mg	IV: <30 min PO onset: 30 min	Sedation, antiemetic, anticholinergic, antipruritic	4–6 h	Liver/kidney	Orthostatic hypotension	
Other Sedative-Hypnotics and Tranquilizers									
Chloral hydrate	Aquachloral	PO	Adult: hypnotic 500–1,000 mg; sedative 250 mg Children: hypnotic 50 mg/kg up to 1 g; sedative: 25 mg/kg	15–30 min	Sedation, hypnosis, adjunct to pain medications	7–10 h	Liver/kidney	Yes	Rarely used today as there are better and safer choices

IM, intramuscularly; IV, intravenously; PO, by mouth; SL, under the tongue.

Table 1-14 Narcotic Premedicants

Drug	Trade Name	Route of Administration	Adult Dosage	Onset of Clinical Effects	Duration of Effect	Elimination Half-life	Metabolism	Notes
Morphine	Astromorph, Duramorph	IV, IM, SQ, PO	IM: 10 mg (0.1 mg/kg) IV/SQ: 0.05–0.1 mg/kg PO: 10–30 mg	IV: 5 min (20 min for peak effects) IM: 30–60 min PO: 1 hour	4–5 hours	1.7–3.3 h	Liver	Has active metabolites; should be used with caution in patients with renal failure
Meperidine	Demerol	IV, IM, SQ, PO	IV: 0.25–1mg/kg IM: 1–1.5 mg/kg	5 min 10–15 min	2–4 h	3–5 h	Liver	Has active metabolites; has vagolytic properties, unlike other narcotics which are vagotonic
Codeine	Codeine sulfate Codeine phosphate	PO, IM	PO: 50–60 mg IM: 120 mg	PO: 30–60 min IM: 10–30 min	4–6 hours	3–4 h	Liver	
Methadone	Dolophine	IV, IM, PO	IV: 0.1 mg/kg; PO: 0.2 mg/kg	IV: 10–20 min; PO: 30–60 min	4–6 hours;	35 h	Liver	
Fentanyl	Sublimaze	IV, IM	IV: 0.5–1.0 µg/kg;	IV: 1–3 min	1–2 hours	3.1–6.6 h	Liver	
Alfentanil	Alfenta	IV, IM	IM: 12.5 µg/kg for sedation before regional blocks	IV: 1 min IM: <5 min	<1 hr	1.4–1.5 h	Liver	

IM, intramuscularly; IV, intravenously; PO, by mouth, SQ, subcutaneously.

Table 1-15	Comparative Effects of Anticholinergics Administered Intramuscularly as Premedication		
	Glycopyrrolate	**Scopolamine**	**Atropine**
Antisialagogue effect	++	+++	+
Sedative & amnestic effect	0	+++	+
CNS toxicity	0	++	+
Increased gastric fluid pH	0	0	~
Relaxation of lower esophageal sphincter	++	++	++

Box 1-12 and Tables 1-10 and 1-18 list the agents that may be used for the preoperative prophylactic treatment of aspiration. In general, patients at risk for aspiration are treated with a dose of an H_2-blocker the night before surgery and on the morning of surgery. The morning dose of the H_2-blocking agent may be combined with a gastric stimulant such as metoclopramide for maximum benefit. Nonparticulate antacids may be substituted for the above in selected "at risk" patients but must be given 30 minutes before induction.

Preoperative Administration of Medications Taken for Medical Illness

In general, all necessary medications prescribed for the patient should be continued up through the morning of surgery. The morning medications should be taken with a small sip of water. Patients taking diuretics may hold these medications on the morning of surgery, although, if they are taken, very little clinical harm results. Diabetic patients requiring insulin therapy should either hold their morning dose of insulin or administer one-third of their total morning dose of insulin as NPH (see endocrine section, later).

Preoperative Approach to Patients Receiving Glucocorticoids

Patients who have taken supraphysiologic doses of glucocorticoids for more than 2 weeks during the past year are at risk for perioperative adrenal insufficiency and should receive perioperative supplemental corticosteroid administration (see endocrine section, below).

Preoperative Nil-by-mouth Status

Pulmonary aspiration is an infrequent complication of anesthesia but when it does occur it is a very serious and life-threatening event. The statistical risk of clinically apparent perioperative aspiration is 1 in 3,886 for anesthetics administered for elective surgery and 1 per 895 anesthetics administered for emergency surgery. Overall, the risk of pulmonary aspiration for all administered anesthetics is 1.4:10,000, and is more common in certain risk groups (see Box 1-11). Patients who aspirate and develop symptoms of pulmonary aspiration (36%) usually do so within 2 hours of the presumed event, although the majority of patients with presumed aspiration (64%) never develop clinical symptoms. The validity of traditional risk criteria for aspiration – gastric fluid volume >25 mL (0.4 mL/kg) and gastric fluid pH <2.5 – is debated. There is no evidence that existing gastric fluid volume increases the risk of pulmonary aspiration in patients undergoing elective operations. In fact, normal patients given unlimited access to water until 2 hours before the induction of anesthesia do not have an altered gastric fluid volume or pH compared with adult patients fasted in the traditional manner. Recently, the ASA published practice guidelines for preoperative fasting status and aspiration prophylaxis (Tables 1-19 and 1-20). It is important to note that these recent guidelines are for relatively healthy individuals without risk factors for delayed gastric emptying. Stressed patients undergoing emergency surgery or patients with predisposing factors for delayed gastric emptying (diabetic patients, patients taking narcotics, morbidly obese patients) should follow more traditional nil-by-mouth (NPO) guidelines.

Herbal Medicines

Herbal supplementation is an increasingly common form of alternative medical therapy. In fact, 12% of the adult population in the United States has used herbal medicines in the last year. Total out-of-pocket expenditures for users of alternative therapies in 1997 was estimated at $27 billion, with nearly $10 billion/year spent on herbal products alone. Herbal supplements are used most commonly for back problems, anxiety, depression, and headaches. Because most herbal medicines are considered dietary aids, they are not regulated by the Food and Drug Administration (FDA). Quality control of these preparations is thus a problem as there are no minimum standards to meet before releasing the agents into the market. Consequently, the safety of these medicines, particularly if used to excess, is poorly understood. About 15 million people in the United States who use herbal medicines are thus at risk of adverse reactions. Reports of

Table 1-16 Anticholinergic Premedicants

Drug	Trade Name	Route of Administration	Adult Dosage	Onset of Clinical Effect	Clinical Effects	Duration of Effects	Metabolism	Notes
Scopolamine	Scopolamine HBr	IV, IM, SQ, PO	IV/IM: 0.2–0.65 mg PO: 0.4–0.8 mg	IV: Immediate IM/PO: 30 min	Sedation, amnesia, antisialagogue	IV: 2 h IM/PO: 4–6 h	Hepatic/renal	"Central anticholinergic syndrome"
Glycopyrrolate	Robinul	IV, IM, SQ, PO	IV/IM/SQ: 0.1–0.2 mg PO: 50 μg/kg	IV: <1 min IM/SQ: 15–30 min PO: 1 hr	Antisialagogue, mild vagolysis	IV: 2–3 h PO: 8–12 h	Hepatic/renal	Does not cross the blood–brain barrier; ↓ LES tone
Atropine	Atropine sulfate	IV, IM, PO	IV/IM: 0.4–1.0 mg PO: 0.4–0.6 mg Children: IV: 10–20 μg/kg	IV: 45–60 sec IM: 5–40 min PO: >30 min	Anticholinergic (vagolysis), bronchodilator, antiulcer	IV/IM vagolysis: 1–2 h IV/IM antisialagogue: 4 h	Hepatic/renal	"Central anticholinergic syndrome"; ↓ LES tone

IM, intramuscularly; IV, intravenously; ↓LES, lower esophageal sphincter; PO, by mouth; SQ, subcutaneously.

Box 1-10 Antiemetics for Postoperative Nausea and Vomiting

BUTYROPHENONES
Droperidol (Inapsine)

SEROTONERGIC (5-HT) ANTAGONISTS
Ondansetron
Dolasetron
Granisetron

PROKINETICS
Metoclopramide
Domperidone
Anticholinergics
Scopolamine
Atropine

ANTIHISTAMINES
Cyclizine
Dimenhydrinate
Diphenhydramine

PHENOTHIAZINES
Promethazine
Prochlorperazine
Perphenazine

---

toxicity and drug interactions are increasing but are still primarily limited to case reports.

Unfortunately, 70% of herbal medicine users fail to inform their physician about herbal use, many because, as these products are considered supplements and not medicines, they feel they are completely safe. During the preoperative assessment process, therefore, specific questioning regarding the use of herbal supplements and other alternative therapies is essential. Table 1-21 lists the more common herbal supplements on the market along with common side effects or interactions.

PREOPERATIVE CARDIAC ASSESSMENT

Nearly 30 million patients undergo surgical procedures each year. Of these patients, 30–40% have known coronary artery disease or the risk factors for it and, of these individuals, 10–15% will suffer a perioperative cardiac complication, including 0.5–1% with a myocardial infarction. In particular, patients undergoing vascular surgery comprise a particularly high-risk group of patients with a prevalence of asymptomatic coronary artery disease approaching 60%.

The main goals of the preoperative assessment of the cardiac patient for noncardiac surgery are risk stratifica-

tion and the potential reduction of this risk by preoperative interventions. These interventions may include modifying drug therapy or the surgical approach, more intensive intraoperative monitoring, altering anesthetic techniques, and, in selected cases, preoperative myocardial revascularization. In assessing cardiac risk before noncardiac surgery, it is thus important to follow an organized approach to clinical evaluation. Such an approach includes a focused but complete history and physical examination, necessary laboratory testing, and an electrocardiogram. Particular attention is focused on the identification of those risk factors associated most with increased perioperative cardiac risk (Box 1-13).

In addition to identification of cardiac disease, it is also important to define disease severity, stability, and prior treatment. Based upon the findings of this initial evaluation, a risk assessment is made regarding the likelihood of perioperative cardiac complications. This is often accomplished by the use of one or more risk indices. These risk indices have been incorporated into clinical algorithms that guide the preoperative cardiac assessment process (Figures 1-2 through 1-4). The appropriate use of a risk index will assist in placing the patient into one of three categories of perioperative cardiac risk: low-risk, intermediate-risk, and high-risk (Tables 1-22 through 1-24). Low-risk patients generally require no further testing; high-risk patients require postponement of all but truly emergency surgery; and intermediate-risk patients often require additional preoperative testing in order to further refine cardiac risk.

History

Obtaining an accurate preoperative history is fundamental in estimating perioperative risk and guiding further therapy. A number of cardiac diseases are associated with an increased perioperative risk and a brief discussion of each of these diseases is appropriate.

Preoperative Cardiac Risk Factors

Previous Myocardial Infarction

Patients with a prior myocardial infarction (Table 1-24) have a 10-fold relative increase in risk of cardiac complications compared with patients who do not have coronary disease. Even though the 10-fold increase in risk still corresponds to a relatively low absolute risk of approximately 4% for a myocardial infarction, if a perioperative infarction occurs, the mortality rate is 36–70%. The risk of reinfarction, however, diminishes with time since the original myocardial infarction. In contrast to older studies, more recent studies demonstrate that, with appropriate

Table 1-17 Antiemetic Premedicants

Drug	Trade Name	Route of Administration	Adult Dose	Time to Clinical Effects	Elimination Half-life	Metabolism	Comments
Ondansetron	Zofran	IV, PO	IV: 4 mg PO: 8–16 mg	IV: 15–30 min PO: >30 min	4 h	Liver	Headache, tachycardia
Dolasetron	Anzemet	IV, PO	IV: 12.5 mg (up to 50 mg) PO: 50–100 mg; Children>2 years, 0.35 mg/kg	IV: 15 min PO: 1 h	7–8 h	Liver	Reversible ECG changes ($\uparrow$ PR duration, $\uparrow$ QRS, $\uparrow$ QT)
Droperidol	Inapsine	IV, IM	IV: 0.625–1.25 mg (15 μg/kg)	IV: 3–10 min	2 h	Liver	Feelings of impending death
Metoclopramide	Reglan	IV, IM, PO	IV/IM/PO: 10 mg	IV/IM: <1 hr PO: <1–2 h	4–7 h	Renal	Avoid with MAOIs, Htn, pediatrics

Htn, hypertension; IM, intramuscularly; IV, intravenously; MAOI, monoamine oxidase inhibitor; PO, by mouth.

Box 1-11 Risk Factors Associated with Pulmonary Aspiration

Acute abdominal disorders
Esophageal reflux disease
Diabetes mellitus
Hiatal hernia (with symptoms of reflux)
Morbid obesity
Pregnancy (>12 weeks estimated gestational age)
Nasogastric tubes
Closed head injury with Glasgow Coma Scale Score ≤8
Coma (Glasgow Coma Scale Score ≤8)
Major stroke
Ascites
Alcohol or drug overdose
Scleroderma
Seizures
Multitrauma
Very young age

---

precautions and an increased use of perioperative monitoring, patients with a myocardial infarction less than 3 months before have about a 6% reinfarction rate, while those with a myocardial infarction between 3–6 months prior to surgery have a reinfarction rate of 2–3%. During recovery from a myocardial infarction, risk stratification

---

Box 1-12 Premedicants Used for Aspiration Prophylaxis

GASTROINTESTINAL STIMULANTS
Metoclopramide

GASTRIC ACID SECRETION BLOCKERS
Cimetidine
Famotidine
Ranitidine
Omeprazole

ANTACIDS
Sodium citrate

ANTIEMETICS
Droperidol
Ondansetron
Dolasetron

ANTICHOLINERGICS
Atropine
Glycopyrrolate
Scopolamine

COMBINATIONS OF THE ABOVE

---

is typically performed using cardiac ischemic testing. If ischemic testing does not indicate residual myocardium at risk, elective noncardiac surgery may be performed 4–6 weeks after the myocardial infarction with a low risk of reinfarction.

Angina

Patients with angina have an increased incidence of perioperative cardiac complications. During the interview process, it is important to categorize the angina into one of four classes (Table 1-25) based upon the amount of activity required to produce angina. If the history is reliable, and it is determined that the patient has class I or II stable angina, then the perioperative risk of cardiac events is fairly low. If the history is unreliable or unhelpful, then cardiac ischemic testing should be performed before surgery.

In patients determined to have severe class III or IV unstable angina, all elective noncardiac surgery should be postponed until medical stabilization is achieved, as the risk of an adverse perioperative cardiac event is very high (≥30%).

Congestive Heart Failure

There are about 2 million patients in the United States with CHF. Patients undergoing major surgery who have left ventricular dysfunction or clinical evidence of CHF have a very high risk of developing perioperative pulmonary edema (15%), whereas those with medically controlled CHF have a much lower risk (approximately 5%). A careful history and physical examination is essential in detecting previously unsuspected CHF. In addition, the identification of the etiology of CHF is important as different etiologies of heart failure have differing perioperative implications. For instance, prior CHF due to hypertensive heart disease affects risk differently than CHF resulting from coronary artery disease. In fact, 50% of patients with a history of CHF have normal left ventricular function and have heart failure on the basis of diastolic dysfunction. Adequate preoperative preparation, therefore, depends upon an understanding of the pathophysiology of the myopathic process, and every effort should be made before surgery to determine the cause of the heart failure. Patients with hypertrophic obstructive cardiomyopathy develop hemodynamic deterioration in the setting of hypovolemia as a result of an increase in outflow obstruction. In addition, sympathomimetic agents should be avoided because they also increase the degree of dynamic obstruction as well as decrease diastolic filling. Because of these considerations, patients with a history or signs of CHF should undergo preoperative echocardiographic examination to assess left ventricular function and to quantify the severity of systolic and diastolic dysfunction.

Valvular heart disease

Cardiac murmurs are common in patients scheduled for noncardiac surgery. It is important to distinguish

Table 1-18   Aspiration Pneumonitis Prophylaxis

Drug	Trade Name	Route of administration	Adult Dosage	Clinical Effects	Time to Clinical Effect	Elimination Half-life	Metabolism	Notes
Cimetidine	Tagamet	PO, IV	PO: 400 mg hs, am IV: 300 hs, am	↑ gastric pH	PO: 1–2 h IV: <45 min	PO/IV: 2 h	Liver microsomes	Inhibits liver microsome P450, elevating certain drug levels
Ranitidine	Zantac	PO, IV	PO: 150 mg hs, am IV: 50 mg hs, am	↑ gastric pH	IV:15 min PO: 30 min	IV: 6–8 h PO: 8–12 h	Liver	
Famotidine	Pepcid	PO/IV	PO: 40 mg hs, am IV: 20 mg hs, am	↑ gastric pH	IV: 15 min PO: 30–60 min	PO/IV: 10–12 h	Liver	
Nonparticulate antacids (sodium citrate)	Bicitra	PO	30 mL	Neutralize stomach pH; less toxic if aspirated	30 min			
Omeprazole	Prilosec	PO	20–40 mg	↓ gastric acid production, ↑ gastric pH	1 h	30–60 min	Hepatic	Inhibits gastric acid secretion by inhibition of parietal cell H⁺ ion pump
Misoprostol	Cytotec	PO	200 mg		<15 min	20–40 min	Liver	Prostaglandin E₁ analog with gastric acid antisecretory activity
Cisapride	Propulsid	PO	10 mg 4 × daily 15 min before meals	Indicated for GERD, gastroparesis, prevention of acid aspiration pneumonitis, nonulcer dyspepsia	0.5–1 h	6–12 h	Liver	Increases gut motility
Metoclopramide*	Reglan	IV, IM, PO	10 mg		IV/IM: <1 h PO: <1–2 h	4–7 h	Renal	Avoid with MAOIs, Htn, pediatrics

*Refer to antiemetic data sheet. am, in the morning; hs, at night; Htn, hypertension; IM, intramuscularly; IV, intravenously; MAOI, monoamine oxidase inhibitor; PO, by mouth.

Table 1-19   Summary of Fasting Recommendations to Reduce the Risk of Pulmonary Aspiration in Healthy Patients Undergoing Elective Surgery

Ingested Material	Minimum Fasting Period
Clear liquids (water, fruit juices without pulp, carbonated beverages, clear tea, black coffee)	2 hours
Breast milk	4 hours
Infant formula	6 hours
Non-human milk	6 hours
Light meal (toast and clear liquids)	6 hours
Regular meal (all other solids)	8 hours

These recommendations apply only to healthy patients undergoing elective procedures and are not intended for women in labor. Practice guidelines for preoperative fasting and the use of pharmacologic agents to reduce the risk of pulmonary aspiration: application to healthy patients undergoing elective procedures: a report by the American Society of Anesthesiologists Task Force on Preoperative Fasting. *Anesthesiology* 1999;90:896–905.

significant from insignificant murmurs as this may impact upon the perioperative treatment plan (see Table 1-26).

Aortic valve disease

Aortic stenosis is the most common cardiac valve lesion in the United States. Patients with aortic stenosis are at much greater risk of postoperative mortality than patients without aortic stenosis, with severe aortic steno-

Table 1-20   Summary of Pharmacologic Recommendations to Reduce the Risk of Pulmonary Aspiration

Medication Type	Recommendation
Gastrointestinal stimulants (metoclopramide)	No routine use
Gastric acid secretion blockers (cimetidine, famotidine, ranitidine, omeprazole, lansoprazole)	No routine use
Antacids (sodium citrate, sodium bicarbonate, magnesium trisilicate)	No routine use
Antiemetics (droperidol, ondansetron)	No routine use
Anticholinergics (atropine, scopolamine, glycopyrrolate)	No use
Combinations of the above medications	No routine use

Practice guidelines for preoperative fasting and the use of pharmacologic agents to reduce the risk of pulmonary aspiration: application to healthy patients undergoing elective procedures: a report by the American Society of Anesthesiologists Task Force on Preoperative Fasting. *Anesthesiology* 1999;90:896–905.

sis presenting the greatest risk with noncardiac surgery. Aortic stenosis is first suggested by the finding of a systolic ejection murmur at the right upper sternal border with radiation to the neck. The classic symptoms of aortic stenosis are angina, syncope, and CHF. Angina develops in aortic stenosis because of the combination of a reduced coronary flow reserve and increased myocardial oxygen demand caused by high afterload. Heart failure in aortic stenosis can be caused by diastolic dysfunction, systolic dysfunction, or both. Diastolic dysfunction results primarily from left-ventricular hypertrophy while systolic dysfunction results from excess afterload, decreased contractility, or a combination of these factors.

Echocardiography with Doppler flow is indicated for the initial evaluation in all patients suspected of aortic valvular disease and should include an assessment of the transvalvular gradient and the area of the aortic valve, the extent of left ventricular hypertrophy, and an estimation of left ventricular function. In general, hemodynamics are minimally affected as the valve area is reduced from the normal 3–4 cm^2 to 1.5–2 cm^2. Indeed, asymptomatic patients, even those with severe disease, generally have an excellent prognosis without aortic valve replacement, whereas patients with symptomatic aortic stenosis generally have an expected survival of less than 3 years. Symptomatic patients, therefore, should undergo aortic valve replacement.

In general, clinical symptoms due to aortic stenosis occur if the mean aortic-valve gradient exceeds 50 mm Hg or the aortic valve area is less than 1 cm^2. As there is no proven medical therapy for aortic stenosis, the only effective relief is aortic valve replacement, with the decision to replace the valve based upon the presence of the classic symptoms of aortic stenosis combined with a severely stenotic valve. In patients with documented aortic stenosis scheduled for noncardiac surgery, the presence or absence of symptoms is the key factor. In general, patients with severe but asymptomatic aortic stenosis, especially if they are active, tolerate noncardiac surgery well, provided intraoperative hemodynamics are closely monitored. If the aortic stenosis is severe and symptomatic, elective noncardiac surgery should generally be postponed or canceled, as these patients require aortic valve replacement before elective noncardiac surgery. In patients with severe aortic stenosis who refuse cardiac surgery or are otherwise not candidates for aortic valve replacement, noncardiac surgery can be performed with a mortality risk of approximately 10%.

Patients with aortic valvular regurgitation tolerate surgery much better than those with aortic stenosis. These patients can typically be medically stabilized prior to surgery, while the valve repair, if indicated, may be delayed until after the noncardiac surgery. Exceptions may include severe valvular regurgitation with reduced left ventricular function; in these situations, the overall hemo-

Table 1-21   Commonly Used Herbal Medicines and Potential Adverse Interactions

Herbal medicine	Common use	Potential adverse effects
St John's wort	Anxiety and depression	Photosensitivity, interactions with monoamine oxidase inhibitors, prolonged effects of anesthesia
Ginkgo	Circulatory stimulant; used for dementia, intermittent claudication, tinnitus	Enhanced bleeding in patients on anticoagulants and antithrombotic therapy (i.e., aspirin, nonsteroidal anti-inflammatory drugs, warfarin)
Ginseng	Energy booster (especially athletes); antioxidant	Additive effects with other stimulants, hypertension, insomnia, hypertonia, edema, postmenopausal bleeding
Echinacea	Prevention and treatment of common cold, UTI, cough	Hepatotoxicity (especially when used with other hepatotoxins), ↓ effectiveness of corticosteroids
Garlic	Hypercholesterolemia, hypertension, antioxidant	Potentiates warfarin effect (↑ INR)
Feverfew	Prevention of migraines, antipyretic	↓ platelet activity and ↑ bleeding; avoid in patients on warfarin; rebound headache with abrupt discontinuation; gastrointestinal tract irritation
Kava	Anxiety	Fulminant hepatic failure; potentiates sedatives and alcohol; ↑ suicide risk in patients with depression
Valerian root	Insomnia, anxiety	Potentiates barbiturates
Hawthorn leaf	Heart failure	May interact with drugs used for hypertension, hypotension, cardiac disorders; nausea, fatigue, sweating, rash; ↑ uterine activity
Saw palmetto	Benign prostatic hypertrophy; antiandrogen	Additive effects with other hormone therapies (e.g. birth control pills, estrogen replacement therapy)
Ephedra (*ma huang*)	Antitussive	Interacts with cardiac glycosides → dysrhythmias; ↑ sympathomimetic effects with monoamine oxidase inhibitors, oxytocin; seizures, psychosis, coma
Cayenne	Muscle spasm or soreness	Hypothermia with overdose; skin ulceration and blistering with prolonged use
Goldenseal	Diuretic, anti-inflammatory, laxative, hemostatic	↑ edema, ↑ blood pressure, ↑ free water excretion

UTI, urinary tract infection; INR, international normalized ratio.

dynamic reserve is so limited that destabilization during perioperative stresses is likely.

Mitral Valve Disease

Preoperative identification of mitral valve stenosis is important as perioperative control of heart rate is essential. Tachycardia is poorly tolerated in significant mitral stenosis as diastolic filling is negatively impacted, resulting in severe pulmonary edema. Preoperative surgical correction of mitral valve disease is typically performed after noncardiac surgery unless the repair is indicated to prolong survival and prevent complications unrelated to the proposed noncardiac surgery. Patients with severe mitral regurgitation generally tolerate surgery well; however, benefit is achieved with afterload reduction. Patients with mitral valve disease, including those with mitral valve prolapse who have clinical or echocardiographic evidence of mitral valve regurgitation, should receive perioperative endocarditis prophylaxis. Moreover, patients with a mechanical prosthetic valve should receive endocarditis prophylaxis as well as careful anticoagulation management.

Dysrhythmias

Frequent premature ventricular contractions or non-sinus rhythm (e.g., atrial fibrillation) occurring in patients with cardiac disease, especially left ventricular failure, are predictive of perioperative cardiac morbidity in noncardiac surgery. The presence of complete (third-degree) heart block, second-degree heart block (Mobitz II), and left bundle branch block also increase perioperative risk. The indications for antidysrhythmic therapy and cardiac pacing are the same as those in the nonoperative setting, and are only initiated for symptomatic or hemodynamically significant dysrhythmias. Conversely, patients with dysrhythmias but without underlying heart disease do not have an increase in perioperative cardiac risk; therefore, the addition of new, antidysrhythmic medications in the asymptomatic patient is not warranted.

Diabetes Mellitus

Patients with diabetes mellitus (especially those who have taken insulin for more than 5 years) have an increased incidence of coronary artery disease, including a higher incidence of silent myocardial ischemia and

---

Box 1-13   Risk Factors for Perioperative Cardiac Complications

DEFINITE CARDIAC DISEASE

Coronary artery disease
• Myocardial infarction
• Angina
Congestive heart failure
Symptomatic dysrhythmias (frequent premature atrial contractions, atrial fibrillation, second-degree heart block, third-degree heart block, premature ventricular contractions)
Left ventricular hypertrophy
Valvular heart disease (especially critical aortic stenosis)
Presence of pacemaker or implantable cardioverter-defibrillator

INCREASED RISK OF CARDIAC DISEASE

Diabetes
Renal insufficiency
Hypertension
Peripheral vascular disease
Age >70 years

OTHER RISK FACTORS

High-risk surgery (vascular, thoracic, upper abdominal)
Poor functional status
Anemia
Cerebrovascular disease

---

infarction when compared to the general population. The presence of coronary artery disease correlates with an increased incidence of postoperative myocardial ischemia, CHF and wound infections. Diabetic patients also have an increased incidence of renal insufficiency.

Age

Advanced age (>70 years) has been clearly shown to be an independent predictor of perioperative cardiac risk, even after controlling for the severity of cardiac disease and other diseases. Older patients have reduced exercise levels and this may mask the presence of limited physiologic reserve as well as underlying cardiac disease.

Hypertension

Long-standing hypertension is associated with coronary artery disease; hence, in patients undergoing therapy for hypertension, the physical examination should include a search for end-organ damage and evidence of associated cardiovascular pathology. If the initial evaluation establishes hypertension as mild or moderate and no associated metabolic or cardiovascular abnormalities are detected, then surgery may proceed as planned.

There is benefit in effective preoperative blood pressure control among patients with established hypertension, so antihypertensive medications should be continued during the perioperative period. Patients should not have beta-blocker or clonidine therapy withheld, because of potential heart rate or blood pressure rebound. In patients unable to take oral medications, parenteral beta-blockers and transdermal clonidine may be substituted. For patients with newly diagnosed mild hypertension, initiating therapy after surgery is appropriate. Patients with significant elevations of blood pressure (i.e., systolic blood pressure >180 mm Hg and/or diastolic blood pressure >110 mm Hg) should have their blood pressure controlled before surgery. Patients with poorly controlled preoperative hypertension are known to have perioperative blood pressure lability, with associated electrocardiographic evidence of myocardial ischemia. Instituting effective preoperative treatment of poorly controlled hypertension can reduce hemodynamic lability. In particular, studies have demonstrated that introduction of preoperative beta-adrenergic blockers leads to more effective control of blood pressure fluctuations and a reduction in the number and duration of perioperative coronary ischemic episodes. The administration of beta-adrenergic blocking agents to patients with known coronary artery disease or risk factors for coronary artery disease who are undergoing noncardiac surgery can reduce cardiovascular morbidity and mortality during the perioperative period.

Renal Insufficiency

Pre-existing renal disease (preoperative serum creatinine levels >1.4 mg/dL) has been identified as a risk factor for postoperative renal dysfunction and increased long-term morbidity and mortality compared with patients without renal disease. A recent study identified a preoperative creatinine level greater than 2 mg/dL as an independent risk factor for cardiac complications after major noncardiac surgery. Preoperative evaluation of a patient with end-stage renal disease on dialysis or after renal transplantation should focus upon the association with coronary artery disease, as well as the fluid, electrolyte, and acid–base problems found in these conditions. Patients with end-stage renal disease should have dialysis within 24 hours of surgery in order to reduce the incidence of perioperative pulmonary edema and coagulopathy seen with uremia. Pre-existing renal disease has been identified as a risk factor for postoperative renal dysfunction and increased long-term morbidity and mortality compared with patients without renal disease.

Surgical Risk

The surgical risk of noncardiac surgery is related to two main factors: first, the type of surgical procedure being planned may identify a subset of patients with a greater likelihood of underlying heart disease (e.g., vascular surgery); second, the degree of hemodynamic cardiac stress associated with the particular surgical procedure is important, as certain types of procedures are associated with major alterations in blood volume, blood pressure, heart rate, coagulation status, oxygenation, and

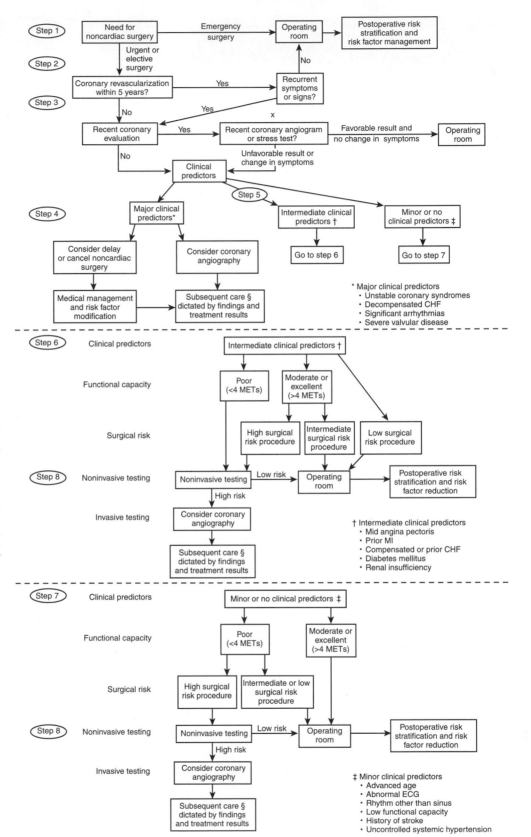

Figure 1-2 Stepwise approach to preoperative cardiac assessment. The steps are discussed in the text. § Subsequent care may include cancellation or delay of surgery, coronary revascularization followed by noncardiac surgery, or intensified care. CHF, congestive heart failure; ECG, electrocardiogram; MET, metabolic equivalent; MI, myocardial infarction. (Redrawn from ACC/AHA Guideline update for perioperative cardiovascular evaluation for noncardiac surgery – executive summary: a report of the American College of Cardiology/American Heart Association Task Force on Practice Guidelines (Committee to Update the 1996 Guidelines on Perioperative Cardiovascular Evaluation for Noncardiac Surgery). *J Am Col Cardiol* 2002;39:542–553.

Table 1-22   Detsky's Modified Multifactorial Risk Index

	Points
Coronary artery disease	
Myocardial infarction <6 months	10
Myocardial infarction > 6 months	5
Canadian Cardiovascular Society angina*	
Class III	10
Class IV	20
Alveolar pulmonary edema	
Within 1 year	10
Ever	5
Valvular disease	
Suspected critical aortic stenosis	20
Arrhythmias	
Rhythm other than sinus	5
More than five PVCs before surgery	5
Poor general medical status	5
Age >70 years	5
Emergency operation	10
Total score	**(0–120)**

Class I: 0–15 points, cardiac risk <3%; class II: 20–30 points, cardiac risk 3–15%; class III: >30 points, cardiac risk >15%.
* Canadian Cardiovascular Society classification of angina: 0, asymptomatic; I, angina with strenuous exercise; II, angina with moderate exertion; III, angina with walking one to two level blocks or climbing one flight of stairs or less at a normal pace; IV, inability to perform any physical activity without development of angina. (See Detsky *et al.*, 1986.)

neurohumoral activation. The magnitude of these changes affects the incidence of perioperative cardiac events. Emergency surgery as well as operations lasting greater than 3 hours significantly increases the risk of perioperative cardiac complications. Examples of noncardiac surgeries and their surgery-specific risks are given in Table 1-27.

Table 1-23   Low-risk Variables

Criteria of Eagle	Criteria of Vanzetto
Age >70 years	Age >70 years
History of angina	History of angina
Diabetes mellitus	Diabetes mellitus
Q waves on ECG	Q waves on ECG
History of ventricular ectopy	History of myocardial infarction
	ST-segment ischemic changes on resting ECG
	Hypertension with severe left ventricular hypertrophy
	History of congestive heart failure

ECG, electrocardiogram.
(See Eagle *et al.*, 1989; Vanzelto *et al.*, 1996.)

Table 1-24   Risk of Perioperative Cardiac Events

Variables		Risk of Cardiac Events (%)
Eagle	0	0–3
	1–2	6–16
	>3	29–50
Vanzetto	0	2
	1	4
	2–4	4
	>5	16

Activity

The activity level predicts postoperative cardiac risk in patients undergoing noncardiac surgery. In one study, patients more than 65 years of age undergoing major abdominal or thoracic noncardiac surgery who were unable to reach a heart rate of 100 beats/min or more with supine bicycle exercise showed better prediction of perioperative complications than predicted by the rest or exercise electrocardiogram or radionuclide ejection fraction. In another study of vascular surgery patients, complication rates were substantially lower in patients who could reach 85% of their maximal predicted heart rate than in patients who could not; exercise capacity appeared to be more important than the amount of ST-segment depression at peak exercise. In a very recent study, the inability to climb one flight of stairs was highly predictive of perioperative cardiopulmonary complications in patients undergoing major thoracic or abdominal surgery. Functional capacity should be expressed in metabolic equivalent (MET) levels (Table 1-28). Multiples of the baseline MET value can be used to express aerobic demands for specific activities. Perioperative cardiac and long-term risks are increased in patients unable to meet a 4-MET demand during most normal daily activities.

Underlying Medical Diseases

Patients with coexisting medical problems, such as underlying pulmonary disease (e.g., hypoxemia, hypercapnia), hypokalemia, acidosis, serious liver disease, or other disease states, also have a higher risk of cardiac complications, again presumably because their lack of physiologic reserve puts added stress on the cardiovascular system.

Implantable Cardiac Defibrillators

The preoperative evaluation of patients with implantable cardiac defibrillators (ICDs) is outlined in Box 1-14. The patient with an ICD typically has severe depression of left ventricular function, most commonly due to ischemic disease. The patient usually has a history of sudden death or hemodynamically significant

---

Table 1-25   Classifications of Angina Pectoris

Canadian Cardiovascular Society	New York Heart Association
Class I Ordinary physical activity without angina	Class I No symptoms with ordinary activity
Class II Slight limitation with ordinary activity	Class II Symptoms with ordinary activity; slight limitation of activity
Class III Marked limitation of ordinary activity	Class III Symptoms with less than ordinary activity; marked limitation of activity
Class IV Inability to carry on any physical activity without discomfort	Class IV Symptoms with any physical activity or even at rest

ventricular tachydysrhythmias and is taking multiple medications. Similar to a patient with a pacemaker, a patient with an ICD has significant coexisting disease and therefore appropriate medical optimization before surgery is essential. All patients should undergo preop-erative device testing in order to provide information about the frequency of ICD activation, therapies delivered by the ICD, and responses exhibited by the patient (e.g., number of shocks required and what the effective output typically is). The device should be inactivated

---

Table 1-26   Differentiation of Pathologic from Non-pathologic Cardiac Murmurs

Pathologic (organic) murmurs

Systolic murmurs	Loud (≥ grade 3) murmur
	Holosystolic or late systolic murmur, especially at the left sternal border or apex
	Systolic murmur that becomes louder with the Valsalva maneuver (e.g., hypertrophic obstructive cardiomyopathy, mitral valve prolapse)
	Other systolic murmurs in patients with the clinical findings suggesting infective endocarditis
	Systolic murmur that is accompanied by an abnormal electrocardiogram
	Systolic murmur that is accompanied by the signs or symptoms of cardiac disease

Diastolic murmurs
Continuous murmurs

Non-pathologic (innocent) murmurs
Grade 1 or 2 midsystolic murmurs without other clinical manifestations of cardiac disease

Clinical findings	Normal activity level
	Absence of cardiac symptoms
	Normal electrocardiogram
	Normal chest radiograph

Causes	Murmur heard best at second left intercostal space	Due to rapid ejection into a normal aortic root	Fever Pregnancy Thyrotoxicosis Anemia
		Aortic sclerotic murmur (older adults)	Due to fibrous or fibrocalcific thickening of the bases of otherwise normal aortic cusps as they insert into the sinuses of Valsalva
	Murmur heard best at lower left sternal edge or cardiac apex (Still murmur)	Due to vibrations of normal pulmonary valve leaflets at their attachments or periodic vibrations of a left ventricular false tendon	
	Murmur heard best at second right intercostal space	Due to exaggeration of the normal ejection vibrations within the pulmonary trunk	Children Adolescents Young adults Thin-chested individuals with reduced anterior–posterior diameter

Pathologic murmurs require cardiac echocardiography; nonpathologic murmurs require no further work up.

Table 1-27 Cardiac risk stratification for noncardiac surgical procedures

Cardiac risk	Type of surgery	Complication rate* (%)
High-risk	Aortic surgery Peripheral vascular surgery Surgeries with major blood loss or fluid shifts involving the chest or abdomen	>5%
Intermediate-risk	Uncomplicated abdominal Head and neck Orthopedic (e.g. hip, major back) Thoracic Urologic (e.g. radical prostatectomy)	1–5%
Low-risk	Cataract removal Endoscopic procedures Breast surgery Dermatologic procedures	<1%

*Combined incidence of cardiac death and nonfatal myocardial infarction.

just prior to surgery and then reactivated after the operation.

Previous Revascularization Procedures

Patients who have undergone a previous coronary revascularization have a perioperative risk of cardiac complications similar to those without known cardiac risk factors. However, the practice of performing a preoperative coronary artery bypass graft (CABG) in patients at high risk of perioperative cardiac complications is very debatable. Two decision analyses have addressed the short-term benefit of prophylactic coronary artery bypass surgery among patients with vascular disease (high-risk group) and both studies suggest that proceeding directly to surgery results in better short-term outcomes than performing a coronary angiogram followed by CABG and then the originally scheduled surgery. Similarly, prophylactic coronary revascularization is less beneficial among patients undergoing lower-risk surgery.

Conversely, patients with unstable angina refractory to medication, with left main coronary artery stenosis, with triple-vessel disease and impaired left ventricular function, and with the possibility of two-vessel coronary artery disease with proximal left anterior descending involvement (and left ventricular dysfunction) have a need for coronary revascularization that is independent of the scheduled noncardiac procedures. In these patients, the coronary revascularization is performed to reduce short- and long-term mortality. In short, the indications for preoperative CABG remain the same as in the nonoperative setting and, therefore, CABG is rarely indicated merely to get the patient through surgery. In patients who have undergone previous percutaneous coronary interventions such as angioplasty or coronary stent placement, the reductions in perioperative cardiac morbidity and mortality appear to be similar to those seen after CABG. However, the same recommendations apply to these procedures as to preoperative CABG; that is, since these procedures are associated with complications of their own, preoperative indications for these procedures are the same as in the nonoperative setting. In those patients who have undergone percutaneous coronary interventions however, delaying surgery for at least 1 week after balloon angioplasty to allow for healing of the vessel injury and at least 2 weeks (and ideally 4–6 weeks) after placement of a coronary stent is recommended.

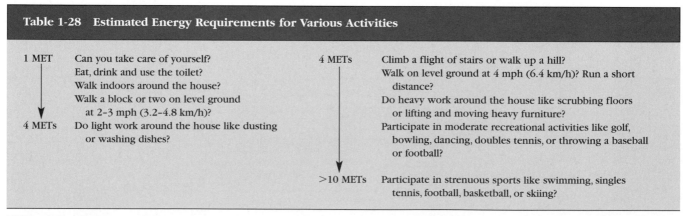

Table 1-28 Estimated Energy Requirements for Various Activities

1 MET	Can you take care of yourself?	4 METs	Climb a flight of stairs or walk up a hill?
	Eat, drink and use the toilet?		Walk on level ground at 4 mph (6.4 km/h)? Run a short distance?
	Walk indoors around the house?		Do heavy work around the house like scrubbing floors or lifting and moving heavy furniture?
	Walk a block or two on level ground at 2–3 mph (3.2–4.8 km/h)?		Participate in moderate recreational activities like golf, bowling, dancing, doubles tennis, or throwing a baseball or football?
4 METs	Do light work around the house like dusting or washing dishes?		
		>10 METs	Participate in strenuous sports like swimming, singles tennis, football, basketball, or skiing?

MET, metabolic equivalent.
From ACC/AHA Guideline update for perioperative cardiovascular evaluation for noncardiac surgery – executive summary: a report of the American College of Cardiology/American Heart Association Task Force on Practice Guidelines (Committee to Update the 1996 Guidelines on Perioperative Cardiovascular Evaluation for Noncardiac Surgery). *J Am Col Cardiol* 2002;39:542–553.

Box 1-14 Preoperative Management of a Patient with an Implantable Cardiac Defibrillator

1. Identify the defibrillator manufacturer, date and indication for placement
2. Optimize medical therapy for any associated medical diseases
3. Continue all antidysrhythmic therapy
4. On the day of surgery, have a cardiologist disable the ICD functions just prior to surgery
5. Perform the surgical procedure
6. Reactivate the ICD functions postoperatively

Physical Examination

The preoperative cardiovascular examination should include an assessment of vital signs (including measurement of blood pressure in both arms), carotid pulse and bruits, auscultation of the lungs, precordial auscultation, and an examination of the extremities for edema. The presence of an implanted pacemaker or ICD should also be confirmed. Additionally, the general appearance of the patient provides important information regarding the patient's overall status. Cyanosis, pallor, dyspnea at rest or with minimal activity, poor nutritional status, and morbid obesity should be noted during the preoperative assessment. Cardiac auscultation may provide evidence of underlying cardiac disease. If a murmur is present, a decision should be made about whether or not it represents significant valvular disease and thus warrants further diagnostic attention.

Cardiac Risk Stratification and Appropriate Use of Cardiac Testing

As part of the presurgical clinical assessment, it is important to risk-stratify patients in order to estimate perioperative cardiac morbidity. This is best accomplished using published clinical algorithms. These algorithms incorporate the clinical risk profile with the type of surgery to arrive at a perioperative risk profile. Although a number of preoperative cardiac evaluation algorithms have been published, two algorithms in particular are used most often – the American College of Cardiology (ACC)/American Heart Association (AHA) clinical algorithm (see Figure 1-2), and the algorithm published by the American College of Physicians (ACP).

The ACP algorithm (see Figures 1-3 and 1-4) incorporates an evidence-based approach to making recommendations. It uses both the Detsky multifactorial risk index and the Eagle clinical risk model to determine periopera-

Table 1-29 Goldman's Cardiac Risk Index for Noncardiac Surgery

Clinical Variable	Point Assignment
History	
Age >70 years	5
Recent myocardial infarction (<6 months)	10
Physical examination	
Ventricular gallop or jugular venous pressure ≥12 cm water	11
Significant valvular aortic stenosis	3
Electrocardiogram	
Rhythm other than sinus or atrial ectopy on preoperative tracing	7
More than 5 per minute ectopic ventricular beats on any tracing before surgery	7
Poor general medical condition (any two of the following): <60 mm Hg or P_aCO_2 >50 mmHg	3
Serum potassium <3.0 mEq/L or bicarbonate <20 mEq/L	
Blood urea nitrogen >50 mg/dL or creatinine >3.0 mg/dL	
Chronic liver disease	
Noncardiac debilitation	
Surgical procedure	
Intraperitoneal, intrathoracic, aortic	3
Emergency	4
Maximum score	**53**

From Goldman L, Caldera DL, Nussbaum SR, *et al*. Multifactorial index of cardiac risk in noncardiac surgical procedures. *N Engl J Med* 1977;297:845–850.

tive risk and the need for further testing. The Detsky risk index is a modification of the original cardiac risk index proposed by Goldman in 1977. In the original Goldman risk index, 1,001 consecutive patients more than 40 years of age undergoing major noncardiac surgery were prospectively studied for the occurrence of postoperative cardiac complications. Using multivariate discriminant analysis, nine independent significant correlates of life-threatening and fatal cardiac complications were identified (Table 1-29). Patients were divided into four risk classes according to their total number of points. Each risk class had a progressively higher perioperative complication rate.

The original cardiac risk index was later modified by Detsky and colleagues. They prospectively studied 455 consecutive patients referred to a general medical consultation service for cardiac risk assessment before noncardiac surgery. In essence, these patients comprised a more defined group of individuals at greater perioperative cardiac risk since they were undergoing preoperative consultation for cardiac issues: previous myocardial infarction, angina, known coronary artery disease, cardiomyopathy, CHF, arrhythmia, valvular heart disease, and abnormal electrocardiogram. Detsky and colleagues then modified the original cardiac risk index to reflect new factors that they felt to be more important (angina classification, remote myocardial infarction, suspected critical aortic stenosis, and alveolar pulmonary edema) and simplified the scoring system into three classes of risk (see Table 1-22), instead of Goldman's four classes. Detsky's revised index included 12 clinical risk factors (each assigned a point total) divided into eight categories. Based upon the total number of points, patients were categorized into low-, intermediate-, or high-risk perioperative cardiac risk categories.

The other clinical risk profile used by the ACP in their algorithm is the Eagle clinical risk model (see Tables 1-23 and 1-24). In this study, 200 patients were retrospectively examined to determine whether clinical markers and preoperative dipyridamole–thallium imaging (DPT) were each useful in predicting ischemic events after vascular surgery. Five clinical predictors were found to be independent predictors of perioperative cardiac risk in this population of vascular surgery patients: Q waves, history of ventricular ectopic activity, diabetes mellitus, advanced age (>70 years), and angina. In particular, those patients without any clinical predictors did well with surgery irrespective of the DPT test, while those with three or more clinical predictors had a high incidence of cardiac events, again irrespective of the DPT result. In those patients with one or two clinical predictors (intermediate-risk group of patients), a positive DPT result was highly correlated with perioperative cardiac events, while a negative result on DPT correlated with a low risk of cardiac events.

The conclusion of the study was that preoperative DPT imaging appeared to be most useful in stratifying vascular patients at intermediate risk by clinical evaluation, particularly for patients with one or two clinical predictors where a thallium redistribution correlated with substantial change in probability of cardiac events.

Finally, the other clinical risk model referred to in the ACP algorithm is that of Vanzetto and associates. This study was prospectively designed to investigate whether reinjection thallium-201 single-photon-emission computed tomography (SPECT) had a significant additive predictive value for the occurrence of perioperative cardiac events in clinically selected patients at high cardiac risk undergoing abdominal aortic surgery. From an original group of 517 consecutive patients referred for imaging, 134 had two or more of the clinical or electrocardiographic cardiac risk variables outlined in Tables 1-22 and 1-23. When all the cardiac events were taken into consideration, all the above variables, as well as Q waves and ischemic ST abnormalities on the ECG, showed significant predictive value for the occurrence of cardiac events upon statistical analysis. Furthermore,

thallium SPECT imaging had an additive predictive value for major cardiac events over clinical and electrocardiographic risk factors alone. The conclusion was that, when performed on clinically selected patients at high cardiac risk undergoing major vascular surgery, thallium SPECT demonstrated significant prognostic value for cardiac events over that provided by clinical variables alone.

In summary, roughly 10% of patients will be considered to be at high surgical risk after clinical preoperative assessment. Among unselected patients undergoing vascular surgery, an additional 9–20% may be reclassified as high-risk by noninvasive testing. The algorithm issued by the ACP uses an evidence-based approach; thus intermediate-risk patients undergoing nonvascular surgery are generally not tested because of the lower risk of cardiac complications with this type of surgery. Using the ACP algorithm, fewer patients will be tested preoperatively compared to the algorithm proposed by the ACC.

The ACC/AHA guidelines are similarly based on a review of the medical literature and a best evidence search; however, the guidelines rely more heavily upon expert opinions and observational or retrospective studies to formulate the algorithm compared to the algorithm recommended by the ACP. The ACC/AHA algorithm does not so clearly divide patients into nonvascular and vascular surgical groups when assessing risk. More patients, therefore, will be tested following this algorithm.

No matter which algorithm is chosen to evaluate perioperative cardiac risk, successful use of the algorithms requires an appreciation of the different levels of risk attributable to certain clinical conditions, levels of functional capacity, and types of surgery. Approached in this manner, low-risk patients can generally undergo the planned procedure without additional testing, whereas high-risk patients should have the proposed surgery either postponed or modified substantially. Intermediate-risk patients (especially those undergoing vascular surgery) should generally undergo additional cardiac testing to further assess risk, particularly if scheduled for major vascular surgery. This is best accomplished by either exercise stress testing or pharmacologic stress tests (either MPI or DSE). Depending upon the results of these tests, patients can be placed into an appropriate perioperative risk category – high-risk (cardiac event rate >5%), intermediate-risk (cardiac event rate <5%), or low-risk (cardiac event rate <1%).

Preoperative Cardiac Testing

Basic preoperative testing of patients with risk of cardiac disease should include an electrocardiogram, hemoglobin, electrolytes, blood urea nitrogen and creati-

Table 1-30 Basic Preoperative Testing in Patients with Cardiac Disease or Cardiac Risk Factors

Test	Indications
Electrocardiogram	Abnormalities seen in over 50% of patients
Hemoglobin	Rule out anemia
Electrolytes, blood urea nitrogen, creatinine	Diabetes, renal insufficiency, diuretics, hypertension, vascular disease
Glucose	Diabetes
Liver function tests	Congestive heart failure, right heart failure, pulmonary hypertension
Chest radiograph	Coronary artery disease, valvular heart disease, clinical evidence cardiopulmonary disease
Urinalysis	Diabetes, urinary tract infection

nine, and possibly a chest radiograph. Additional testing may include cardiac stress testing, echocardiography, and a coronary angiogram (Table 1-30).

Preoperative Electrocardiogram

In patients at risk for cardiac disease, electrocardiographic abnormalities are found in up to 50% of patients, while those patients with known coronary artery disease reveal abnormalities about 70% of the time. Changes involving ST segments or T-wave abnormalities are the most common (up to 90%). The indications for a preoperative electrocardiogram are listed in Box 1-15.

Chest Radiography

Preoperative chest radiography should be obtained in patients scheduled for moderate to major surgery who show evidence of cardiopulmonary disease by his-

tory or examination. Patients with valvular or ischemic heart disease or a history of CHF should have a recent (less than 1 month) chest radiograph. Radiographic evidence of cardiomegaly is associated with a left ventricular ejection dysfunction (ejection fraction <40%) in 70% of patients and is a predictor of perioperative cardiac morbidity.

Evaluation of Left Ventricular Function and Anatomy

Preoperative assessment of left ventricular function is most commonly determined by transthoracic echocardiography or radionuclide imaging. The clinical indications for preoperative assessment of cardiac function and anatomy are outlined in Box 1-16. Although left ventricular function is predictive of postoperative CHF, it is not predictive of postoperative ischemic risk (myocardial infarction, angina, cardiac death). Patients with aortic stenosis suspected by examination or history should be evaluated before all but minor surgical procedures.

Ambulatory Ischemia Monitoring (Holter Monitoring)

Both asymptomatic preoperative and postoperative ischemia have been shown to be predictive of postoperative cardiac complications in patients with known cardiac disease or risk factors for cardiac disease. Postoperative ischemia is especially important if it persists for 4 or more hours. Although ambulatory ischemia monitoring is useful in prediction of perioperative cardiac complications, it has not yet been found to be clinically superior to pharmacologic stress testing in perioperative risk prediction.

Box 1-15 Recommendations for Preoperative 12-Lead Resting Electrocardiogram

All patients >50 years of age.
Asymptomatic patient more than 45 years old with two or more atherosclerotic risk factors
Recent episode of chest pain or ischemic equivalent in clinically intermediate- or high-risk patients scheduled for an intermediate- or high-risk operative procedure
Asymptomatic patients with diabetes mellitus
Patients with prior coronary revascularization
Prior hospital admission for cardiac causes

Box 1-16 Indications for Preoperative Echocardiography in Patients Scheduled for Intermediate- to High-risk Surgery

History of a myocardial infarction (by history or electrocardiogram)
History of congestive heart failure (by personal account or on the medical record) – if previous evaluation has documented severe left ventricular dysfunction, repeat preoperative testing may not be necessary
Cardiomegaly on chest radiograph without previous documentation of cardiac disease
A patient with a loud heart murmur, especially if aortic stenosis is suspected
A patient with dyspnea of unknown etiology
Significant left ventricular hypertrophy on electrocardiogram

Coronary Angiography

The indications for preoperative coronary angiography are the same as exist for patients in the nonoperative setting (Box 1-17).

Revascularization Procedures

Coronary Artery Bypass Grafting

As previously discussed, the preoperative clinical indications for CABG are identical to those for patients in the nonoperative setting. Patients who have previously undergone CABG and who have no symptoms of cardiac disease can safely undergo noncardiac surgery with a perioperative risk of complications similar to that of patients without cardiac risk factors.

Percutaneous Transluminal Coronary Angioplasty

Although the perioperative cardiac death rate is reduced in patients who have undergone preoperative percutaneous transluminal coronary angioplasty (PTCA), several studies have also demonstrated a number of complications from angioplasty, including emergency CABG in some. Therefore, the preoperative clinical indications for PTCA in the perioperative setting are the same as in the nonoperative setting, irrespective of the surgical procedure planned.

Box 1-17   Recommendations for Coronary Angiography in the Perioperative Evaluation

Patients with suspected or known coronary artery disease who have:

- Evidence for high risk of adverse outcome based on noninvasive test results (left main or three-vessel coronary artery disease)
- Angina unresponsive to adequate medical therapy
- Unstable angina, particularly when facing intermediate- or high-risk noncardiac surgery
- Equivocal noninvasive test results in high-risk patients undergoing high-risk surgery
- Multiple markers of intermediate clinical risk and planned vascular surgery (noninvasive testing should be considered first)
- Moderate to severe ischemia on noninvasive testing but without high-risk features and lower left ventricular ejection fraction
- Nondiagnostic noninvasive test results in patients at intermediate clinical risk undergoing high-risk noncardiac surgery
- Urgent noncardiac surgery while convalescing from acute myocardial infarction
- Perioperative myocardial infarction

Preoperative Cardiac Stress Testing

The decision regarding whether or not to have a patient undergo preoperative stress testing should be based upon the presence of clinical risk factors, the patient's functional status, and the type of surgery scheduled (see Figures 1-2 to 1-4). Although exercise electrocardiography (treadmill) testing is the standard test in patients able to exercise, exercise stress testing is not possible in a significant proportion of patients who are undergoing vascular surgery or in patients with diseases that restrict ambulation (i.e., stroke and hip disease). Additionally, the exercise stress test has shown a poor predictive value for patients having major surgery. Therefore, for identifying ischemic risk preoperatively, either myocardial perfusion imaging (MPI) or dobutamine stress echocardiography (DSE) should be performed.

Myocardial Perfusion Imaging

Myocardial perfusion imaging is most helpful primarily with intermediate-risk patients, among whom those with one or two risk factors and a positive scintiscan have a 30% complication rate, while those with one or two factors and a negative thallium scintiscan have just a 3% complication rate, similar to patients with no clinical factors. Patients with cardiac risk factors by Eagle's criteria (Table 1-23) or who are class I on the Detsky multifactorial index (Figures 1-3 and 1-4) and have no prior history of known coronary heart disease are at low risk for complications regardless of the MPI result and, therefore, should not be tested.

At the other extreme, patients with three or more of the factors reported by Eagle or who are known to be class III on the multifactorial index are at high risk regardless of the MPI result (see Box 1-13 and Tables 1-22 and 1-23). These patients should generally undergo an aggressive cardiac investigation with angiography followed by a revascularization procedure.

Myocardial perfusion imaging involves the administration of a coronary arteriolar vasodilator (dipyridamole or adenosine) followed by radionuclide imaging (usually either thallium or technetium-99m sestamibi). Coronary artery vasodilators are capable of inducing myocardial ischemia in areas that rely on collateral perfusion. After administration of the coronary vasodilator tracers labeled with a radionuclide, the subsequent redistribution images obtained 3–4 hours later reflect myocardial viability. A myocardial defect on an initial scan that subsequently resolves is an indication of viable myocardium. A defect that is apparent on both scans suggests a region of myocardium that has infarcted. Whether using dipyridamole–thallium or adenosine–technetium sestamibi (cardiolyte), the sensitivity and specificity are nearly equal. The sensitivity of MPI is 83–97% with a specificity

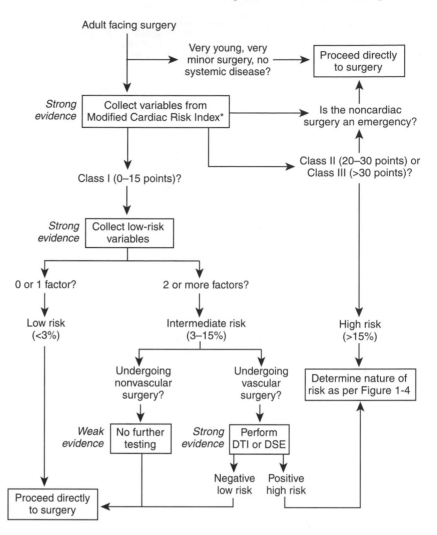

Figure 1-3   Suggested algorithm for the risk assessment and management of patients at low or intermediate risk for perioperative cardiac events (usually myocardial infarction and death). * Boxed phrases indicate recommended actions. The italicized words indicate the level of evidence supporting the recommendation. (Redrawn from Clinical guideline, Part I: Guideline for assessing and managing the perioperative risk from coronary artery disease associated with major noncardiac surgery. *Ann Intern Med* 1997; 127:309–312.) See Table 1-23.

of 38–94%. The positive predictive value of a positive MPI scan is 20–30% with a negative predictive value of more than 95%.

Positive Myocardial Perfusion Imaging and the Extent of Myocardium at Risk

The clinical significance of a positive MPI scan appears to be related to the degree of positivity rather than whether it is merely positive or negative. In other words, the key factor is how much myocardium is at risk (i.e., the number of segments with reversible perfusion defects). For example, in one study, patients with perfusion defects in clinically significant areas of myocardium (anterior, inferior, or posterolateral segments) were associated with the highest cardiac event rate (52%) in comparison to those patients who had redistribution of flow involving only minor segments (septal, inferoapical, true apical), who had event rates of 3%. Interestingly, fixed defects on MPI are not benign either, as it has been shown that fixed defects are associated with adverse perioperative outcome in 25% of patients with fixed defects of the anterior wall and 33% of patients with

fixed defects of other walls suffering a major perioperative event. Thus, although there may be little that can be done for these patients preoperatively (at least surgically), these really are high-risk patient groups with a high perioperative event rate. Proper interpretation of MPI studies can therefore be used for additional risk discrimination to that provided by the clinical evaluation alone.

Dobutamine Stress Echocardiography

Preoperative cardiac stress testing can also be performed using stress echocardiography. Stress echocardiography commonly involves either the use of exercise or pharmacologic agents, with dobutamine being the most frequently utilized pharmacologic stressor. Dobutamine is a beta-adrenergic agonist that causes an increase in myocardial oxygen demand by its inotropic and chronotropic effects and therefore induces myocardial ischemia in patients with coronary artery disease. It can be used as an alternative to dipyridamole, adenosine, or exercise testing. Dobutamine is infused starting at 5–10 μg/kg/min and increased every 3 minutes until either the

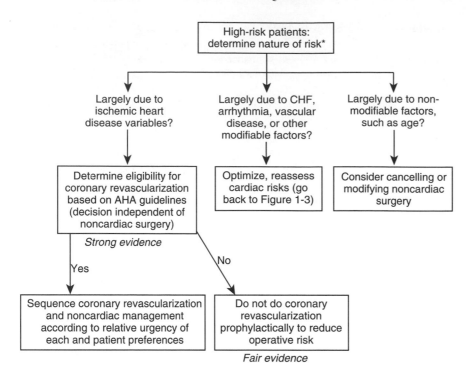

Figure 1-4 Suggested algorithm for the management of patients at high risk for perioperative cardiac events. *Boxed phrases indicate recommended actions. The italicized words indicate the level of evidence supporting the recommendation. (Redrawn from Clinical guideline, Part I: Guideline for assessing and managing the perioperative risk from coronary artery disease associated with major noncardiac surgery. *Ann Intern Med* 1997; 127:309–312.)

infusion reaches 40 μg/kg/min or the heart rate reaches more than 85% of predicted, or serious side effects occur. Echocardiographic imaging is viewed throughout the infusion and then at rest again. The images are stored and then reviewed. Typically, the cardiac images are divided into multiple segments and subsequently reviewed for evidence of any new wall-motion changes. A test is considered positive if wall-motion abnormalities develop with stress in previously normal vascular territories or worsen in a segment that was abnormal at baseline. Stress echocardiography provides information on the location and extent of jeopardized myocardium. In addition, this test provides insight into left ventricular and cardiac valve function. Overall, the sensitivity and specificity of DSE compares very favorably with MPI

(Table 1-31). The positive predictive value is similar to MPI at 20–30%, with a negative predictive value of 99% (i.e., the likelihood of a perioperative cardiac event is very low in the presence of a negative preoperative DSE). The test has a higher sensitivity for multivessel disease (about 90%) than for single-vessel disease (56%). A negative exercise echocardiogram is associated with rates of survival without cardiac events of 99.2% at 1 year and 97.4% at 3 years.

As outlined in Table 1-31, DSE and MPI have a similar diagnostic accuracy; therefore the choice of imaging test (echocardiography versus radionuclide imaging) should take into consideration the test that is most reliable and valid at a given institution.

Risk Stratification Using Dobutamine Stress Echocardiography

Like MPI, DSE can be used for further cardiac risk stratification before major surgery. In a study of patients undergoing infrarenal aortic surgery who underwent preoperative DSE, patients with normal DSE, those with abnormal DSE with changes of ischemia during testing, and those with abnormal DSE representing small areas of ischemic myocardium were allowed to proceed to surgery, while surgery was postponed in patients with abnormal DSE representing large areas of ischemic myocardium. Perioperative outcome was excellent among those patients who proceeded to aortic repair. Once again, it is the degree of test positivity (i.e., amount of myocardium at risk) that is most important when estimating risk assessment before surgery.

Table 1-31	Sensitivity and Specificity of Noninvasive Tests for the Detection of Coronary Artery Disease	
Diagnostic Test	**Sensitivity (Range) %**	**Specificity (Range) %**
Exercise electrocardiography	68	77
Radionuclide scintigraphy (SPECT)	88 (73–98)	77 (53–96)
Stress echocardiography	76 (40–100)	88 (80–95)

SPECT, single-photon emission computed tomography. From Lee TH, Boucher CA. Noninvasive tests in patients with stable coronary artery disease. *N Engl J Med* 2001;344:1840–1845.

Stress Tests in Patients who are not Candidates for Preoperative Revascularization

Should stress tests (MPI, DSE) be performed in patients who are unlikely to undergo preoperative revascularization procedures (e.g., patients undergoing cancer surgery)? The answer to this question is yes in selected situations. For example, the additional risk stratification offered by the information obtained from these tests could assist in planning the perioperative treatment plan. Such information could be used such that:

- markedly abnormal tests might stimulate a re-examination of the scheduled procedure or perhaps the need to alter the surgery accordingly
- depending upon the degree of abnormality found, a more aggressive perioperative treatment regimen might be indicated starting with preoperative addition of cardiac medications (e.g., nitrates, beta-blockers), and involving more aggressive intraoperative monitoring
- more intensive monitoring in an intensive care unit environment is provided for at least 48–72 hours postoperatively.

Moreover, information from a test such as the DSE regarding the patient's "ischemic threshold" would serve as a guide for intraoperative control of hemodynamics. Such an approach was utilized in one study in which patients with abnormal scans (both fixed and redistribution defects) had intensified anti-ischemic therapy preoperatively. These patients had a reduction in the perioperative death rate and myocardial infarction rate from 37% to 6%, and for all cardiac event rates from 47% to 8%, compared to patients with abnormal scans who did not have intensified preoperative anti-ischemic therapy.

Preoperative Cardiac Medications

Patients taking cardiac-related medications should continue to receive these drugs up to the morning of surgery and throughout the perioperative period. Patients taking antianginal medications such as beta-adrenergic blocking drugs, the calcium-channel blocking agents, and nitrates should have these medications maintained throughout the entire perioperative period to avoid withdrawal effects and to prevent perioperative ischemia. Similarly, patients on antihypertensive treatment should also have such treatment continued throughout the perioperative period. The use of perioperative beta blockade therapy to decrease the perioperative cardiac risk in high-risk patients is highly encouraged. Two randomized studies, in particular, have demonstrated that the administration of perioperative beta-blockade to patients with known cardiac disease (history of myocardial infarction, angina, CHF) or cardiac risk factors (diabetes, hypertension, age >70 years, poor functional status, high cholesterol, smoking) who are undergoing major noncardiac surgery have a decreased incidence of perioperative ischemia, including a decreased perioperative risk of myocardial infarction or cardiac death, and a decreased long-term risk of cardiac death. In these studies, the beta-blockers were started preoperatively and continued postoperatively. Therapeutic endpoints included target heart rates below 60 beats/min with a systolic blood pressure of more than 100 mm Hg. From the results of these studies, beta-blocker therapy should be administered to all patients at high risk for coronary events who are scheduled to undergo noncardiac surgery. High-risk patients are those with a history of one or more of:

- myocardial infarction
- angina
- heart failure
- diabetes

especially if the proposed surgery is itself associated with an elevated risk, as is the case for vascular, thoracic, and major abdominal procedures. Ideally, beta-blocker therapy should be initiated several days or weeks preoperatively so that the dose can be adjusted to achieve a resting heart rate of no more than 60 beats/min. In emergency situations, intravenous beta-blockers may be substituted. The perioperative use of beta-adrenergic agonists (e.g., mivazerol) in patients undergoing major vascular or orthopedic procedures has demonstrated that, in the subgroup of patients with known coronary artery disease, mivazerol is associated with a significantly lower incidence of myocardial infarction and death from cardiac causes.

Eligibility for Beta-blocker Use

Criteria used by Mangano and colleagues to define eligibility for beta-blocker use were coronary artery disease (defined as a previous myocardial infarction, typical angina, or atypical angina with positive results on a stress test) or risk for coronary artery disease (defined as the presence of at least two of the following: age >65 years, hypertension, current smoking, serum cholesterol level >240 mg/dL, and diabetes mellitus). Administration of the drug at each time point required that the heart rate be at least 55 beats/min and the systolic blood pressure at least 100 mm Hg with no evidence of CHF, third-degree heart block, or bronchospasm. Patients received two 5 mg doses administered as intravenous atenolol, each over 5 minutes given 30 minutes before surgery, and again immediately after surgery. After surgery, patients were given oral atenolol, 100 mg (if heart rate was >65 beats/min) or 50 mg (if heart rate was >55 beats/min). If the patient was unable to take oral medication, two 5 mg doses were given intravenously every 12 hours. Atenolol was given until hospital discharge (maximum, 7 days).

Endocarditis Prophylaxis

Endocarditis is an infection of the heart resulting in substantial morbidity and mortality. Endocarditis usually develops in individuals with underlying structural cardiac

Table 1-32 Cardiac Conditions Associated with Endocarditis

Endocarditis Prophylaxis Recommended	Endocarditis Prophylaxis Not Recommended

High-Risk Category
Prosthetic cardiac valves, including bioprosthetic and homograft valves
Previous bacterial endocarditis
Complex cyanotic congenital heart disease
  (e.g., single ventricle states, tetralogy of Fallot)
Surgically corrected systemic
  pulmonary shunts or conduits
	Isolated secundum atrial septal defect
	Surgical repair of atrial septal defect, ventricular septal
	  defect, or patent ductus arteriosus
	Previous coronary artery bypass graft
	  surgery
	Mitral valve prolapse without valvular regurgitation

Moderate-Risk Category
Most other congenital cardiac malformations
  (other than above and below)
Acquired valvular dysfunction
  (e.g., rheumatic heart disease)
Hypertrophic cardiomyopathy
Mitral valve prolapse with valvular regurgitation
  and/or thickened valve leaflets
	Physiologic, functional, or innocent heart
	  murmurs
	Previous rheumatic fever without valve
	  dysfunction
	Cardiac pacemakers and implanted defibrillators

defects who develop bacteremia with organisms likely to cause endocarditis (Table 1-32). Some surgical and dental procedures and instrumentations, in particular, cause transient bacteremia that may infect abnormal heart valves or the endocardium near anatomic defects, resulting in bacterial endocarditis (Table 1-33). Certain cardiac conditions are associated with endocarditis more often than others; consequently, in individuals who have an elevated risk for developing endocarditis, endocarditis prophylaxis should be administered just prior to the operation. The antibiotic doses should be sufficient to assure adequate antibiotic blood levels and continued for a brief period after surgery (i.e., 6–8 hours; Tables 1-34 and 1-35). Procedures for which antimicrobial prophylaxis is not recommended are listed in Table 1-33. Mitral valve prolapse is common and the need for prophylaxis for this condition is controversial, as only a small percentage of patients with mitral valve prolapse develop complications. An approach to determination of the need for prophylaxis in individuals with suspected mitral valve prolapse is illustrated in Figure 1-5.

Antimicrobial Regimens for Dental, Oral, Respiratory Tract, or Esophageal Procedures
Streptococcus viridans (beta-hemolytic streptococci) is the most common cause of endocarditis following dental or oral procedures, certain upper respiratory tract procedures, bronchoscopy with a rigid bronchoscope, surgical procedures that involve the respiratory mucosa, and esophageal procedures. Prophylaxis should therefore select antibiotic agents effective against these organisms (see Table 1-32).

Regimens for Genitourinary and Nonesophageal Gastrointestinal Procedures
Bacterial endocarditis that occurs following genitourinary and gastrointestinal tract surgery or instrumentation is most often caused by *Enterococcus faecalis* (enterococci); therefore, antibiotic prophylaxis should target enterococci.

Summary of Preoperative Cardiac Assessment

In summary, preoperative cardiac assessment involves acquisition of pertinent cardiac history, performance of a focused physical examination, and a review of indicated preoperative testing. This information is then utilized to place the patient into a perioperative cardiac risk category. Patients at intermediate risk who are scheduled for intermediate- to high-risk surgery should undergo further ischemic testing, particularly if scheduled for major vascular surgery. Finally, perioperative beta-blockade is emphasized for patients with known cardiac disease or the risk factors for it.

PREOPERATIVE ASSESSMENT OF PATIENTS WITH HYPERTENSION

Background

It is estimated that one fourth of all adults in the United States, or roughly 60 million individuals, have hypertension, with the majority of these individuals at an increased risk of cardiovascular disease. Essential hypertension is the etiologic cause in 95% of the cases, and results from pathogenetic factors including genetic disorders, sodium and water retention disorders, inherited cardiovascular risk factors (hypercholesterolemia, obesity, diabetes), and altered renin–angiotensin–aldosterone

Table 1-33   Surgical Procedures and Endocarditis Prophylaxis

Endocarditis Prophylaxis Recommended	Endocarditis Prophylaxis Not Recommended
Dental Procedures	**Dental Procedures**
Dental extractions	Restorative dentistry (operative and prosthodontic)
Periodontal procedures	with/without retraction cord
Dental implants	Intracanal endodontic treatment; post placement and buildup
Endodontic (root canal) instrumentation	Postoperative suture removal
Initial placement of orthodontic bands but not brackets	Placement of removable prosthodontic or orthodontic
Intraligamentary local anesthetic injections	appliances
Prophylactic cleaning of teeth or implants where bleeding is	Taking of oral impressions
anticipated	Fluoride treatment
Respiratory tract	**Respiratory Tract**
Tonsillectomy and/or adenoidectomy	Endotracheal intubation
Surgical operations that involve respiratory mucosa	Bronchoscopy with a flexible bronchoscope,
Bronchoscopy with a rigid bronchoscope	with or without biopsy
	Tympanostomy tube insertion
Gastrointestinal Tract	**Gastrointestinal Tract**
Sclerotherapy for esophageal varices	Transesophageal echocardiography
Esophageal stricture dilation	Endoscopy with or without gastrointestinal biopsy
Endoscopic retrograde cholangiography with biliary obstruction	
Biliary tract surgery	
Surgical operations that involve intestinal mucosa	
Genitourinary Tract	**Genitourinary Tract**
Prostatic surgery	Vaginal hysterectomy
Cystoscopy	Vaginal delivery
Urethral dilation	Cesarean section
	Procedures in uninfected tissue:
	Urethral catheterization
	Uterine dilatation and curettage
	Therapeutic abortion
	Sterilization procedures
	Insertion or removal of intrauterine devices
	Other
	Cardiac catheterization, including balloon angioplasty
	Implanted cardiac pacemakers, implanted defibrillators,
	and coronary stents
	Circumcision

system reactivity. Millions of American citizens scheduled for surgery each year have mild to severe hypertension and it is therefore essential that an organized approach to the preoperative assessment of the hypertensive patient is followed.

Diagnosis

Hypertension is diagnosed when at least two separate readings 1–2 weeks apart are above 140/90 on average, and is commonly classified into four stages, as illustrated in Table 1-36. The decision to perform further diagnostic testing is dependent upon the presence of associated cardiovascular risk factors, activity level, and the type of surgical procedure planned.

Treatment

In performing a preoperative assessment of the hypertensive patient, it is important to understand the current treatment strategies utilized for controlling blood pressure. The goal for the treatment of hypertension is prevention of the cardiovascular complications of high blood pressure, including coronary artery disease, stroke, CHF, arterial aneurysms, and renal disease. The reduction of blood pressure by the use of pharmacologic agents reduces mortality from cardiovascular disease by 21%, reduces strokes by 38%, and reduces coronary artery disease by 16% in those taking beta-blockers or diuretics. Successful treatment of hypertension decreases the incidence of left ventricular hypertrophy and the development

Table 1-34 Prophylactic Regimens for Dental, Oral, Respiratory Tract, or Esophageal Procedures

Situation	Agent	Regimen
Standard general prophylaxis	Amoxicillin	Adults: 2.0 g; children: 50 mg/kg PO 1 hr before procedure
Unable to take oral medications	Ampicillin	Adults: 2.0 g IM or IV; children: 50 mg/kg IM/IV 30 min before procedure
Allergic to penicillin	Clindamycin or	Adults: 600 mg; children: 20 mg/kg PO 1 hr before procedure
	Cephalexin* or cefadroxil or	Adults: 2.0 g; children: 50 mg/kg PO 1 hr before procedure
	Azithromycin or clarithromycin	Adults: 500 mg; children: 15 mg/kg PO 1 hr before procedure
Allergic to penicillin and unable to take oral medications	Clindamycin or	Adults: 600 mg; children: 20 mg/kg IV within 30 min before procedure
	Cefazolin*	Adults: 1 g; children: 25 mg/kg IM or IV within 30 min before procedure

* Cephalosporins should not be used in individuals with immediate-type hypersensitivity reaction (urticaria, angioedema, or anaphylaxis) to penicillins.
IM, intramuscularly; IV, intravenously; PO, by mouth.

of CHF. Current information supports aggressive treatment of hypertension, especially for the elderly. Data conclusively indicate that the natural history of the complications of hypertension can be altered with currently available antihypertensive drugs, of which there are over 100 from seven drug classes (Box 1-18). The following algorithm illustrates the clinical approach to therapy for essential hypertension (Figure 1-6).

Specific patient groups tend to benefit from a particular drug or drug combination (Table 1-37). For example, diabetic patients with hypertension tend to benefit from angiotensin converting enzyme inhibitors either alone or added to a combination regimen. These agents are particularly useful in delaying the progression of renal dysfunction.

Preoperative Assessment of Patients with Hypertension

The preoperative assessment of patients with essential hypertension involves four basic concerns:

- a familiarity with the medical approach used in treating hypertension (see Figure 1-6), including the classes of drugs prescribed and the important side effects of the antihypertensive agents (see Table 1-37)
- an assessment of end-organ damage
- an accurate estimation of fluid volume status
- a determination regarding whether surgery should proceed in the presence of poorly-controlled hypertension.

The medical treatment of hypertension has already been discussed. Most of the currently available anti-

Table 1-35 Prophylactic Regimens for Genitourinary/Gastrointestinal (Excluding Esophageal) Procedures

Situation	Agent	Regimen
High-risk patients	Ampicillin plus gentamicin	Adults: ampicillin 2.0 g IM or IV plus gentamicin 1.5 mg/kg (not to exceed 120 mg) 30 min before procedure; 6 hr later, ampicillin 1 g IM/IV or amoxicillin 1 g PO
		Children: ampicillin 50 mg/kg IM/IV (not to exceed 2.0 g) plus gentamicin 1.5 mg/kg 30 min before procedure; 6 hr later, ampicillin 25 mg/kg IM/IV or amoxicillin 25 mg/kg PO
High-risk patients allergic to ampicillin/amoxicillin	Vancomycin plus gentamicin	Adults: vancomycin 1.0 g IV over 1 hr, plus gentamicin 1.5 mg IV/IM (not to exceed 120 mg); complete injection/infusion within 30 min of starting procedure
Moderate-risk patients	Amoxicillin or ampicillin	Adults: amoxicillin 2.0 g 1 h before procedure, or ampicillin 2.0 g IM/IV 30 min before procedure
		Children: amoxicillin 50 mg/kg PO 1 hr before procedure, or ampicillin 50 mg/kg IM/IV 30 min before procedure
Moderate-risk patients allergic to ampicillin/amoxicillin	Vancomycin	Children: vancomycin 20 mg/kg IV over 1 hr; infusion to be completed 30 min before procedure
		Children: vancomycin 20 mg/kg IV over 1 hr; infusion to be completed 30 min before procedure

IM, intramuscularly; IV, intravenously; PO, by mouth.

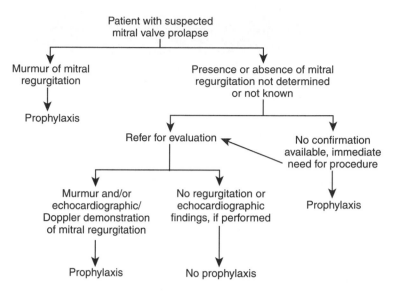

Figure 1-5 Clinical approach to the determination of the need for prophylaxis in patients with suspected mitral valve prolapse. (Redrawn from Dajani A, Taubert K, Wilson W, *et al*. Prevention of bacterial endocarditis: recommendations by the American Heart Association. *Circulation* 1997;96:358–366.)

hypertension agents are listed in Table 1-38. The detection of end-organ damage is important as it gives an estimate of the severity of hypertension as well as the effectiveness of the medications prescribed. Estimation of volume status is of value as actual or relative hypovolemia is common, particularly with use of diuretics and vasodilators. Both the detection of end-organ damage and assessment of volume status are facilitated by a good history, physical examination, detecting postural blood pressure changes, and a review of pertinent laboratory tests (BUN, creatinine, electrolytes, liver function tests, serum glucose, electrocardiogram, and a chest radiograph (cardiomegaly).

Surgery should be postponed in all but true emergency cases when the diastolic blood pressure exceeds 110 mm Hg. It is probably acceptable to proceed with surgery if diastolic pressures are below this level as studies have not shown an independent association with postoperative cardiac or renal complications. Note, however, that patients with preoperative hypertension (treated or untreated) tend to have exaggerated blood pressure responses perioperatively with marked hypertensive responses to laryngoscopy and anesthetic emergence, and hypotensive responses to anesthetic maintenance. Patients who have poorly controlled blood pressure preoperatively demonstrate more hemodynamic lability during the intraoperative period

compared to patients with well-controlled hypertension. Although there is little direct correlation between preoperative hypertension and outcome, the hemodynamic lability may lead to an increase in perioperative cardiac morbidity.

PREOPERATIVE PULMONARY ASSESSMENT

The main purpose of preoperative assessment of patients with pulmonary disease is to identify patients at risk of postoperative pulmonary complications and to institute appropriate perioperative therapy (Figure 1-7). During the evaluation process, the main goals in assessing pulmonary risk are:

- a basic understanding of the pathophysiology of the pulmonary disease
- recognition of patients at high risk for postoperative pulmonary complications, including those undergoing lung surgery

Table 1-36 Stages of hypertension		
Stage	**Systolic Pressure (mm Hg)**	**Diastolic Pressure (mm Hg)**
1 (mild)	140–159	90–99
2 (moderate)	160–179	100–109
3 (severe)	180–209	110–119
4 (very severe)	≥210	≥120

Box 1-18   Drug Classes for the Treatment of Hypertension

Diuretics
Sympatholytics
- Centrally acting
- Peripherally acting agents
- Beta-adrenergic blocking agents
- Alpha-adrenergic blocking agents
Angiotensin-converting enzyme inhibitors
Angiotensin II receptor antagonists
Calcium channel blocking agents
Direct vasodilators
Combination agents

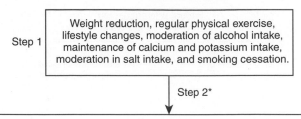

Step 1 | Weight reduction, regular physical exercise, lifestyle changes, moderation of alcohol intake, maintenance of calcium and potassium intake, moderation in salt intake, and smoking cessation.

Step 2*

- Continue lifestyle changes, add initial pharmacologic agent
- Diuretics (elderly, blacks) or beta blockers are usual first-line choices; they have been shown to be effective in reducing risk of stroke and cardiovascular complications, but have adverse metabolic side effects
- ACE inhibitors (CHF, diabetics), calcium channel blockers (LVH), alpha-adrenergic blockers, and angiotensin II type 1 receptor blockers may be chosen instead as first-line therapy; they have favorable metabolic profiles and cardiac, vascular, and renal protective effects but less evidence exists regarding ability to reduce long-term cardiovascular morbidity and mortality

Step 3

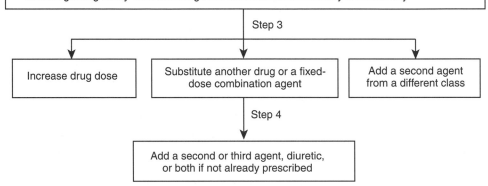

| Increase drug dose | Substitute another drug or a fixed-dose combination agent | Add a second agent from a different class |

Step 4

Add a second or third agent, diuretic, or both if not already prescribed

Figure 1-6 Stepped-care approach to the treatment of essential hypertension. * Step 2 is indicated for patients with either stage 1 hypertension with evidence of end-organ damage or stage 2 hypertension; steps 3 and 4 are therapeutic options for continued poorly controlled hypertension. ACE, angiotensin converting enzyme; CHF, congestive heart failure; LVH, left ventricular hypertrophy.

- modification of risk factors for postoperative pulmonary complications and optimization of preoperative status (i.e., smoking cessation, respiratory therapy, and treatment of preoperative bronchospasm)
- facilitation of postoperative recovery through effective pain management techniques.

The most commonly encountered pulmonary diseases include chronic obstructive pulmonary disease (COPD) and reactive airway disease (i.e., asthma). The designation COPD includes chronic bronchitis and emphysema. Chronic bronchitis is defined clinically by patients who have a chronic productive cough (for ≥3 months of the year for ≥2 years) due to excess bronchial mucus secre-

tion leading to a severe reduction in expiratory flow rates. Chronic bronchitis pathologically includes large airway mucus gland hyperplasia, airway inflammation and obstruction of small airways. Cigarette smoking is the most common etiologic factor in chronic bronchitis.

Emphysema is characterized by abnormal permanent enlargement of the airspaces distal to terminal bronchioles, accompanied by destruction of lung parenchyma. Pulmonary function tests disclose a decreased diffusing capacity (for carbon monoxide) and chest radiography shows a hyperexpansion of the lungs with flattened diaphragms and reduced lung parenchymal density (hyperlucency). The dominant clinical and pathophysiologic

Table 1-37 Selected Patient Group with Indicated Antihypertensive Drug Class

Patient Group	Indicated Drug Class	Drug Classes to Avoid
Elderly or blacks	Diuretics or CCB	Sympatholytics (including beta-blockers)
Congestive heart failure	ACE inhibitors, diuretics	Beta-blockers, verapamil, diltiazem
Coronary artery disease	Beta-blockers, ACE inhibitors (especially post myocardial infarction, or with ↓ ejection fraction)	
Left ventricular hypertrophy	ACE inhibitors, CCB, beta-blockers, sympatholytics	Diuretics, vasodilators
Diabetics or hyperlipidemia	ACE inhibitors, CCB, alpha-1-blockers	Beta-blockers, diuretics
COPD or PVD		Beta-blockers

ACE, angiotensin-converting enzyme; CCB, calcium channel blockers; COPD, chronic obstructive pulmonary disease; PVD: peripheral vascular disease.

Table 1-38 Antihypertensive Fact Sheet

Drug Class	Generic Name	Trade Name	Mechanism of Action	Common Side Effects	Anesthetic Interactions
Diuretics					
Thiazide diuretics	Chlorothiazide Hydrochlorothiazide Indapamide Methyclothiazide Chlorthalidone Metolazone	Diuril Oretic, HydroDIURIL, Esidrix Lozol Aquatensen, Enduron Hygroton Zaroxolyn	Increase urinary excretion of sodium and chloride by inhibiting reabsorption of Na^+ and Cl^- in the cortical thick ascending limb of Henle and early distal tubule	Hypokalemia, hypochloremia, alkalosis, hyperglycemia, hyperuricemia, hypercholesterolemia, hypercalcemia	Low plasma volume → increased hemodynamic sensitivity to anesthetic agents Hypokalemia – potentiation of muscle relaxants (with prolongation of respiratory depression); dysrhythmias such as APCs, PVCs, atrial flutter, ventricular bigeminy, torsade de pointes); digitalis – toxicity
Loop diuretics	Furosemide Bumetanide Ethacrynic acid Torsemide	Lasix Bumex Edecrin Demadex	Inhibit reabsorption of Na^+ and Cl^-, not only in proximal and distal tubules but in the thick ascending limb of Henle		
Potassium-sparing diuretics	Spironolactone Triamterene Amiloride	Aldactone Dyrenium Midamor	Interfere with Na^+ reabsorption in the distal tubule, thus ↓ K^+ secretion. Weak diuretics and antihypertensives	Elevated potassium, nausea and vomiting, gastrointestinal disturbances	Hyperkalemia → bradyarrhythmias
Sympatholytics					
Beta-adrenergic blockers	Propranolol Propranolol SR Atenolol Metoprolol Nadolol Timolol Pindolol Acebutolol Bisoprolol Betaxolol	Inderal Inderal LA Tenormin Lopressor; Toprol XL Corgard Blocadren Visken Sectral Zebeta Kerlone	Competes with beta-adrenergic agonists for available binding sites (β_1-cardiac muscle, β_2-bronchial and vascular musculature). Antihypertensive effects due to competitive antagonism of catecholamines at cardiac adrenergic sites (↓ CO), central effect with ↓ sympathetic outflow to periphery	Bronchospasm, cardiac depression → CHF; bradycardia, claudication (ASVD), Raynaud's phenomenon, paresthesias, fatigue, depression, increased triglycerides, increased cholesterol, withdrawal syndrome – less likely with labetalol	Decreased ischemic episodes intraoperatively (in patients with ischemic heart disease); cardiac depression; bradycardia; poor response to sympathomimetic amines; bronchospasm
Beta- and alpha-blocker	Labetalol	Trandate, Normodyne	Blocks beta-receptors responsible for renin release in the kidneys.		
Centrally-acting agents	Methyldopa Clonidine tablets Clonidine patch Guanfacine Guanabenz	Aldomet Catapres Catapres TTS Tenex Wytensin	Stimulate central inhibitory alpha-adrenergic receptors activity → decreasing sympathetic outflow to periphery. Also ↓ renin activity. ↓ tissue concentrations of serotonin, norepinephrine, and epinephrine	Methyldopa: sedation, bradycardia, ↑ LFTs Clonidine: CHF, orthostasis, tachycardia, bradycardia, conduction disturbances, withdrawal syndrome (24 h)	Methyldopa: ↓ MAC of halothane; Clonidine: continue use up to 4 hours preop, and begin ASAP after surgery. Treat ↑ BP with NTG, phentolamine, prazosin, or ACE inhibitor

Continued

Table 1-38 Antihypertensive Fact Sheet—cont'd

Drug Class	Generic Name	Trade Name	Mechanism of Action	Common Side Effects	Anesthetic Interactions
Alpha-adrenergic blockers	Prazosin Terazosin Doxazosin	Minipress Hytrin Cardura	Postsynaptic alpha-1-receptor blockers; dilates resistance and capacitance vessels – greatest effect on diastolic blood pressure	First-dose effect (postural hypotension); headache, drowsiness, palpitations, dizziness, nausea	Verapamil increases prazosin levels → hypotension; Alpha-blockers ↓ effect of clonidine
Calcium Channel Blockers	Verapamil Verapamil (extended release) Diltiazem Nifedipine Isradipine Amlodipine Felodipine Nicardipine Nisoldipine	Calan, Isoptin, Verelan, Calan SR, Isoptin SR, Covera-HS Cardizem (SR, CD), Dilacor XR Procardia (XL), Adalat (CC) DynaCirc Norvasc Plendil Cardene (SR) Sular	Inhibit intracellular transport of Ca^{2+} through specific calcium channels located in specialized cardiac conduction cells and vascular smooth muscle cells; Verapamil inhibits hepatic cytochrome P450 enzymes	Additive cardiac depressive effects with beta-blockers; ↑ digoxin levels with verapamil; tachycardia, edema, flushing (nifedipine, amlodipine, nicardipine); withdrawal syndrome if abruptly stopped (rebound coronary spasm)	↑ anesthetic effects of etomidate (respiratory depression, apnea); Potentiates narcotic effects (hypotension, ↑ fluid requirements); additive effects of benzodiazepines (verapamil) Potentiates nondepolarizing relaxants (verapamil);
Angiotensin Converting Enzyme Inhibitors	Captopril Enalapril Lisinopril Benazepril Quinapril Ramipril Fosinopril Moexipril Perindopril	Capoten Vasotec Zestril, Prinivil Lotensin Accupril Altace Monopril Univase Aceon	Suppression of renin–angiotensin–aldosterone system by inhibiting angiotensin I → angiotensin II. May also inhibit local angiotensin II at vascular and renal sites and attenuate release of catecholamines from adrenergic nerve endings	First dose hypotensive effect (esp. with CHF; hypovolemia); cough, headache, dizziness; angioedema; hyperkalemia (esp. with CHF); renal insufficiency/failure	Exaggerated hypotensive effects with use of anesthetics (treat with fluid); Hyperkalemia possible in patients on ACE inhibitors, especially those with CHF, renal insufficiency, and diabetes mellitus
Angiotensin II Receptor Antagonist	Losartan Valsartan Irbesartan	Cozaar Diovan Avapro	Blocks effects of angiotensin II at tissue sites by competitive binding to angiotensin II receptor	Similar profile to ACE inhibitors	Similar profile to ACE inhibitors
Direct Vasodilators	Hydralazine Minoxidil	Apresoline Loniten	Direct relaxation of vascular smooth muscle (alters cellular calcium metabolism interfering with Ca^{2+} movement within the vascular smooth muscle cell)	Hyperdynamic circulation; palpitations, headache, nausea and vomiting; fluid retention; lupus-like syndrome	Resting tachycardia may precipitate angina, cardiac ischemia; concurrent use with beta blockers increases serum levels of both

Table 1-38 Antihypertensive Fact Sheet—cont'd

Drug Class	Generic Name	Trade Name	Mechanism of Action	Common Side Effects	Anesthetic Interactions
Combination Agents			For mechanism of action, side effects, and anesthetic concerns, refer to individual drug categories		
Diuretic combinations	HCTZ/amiloride	Moduretic			
	HCTZ/spironolactone	Aldactazide			
	HCTZ/triamterene	Maxzide, Dyazide			
ACE inhibitor and diuretic	Benazepril/HCTZ	Lotensin HCT			
	Captopril/HCTZ	Capozide			
	Enalapril/HCTZ	Vaseretic			
	Lisinopril/HCTZ	Zestoretic			
Beta blocker and diuretic	Atenolol/chlorthalidone	Tenoretic			
	Propranolol/HCTZ	Inderide			
	Propranolol LA/HCTZ	Inderide LA			
	Timolol/HCTZ	Timolide			
	Bisoprolol/HCTZ	Ziac			
Calcium channel blocker and ACE inhibitor	Amlodipine/benazepril	Lotrel			
	Diltiazem/enalapril	Teczem			
	Felodipine/enalapril	Lexxel			
Vasodilator and diuretic	Hydralazine/HCTZ	Apresazide			
	Prazosin/polythiazide	Minizide			
Centrally-acting agent and diuretic	Clonidine/chlorothiazide	Combipress			
	Methyldopa/chlorothiazide	Aldoclor			
	Methyldopa/HCTZ	Aldoril			
	Reserpine/HCTZ	Hydropres			
	Reserpine/hydroflumethiazide	Salutensin-Demi, Salutensin			

MAC, minimum alveolar anesthetic concentration.

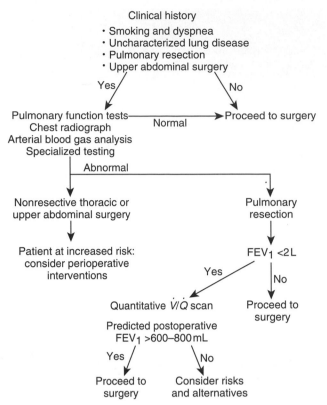

Figure 1-7   Algorithm for preoperative pulmonary risk assessment. (Redrawn from Sheperd K, Hurford W. Pulmonary disease. In: Sweitzer BJ, ed. *Handbook of preoperative assessment and management.* Philadelphia: Lippincott Williams & Wilkins, 2000:97–125.)

Box 1-19   Risk Factors Implicated in Postoperative Pulmonary Complications

Age >60 years
Gender (male > female)
Chronic obstructive pulmonary disease
Coexisting medical diseases (diabetes, hypertension, ischemic cardiac disease, renal and hepatic disease, cancer, stroke)
Smoking history (>10 pack-years)
Preoperative wheezing or unexplained dyspnea
History of acute upper or lower respiratory tract infection requiring treatment in the last 14 days
Impaired exercise capacity
Impaired preoperative cognitive function
Impaired postoperative mobility status
Obesity (body mass index ≥27)
Prolonged preoperative length of stay (days)
ASA physical status (>ASA II)
Duration of anesthesia (>3 hours)
Surgical incision site (upper abdomen, both upper and lower abdomen)
Absence of preoperative education regarding deep breathing, incentive spirometry
History of cancer

---

feature of both types of COPD is limitation of expiratory airflow rates. Patients with COPD typically present with dyspnea, cough, wheezing, sputum production, and recurrent respiratory infections.

Asthma is a chronic inflammatory airway disease process the major characteristics of which include variable degrees of airflow obstruction, bronchial hyperresponsiveness, and airway inflammation. Cellular and chemical mediators augment airway inflammation, bronchial smooth muscle tone, and the airway bronchoconstrictor responsiveness. The typical clinical hallmark of asthma is the episodic occurrence of bronchospasm characterized by wheezing and shortness of breath (with improvement after the use of bronchodilators).

Identifying Preoperative Risk Factors for Postoperative Pulmonary Complications

Postoperative pulmonary complications are an important part of the risk of surgery and often significantly prolong the hospital stay. Postoperative pulmonary complications generally include pneumonia, respiratory failure with prolonged mechanical ventilation, bronchospasm, atelectasis, and exacerbation of underlying chronic lung disease. Patient-related risk factors that may contribute to the risk of postoperative pulmonary complications are listed in Box 1-19. In the presence of such risk factors, the incidence of postoperative pulmonary complications increases by two- to fourfold when compared with patients without such risk factors.

When evaluating perioperative pulmonary risk, the surgical site is the most important predictor of pulmonary risk. Risk increases as the incision approaches the diaphragm. Upper abdominal and thoracic surgery entail the greatest risk of postoperative pulmonary complications, ranging from 10% to 40%. Reductions in functional residual capacity and vital capacity after upper abdominal surgery may persist for 5–7 days. Postoperative pulmonary complications are much less after operations outside the chest or abdomen.

Reduced exercise capacity is another predictor of increased perioperative risk. In a study of patients over 65 years of age who were undergoing abdominal or nonresective thoracic surgery, the inability to perform 2 minutes of supine bicycle exercise sufficient to raise the heart rate to 99 beats/min was the strongest predictor of pulmonary complications.

History

Preoperative history taking should elicit background features and specific symptoms referable to the pulmonary system (Box 1-20). If positive responses are obtained to questions about the symptoms listed, then a more detailed questioning should occur. In particular, questioning should attempt to elicit the clinical features of asthma or other types of COPD (e.g., bronchitis, emphysema). Information regarding exercise tolerance and the presence or absence of dyspnea is important. In addition, determining whether recent changes have occurred in these symptoms is vital. Given the nonspecificity of symptoms, however, further tests of respiratory and cardiac function are frequently indicated.

Patients with asthma are a particularly high-risk group of patients and have an increased risk of perioperative complications. Although early studies reported increased overall rates of postoperative complications of 24% in asthmatic patients versus 14% in controls, more recent studies have confirmed much lower risk. For example, in a recent study of patients with asthma, 33% of whom had received bronchodilators within the previous 30 days, the overall incidence of perioperative bronchospasm was only 1.7%. The most important historical questions relate to wheezing, coughing, and sputum production. A history of severe asthma requiring corticosteroid therapy, emergency department visits or hospitalizations, the need for mechanical ventilation, and severe bronchospasm with a previous anesthetic substantially increases the risk for perioperative complications. For patients with bronchitis, important information relates to the presence of wheezing, coughing, and the quantity of sputum production. Patients who produce sputum daily and especially those with a recent increase in the quantity of purulent sputum have an increased risk of postoperative pulmonary complications. Unexplained dyspnea is a serious complaint and can be caused by a wide spectrum of pulmonary and nonpulmonary causes, restrictive disorders, pulmonary vascular disease, and obstructive airway diseases; and should always stimulate further questioning and investigation.

Patients with sleep apnea syndrome may present perioperative challenges, especially with airway management. Sleep apnea, defined as repeated episodes of obstructive apnea during sleep together with daytime sleepiness, mood changes, and altered cardiopulmonary function, is common. It is estimated that 2–4% of middle-aged adults are affected with this disorder. The sleep apnea syndrome is frequently identified in patients with obesity. Patients with sleep apnea have an increased risk of diurnal hypertension, nocturnal dysrhythmias, pulmonary hypertension, right and left ventricular failure, ischemic cardiac disease, and stroke.

Box 1-20   Important Points in Preoperative Pulmonary Assessment

BACKGROUND FEATURES

Smoking (>10 pack-years)
Recent infections
Current medication
Allergies
Site of surgery
Type of surgery
Anticipated length of surgery and anesthesia

CLINICAL SYMPTOMS

Cough
Sputum character and amount
Wheezing
Dyspnea
Exercise tolerance
Chest tightness and pain

SPECIFIC PULMONARY DISEASE STATES

Asthma
Recent wheezing, coughing, sputum production
Recent upper respiratory infection with symptoms
Use of corticosteroids (current, ever)
Emergency department visits (date of most recent)
Hospitalizations requiring mechanical ventilation
Previous bronchospasm with anesthesia
Chronic obstructive pulmonary disease
Wheezing, coughing, quantity of sputum production
Increased dyspnea
Recent URI with symptoms
Recent change in sputum quantity and quality
Sleep apnea syndrome
Obesity
History of snoring, choking while sleeping
Daytime sleepiness
Difficulty concentrating
Changes in personality

Physical Examination

While performing the physical examination, the clinical appearance of the patient is important. An assessment should be made as to the presence of labored breathing (neck accessory or intercostal muscles). If the breathing is unlabored, then it is likely that the patient is at their clinical baseline. However, the presence of inspiratory crackles (interstitial edema, atelectasis), rhonchi (large airway secretions), and decreased localized breath sounds (consolidation) should be noted. Expiratory wheezing generally occurs in the presence of bronchospasm and is an important finding in asthma. For patients with sleep apnea, no specific physical findings are diagnostic. However, morbid obesity, a short neck with limited range of motion, advanced age, and a high Mallampati classification may raise suspicion. Patients with COPD who, before surgery, have clinical findings of airflow obstruction (wheezing), who are not at their baseline symptomatically, and who have increased dyspnea with activity should be aggressively treated. Elective surgery should be postponed in these situations and pulmonary treatment initiated. Combinations of bronchodilators, physical therapy, antibiotics, smoking cessation, and corticosteroids reduce the risk of postoperative pulmonary complications.

Preoperative Pulmonary Testing

Pulmonary testing, when appropriate, can provide important information about the character and severity of the lung disease. Such testing, however, should be limited to specific clinical scenarios. Arterial blood gases, for example, are indicated in a very few selected clinical situations (Table 1-39). Similarly, preoperative chest radiographs are no longer routinely recommended before surgery: they should only be obtained in patients who have clinical evidence of pulmonary disease (e.g., wheezing, rales, consolidation, recent development of a productive cough) or cancer, or who are scheduled for thoracic surgery. Spirometry is indicated primarily for patients with significant clinical symptoms of lung disease in order to provide a diagnosis, follow therapy, or in patients scheduled for abdominal or thoracic surgery. Ventilation/perfusion ($\dot{V}/\dot{Q}$) scanning is indicated for patients scheduled for lung resection who have severe spirometric abnormalities on preoperative testing. The pulmonary tests encountered most often and the indications for such tests are listed in Table 1-39.

Spirometry

Spirometry is useful in certain preoperative situations (see Table 1-39). Although spirometry facilitates the diagnosis of lung disease and estimates disease severity, it is not useful in estimating perioperative risk. Clinical identification of underlying pulmonary disease is as reliable as pulmonary function testing in assessing a patient's risk of developing perioperative pulmonary complications. There are occasions, however, when preoperative spirometry has clinical usefulness and a brief discussion of the test is, therefore, appropriate. Spirometry is based on a vital capacity or forced vital capacity (FVC) maneuver (Figure 1-8).

The patient inhales as deeply as possible, and then exhales completely and as forcefully as possible. Volume is recorded as a function of time and therefore allows an assessment of flow rates. The FVC is the maximum

Test	Indications
Arterial blood gas	History and/or physical examination indicating severe pulmonary disease
	Severe spirometric abnormalities
	Pulmonary resection
Chest radiography	No routine requirement
	Clinical evidence of disease (wheezing, rales, consolidation, recent onset productive cough)
	Thoracic surgery
Spirometry	Clinical symptoms of lung disease, especially if undergoing cardiac, thoracic, and upper abdominal surgery
	Assessment of baseline function in patients with asthma or COPD
	Determine degree of reversibility of pulmonary disease
	Investigation of unexplained dyspnea
	Smoking history in patient scheduled for thoracic or upper abdominal surgery
	Pulmonary resection
Quantitative $\dot{V}/\dot{Q}$ scanning	Performed in patients scheduled for pulmonary resection with severe reductions in spirometric values in order to predict postoperative pulmonary function

Table 1-39   Preoperative Pulmonary Testing and Indications

COPD, chronic obstructive pulmonary disease, $\dot{V}/\dot{Q}$, ventilation/perfusion.

amount of gas that can be exhaled after a maximal inhalation. The amount of gas exhaled in the first second of the FVC is known as the forced expiratory volume in 1 second (FEV_1). Persons with normal lungs should be able to exhale 75–80% of FVC within this time, whereas those with increased airway resistance will exhibit a reduction in airflow rate and a decrease in both FEV_1 and the FEV_1:FVC ratio. Normal adult spirometric values are listed in Table 1-40.

The early portion of the FVC curve is more effort-dependent (FEF 200–1200; see Figure 1-8); while the mid-portion of the curve, measured between the first and last quarters of the FVC measurement is considered the most effort-independent portion (FEF 25%–75%) and is the most sensitive indicator of small airways obstruction (e.g., asthmatic patient). The FEV_1 or $FEF_{25\%-75\%}$ values can be used to estimate the degree of pulmonary obstructive lung disease (Table 1-41).

Expiratory flow parameters are the best spirometric predictors of postoperative pulmonary complications. Perioperative risk is increased in abdominal and thoracic surgical procedures. For abdominal surgery, an FEV_1 of less than 2 L (or < 50% of predicted) suggests that the patient is at increased risk for pulmonary complications.

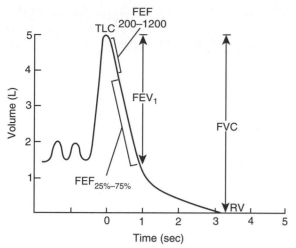

Figure 1-8   Typical spirometric flow diagram. See p. 50 for explanation. FEF, forced expiratory flow; RV, residual volume; TLC, total lung capacity.

For lung resection, an increased risk of pulmonary complications is associated with a reduction in FEV_1 or FVC of ≤70% of predicted, or a ratio of FEV_1 to FVC of ≤65%. For patients undergoing pulmonary resection surgery, an FEV_1 of ≥2 liters (or ≥60% of the predicted normal value) is desired for a pneumonectomy, while an FEV_1 of 1.5 L is preferred for a lobectomy.

Arterial blood gases are indicated preoperatively in patients with severe abnormalities on pulmonary function testing and in those being evaluated for lung resection. Quantitative ventilation/perfusion lung scanning is indicated in patients who are scheduled for major lung resection and show severe abnormalities on spirometric testing.

Quantitative ventilation/perfusion lung scanning involves the use of inhaled and intravenously injected radionuclides. The total amount of radioactivity is quantified and the percentages of ventilation and perfusion to

Table 1-40	Normal Spirometric Values for Adult 70 kg Male, Sitting Position

Test	Value
FVC	4.7 L
FEV_1	3.9 L
FEV_1/FVC	83%
MMF	3 L/sec
FRC	2.7 L

FEV_1, forced expiratory volume in 1 second; FRC, functional residual capacity; FVC, forced vital capacity; MMF, mid-maximal flow rate ($FEF_{25\%-75\%}$).
From Frost E. Preanesthesia assessment of the patient with respiratory disease. *Anesthesiol Clin North Am* 1990;8:657-675.

Table 1-41	Values of FEV_1 or $FEF_{25\%-75\%}$ and Severity of Obstructive Lung Disease

FEV_1 or $FEF_{25\%-75\%}$ (% predicted)	Degree of Obstruction
75	Normal
65-75	Mild obstruction
50-65	Moderate obstruction
<50	Severe obstruction

each lung are determined. Residual FEV_1 is then predicted by multiplying the FEV_1 by the percentage of radioactive counts from the nonoperative lung (or lung region). A calculated predicted postoperative FEV_1 of at least 0.8 L (or more than 40% of the predicted normal value) is considered to be sufficient lung tissue for lung resection.

Overall, postoperative pulmonary complications occur in 29% of patients with severe COPD as defined by an FEV_1 of ≤50% of the predicted value and a ratio of FEV_1 to FVC of ≤70%. Although spirometric abnormalities may suggest increased perioperative pulmonary risk, clinical findings remain the most accurate in the prediction of perioperative pulmonary complications.

Preoperative Management

Overall, the goal of preoperative assessment is to detect (and modify) risk factors for postoperative pulmonary complications. Appropriate use of preoperative pulmonary testing may be warranted as part of the risk assessment (see Figure 1-7). Interventions that may lessen the likelihood of perioperative complications are listed in Box 1-21. Table 1-42 lists the therapeutic agents commonly used in bronchospastic lung disease.

Patients with symptomatic COPD should be treated with inhaled bronchodilators. Inhaled anticholinergic agents such as ipratropium should be tried first, while inhaled beta-adrenergic receptor agonists, used up to four times daily, should be added as needed for symptoms. The two agents have an additive effect and are available as a combination inhaled therapy (Combivent™). Smoking cessation for at least 8 weeks before elective surgery is also strongly advised. A short (1-2 week) preoperative course of systemic corticosteroids is reasonable for patients who continue to have symptoms despite bronchodilator therapy and who are not at their personal baseline level as determined by symptoms, chest examination, and spirometry. Preoperative antibiotics should be used for patients in whom the presence of infection is suggested by a change in the character or amount of sputum.

Box 1-21 Interventions Used Preoperatively to Decrease Risk of Perioperative Respiratory Complications in Patients with Lung Disease

Treat airflow obstruction (chronic obstructive pulmonary disease, asthma)
- Oral or inhaled bronchodilators
- Oral or inhaled corticosteroids
- Antibiotics

Smoking cessation (8 weeks preoperatively)
Weight loss
Prevention of aspiration
Lung expansion techniques
- Chest physiotherapy
- Deep breathing and coughing
- Incentive spirometry
- Mask continuous positive airway pressure

Similarly, asthmatic patients are at increased risk of postoperative pulmonary complications, especially if they have difficult-to-control asthma, have had a recent attack, or have had a recent upper respiratory infection. Airway hyperreactivity persists for several weeks after an episode of asthma, and an improvement in asthma symptoms does not preclude the development of bronchospasm in response to various stimuli. In addition to usual bronchodilator therapy, patients with asthma should be treated with prednisone (40 mg) starting 24–48 hours before surgery and continued for 1–2 days after surgery. Intravenous hydrocortisone (e.g., 100 mg every 8 hrs) may be given in those unable to take medication orally. Preoperative steroid therapy is particularly recommended for asthmatics with an FEV_1 less than 80% of predicted. Steroid therapy can be tapered off during the first week, postoperatively. A short course of perioperative corticosteroids does not increase the incidence of infection or other postoperative complications in patients with asthma. The addition of inhaled anticholinergic agents may be beneficial, although these drugs are generally more effective in patients with COPD.

Finally, preoperative maneuvers that increase lung volume (lung volume expansion techniques) reduce the incidence and severity of postoperative pulmonary complications in high-risk patients. The most beneficial expiratory maneuver is coughing. Incentive spirometry has been shown to reduce the frequency of both radiological and clinical complications after abdominal surgery but deep breathing is equally effective in motivated patients. Patients should perform either maneuver as often as possible during the first 3–4 postoperative days. Application of continuous positive airway pressure

should be employed for patients who are unable to perform lung expansion techniques because of lack of cooperation or severity of illness.

PREOPERATIVE RENAL ASSESSMENT

Five percent of adults in the United States suffer from renal disease. Further increases in the life expectancy of patients with end-stage renal disease will only add to these numbers as continuing advances in medical treatments and transplantation surgery occur. Renal dysfunction is known to increase the risk of anesthesia and postoperative renal failure is a leading cause of perioperative morbidity and mortality. Preoperative identification of patients with renal dysfunction requires a review of the patient's medical history, identification of risk factors associated with renal dysfunction, and appropriate preoperative testing. Appropriate preoperative management and perioperative planning can preserve renal function and improve perioperative outcome.

Risk Factors

A number of factors should be considered in assessing renal risk in the perioperative period (Box 1-22). These include pre-existing renal reserve, factors associated with surgical procedures, and other renal insults to which the patient might be exposed during the perioperative period. Preoperative testing of renal function is essential in selected patients.

The major factor determining renal risk is pre-existing renal reserve. Indeed, looking at perioperative renal function, the only factor consistently predictive of postoperative renal failure is preoperative renal dysfunction. Renal function decreases with age with total nephron number declining by 50% at 70 years of age. Age is also associated with an increased frequency of diseases affecting the kidney, including atherosclerosis and hypertension. Indeed, age has been shown to be an independent risk factor for postoperative renal dysfunction independent of underlying renal function or other coexisting diseases. Pre-existing disease states such as cardiac disease, diabetes, and peripheral vascular disease increase renal risk in the perioperative period. Long-standing diabetes has been demonstrated to be an independent risk factor for renal dysfunction regardless of level of renal reserve. Hepatic failure is associated with increased renal risk.

Surgical procedures also increase the risk of perioperative renal dysfunction. Such procedures include cardiopulmonary bypass, aortic cross-clamping, surgery for transplantation of the liver or kidney, and any procedure involving large fluid shifts, which may cause a reduction or interruption of the renal circulation resulting in

Table 1-42 Preoperative Pulmonary Medications and Common Dosing

Drug Class	Drug	Trade Name	Action	Dose	Side Effects
Inhaled beta-2-adrenergic agonists	Albuterol Salmeterol Pirbuterol	Proventil Serevent Maxair	Augment cAMP-mediated relaxation of bronchial smooth muscle Beneficial effects on mucociliary function	2 inhalations every 4-6 hrs	Cardiac (dysrhythmias, tachycardia); hypokalemia; headache; bronchitis; cough; URI; ECG changes (ST segment depression)
Anticholinergic agonists	Ipratropium bromide	Atrovent	Bronchodilate by blocking action of cGMP Inhibit reflex bronchoconstriction with intubation	2 puffs from metered-dose inhaler every 6-8 hrs	Headache; dry mouth; nausea; URI; constipation; bronchitis; dyspnea
Combination: inhaled beta-2-adrenergic agonists and anticholinergic agonists	Albuterol and ipratropium bromide	Combivent	Combine actions of both classes together in one drug	2 inhalations qid	Same side effects as individual drugs
Methylxanthines (aminophylline, theophylline)	Aminophylline Theophylline	Generic only Elixophyllin	Inhibition of phosphodiesterase isoenzymes	IV load: 4-5 mg/kg; Infusion: 0.4-0.8 mg/kg/hr	Tremulousness; tachycardia; dysrhythmias; vomiting; seizures; tremors
Corticosteroids	Prednisone Prednisolone Hydrocortisone	Detasone (oral) Delta-Cortef (oral) Nutracort (oral) Solu-Cortef (IV)	Reduce airway inflammation and hyperresponsiveness, mucous secretion, smooth muscle constriction, edema; inhibit formation of inflammatory leukotrienes	PO: prednisone 40 mg/day 2-7 days preoperatively IV: perioperative dose: 25-100 mg hydrocortisone	Hyperglycemia; hypertension; salt retention; changes in affect; decreased wound healing; fluid retention; peptic ulcers
	Beclomethasone dipropionate	Beclovent, Vanceril, Vancenase (inhaled)		Inhaled: 1-2 inhalations intranasally bid	

bid, twice a day; cAMP, cyclic adenosine monophosphate; qid, four times a day.

prolonged prerenal ischemia. In the case of major thoracic or thoracoabdominal aortic surgery, acute postoperative renal insufficiency is a common complication, occurring in 25% of patients with 8% requiring hemodialysis. Age more than 50 years, preoperative renal dysfunction, duration of renal ischemia, and the amount of blood transfusion therapy (>5 units) are all significant predictors of postoperative renal dysfunction.

Preoperative Assessment

Renal function is often estimated by obtaining serum creatinine and BUN measurements. Unfortunately, more than 50% of renal function must be lost before the serum creatinine begins to rise. Although patients with only 20–40% of normal kidney function and increased BUN and creatinine levels may remain well compensated under normal conditions, limited renal reserve is present and perioperative stress may contribute toward a marked deterioration in renal function.

The preoperative approach to patients with renal disease should be well planned. Risk factors for renal dysfunction, as mentioned, should be kept in mind (Box 1-22). Patients with laboratory evidence of renal dysfunction or

---

Box 1-22   Factors Predisposing to New-onset or Worsened Perioperative Renal Dysfunction

PRE-EXISTING RENAL RESERVE

Elderly

Diuretics

Comorbid diseases
- Pre-existing renal insufficiency
- Left ventricular dysfunction
- Diabetes mellitus
- Hypertension
- Peripheral vascular disease
- Hepatic dysfunction
- Sepsis

SURGICAL PROCEDURE

Vascular operations with aortic cross-clamping

Cardiopulmonary bypass

Excessive length of surgical procedure

Major blood loss

Procedures with major fluid shifts

INTRAOPERATIVE FACTORS

Hypotension

Hypovolemia

Antibiotics (e.g., aminoglycosides)

Radiocontrast agents

---

known renal disease should have the etiology of the renal dysfunction determined preoperatively whenever possible. In assessing patients with renal dysfunction, division is made into three basic types: acute, chronic, and acute on chronic renal failure (Table 1-43).

Acute renal failure (ARF), usually a recent diagnosis, is divided into three categories: prerenal, intrarenal, and postrenal failure. Conversely, chronic renal failure (CRF) is a disease that is either well known to the patient or is well documented in the medical record. In some instances, however, the patient does not know the etiology of the CRF and the preoperative records are limited. In these situations, the etiology of the renal dysfunction should be determined before proceeding with elective surgery. Finally, acute on chronic renal failure is a clinical situation where acute deterioration of renal function occurs in the setting of CRF.

Acute Renal Failure

Acute renal failure is a disease due to a variety of insults and is defined as an acute loss of renal function occurring over a period of hours to several days. Typical abnormalities seen include disturbances of extracellular fluid balance, acid base metabolism, and serum electrolytes. The diagnosis of ARF is primarily determined by increasing levels of serum creatinine and/or BUN, usually associated with a decline in urine production. The diagnosis of ARF should be considered whenever there is an increase in the serum creatinine level of more than 0.5 mg/dL or an increase of 50% or more in the baseline serum creatinine. ARF occurs in approximately 1% of hospitalized patients, in 20% of patients treated in intensive care units, and as many as 4–15% of patients after cardiovascular surgery. Some 40% of the cases of perioperative renal dysfunction are due to renal hypoperfusion and of those patients who develop ARF approximately 30% will require dialysis.

The approach to patients with ARF should begin with an accurate history followed by a thorough medical chart review, physical examination, and laboratory testing in order to determine the cause of ARF. The recommended approach begins by placing the patient into one of three diagnostic categories: prerenal, postrenal, and intrinsic renal failure (Table 1-44). Intravascular volume status is perhaps the most important factor in the evaluation of ARF, with 60% of the cases of community-acquired ARF being due to prerenal conditions. Common scenarios include excessive, nonreplaced fluid deficits due to gastrointestinal, renal, or cutaneous losses. The physical examination often reveals signs of volume depletion such as tachycardia, postural blood pressure changes, poor skin turgor, dry mucous membranes, and hypotension. Laboratory testing should include serum electrolyte determination, urinary electrolytes, and a urinalysis.

Table 1-43	Types of Renal Failure		
		Clinical disorders	*Causes*
Acute	Prerenal (absolute or effective reduction in plasma volume)	Hypovolemia	Diuretics Vomiting Gastrointestinal losses (diarrhea, bowel preps)
		Congestive heart failure Nephrotic syndrome Cirrhosis Sepsis Nonsteroidal anti-inflammatory drugs Antihypertension medications (e.g., angiotensin-converting enzyme inhibitors) Cyclosporine Amphotericin B	
	Intrarenal	Tubular disorders Vascular related	Acute tubular necrosis Atheroembolic disease Scleroderma Malignant hypertension Hemolytic–uremic syndrome Acute cortical necrosis
		Interstitial disease	Allergic interstitial nephritis Antibiotics Nonsteroidal anti-inflammatory drugs Thiazide diuretics Cimetidine Phenytoin Chinese herb teas
		Glomerulonephritis	
	Postrenal	Prostatism Ureteral stones Retroperitoneal disease Medication-induced crystalluria Bladder neoplasm	
Chronic		Diabetes mellitus Hypertensive nephrosclerosis Chronic glomerulonephritis Chronic interstitial nephritis Analgesic nephropathy Polycystic kidney disease	
Acute on chronic		Combination of above disorders	Any combination of the above

In determining the cause of ARF, the most important tests are the urinary studies (i.e., the urinalysis, examining the urinary sediment, and urinary electrolytes). These tests are reviewed in order to determine whether tubular function is intact. A low fractional excretion of sodium (<1%) suggests that oliguria (and perhaps azotemia) is probably due to decreased renal perfusion, and the nephron is responding appropriately by decreasing the excretion of filtered sodium to improve plasma volume and perfusion. A low urinary osmolality (<300 mosmol/kg), a fractional excretion of sodium above 1%, and a urinary sodium higher than 20 mEq/L suggest tubular dysfunction, which is consistent with intrinsic renal parenchymal disease (i.e., acute tubular necrosis). The various serum and urinary findings used in diagnosing the major causes of ARF are shown in Table 1-44.

If the etiology is still unclear, a renal ultrasound looking for evidence of urinary obstruction and perhaps a renal biopsy should be considered to rule out glomerular diseases. Clearly, patients with newly diagnosed renal failure should have elective surgery postponed until the complete assessment is completed.

Chronic Renal Failure

Chronic renal failure is defined as a persistent impairment of kidney function. Clinically, it often involves a progressive loss of kidney function and may result in

Table 1-44 Laboratory Evaluation of Renal Failure

Test	Prerenal	Intrinsic Renal	Postrenal
BUN/Cr ratio	>20	10–20	10–20
Uosm (mosmol/kg)	>350	≤300	>400 early; ≤300 late
Urine Na (mEq/L)	<20	>40	<20 early, >40 late
FeNa (%)	<1	>2–3	<1 early; >3 late
Urine specific gravity	>1.020	≤1.010	>1.010 early, <1.010 late
Urine sediment	Normal, hyaline casts	Dark granular casts, hyaline casts, epithelial casts, RBC casts, WBC casts	Normal, hyaline granular casts

BUN, blood urea nitrogen; Cr, creatinine; FeNa, fractional excretion of sodium (calculated as UNa/PNa × PCr/UCr × 100); RBC, red blood cells; Uosm, urinary osmolality; WBC, white blood cells.
From Albright R. Acute renal failure: a practical update. *Mayo Clin Proc* 2001;76:67-74.

complete renal failure, necessitating renal replacement therapy (i.e., dialysis or transplantation). When renal replacement therapy is required, the condition is termed end-stage renal disease. End-stage renal disease develops in more than 80,000 people a year in the United States. In the early stages of CRF, when the glomerular filtration rate is still about 35–50% of normal, patients typically remain symptom-free, although renal reserve is reduced. At this stage, most kidney functions remain intact, and BUN and serum creatinine levels may be normal or only slightly elevated. As the glomerular filtration rate declines to around 20–35% of normal, azotemia occurs, and the initial manifestations of renal insufficiency usually appear. Although patients remain relatively asymptomatic, renal reserve is significantly reduced and any stressor such as infection, dehydration, and urinary obstruction may contribute toward a more rapid deterioration in renal function, inducing the signs and symptoms of uremia. With further reductions in glomerular filtration rate to less than 20% of normal, the patient develops the signs and symptoms of overt renal failure, referred to as uremia (Box 1-23). Uremia occurs when glomerular filtration rate is less than 10% of normal and patients usually begin hemodialysis. In patients with uremia, disorders of electrolytes (hyperkalemia, hyponatremia, acidosis), endocrine (hyperparathyroidism), neuromuscular (asterixis, cramps, lethargy), cardiopulmonary (hypertension, CHF), gastrointestinal (peptic ulcer disease, gastrointestinal bleeding, nausea, vomiting), and hematologic (anemia, bleeding) systems are present (Box 1-24).

Acute on Chronic Renal Failure

Patients with acute on chronic renal failure present with an acute deterioration superimposed on an already diminished baseline renal function. They are at high risk for perioperative renal deterioration, and any insult to the kidneys is magnified. The general diagnostic approach used for patients with ARF should be followed and all but emergency surgery postponed.

Kidney Transplantation

More than 100,000 patients have received renal transplants, with the majority of patients returning to a relatively normal lifestyle. Slightly over half of the transplant patients are still alive, although one-third have returned to dialytic therapy. The advantages of transplantation, in addition to increased survival, include improvement of the anemia, normalization of endocrine and sexual functions, and a reduction in the chronic fatigue commonly associated with uremia. Patients with kidney transplants are maintained on combinations of immunosuppressive agents including prednisone, azathioprine, cyclosporine, and tacrolimus. Side effects of these agents include bone marrow suppression (azathioprine), hyperglycemia, gastrointestinal ulcers,

Box 1-23 Signs and Symptoms of Chronic Renal Failure

Proteinuria
Hypertension
Nocturia
Secondary hyperparathyroidism
Anemia
Acidosis
Itching
Hyperkalemia

Box 1-24   Abnormalities in End-stage Renal Disease

CARDIOVASCULAR

Hypertension
Congestive heart failure
Pulmonary edema
Accelerated atherosclerosis
• Coronary
• Cerebral
• Peripheral vascular disease
Pericarditis

HEMATOLOGIC

Normochromic normocytic anemia
Platelet dysfunction

GASTROINTESTINAL

Gastroesophageal reflux disease
Gastritis, duodenitis
Hypoalbuminemia

METABOLIC

Malnutrition
Hypertriglyceridemia

FLUIDS AND ELECTROLYTES

Metabolic acidosis
Hypervolemia
Hyperkalemia
Hyponatremia
Hyperphosphatemia
Hypocalcemia
Renal osteodystrophy

NEUROLOGIC

Uremic encephalopathy
Mixed sensory and motor neuropathy
Seizures
Coma

INFECTIOUS

Defects in function of macrophages, neutrophils, and monocytes

dysfunction. Once it is determined to proceed with surgery, meticulous attention to intraoperative renal function will avoid renal deterioration in many instances and reduce perioperative morbidity and mortality. Acute postoperative renal failure is most likely to occur in those patients who have renal insufficiency before surgery, are older than 60 years, and have preoperative left ventricular dysfunction. Therefore, obtaining a normal intravascular fluid volume preoperatively and assuring perioperative hemodynamic stability (with the use of invasive hemodynamic lines as needed) is essential in limiting further renal deterioration. Patients with end-stage renal disease should have a careful review of any associated medical diseases such as poorly controlled hypertension, ischemic cardiac disease, CHF, and level of anemia, and should have a careful preoperative determination of clinical fluid status and electrolyte levels. In general, patients should be dialyzed within 24 hours of the surgical procedure. Longer periods risk fluid overload, worsening metabolic acidosis, and hyperkalemia. Kidney transplant patients presenting for surgery should have their corticosteroids continued as well as their immunosuppressants. If the patient is scheduled for a major surgical procedure, then additional steroid coverage may be required. It is particularly important to assure adequate fluid status perioperatively as the transplanted kidney has little reserve to tolerate hypovolemic states.

PREOPERATIVE EVALUATION OF HEPATIC DISEASE

Preoperative assessment of patients with known and unsuspected liver disease is not uncommon. In fact, up to 10% of patients with end-stage liver disease have undergone surgery during the last 2 years of life. In patients with hepatic disease, an appreciation of the risks of surgery is essential for optimal preoperative evaluation. The risk of perioperative mortality and morbidity in patients with liver disease depends on the type of surgery, nature and severity of the underlying hepatic disease, and extent of hepatic dysfunction. In obtaining the history, it is important to elicit the presence of risk factors for chronic liver disease as well as any clinical symptoms attributable to liver disease (Table 1-45). The physical examination should seek to ascertain any evidence of liver dysfunction (Box 1-25). In general, routine liver-related tests are not recommended unless underlying liver disease is clinically suspected. If, however, abnormalities are noted on liver-related test results, elective procedures should be deferred until an evaluation has been done for the presence, nature, and severity of the liver disease (Table 1-46).

delayed wound healing (corticosteroids), and hepato- and renal toxicity (cyclosporine, tacrolimus). Because of these associated side effects, preoperative tests should include a complete blood count, glucose, serum electrolytes, and a BUN and creatinine.

In summary, appropriate preoperative preparation of patients with renal insufficiency is essential in order to preserve kidney function. It is important to determine the etiology of the renal failure, especially if it is acute, and to correct those factors contributing to renal

Table 1-45 Preoperative Historical Factors Suggestive of Hepatic Disease	
Hepatitis	**Cirrhosis**
Jaundice	History of hepatitis
Anorexia	Alcohol abuse
Nausea and vomiting	Intravenous drug use
Abdominal pain	Sexual contacts
Pruritus	Tattoos
Fever	Blood transfusion
Intravenous drug use	Jaundice
Blood transfusion	Increased abdominal girth
Sexual contacts	Easy bruisability
Tattoos	Muscle wasting
Alcohol abuse	Peripheral edema
Drug or toxin exposure	Mental status changes
Travel to foreign countries	Gastrointestinal bleeding

Box 1-25 Physical Examination Findings Suggestive of Severe Hepatic Disease

Jaundice
Peripheral edema
Muscle wasting
Generalized cachexia
Petechia and ecchymoses
Hyperdynamic precordium
Reduced breath sounds in lung bases (pleural effusions)
Spider angiomas
Caput medusae (dilated veins over abdominal wall)
Abdominal tenderness on percussion (peritonitis, congested liver)
Hepatomegaly
Splenomegaly

Hepatitis

Hepatitis is nonspecific inflammation of the liver (see Table 1-46). The pathophysiology involves direct hepatocellular damage, which may progress to hepatocyte necrosis and loss of liver function. Most commonly, hepatitis is the result of a viral infection, although exposure to hepatotoxins such as alcohol and/or drugs can also cause hepatitis. Six viral agents, designated hepatitis A, B, C, D (Delta), E, and G are the etiologic causes in the majority of hepatitis cases. Hepatitis G virus (HGV) is seen primarily outside the United States and does not appear to be pathogenic. Other viral agents, including herpesvirus, Coxsackievirus, and Epstein–Barr virus, may rarely produce the clinical syndrome of hepatitis. Hepatitis viruses A–E are similar and cannot be distinguished reliably by clinical features or routine laboratory tests. Infection may either occur asymptomatically or be associated with nonspecific flu-like symptoms; up to half of patients experience jaundice. The typical laboratory abnormality in acute hepatitis is a marked elevation in the serum aminotransferase levels, occasionally as high as 3,000 IU/L.

Acute hepatitis

The most common viruses responsible for hepatitis and their corresponding clinical attributes are listed in

Table 1-46 Major Types of Liver Disease, Histopathology, and Laboratory Findings

Hepatic Disorder	Etiology	Histopathology	Laboratory
Hepatitis	Viral	Panlobular infiltration with	↑ ↑ ALT, AST
Acute	Alcohol	mononuclear cells, hepatic	↑ AP
	Drugs	cell necrosis, hyperplasia of	↑ ↑ Total bilirubin
		Kupffer cells, cholestasis	↓ Albumin
Chronic	Viral	Periportal necrosis	↑ to ↑ ↑ AST, ALT >6 months
	Alcohol	(piecemeal and/or bridging	↑ → Alkaline phosphatase
	Autoimmune	necrosis), intralobular	↑ Bilirubin
	NASH	necrosis, portal	↑ gamma-GTP
	Idiopathic	inflammation and fibrosis	
Cirrhosis			
	Viral	Nodules of liver cells	↑ → ALT, AST
	Alcohol	separated by dense broad	↑ → AP
	Biliary	bands of fibrosis. Large	↑ Total bilirubin
	Cardiac	amounts of connective tissue	↓ ↓ Albumin
	Idiopathic		↑ Prothrombin time

↑, increased; ↓, decreased; →, unchanged; ALT, serum alanine aminotransferase; AP, alkaline phosphatase; AST, serum aspartate aminotransferase; GTP, glutamyl-transpeptidase; NASH, nonalcoholic steatohepatitis.

Table 1-47. No distinct clinical features distinguish one virus from another. Most cases remain entirely asymptomatic and anicteric, the diagnostic suspicion being raised only because of elevated transaminase levels. In the case of clinically obvious acute hepatitis (whether A, B, or C), the onset may be gradual or sudden, with symptoms of increased fatigue, malaise, dark urine, anorexia, nausea, vomiting, and eventually jaundice. Examination may disclose an enlarged tender liver, and the patient may have ascites, peripheral edema, and asterixis.

Most patients have mild anemia and relative lymphocytosis. The white blood cell count is usually normal but may be over 12,000/mm³. Liver transaminases (serum alanine aminotransferase, ALT; serum asportable aminotransferase, AST) increase 7–14 days before the clinical onset of jaundice, and begin to decrease shortly after jaundice appears. The degree of aminotransferase elevation does not necessarily parallel severity, but levels less than 500 IU/L usually reflect mild illness. The alkaline phosphatase level is slightly increased but may be markedly elevated in the few patients in whom prominent cholestasis develops later in the course of acute illness. Serum gamma-globulin levels are normal or slightly elevated; concentrations greater than 3 g/dL suggest chronic active hepatitis rather than acute viral hepatitis. The serum albumin level and prothrombin time reflect the liver cells' synthetic capacity and are reduced in patients with severe, acute viral hepatitis. The serum bilirubin level generally does not exceed 15–20 mg/dL, although levels greater than 30 mg/dL have been observed and imply severe disease or associated hemolysis. The specific etiology of viral hepatitis is determined by serologic testing. The treatment of individuals with acute hepatitis is symptomatic and supportive in all cases.

Elective surgery in patients with acute viral hepatitis is associated with a very high morbidity (11%) and mortality (10%). Consequently, patients with acute, symptomatic liver disease should have elective surgery postponed, if possible, until they have recovered. It is recommended to delay elective surgery until 4 weeks or more after blood tests have normalized. The decision to proceed with urgent or emergency surgery in the patient with acute hepatitis is based on an assessment of the benefits of surgical treatment versus the substantial risk of an adverse outcome in patients with acute hepatitis. If surgery is necessary because of life-threatening illness, it should be performed only with close intraoperative hemodynamic monitoring.

Chronic hepatitis

Chronic hepatitis is a diverse clinical and pathologic syndrome that may be caused by a variety of different diseases characterized by long-term elevation of liver function tests and the finding of hepatic inflammation on liver biopsy (see Table 1-46). The term chronic hepatitis is applied to disease that has lasted for 6 months or longer, although the diagnosis can be established earlier. The most important groups of diseases that cause chronic hepatitis are chronic viral hepatitis and autoimmune hepatitis. Less commonly, chronic hepatitis can be due to drugs, Wilson's disease, alpha-1-antitrypsin deficiency, early-stage primary biliary cirrhosis, primary sclerosing cholangitis, or an unknown etiology (termed idiopathic).

Table 1-47 Characteristics of Hepatitis Viruses

Virus	Viral Type	Symptoms	Transmission	Tests	Carrier State
Hepatitis A	ssRNA	Constitutional; jaundice 50%	Food borne; water borne	IgM Anti-HAV (acute); IgG Anti-HAV (chronic)	No
Hepatitis B	DNA picornavirus	Constitutional; jaundice 50%	Parenteral; body fluids; sexual transmission	HBsAg; HBeAg; Anti-HBc; Anti-HBAg; DNA-polymerase	5–10%
Hepatitis C	ssRNA	Constitutional; jaundice 25%	Parenteral; sexual transmission	Anti-HCV; PCR; HCV-RNA	60%
Hepatitis D	Incomplete RNA	Constitutional	Requires HBV for clinical disease	IgM Anti-HD (acute); IgG Anti-HG (life immunity)	?most
Hepatitis E	ssRNA	Constitutional	Fecal-oral (more common outside the US)	IgM Anti-HE (acute); IgG Anti-HE (chronic)	Does not progress to cirrhosis

HAV, hepatitis A virus; HBc, hepatitis B virus core; HBsAg, hepatitis B surface antigen; HBV, hepatitis B virus; HCV, hepatitis C virus; HD, hepatitis D virus; HE, hepatitis E virus; PCR, polymerase chain reaction.

Hepatitis B and C are the leading causes of chronic hepatitis worldwide, accounting for more than 75% of cases. Unlike hepatitis C virus infection, in which up to 80% of patients develop chronic hepatitis, only 10% of individuals infected with hepatitis B virus develop chronic hepatitis. The persistence of hepatitis B surface antigen (or anti-hepatitis B virus core) for more than 6 months is an indication of the hepatitis B virus chronic carrier state. Although only about 3–6% of chronic hepatitis B virus carriers develop progressive liver disease, 20–35% of chronic hepatitis C patients develop cirrhosis over a 20-year period. The presence of anti-hepatitis B virus core antibody may signify either recent acute or chronic hepatitis and confers no immunity.

The clinical manifestations of chronic hepatitis range from an asymptomatic stable disease with only mild elevations in serum aminotransferase levels to a severe, rapidly progressive clinical course with fulminant hepatic failure. The most common symptoms of chronic hepatitis are fatigue, malaise, and mild abdominal pain. Patients with mild forms of chronic hepatitis are usually asymptomatic or have minimal symptoms with few clinical indicators of chronic liver disease on physical examination. In more advanced cases, the symptoms and signs of chronic hepatitis include anorexia, jaundice, palmar erythema, ascites, edema, hepatomegaly, and encephalopathy. Extrahepatic manifestations of chronic hepatitis are common and include arthralgias, arthritis, glomerulonephritis, skin rashes, amenorrhea, acne, hirsutism, and thyroiditis. ALT and AST levels are usually elevated in patients with chronic hepatitis, although a small number of patients with histologic chronic hepatitis have transiently normal aminotransferase levels. Even a mild elevation of aminotransferase levels (5–10 IU/L higher than the upper limit of normal) should lead to the suspicion of the presence of chronic hepatitis. Elevations of more than 400 IU/L are common in cases of untreated autoimmune hepatitis and severe chronic viral hepatitis. The serum bilirubin level is usually normal (≤ 1.0 mg/dL) in chronic viral hepatitis but may be more than 3 mg/dL in patients with moderately severe autoimmune hepatitis. In the most severe forms of chronic hepatitis, a low serum albumin level and prolongation of the prothrombin time signify impaired hepatic synthetic function.

Echocardiographic studies of the abdomen show variable degrees of hepatomegaly with or without splenomegaly, irregularity of liver density or contour, and evidence of portal hypertension with ascites, an increased number of portal collateral vessels, or both.

The specific etiology of chronic hepatitis is usually determined by clinical evaluation combined with immunologic and serologic testing, but liver biopsy may be required in order to confirm certain diagnoses and establish histologic grading and staging. Patients with known or suspected chronic hepatitis require preopera-

---

Box 1-26 Preoperative Tests in Patients with Liver Disease

Alanine aminotransferase (ALT)
Aspartate aminotransferase (AST)
Alkaline phosphatase
Total bilirubin
Serum albumin
Prothrombin time (PT)
Partial thromboplastin time (PTT)
Platelet count
Complete blood count
Serum electrolytes
Serum glucose
Blood urea nitrogen (BUN)
Serum creatinine

---

tive blood tests including the tests of liver function outlined in Box 1-26. Serum AST and ALT levels correlate with severity of histologic damage in most forms of hepatitis. In hepatitis C, the history and physical examination along with a serum albumin and clotting studies are often more useful than hepatocellular enzyme determinations in assessing disease severity.

Cirrhosis

Cirrhosis of the liver is caused by a variety of progressive insults to the liver (see Table 1-45). On histologic tissue examination, marked disruption of hepatic architecture is noted with the presence of fibrous tissue and scarring together with nodular areas of attempted regeneration of liver parenchyma. The fibrosis tissue and scarring result in an increased resistance to blood flow through the liver, leading to an elevation of portal vein pressures termed portal hypertension.

As hepatic vascular resistance increases, venous blood is diverted around the fibrotic liver via collateral vascular channels, or portosystemic shunts. Esophageal vascular channels, termed esophageal varices, are a consequence of portal hypertension and spontaneous bleeding may occur resulting in frequent bouts of upper gastrointestinal tract hemorrhage. Congestion of the portal vein is frequently associated with splenomegaly and the development of peripheral thrombocytopenia due to platelet sequestration in an enlarged spleen. Portal hypertension is also associated with the formation of ascites. Ascites may be massive at times and result in respiratory difficulties (pleural effusion, decreased diaphragmatic excursion) and hypoxemia.

Spontaneous infection of the peritoneal cavity is seen, termed spontaneous bacterial peritonitis. Hypoxemia occurring in the setting of severe hepatic cirrhosis and a normal chest radiograph is termed the hepatopulmonary syndrome and is in part due to pulmonary arteriovenous shunting. Renal dysfunction occurring in patients with cirrhosis has been termed the hepatorenal syndrome. This form of renal failure is poorly understood but appears much like prerenal azotemia, is characterized by severe renal vasoconstriction and poor clinical response to therapy, and is associated with a very high mortality.

Elective surgery in patients suspected to have chronic liver disease should be delayed until the cause and severity of the liver disease are established. In the absence of cirrhosis, elective surgery is reasonable, although meticulous hemodynamic and fluid management is essential. If cirrhosis is present, a determination of hepatic function and an assessment of perioperative risk are necessary.

The Child–Pugh score will help stratify risk in cirrhotic patients (Table 1-48). In patients with poorly controlled or decompensated liver disease, a high risk of perioperative morbidity and mortality is seen. In a recent retrospective study of patients with cirrhosis undergoing surgery, the perioperative mortality within 30 days of surgery was 11.9%, and the perioperative complication rate was 30.1%. Perioperative complications and mortality were related to the preoperative presence of a high Child–Pugh score, the presence of ascites, a diagnosis of cirrhosis other than primary biliary cirrhosis, an elevated creatinine concentration, the diagnosis of COPD, preoperative infection, preoperative gastrointestinal bleeding, a high American Society of Anesthesiologists physical class score, surgery on the respiratory system, and the presence of intraoperative hypotension. In another recent report, there was a 28% perioperative mortality rate for patients with chronic liver failure who underwent nonhepatic surgery. With the exception of procedures aimed at correcting the liver disease or its consequences (e.g., transplantation or hepatic shunt coplacement), surgery should be deferred, if possible, until the patient's medical condition is optimized. Nonoperative or less invasive management should be considered in these instances.

Liver Transplantation

There are an increasing number of liver transplant recipients undergoing surgery, consequently, a familiarity with the preoperative assessment of such patients is mandatory. Reviewing the medical record and performance of the physical examination should allow a reasonably accurate assessment of current liver function. If the patient is active, appears healthy, and discloses few complaints, then the patient is probably medically optimized. A review of preoperative laboratory tests will help confirm normal or near-normal hepatic function.

Transplant patients are chronically maintained on immunosuppressant therapy, with attendant side effects. Cyclosporine may cause nephrotoxicity and hypertension, and accelerate atherosclerotic coronary artery disease, while azathioprine causes myelosuppression. Adverse effects of corticosteroids include gastric ulceration, glucose intolerance, glaucoma, skin atrophy, and poor wound healing.

The patient who has undergone previous liver transplantation and who is scheduled for moderate to major surgery should undergo preoperative liver function tests (see Box 1-26). Because immunosuppressants such as cyclosporine (and the newer agent tacrolimus) have serious potential for renal toxicity, BUN and serum creatinine should be evaluated preoperatively. A complete blood count is also required in patients taking azathioprine, as it is a bone marrow suppressant. Also, preoperative serum electrolytes are necessary in patients on corticosteroids, as sodium retention, edema, hypokalemia, alkalosis, and hyperglycemia are seen.

Evaluation of Abnormal Liver Enzyme Results in Asymptomatic Patients

There are occasions when abnormal liver enzyme tests are found in an asymptomatic patient. The dilemma that arises is to decide what should be done at this point. Is it appropriate to proceed with surgery or should elective surgery be postponed until further investigation is completed? The first step in the evaluation of a patient with elevated liver enzyme levels but no symptoms is to repeat the test to confirm the result. If the result is still abnormal, the degree of the elevation should be noted. A minor elevation (less than twice the normal value) may be of no clinical importance if the disorders listed in Box 1-27 have been ruled out. For patients undergoing minor peripheral procedures, proceeding with surgery is safe.

Table 1-48 Modified Child–Pugh Score*			
Presentation	1	2	3
Albumin (g/dL)	>3.5	2.8–3.5	<2.8
Prothrombin time			
Seconds prolonged	<4	4–6	>6
INR	<1.7	1.7–2.3	>2.3
Bilirubin (mg/dL)	<2	2–3	>3
Ascites	Absent	Slight–moderate	Tense
Encephalopathy	None	Grade I–II	Grade III–IV
Perioperative			
mortality (%)	0–10	4–31	19–76

Class A, 5–6 points; class B, 7–9 points; class C, 10–15 points. INR, international normalized ratio.
From Pugh R, Murray-Lyon I, Dawson J, *et al*. Transection of the oesophagus for bleeding oesophageal varices. Br J Surg 1973;60:646-649.

Box 1-27   Causes of Chronically Elevated Aminotransferase Levels

HEPATIC CAUSES

Alcohol abuse

Medication
- Non steroidal anti-inflammatory drugs
- Antibiotics
- Antiepileptic drugs
- Antituberculosis drugs
- Herbal preparations
- Illicit drugs or substances

Chronic hepatitis B and C

Steatosis and nonalcoholic steatohepatitis

Autoimmune hepatitis

Hemochromatosis

Wilson's disease (in patients <40 years)

Alpha-antitrypsin deficiency

NONHEPATIC CAUSES

Celiac sprue

Inherited disorders of muscle metabolism

Acquired muscle diseases

Strenuous exercise

If the results of repeated tests remain abnormal and the patient is scheduled to undergo moderate to major surgery, further evaluation is indicated (Figure 1-9). Obtaining a more detailed history is of value in order to identify the most common causes of elevated aminotransferase levels, such as alcohol-related liver injury, chronic hepatitis B and C, autoimmune hepatitis, hepatic steatosis (fatty liver), and nonalcoholic steatohepatitis. In asymptomatic patients with elevated alanine aminotransferase levels who have undergone a liver biopsy, a fatty liver is the most common finding (56%). The concern regarding proceeding with surgery in asymptomatic patients with elevation of liver enzymes is that these patients may be harboring early cirrhosis, particularly those with alcoholic cirrhosis or chronic hepatitis C cirrhosis. In these situations, the hemodynamic stresses of surgery may result in rapid postoperative deterioration in liver disease with an increased risk of perioperative mortality.

In short, the preoperative assessment of patients with liver disease (or with risk factors for it) relies upon a good history and physical examination. Preoperative liver biochemistries are indicated in certain patient groups. Understanding the underlying pathophysiology of a patient's liver dysfunction is important in facilitating optimal perioperative management and reducing morbidity and mortality.

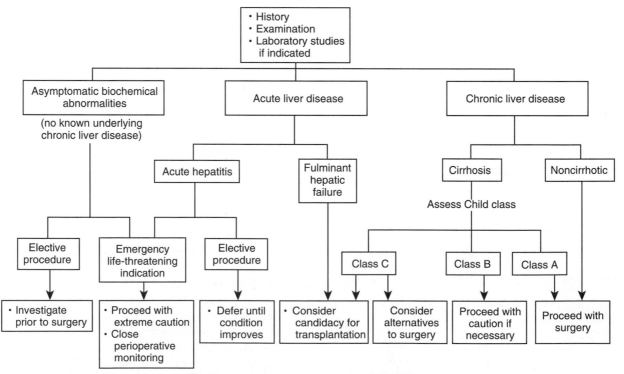

Figure 1-9   Preoperative approach to patients with known or suspected liver disease. (Redrawn from Patel T. Surgery in the patient with liver disease. *Mayo Clin Proc* 1999;74:593–599.)

PREOPERATIVE ASSESSMENT OF PATIENTS WITH GASTROINTESTINAL DISORDERS

Patients with gastrointestinal disease (Box 1-28) who are scheduled for surgery require a careful preoperative evaluation focusing upon intravascular fluid volume, electrolyte concentrations, cardiac function, and nutritional status. Patients with acute gastrointestinal disease (e.g., bowel obstruction, peritonitis, trauma) are often critically ill with hemodynamic instability. Aggressive preoperative fluid administration, blood transfusions, antibiotics, and vasoactive medications may be required. Hemodynamic monitoring is indicated in many of these patients to guide fluid management and the administration of vasoactive medications. Elderly patients often harbor underlying cardiopulmonary diseases while younger traumatically injured patients may have cardiopulmonary instability brought on by the initial injury (cardiac contusion) and compounded by the treatments themselves (e.g., massive fluid resuscitation).

Box 1-28   Common Gastrointestinal Diseases Requiring Surgery

CHRONIC DISEASES

Carcinoma
- Esophageal carcinoma
- Gastric carcinoma
- Intestinal carcinoma – small bowel, large bowel, rectum
- Hepatic carcinoma

Esophageal reflux disease
Chronic cholecystitis
Ulcerative colitis
Crohn's disease
Carcinoid tumor

ACUTE DISEASES

Acute cholecystitis
Acute appendicitis
Perforated viscus
- Gastric-duodenal perforation
- Intestinal perforation
- Ruptured diverticulum

Bowel obstruction
Pancreatic abscess
Traumatic injuries
- Spleen
- Liver
- Bowel
- Vascular structures
- Diaphragm

The assessment of patients with chronic gastrointestinal diseases should include a review of other organ systems, as abnormalities are often found. For example, patients with gastrointestinal tumors may have anemia, coagulopathy, impaired absorption of fat-soluble vitamins, renal insufficiency, hepatic dysfunction, underlying cardiac ischemic disease, and chronic pulmonary disease. Identification and optimization of these diseases prior to planned surgery will limit perioperative morbidity and mortality. Finally, care must be taken during induction of anesthesia with the rapid administration of drugs combined with application of cricoid pressure to guard against reflux of gastric contents and potential pulmonary aspiration. Preoperative nasogastric suctioning, or preoperative use of histamine receptor-blocking agents may be appropriate. Two gastrointestinal diseases, in particular, present challenges in preoperative assessment and therefore will be discussed in more detail.

Pancreatitis

Acute pancreatitis is an inflammation of the pancreas, which results when inactive (precursor) pancreatic proteolytic enzymes, such as trypsinogen, are activated within the pancreas. The clinical findings include moderate to severe epigastric pain, fever, nausea, and vomiting. The disease may remain confined to the pancreas or the inflammatory state may spread to involve other organs, thus becoming a multisystem disease. The pathologic findings include pancreatic interstitial edema, fat necrosis, and areas of peripancreatic necrosis and hemorrhage. Alcoholism and biliary tract disease are responsible for the majority of cases. Other etiologic factors include drugs, and hereditary or idiopathic factors.

Pancreatitis may be mild and self-limited, or may be extensive with a necrotizing course. The serum amylase and lipase levels are typically elevated, although lipase elevation is more specific because amylase has non-pancreatic sources. The systemic manifestations of acute pancreatitis include hypotension, anemia, metabolic acidosis, hypocalcemia, hypomagnesemia, and sepsis. Acute pancreatitis is typically managed nonoperatively, with fluid resuscitation, bowel rest, antibiotic administration, nutritional therapy, and other supportive treatments. At times, however, radiologic drainage of infected intra-abdominal fluid collections is required. Surgery may be indicated in the more seriously ill patients who develop pancreatic necrosis and sepsis.

Chronic pancreatitis is characterized by recurrent bouts of acute pancreatitis; or a more chronic, smoldering pattern of pancreatic inflammation. Pathologic findings show a patchy and focal pancreatic involvement with atrophic acinar cells with decreased or absent zymogen granules, ductular hyperplasia with strictures, squamous and goblet cell metaplasia, and intraductal calculi. In the late stages of chronic pancreatitis, the gland is atrophic with adherence to adjacent organs. The causes of chronic pancreatitis are similar to those of acute pancreatitis, but idiopathic causes play a greater role.

Patients with acute pancreatitis may present to the operating room for surgical debridement of an infected necrotic pancreas or for drainage of a pancreatic abscess. Morbidity and mortality rates are significant; thus, percutaneous radiologically guided drainage procedures are increasingly used for approachable abscesses. For those patients with severe acute pancreatitis caused by gallstones, papillotomy guided by endoscopic retrograde cholangiopancreatography (ERCP) may be a technique necessitating anesthesia. Patients in remission from acute pancreatitis or those with chronic pancreatitis may require operative intervention for drainage of pseudocysts. Pseudocysts are collections of fluid, dead tissue, pancreatic enzymes, and blood that may complicate pancreatitis and require intervention because of chronic pain, intestinal obstruction, infection, or large or increasing size with risk of rupture. Patients with chronic pancreatitis unresponsive to medical management may present for pancreatectomy or Whipple's resection (pancreaticoduodenectomy).

Preoperative approach

The patient for whom surgical treatment has been chosen has usually failed other methods of treatment. This selects out patients with a more complicated course who thus have a higher risk for morbidity and mortality. Although no specific predictors of perioperative risk have been identified for the patient with acute pancreatitis, the traditional Ranson's criteria (Box 1-29) have been used extensively in evaluating medical patients to describe mortality from the disease. Patients meeting fewer than three of Ranson's criteria after 48 hours have a more benign disease course, whereas those with three or more risk factors have a significantly increased mortality, on the order of 20% to 30%.

The perioperative risk of patients with chronic pancreatitis is unknown but, with a standard, careful preoperative evaluation and appropriate anesthetic technique, many of these patients have undergone successful surgical procedures with a reasonably good outcome.

Carcinoid Syndrome

Carcinoid tumors account for 75% of gastrointestinal endocrine tumors, being derived from enterochromaffin and argentaffin cells within the digestive tract. These neuroendocrine cells are capable of secreting a large variety of peptides and biogenic amines as well as hormones and neurotransmitters. Carcinoid tumors arise from a number of locations, although 95% of carcinoids originate in the appendix, small bowel, and rectum (Box 1-30).

Box 1-29 Ranson's Criteria for Predicting the Severity of Acute Pancreatitis

ON ADMISSION

Age >55
Serum glucose >200 mg/dL
WBC >16 000/mm^3
LDH >350 IU/L
AST >250 IU/L

WITHIN 48 HOURS

Serum total calcium <8 mg/dL
P_aO_2 <60 mmHg
Base deficit >4 mEq/L
BUN >5 mg/dL
Hematocrit >10%
Fluid sequestration >6 L

AST, aspartate aminotransferase; BUN, blood urea nitrogen; LDH, lactate dehydrogenase; P_aO_2, arterial pressure of oxygen; WBC, white blood count.

Box 1-30 Location of Carcinoid Tumors

Esophageal
Appendix (most common)
Ileocecal
Rectal
Head and neck
Lung
Gonads
Thymus
Breast
Urinary tract
Cardiac (right-sided valvular)

Carcinoid syndrome is an uncommon disorder seen in fewer than 10% of patients with carcinoid tumor. While occasionally resulting from a large solitary tumor, carcinoid syndrome is usually associated with metastatic disease, typically an ileal carcinoid that has metastasized to the liver. Presumably, the liver clears mediators released from the tumor. Impairment of this clearing ability by the metastatic tumor results in the carcinoid syndrome. The classic triad of carcinoid syndrome is cutaneous flushing, diarrhea, and right-sided valvular heart disease. Tumors less than 1 cm in diameter rarely metastasize while those larger than 2 cm do so more commonly. Clinical features of carcinoid syndrome are listed in Table 1-49.

Carcinoid tumors may produce 5-hydroxytryptophan (5-HTP) as well as insulin, calcitonin, adrenocorticotropic

Table 1-49   Clinical Findings in Carcinoid Syndrome

Symptoms and Signs	Incidence (%)
Flushing	80
Sweating	80
Diarrhea	70
Abdominal pain	70
Bronchospasm and wheezing	30
Dyspnea	30
Myopathy and arthropathy	<10
Dermatitis	<10
Blood pressure lability	<10
Endomyocardial fibrosis of right heart	Rare
Pulmonary stenosis and tricuspid regurgitation	Rare

Box 1-31   Preoperative Management of Carcinoid Syndrome

Preoperative hydration
Correction of electrolyte abnormalities
Cardiac echocardiography
Drug therapy
- Octreotide
- Somatostatin
- Ketanserin
- Cyproheptadine
- Loperamide
- Ondansetron
- H_1- and H_2-blockers
- Beta-blockers
- Corticosteroids
- Aprotinin

hormone (ACTH), vasopressin, glucagon, secretin, gastrin, growth hormone releasing hormone (GHRH) and other biogenic amines. Dopa-decarboxylase, present in midgut carcinoids, converts 5-HTP to 5-hydroxytryptamine (5-HT, or serotonin), which is converted to 5-hydroxyindoleacetic acid (5-HIAA) by monoamine oxidase (MAO). Screening tests typically begin with a 24-hour urine measurement of 5-HIAA.

Medical Management and Preoperative Preparation

The prognosis ranges from a 95% 5-year survival for localized disease to a 20% 5-year survival for those with liver metastasis. Median survival of patients with carcinoid syndrome is 2.5 years from the first episode of flushing. Medical management of carcinoid syndrome involves the use of antagonist drugs to block the peripheral effects of mediators and, more recently, octreotide or somatostatin to inhibit hormone release (Box 1-31). Surgical treatment, however, remains the best therapeutic option for isolated disease and may be considered for metastatic disease.

Most patients with the carcinoid syndrome seen in the perioperative period already carry a biochemical and/or tissue diagnosis of carcinoid and have elements of the various described clinical syndromes. Adequate preoperative preparation requires an attempt to understand the symptom complex. For example, it is important to know whether the patient becomes hypertensive or hypotensive when symptomatic. This knowledge may help prepare for identification and treatment of any such perioperative episodes. Known symptomatology is, unfortunately, only partially helpful, because intraoperative events may occur that were not predicted from preoperative observations.

Octreotide, the long-acting analog of somatostatin, has been shown to be the most effective agent for treatment and for preoperative preparation of the carcinoid syndrome patient. The preferred situation is to operate on a patient who has been treated for several weeks with octreotide and has documented 24-hour urinary 5-HIAA levels in the normal range. There is usually a significant diminution in symptomatology with octreotide therapy in patients who respond. Octreotide is also the first-line drug for use in the event of an intraoperative carcinoid crisis and should be kept in the operating room if the patient is suspected of or known to have a carcinoid tumor.

Other nonspecific measures should also be utilized, including optimal preoperative hydration, histamine blockers, and corticosteroids (see Box 1-31). A thorough preoperative cardiac evaluation is necessary to rule out right-sided heart disease, as this abnormality is seen in a significant percentage of patients with carcinoid syndrome. Preoperative cardiac echocardiography is able to best assess cardiac anatomy in patients with carcinoid syndrome and should be performed.

PREOPERATIVE ASSESSMENT OF ENDOCRINE DISEASE

Diabetes Mellitus

In the United States, nearly 16 million individuals have diabetes mellitus. Many of these patients require surgery at some point in their lives. An understanding of the disease and associated medical complications is essential for appropriate preoperative assessment and preparation.

Diabetes mellitus is a metabolic disease manifested by hyperglycemia due to defects in insulin secretion, insulin action, or both. Important abnormalities in fat and protein metabolism are also present. The diagnosis is dependent upon demonstrating elevated plasma glucose levels. The chronic hyperglycemia of diabetes mellitus is associated with long-term damage and progressive failure of various organs, including the retina, the kidneys, the autonomic nervous system, and the cardiovascular system.

The two main types of diabetes mellitus are type 1 (formerly termed insulin-dependent diabetes – IDDM) and type 2 (formerly termed non-insulin-dependent diabetes – NIDDM). The pathogenesis and treatment of the two types are quite different. Effective treatment of patients with diabetes, no matter what the etiology, includes glucose control and meticulous medical management of the complications of the disease (e.g., control of blood pressure and renal dysfunction).

Type 1 diabetes mellitus is a rare disease, with an incidence of about 2 per 1,000 individuals in the United States, and with an estimated total prevalence of approximately 500,000 individuals. Type 1 diabetes mellitus is due to a progressive autoimmune or inflammatory destruction of β-cells in the islets of the pancreas, which leads to absolute insulin deficiency. There may be a genetic predisposition to the development of type 1 diabetes. Patients appear to be at risk for other autoimmune diseases. Individuals with type 1 diabetes lack endogenous insulin and administration of exogenous insulin is central to treatment. Good glycemic control has been conclusively shown to decrease the impact of chronic complications.

Type 2 diabetes is the more common form of diabetes, accounting for over 90% of the diabetics in the United States with a prevalence of 18% among individuals older than 65 years. Type 2 diabetes occurs in patients with diverse metabolic disturbances that have hyperglycemia as a common feature. Two basic physiologic defects are present in type 2 diabetes: abnormal insulin secretion and resistance to insulin action in target tissues. Obesity is a major risk factor for type 2 diabetes mellitus, with morbidly obese patients having a 15-fold increased risk of developing the disease. Whereas the treatment of type 1 diabetes must include insulin therapy, the treatment of type 2 diabetes is multimodal and includes diet, exercise, drugs that stimulate endogenous insulin secretion (sulfonylureas), drugs that increase insulin sensitivity (metformin, rosiglitazone), and insulin, or a combination of these agents.

Finally, gestational diabetes mellitus constitutes a separate category for cases of diabetes first detected during pregnancy. When diabetes is detected early in pregnancy, it is likely to be type 1 or type 2 diabetes mellitus that is presenting symptomatically and was probably precipitated or worsened by the pregnant state. Gestational diabetes is usually detected in the second and third trimester and is likely to be specific for the pregnant state, to be transient, and to reverse to normal glucose tolerance or to impaired glucose tolerance on follow-up oral glucose tolerance testing 6 weeks after delivery. However, gestational diabetes mellitus is associated with a high risk of future diabetes, especially in women who have impaired glucose tolerance postpartum or who remain obese. Permanent diabetes will develop in approximately 50% of patients within 10 years of gestational diabetes mellitus.

Preoperative assessment

The preoperative evaluation of patients with diabetes is influenced by whether the patient has type 1 diabetes mellitus (and thus at risk for ketoacidosis) or type 2 diabetes mellitus. In patients with type 1 diabetes mellitus, the absence of ketoacidosis should be confirmed by preoperative testing. A focused history and physical examination along with a screening electrocardiogram form the basis of the initial evaluation process. The preoperative assessment should also focus on eliciting evidence of chronic complications of diabetes mellitus, such as myocardial ischemia, renal dysfunction, polyneuropathy, and joint immobility (Table 1-50).

A history of esophageal reflux, diarrhea, and decreased gastric emptying suggests an increased risk of pulmonary aspiration. Autonomic dysfunction should be identified, as recent data indicate that diabetic patients who exhibit signs of autonomic neuropathy, such as early satiety, lack of sweating, lack of pulse rate change with inspiration or orthostatic maneuvers (normal change is >15 beats/min, diabetics with neuropathy often <5 beats/min), and impotence, have a very high incidence of painless myocardial ischemia, perioperative cardiorespiratory arrest (17%), and gastroparesis. Interference with respiration by pneumonia or by anesthetics, including pain medications, or sedative drugs appear to be major precipitating causes in most cases of sudden cardiorespiratory arrest.

A preoperative electrocardiogram is mandatory because of the increased incidence of coronary artery disease in diabetics. Since the greatest cause of morbidity in diabetic patients undergoing surgery is related to coronary artery disease, further testing is guided by the extent of the patient's preoperative cardiac history and the type of surgical procedure planned. Evidence of renal dysfunction such as proteinuria on the urinalysis and elevated blood levels of potassium, creatinine, and blood urea nitrogen should be sought, as intraoperative events (e.g., hypotension, hypovolemia) may further compromise renal function. Many of the chronic diseases seen with long-term diabetes are clinically occult and testing may be useful in identifying early disease.

Table 1-50	Chronic Complications of Diabetes

Complication	Comments
Metabolic Hyperglycemia	Polyuria; hypokalemia; hypophosphatemia; hypomagnesemia; poor leukocyte function with increased infectious risk

Atherosclerosis
Macrovascular disease
  Coronary artery disease
  Peripheral vascular disease
  Cerebrovascular disease
Microvascular disease
Endothelial dysfunction
	The risk of cardiac disease is increased two to five times in type 2 DM. Additive risk factors for cardiovascular disease include obesity, hypertension, hyperlipidemia, and hyperglycemia. Both type 1 and type 2 DM increase the likelihood of cardiovascular events and cerebral vascular disease by 2–3 times and peripheral vascular disease 8–12 times. Patients tend to suffer "silent" myocardial infarctions and this should be considered if sudden perioperative cardiac failure develops

Neurologic
Peripheral sensory neuropathy
Autonomic dysfunction
  Delayed gastric emptying
    (gastroparesis)
    Early satiety
  Orthostatic hypotension
  Resting tachycardia
  Decreased beat-to-beat variability
  Anhidrosis
	Diabetic ulcers, infections; increased incidence of perioperative cardiorespiratory arrest
	Gastroparesis seen in 50% of diabetic patients with long-standing hypertension

Renal Diabetic nephropathy Hypertension	Chronic renal insufficiency; nephropathy seen in 30–40% of type 1 DM and 10% of type 2 DM; microproteinuria seen in early stages of nephropathy; hypertension is common as a result of kidney disease
Microangiopathy Retinopathy	Microaneurysms can be found in more than 90% of insulin-requiring diabetics by 20 years and proliferative retinopathy in more than 60% by 40 years duration; increased incidence of cataracts
Joint–collagen disease Stiff joint syndrome	Associated with type 1 DM; joint immobility and waxy skin; atlantooccipital immobility leads to difficult intubation

DM, diabetes mellitus.

Perioperative control of blood glucose

Maintenance of reasonable glycemic control is essential in diabetics. Since patients are NPO for a time before surgery, an effective regimen that best manages the patient's perioperative blood sugars should be followed (Boxes 1-32 and 1-33). Although many regimens have been proposed to achieve glycemic control in the perioperative period, four general points stand out:

• patients with diabetes type 1 are ketosis-prone and require the presence of exogenous insulin to prevent ketoacidosis; therefore, frequent preoperative glucose determinations (e.g., every 1–2 hrs) are essential

• patients with type 2 diabetes mellitus have enough endogenous insulin to prevent ketoacidosis; therefore less frequent glucose determinations are required (e.g., every 2–4 hrs)

• perioperative glucose levels should be maintained at ≥80 mg/dL but ≤200 mg/dL

• continuous infusions of insulin are better to control glucose levels that are consistently 200 mg/dL or higher; intermittent bolus doses of insulin have been shown to be less effective in controlling hyperglycemia and result in a higher incidence of hypoglycemia.

Box 1-32   Perioperative Glucose Management Guidelines for Type 1 Diabetes Mellitus

- Patients on a *conventional regimen* (i.e., two insulin injections/day) may be managed using either of two approaches:
  - Give one-third to one-half the usual total morning dose of insulin as NPH (or other intermediate-acting insulin) and begin a dextrose infusion of D5W at 80–100 mL/hr (5–10 g/hr dextrose) upon arrival in the preoperative holding area. Check blood sugars every 1–2 hrs perioperatively and treat those ≥200 mg/dL; or
  - Withhold all insulin therapy the morning of surgery. This is especially useful if the patient is scheduled for surgery later in the day. Either method of insulin management is acceptable.
- Patients on a *multiple daily subcutaneous injection regimen* can receive a slightly reduced morning dose of regular insulin every 6 hrs with a glucose infusion started upon arrival in preoperative holding. Glucose checks and treatment as above.
- Patients on a *subcutaneous pump* should have the pumps stopped on the day of surgery and glucose controlled with frequent checks of blood glucose (i.e., every 1–2 hrs).
- In the perioperative period, insulin infusions should be started in any patient with blood glucose levels consistently above 200 mg/dL. Insulin infusions (1 unit regular insulin/mL fluid) are commonly started at 0.025 units insulin/kg/hr.

Box 1-33   Perioperative Management of Type 2 Diabetes Mellitus

- Patient should be NPO after midnight
- The morning dose of the oral hypoglycemic (if patient is taking any) should be held
- Fasting serum glucose should be measured upon arrival in preoperative holding
- An infusion of D5W is set at 80–100 mL/hr for a 70 kg patient. It is appropriate to employ a "no insulin, no glucose" approach preoperatively in managing patients with type 2 diabetes, with changes only in the event that glucose is low or persistently more than 200 mg/dL
- Glucose levels should be monitored every 2–4 hrs intraoperatively (more frequently if values are excessively elevated)
- In patients persistently hyperglycemic (i.e. consistently >200 mg/dL), fluids should be changed to non-insulin-containing solutions, and an insulin infusion should be started. Insulin infusions (1 unit regular insulin/mL fluid) are initiated at 0.025 units insulin/kg/hr and adjusted as needed
- In the postoperative period, serum glucose should be checked every 6 hrs and insulin administered for sugar levels above 200 mg/dL
- Oral hypoglycemic medications should be started only after the patient resumes oral intake

---

Adrenal Disease

Background

The adrenal glands are situated just above each kidney and consist of a cortex and a medulla. The cortex makes steroid hormones and the medulla makes catecholamines. The cortex is composed of three distinct histologic zones: the zona glomerulosa, zona fasciculata, and zona reticularis. Each zone functions independently.

The outermost zona glomerulosa produces aldosterone, the primary mineralocorticoid in humans. Aldosterone regulates sodium balance, primarily acting on the distal tubule of the nephron to increase sodium and water absorption in exchange for potassium and hydrogen ions. The major trophic hormones for aldosterone secretion are renin and ACTH. Renin, in particular, facilitates the formation of angiotensin, which stimulates aldosterone secretion. Other stimuli to aldosterone secretion include an increase in serum potassium, hypovolemia, low serum sodium, and a rise in estrogen levels.

The zona fasciculata produces cortisol, the major glucocorticoid in humans. Glucocorticoid synthesis is controlled by the hypothalamus–pituitary–adrenal axis. The hypothalamus secretes corticotropin-releasing hormone (CRH), which stimulates the pituitary to secrete ACTH; ACTH, in turn, then stimulates the production of cortisol. Normally, 20–30 mg of cortisol is secreted daily in a diurnal pattern. Cortisol plays a vital role in regulating carbohydrate, protein, and lipid metabolism, as well as acting as an intracellular membrane stabilizer. At high doses, cortisol acts as an anti-inflammatory agent by membrane stabilization and inhibition of inflammatory mediator release. At doses exceeding 30 mg, cortisol has increased mineralocorticoid activity, causing increased salt and water retention.

The zona reticularis produces the adrenal androgens.

Disorders of adrenocortical function can be thought of as disorders of overproduction or underproduction of the four classes of steroid hormones produced by the adrenal gland: cortisol, aldosterone, androgen, and estrogen. The diagnosis of disorders of adrenocortical function, like that of other endocrine syndromes, requires a compatible clinical picture, with biochemical confirmation of the associated underlying abnormality. The principal tests used to evaluate adrenal function include measurements of plasma ACTH and cortisol, as well as urinary 17-OHS and 24-hour urinary free cortisol. Resting values of plasma cortisol are 10–25 μg/dL in the morning and 2–10 μg/dL at night.

Finally, the adrenal medulla is responsible for the production of catecholamines in response to neural input. Disorders of the adrenal medulla will be discussed later in this section.

Cushing's Syndrome (Glucocorticoid Excess)

Cushing's syndrome is caused by glucocorticoid excess due to an ACTH-producing pituitary tumor (most common), a non-central-nervous-system tumor with ectopic production of ACTH, or an adrenal tumor. Excess pituitary ACTH with bilateral adrenal hyperplasia (Cushing's disease) accounts for approximately two-thirds of cases of Cushing's syndrome. Pigmentation due to ACTH excess is often noted. Ectopic (nonpituitary) ACTH production can also cause Cushing's syndrome and results from the uncontrolled synthesis and release of ACTH by malignant tumors, most commonly of the lung, thymus, pancreas, and kidney. Hypokalemic alkalosis, weakness, and weight loss are outstanding elements, and the patient seldom has a cushingoid appearance. Adrenal neoplasms, including benign adrenal adenomas that hypersecrete cortisol, account for less than one-third of cases of spontaneous Cushing's syndrome.

Patients with Cushing's syndrome are most commonly scheduled for a transsphenoidal hypophysectomy. If, however, the patient has severe disease with life-threatening complications, or a very large pituitary tumor, or if pituitary treatment has failed, adrenalectomy may be chosen instead.

Preoperative assessment should focus on the signs and symptoms of glucocorticoid excess (Box 1-34). Treatment of electrolyte abnormalities, hypervolemia, or metabolic disturbances should be carried out before surgery. At times, patients with Cushing's syndrome may have undergone a pharmacologic adrenalectomy with drugs such as metyrapone (reduces cortisol production by inhibition of 11-hydroxylase), mitotane (an adrenolytic agent that inhibits cortisol synthesis), or aminoglutethimide (inhibits cortisol synthesis by blocking conversion of cholesterol to D-pregnenolone). These patients should be considered adrenally suppressed and should thus receive full stress-steroid coverage during the perioperative period (i.e., 200–300 mg hydrocortisone/24 hrs).

Adrenal Insufficiency (Glucocorticoid Deficiency)

The most common cause of primary adrenal failure is autoimmune destruction of the adrenal gland, a disease that is often associated with other autoimmune diseases such as Hashimoto's thyroiditis. Additional causes of adrenal insufficiency are listed in (Box 1-35).

In primary adrenal insufficiency, both glucocorticoid and mineralocorticoid production are decreased, and both need to be supplemented. Secondary adrenal insuf-

---

Box 1-34 Signs and Symptoms of Glucocorticoid Excess

Hypokalemia
Metabolic alkalosis
Hypertension
Obesity
Diabetes
Hypervolemia
Muscle weakness
Osteoporosis (history of pathologic fractures)
Poor wound healing
Risk of infection

Box 1-35 Common Causes of Adrenal Insufficiency

Autoimmune destruction
• Hashimoto's thyroiditis
Infection
• Tuberculosis
• Cytomegalovirus
• Human immunodeficiency virus
Tumor
Hemorrhagic necrosis

---

ficiency commonly occurs from withdrawal of chronic glucocorticoid use or from failure of the hypothalamic–pituitary axis, such as occurs in panhypopituitary patients. Patients with secondary adrenal insufficiency present clinically with lethargy, weakness, nausea and vomiting, abdominal pain, hyponatremia, hyperkalemia, and hypotension. Patients with primary adrenal insufficiency will have increased pigmentation caused by elevation of ACTH from the pituitary gland.

For patients with primary adrenal insufficiency who are on high doses of hydrocortisone, no mineralocorticoid supplementation is needed. However, if patients are taking less than 50 mg/day of hydrocortisone, or have hyponatremia and hyperkalemia, then mineralocorticoid supplementation (9α-fluorocortisol 0.05–0.1 mg) is indicated. Other glucocorticoids, such as dexamethasone, can be given, but the low mineralocorticoid activity of these glucocorticoids should be noted. The different glucocorticoid and mineralocorticoid potencies of the various corticosteroid formulations are shown in Table 1-51.

Preoperative stress steroids

Stress steroids are typically administered in the perioperative period to patients who have been on prior glucocorticoid therapy. In general, the patient who has

Table 1-51   Potencies of Various Glucocorticoid Preparations Compared to Hydrocortisone

Agent	Glucocorticoid Potency	Mineralocorticoid Potency	Duration of Action (hr)
Hydrocortisone	1	1	8–12
Methylprednisolone	5	0.5	24–36
Prednisone	4	0.8	12–24
Dexamethasone	25	0	72
Fludrocortisone	10	125	20–24

received 2 weeks or more of supraphysiologic gluco-corticoids (i.e., ≥30 mg hydrocortisone or 7 mg prednisone) within the past year may be at risk of adrenal suppression. Because performing preoperative adrenal reserve testing (ACTH stimulation test) is impractical in the immediate preoperative period, all patients who have been on supraphysiologic glucocorticoids for more than 2 weeks within the previous year should be considered adrenally suppressed during the perioperative period until adrenal response is proven normal.

How much additional steroid coverage should be administered in the perioperative period is dependent upon the type of surgical procedure being performed, combined with nearly a half-century of anecdotal evidence with very limited clinical justification. A recent review concerning the use of stress-dose steroid use in the perioperative period provided little evidence that supraphysiologic doses of corticosteroids are necessary to prevent hemodynamic instability secondary to adrenal insufficiency in the perioperative period. In fact, patients provided with just their usual maintenance doses of steroid tolerated major surgery with no evidence of complications related to adrenocortical insufficiency. An important exception to this finding occurred in critically ill patients – glucocorticoid-dependent patients requiring vasopressors should be started on daily doses of 100–150 mg of intravenous hydrocortisone.

Thus, although chronic corticosteroid administration does depress or eliminate the patient's ability to generate the usual cortisol response to surgical or other traumatic stress, the vast majority of such patients studied have been found to suffer no ill effects, even when no perioperative steroid coverage is provided. Conversely, as the perioperative use of stress-dose steroids has a long history of safe use with few significant side effects, there seems to be no particularly significant justification for abandoning it. Consequently, until conclusive studies indicate otherwise, it would appear prudent to provide modest stress-dose steroid coverage in the perioperative period, as outlined in Table 1-52.

Table 1-52   Perioperative Stress-dose Steroids

Type of Surgery	Steroid Coverage
Major Surgery Esophagectomy Pancreatoduodenectomy Cardiopulmonary bypass	Hydrocortisone or equivalent 100–150 mg/day in divided doses perioperatively for 2–3 days
Moderate Surgery Colon resection Total hip replacement Open cholecystectomy	Hydrocortisone or equivalent 50–75 mg/day for 1–2 days
Minor Surgery Inguinal hernia repair Breast biopsy Peripheral orthopedic surgery	Hydrocortisone or equivalent 25–50 mg/day for 1 day

In uncomplicated postoperative recovery, patients should resume their normal steroid dose by 2–5 days, depending on the magnitude of the surgery

Thyroid Disease

A history of thyroid dysfunction is commonly encountered in patients presenting for surgery. Most commonly, the patient is either taking supplemental thyroid medication (hypothyroidism) or has a history of total or subtotal thyroid gland resection (hyperthyroidism). A basic understanding of thyroid gland physiology is essential to appropriate preoperative assessment of these patients.

Thyroid Gland Physiology

Thyrotropin-releasing hormone (TRH), released from the hypothalamus, stimulates the release of thyroid-stimulating hormone (TSH) from the anterior pituitary. TSH is the primary stimulus of synthesis and secretion of thyroid hormone. Dietary iodine, concentrated in the thyroid gland, combines with tyrosine residues within the thyroglobulin molecule to produce monoiodotyrosine and diiodotyrosine. Oxidative coupling of monoiodotyrosine and diiodotyrosine produces thyroxine (T_4) and triiodothyronine (T_3) bound to thyroglobulin. T_4 and T_3 are secreted as free hormones after hydrolysis from thyroglobulin in the follicular cell lysosomes. T_4 is the major secretory product of the thyroid, although T_3 is the active thyroid hormone. Most of the T_3 (85%) is produced in the peripheral tissues from T_4 deiodination, although a small amount (15%) is secreted directly from the thyroid gland.

Thyroid testing

Traditionally, the biochemical evaluation of thyroid status has been based on measured levels of total T_4, TSH, and calculated free T_4 (termed the free thyroxine index – FT_4I). The FT_4I is calculated from the product of T_4 and a test called the "resin triiodothyronine uptake" (RT_3U). Indeed, the T_4 is elevated in 90% of hyperthyroid patients, and decreased in 85% of hypothyroid patients. The specificity of the T_4 test, however, is much lower. This is because over 99% of T_4 and T_3 is protein-bound and, since only the free unbound hormone is physiologically active, changes in serum binding proteins (primarily thyroid-binding globulin – TBG) affect measured total T_4 levels. Free T_4, however, remains unaffected by protein changes.

Recently, the introduction of sensitive TSH assays (sTSH) has transformed thyroid function testing from thyroxine-based strategies to sTSH-based strategies (Table 1-53).

Currently, the measurement of TSH complemented by the FT_4I represents the best test for the diagnosis and follow-up of most patients with thyroid disease. Since the hypothalamic-pituitary axis is exquisitely sensitive to even the slightest changes in circulating thyroid hormone, small changes in T_4 result in logarithmic changes in the secretion of TSH. In the case of hyperthyroidism, newer sTSH assays are able to detect TSH levels of

Table 1-53	Second-generation Serum Thyroid-stimulating Hormone Concentrations in Various Thyroid Disease States
Clinical State	**Serum TSH Range (μU/mL)**
Normal	0.1–5.0
Hyperthyroid	<0.1
Hypothyroid	
Subclinical	6–16
Overt primary	20–200
Secondary	0.1–5.0
Sick euthyroid syndrome	0.1–5.0
Recovery phase	0.1–15

0.1 μU/mL (second-generation assays) or even lower levels of 0.01 μU/mL (third-generation assays). Because of the improved sensitivity of these newer TSH assays, the initial test of thyroid function should be a second-generation sTSH measurement. From the results of this test, patients may be appropriately categorized into either hyper- or hypothyroid disease states.

Preoperative Assessment of Thyroid Disease

Preoperative assessment of patients with thyroid disease should focus on identification of signs or symptoms that may suggest poorly controlled hyper- or hypothyroidism.

Hyperthyroidism

Hyperthyroidism is primarily a disease of hypermetabolism. Common causes are listed in Box 1-36, and the most commonly encountered clinical symptoms are listed in Box 1-37. The clinical manifestations of hyperthyroidism should be identified preoperatively because clinically overt hyperthyroidism warrants presurgical testing. The risk of proceeding with surgery in an undiagnosed hyperthyroid patient is the increased risk of perioperative thyroid storm, which has a mortality rate of more than 50%.

In patients suspected of clinical hyperthyroidism, a serum sTSH test is indicated. If serum TSH is low, a FTI and RT_3U should be ordered to quantify the severity of the hyperthyroidism. The greatest perioperative risk for patients with overt hyperthyroidism, as mentioned, is

Box 1-36	Common Causes of Hyperthyroidism

Graves' disease (most common)
Multinodular goiter
Subacute thyroiditis
Excessive thyroid hormone intake

Box 1-37   Clinical Manifestations of Hyperthyroidism

Cardiac hypertrophy
Reversible cardiomyopathy
Muscle weakness
Dyspnea
Dysrhythmias (atrial fibrillation)
Heat intolerance
Weight loss
Bone loss
Emotional lability
Difficulty sleeping
Frequent bowel movements

Table 1-54   Treatment of Thyroid Storm

Treatment Modality	Mechanism of Effect

Antithyroid drugs
  Propylthiouracil
  Methimazole
  Carbimazole
	Decrease thyroid hormone synthesis; decrease peripheral conversion of T_4 to T_3

Iodine	Inhibits thyroid hormone release and synthesis; decreases thyroid vascularity
Corticosteroids	Decreases levels of TSH and T_4 and protects against adrenal insufficiency
Beta-blockers	Controls hyperadrenergic symptoms: tachycardia, hypertension, dysrhythmias
Temperature control	Cooling measures control body temperature
Intravenous fluids	Correction of hypovolemia from evaporative losses

T_3, triiodothyronine; T_4, thyroxine; TSH, thyroid-stimulating hormone.

---

that of thyroid storm. Other clinical problems encountered in patients with poorly controlled hyperthyroidism include refractory atrial fibrillation, myocardial ischemia, and prolonged postoperative intubation secondary to muscle weakness. If the surgery is an emergency and can not be postponed, and there is either clinical suspicion of overt hyperthyroidism (compatible clinical history and/or symptoms) or biochemical documentation of such, every effort should be made to prevent thyroid storm by instituting a combination of antithyroid drugs (propylthiouracil), beta-blocking agents, and corticosteroids (which decrease levels of T_4 and TSH and protect against coexisting adrenal insufficiency). Treatment of thyroid storm is outlined in Table 1-54.

Subclinical hyperthyroidism

On occasion, an asymptomatic patient may present for preoperative evaluation in whom thyroid TSH testing has been performed, disclosing a combination of an undetectable serum TSH concentration (<0.1 mU/L) as measured by a sensitive TSH assay, coupled with a normal serum T_3 and T_4 concentrations. This situation is termed subclinical hyperthyroidism. Although obvious symptoms of hyperthyroidism are absent, subtle symptoms or signs of thyrotoxicosis may be present. The most common causes of this condition are listed in Box 1-38. In many of these patients, treatment is unnecessary, but thyroid function tests should be performed every 6 months, with the recognition that a small percentage of patients will progress to overt hyperthyroidism over time (<5% per year). In patients with mild symptoms, a 6-month trial with an antithyroid drug (e.g., methimazole) at a low dose, followed by ablative therapy with iodine-131 is recommended.

Fortunately, elective surgery does not have to be postponed in patients with subclinical hyperthyroidism as they tolerate surgery well. The perioperative use of beta-blockers is appropriate if clinically indicated. If, however, beta-blockers are contraindicated (asthma, CHF), it

---

Box 1-38   Causes of Suppressed TSH Levels

Graves' disease
Nodular goiter
L-thyroxine therapy
Nonthyroidal illness
Drug therapy
• Dopamine
• Corticosteroids
• Amiodarone
Central hypothyroidism

---

would be appropriate to postpone truly elective surgery until the patient is biochemically euthyroid (6–12 weeks after therapy is begun).

Hypothyroidism

Clinical hypothyroidism most commonly occurs after medical treatments for hyperthyroidism (e.g., Graves' disease) or as a result of Hashimoto's thyroiditis. Clinical manifestations are listed in Box 1-39.

The diagnosis of hypothyroidism is made by obtaining a sTSH and FT$_4$I. In subclinical hypothyroidism, the T_4 and FT$_4$I are normal but the TSH is elevated (6–16 μU/mL). In clinical hypothyroidism, the sTSH is usually over 20 μU/mL. Initiation of L-thyroxine treatment for hypothyroidism usually results in normalization of TSH levels over a 4–6 week period.

The perioperative risk of surgery in patients with mild to moderate hypothyroidism is minimal according to

Box 1-39   Clinical Manifestations of Overt Hypothyroidism

Hypotension
Congestive heart failure
Hypovolemia
Hyponatremia
Pleural effusions
Gastrointestinal hypomotility
Electrocardiogram: bradycardia, low voltage
Depressed hypoxic ventilatory drive
Anemia
Mental status changes
Brittle hair
Cold intolerance
Constipation

recent studies. However, in truly elective cases, surgery should be postponed until thyroid tests are normalized. Mild to moderate hypothyroid patients with coronary artery disease who are scheduled for coronary artery bypass surgery may proceed to surgery, as the outcome is quite good and initiating treatment of hypothyroidism might precipitate myocardial ischemia. If urgent surgery is required in patients with mild to moderate hypothyroidism, L-thyroxine in doses of 25 μg daily should be given before and after surgery, increasing by 25 μg every 2 weeks. Doses of 15 μg are recommended for the elderly.

In choosing anesthetics for hypothyroid patients, no good studies have documented unusual sensitivity to inhaled anesthetics or opioids, prolonged recovery from anesthesia and need for postoperative respiratory assistance, or increased incidence of cardiac complications. Since hypothyroid patients may have gastric and intestinal hypomotility, induction using cricoid pressure would be prudent. Drugs should be chosen that minimize cardiac depression, as untreated hypothyroid patients may have limited cardiovascular reserve. Because of the occasional coexistence of adrenal insufficiency (especially in primary hypothyroidism), any unexplained intraoperative hypotension should be considered to be due to concomitant adrenal insufficiency, and supplemental corticosteroids should be administered (100 mg intravenous hydrocortisone).

Myxedema coma is a rare form of severe hypothyroidism presenting as profound lethargy or coma accompanied by hypothermia (temperature <35° C). This condition primarily affects patients over 75 years of age, often in a setting of sepsis, exposure to cold, or ingestion of alcohol or narcotics. The mortality rate is more than 50%. Treatment consists of intravenous thyroxine (300–500 μg bolus followed by 50–200 μg/day).

If emergency surgery is needed for patients with documented or highly suspected overt hypothyroidism, the potential for perioperative cardiovascular instability and myxedema are greatly increased. In this situation, intravenous thyroid medication and steroid supplementation should be administered and inotropic support started as dictated by intraoperative hemodynamics and invasive monitoring.

Subclinical hypothyroidism

Subclinical hypothyroidism, evidenced only by an elevated serum TSH concentration in an apparently asymptomatic individual, is present in about 5% of the population, with a prevalence approaching 15% in women older than 60 years. Debate has continued over whether asymptomatic patients with subclinical hypothyroidism should be treated with supplemental thyroid medication, as many of them feel better on therapy. Two prospective studies indicated that they should be treated (as 3–5% become hypothyroid per year). Although controversial, therapy of such patients is generally recommended except for those having minimal TSH elevation (5–10 μU/mL), the very elderly, and patients with potential or actual cardiac disease. Accordingly, patients may present for surgery on thyroid medication, which was added by their primary care doctor at some point, and have very little history of actual thyroid disease.

Another class of patients includes those with critical illness who demonstrate an array of thyroid function test abnormalities, including lowered T_3, raised rT_3, lowered T_4, and lowered or normal TSH. These patients have what is termed the "sick euthyroid syndrome" and do not benefit from L-thyroxine treatment unless the TSH level is above 20 μU/mL.

Abnormalities of the Parathyroid Gland

Hyperparathyroidism

The term hyperparathyroidism is applied to any condition is which there is an elevated level of parathyroid hormone (PTH). The most common finding in this disorder is hypercalcemia, although the condition can exist in the presence of normal or low serum levels of calcium. Primary hyperparathyroidism is a disease in which excess PTH is produced from the parathyroid gland itself, most typically from a single adenoma (85–90%), parathyroid gland hyperplasia (15%), or parathyroid carcinoma (4%). Familial hyperparathyroidism may exist as part of the multiple endocrine neoplasia (MEN) type I or type II syndromes.

The majority of patients with hyperparathyroidism are asymptomatic and are diagnosed after an initial incidental discovery of mild hypercalcemia. The clinical syndrome of primary hyperparathyroidism is variable; however, typical findings in patients with significant elevations in serum calcium include bone pain, arthralgias, lethargy, confusion, weakness, constipation, loss of appetite, nausea, vomiting, abdominal pain (peptic ulcer disease, pancreatitis), renal failure, and hypertension.

The diagnosis of hyperparathyroidism relies principally on the laboratory findings of an elevated serum calcium level together with an inappropriately elevated level of PTH. Additional confirmation should include single-photon absorptiometry of the wrist, showing cortical bone loss.

The treatment of primary hyperparathyroidism is surgical removal of the parathyroid tissue. For mild disease, initial surgery should involve only one side of the neck. If one parathyroid adenoma and one normal gland are found, the other side of the neck should remain undisturbed. For patients with hyperplastic involvement of all glands, near-total parathyroid gland removal is warranted, perhaps with reimplantation of a portion of the parathyroid gland tissue into the forearm. This approach is usually curative in the majority of cases.

Secondary hyperparathyroidism is a condition seen most commonly in patients with renal failure in whom the reduced levels of calcitriol combined with hyperphosphatemia stimulate parathyroid gland hyperplasia with resulting increases in PTH production. The effects of sustained PTH excess result in bone disease and hypercalcemia that can be difficult to treat. If medical control of the secondary hyperparathyroidism proves unsuccessful, then surgical treatment is indicated. Other diseases which can produce secondary hyperparathyroidism include gastrointestinal malabsorption syndromes involving inadequate absorption of vitamin D, with resulting hypocalcemia.

The preoperative assessment of patients scheduled for parathyroid surgery should include particular attention to the serum calcium level. Severe elevations should be corrected prior to surgery. In addition, assessment of other organ systems should include a neurologic examination (lethargy, psychosis, muscle fatigue, weakness), an assessment for gastrointestinal complaints (nausea, vomiting, pancreatitis), and a cardiac examination with particular attention to the presence of hypertension and volume status, along with a preoperative electrocardiogram (prolongation of the PR interval, widening of the QRS interval, shortening of the ST segment, and a slight flattening of T waves). Laboratory evaluation should include: serum electrolytes, BUN, creatinine, serum phosphate, and hemoglobin.

Hypoparathyroidism

Hypoparathyroidism arises from failure of the parathyroid gland to produce PTH or failure of the tissues to react to it (pseudohypoparathyroidism). The most frequent causes are thyroid surgery (with inadvertent removal of the parathyroid glands), irradiation of the thyroid gland, hemochromatosis, and as part of a polyglandular autoimmune syndrome (adrenal, ovarian, and

---

Box 1-40 Clinical Manifestations of Severe Hypocalcemia

NEUROMUSCULAR

Neuronal membrane irritability
Muscle spasms
Tetany
Seizures

CARDIOVASCULAR

Hypotension
Dysrhythmias
Congestive heart failure
Potentiation of negative inotropy of beta-blockers and calcium channel blockers

---

parathyroid failure). Although hypocalcemia is the most common abnormality found in hypoparathyroidism, other diseases may result in hypocalcemia and should be excluded. Clinical symptoms arise with significant hypocalcemia (ionized calcium ≤0.8 mmol/L) and necessitate prompt therapy (see Boxes 1–40 and 1–41). Acute treatment includes intravenous calcium (either as calcium gluconate or calcium chloride) and correction of any other electrolyte abnormalities. As magnesium is required for proper parathyroid gland function, any hypomagnesemia that is present should be corrected along with the correction of hypocalcemia, otherwise, persistent hypocalcemia will remain.

Pheochromocytoma

Pheochromocytoma is a catecholamine-secreting tumor, typically of the adrenal medulla, that presents as paroxysmal or sustained hypertension in young to middle-aged patients. Pheochromocytomas are derived from chromaffin cells of neural crest origin. Although 90% of these tumors originate in the adrenal glands, extra-adrenal locations also exist, such as in the sympathetic ganglia, carotid body, and aortic chemoreceptors. Some 90% of pheochromocytomas are classified as sporadic or nonsyndromic and 90% are benign. Familial pheochromocytoma occurs in patients with MEN II and von Hippel–Lindau disease. One half of familial tumors tend to be bilateral and/or extra-adrenal.

Symptoms

Most of the signs and symptoms of pheochromocytoma are related to the activity of the released catecholamines (Box 1-42). In addition to hypertension, associated symptoms suggesting the diagnosis include the triad of sweating, headaches, episodic palpitations, as well as hypermetabolism, panic attacks, and CHF caused by myocarditis or focal myocardial necrosis. Postural

Box 1-41 Common Causes of Hypocalcemia

PRIMARY HYPOPARATHYROIDISM
SECONDARY HYPOPARATHYROIDISM

Neck surgery (radical neck, thyroidectomy, trauma)
Sepsis
Liver disease
Hypo- or hypermagnesemia
Burns
Pancreatitis
Aminoglycosides

IMPAIRED VITAMIN D INTAKE OR ABSORPTION

Poor intake
Malabsorption
Hypomagnesemia
Liver disease
Renal failure
Pseudohypoparathyroidism
Sepsis

CALCIUM CHELATION OR PRECIPITATION

Hyperphosphatemia
Citrate
Albumin
Fat embolism
Pancreatitis
Sepsis
Rhabdomyolysis

Box 1-42 Signs and Symptoms of Pheochromocytoma

HYPERTENSION

Sustained (15%)
Paroxysmal (45%)
Sustained and paroxysmal (40%)
Hypertensive crisis (with precipitating events or medications)

CONSTITUTIONAL SYMPTOMS

Headaches
Sweating
Palpitations
Panic attacks
Tachycardia
Postural hypotension
Glucose intolerance
Weight loss

RISK FACTORS

Family history of pheochromocytoma.
Multiple endocrine neoplasia type II
Von Hippel–Lindau disease

Box 1-43 Diagnosis of Pheochromocytoma

SUGGESTIVE CLINICAL SIGNS AND SYMPTOMS
BIOCHEMICAL TESTS

Plasma free metanephrines
24-hour urinary catecholamines
Clonidine suppression test
Glucagon stimulation test

IMAGING STUDIES

Computed tomography
Magnetic resonance imaging
Metaiodobenzylguanidine (MIBG) scintigraphy

hypotension is a common finding on physical examination and is caused partly by a decrease in the plasma volume. An unrecognized pheochromocytoma may lead to death as the result of a hypertensive crisis, arrhythmia, or myocardial infarction.

Diagnosis

The diagnosis of pheochromocytoma is made by a combination of clinical suspicion, blood tests, and imaging studies (Box 1-43). Effective methods for diagnosis and localization are important, as surgical removal can cure pheochromocytoma in up to 90% of cases, whereas, if the tumor is left untreated, long-term survival is poor. Plasma levels of metanephrines have been shown to have a very high sensitivity for detecting pheochromocytoma and are more effective in diagnosing pheochromocytoma than other tests. More than 80% of patients with pheochromocytoma have elevated plasma metanephrine levels that indicate a pheochromocytoma with 100% specificity. Localization of the tumor is achieved using abdominal computed tomography and/or magnetic resonance imaging, followed by scintigraphy using radio-labeled metaiodobenzylguanidine (MIBG) for confirmation.

Preoperative assessment

The definitive treatment for pheochromocytoma is surgical excision of the tumor. Surgery for pheochromocytoma, however, includes a series of potential catecholamine-releasing events, including induction of anesthesia with tracheal intubation, intraoperative manipulation of the tumor, and other stimulating events, which can cause a massive outpouring of catecholamines from the tumor, resulting in a hypertensive crisis, stroke, arrhythmias, or myocardial infarction. To prevent these problems, patients with pheochromocytoma should undergo pharmacologic blockade of catecholamine synthesis or effects before surgery. Such therapy is essential for optimal perioperative outcome and should include afterload reduction with alpha-blockade (phenoxybenzamine), beta-adrenoceptor blockade to oppose the reflex tachycardia that occurs with alpha-blockade, metyrosine (competitive inhibitor of tyrosine hydroxylase, the rate-limiting step in catecholamine biosynthesis) to reduce tumor stores of catecholamines, liberal salt intake and fluids for volume repletion, and an evaluation of cardiac function (history, physical, electrocardiogram, echocardiography) to rule out catecholamine-induced cardiomyopathy.

Cardiac function and electrocardiographic changes (e.g., left ventricular hypertrophy) may improve over time with the use of alpha-blockade. Therapy should begin 10–14 days before surgery and continue up to the time of surgery. Such a regimen leads to better perioperative control of blood pressure and decreases surgical risks. Heavy premedication with benzodiazepines and narcotics is an essential part of the immediate preoperative preparation en route to the operating room. With adequate preoperative therapy and hydration, surgical removal of the pheochromocytoma can be safely performed, with patient survival rates of nearly 100%.

PREOPERATIVE ASSESSMENT OF THE NEUROLOGICAL PATIENT

Performing an accurate history and physical examination should identify nearly all significant neurological disease. Important historical information includes medications being taken for a seizure disorder, psychiatric disease, Parkinson's disease, and patients taking steroids for immunologically related neurological disease. Although preoperative treatment of neurological disorders has not been reported to substantially affect perioperative outcome, knowledge of the pathophysiologic characteristics of these disorders is important in planning intraoperative and postoperative management. Consequently, preoperative knowledge about these disorders and their associated conditions (e.g., cardiac arrhythmias with Duchenne muscular dystrophy or respiratory and cardiac muscle weakness in dermatomyositis) does merit consideration.

In patients with a seizure disorder scheduled for surgery, it is important to make a note of the type of seizure (generalized, partial focal motor, or sensory), how often the seizures occur, whether there has been a recent change in the frequency of the seizures, and the medications prescribed to control them. Although seizures may be related to a variety of insults (tumor, trauma, drug withdrawal), 30% are idiopathic. In general, the epileptic patient requires no special anesthetic management other

than that for the underlying disease. Anticonvulsant medications should be maintained in the therapeutic range, continued up to the time of surgery, and promptly restarted postoperatively.

Parkinson's disease is a degenerative disorder of the central nervous system that results from decreased production of dopamine in the basal ganglia due to the degeneration of the substantia nigra and nerve terminals in the caudate nucleus and putamen. The clinical signs of Parkinson's disease reflect the unopposed effects of cholinergic neurons and include tremors, muscular rigidity, bradykinesia, and postural instability. Therapy is aimed at:

- increasing the neuronal release of dopamine or the receptor's response to dopamine
- stimulating the receptor directly with bromocriptine and lergotrile
- implanting dopaminergic tissue
- decreasing cholinergic activity.

Anticholinergic agents are usually the initial drugs of choice, as they decrease tremor more than muscle rigidity. The dopamine precursor L-dopa (levodopa) in combination with methylhydrazine (carbidopa) is also used. Therapy for Parkinson's disease should be continued through the morning of surgery and reinstituted promptly after surgery. Failure to do so may result in severe rigidity, with difficulty in breathing and protection of the airway. Drugs, such as phenothiazines and butyrophenones (droperidol), that inhibit release of dopamine or compete with dopamine at the receptor should be avoided.

Demyelinating diseases comprise a diffuse group of diseases with unknown causes, including multiple sclerosis and Guillain–Barré syndrome. Demyelinating diseases present with very diverse symptoms, most prominent of which is muscle weakness. There is always the risk of clinical relapse immediately after surgery. Relapse may occur more readily as a result of acute electrolyte and temperature changes in the perioperative period, so such changes should be prevented. Although no form of treatment has been shown to cure these diseases, steroids, plasmapheresis, and beta-interferon may reduce symptoms or shorten a clinical relapse, particularly in diseases such as multiple sclerosis and Guillain–Barré syndrome.

Another neurologically related disease is alcoholism. Alcoholism is associated with acute alcoholic hepatitis, congestive cardiomyopathy, generalized myopathy, cirrhosis, alcohol withdrawal syndromes (including delirium tremens), nutritional disorders, hypoglycemia, alcoholic polyneuropathy, Wernicke–Korsakoff syndrome, and cerebellar degeneration. In alcoholic patients, emergency surgery and anesthesia are not typically associated with worsening liver function. There is, however, a strong association with COPD, as many heavy drinkers are prolific tobacco users. Any patient who has a history of alcohol abuse warrants a careful examination of other organ systems as part of any estimation of preoperative physical status.

Myasthenia gravis is a disorder of clinical muscle weakness caused by immune-mediated disease of the neuromuscular junction. The disease manifestations include ptosis and diplopia, weakness of the pharyngeal and laryngeal muscles, asymmetric peripheral skeletal muscle weakness, cardiomyopathy, and hypothyroidism. The muscle weakness worsens with repetitive use and improves with rest. There is a beneficial response to anticholinergic drugs. Other treatment modalities for severe disease include corticosteroids, immune suppressants, surgical thymectomy, and plasmapheresis. It has been recommended that withholding all anticholinergic drugs for 6 hours prior to surgery with reinstitution of the medicines early in the postoperative period is beneficial. Myasthenic patients may require postoperative mechanical ventilation; this is especially common in patients with myasthenia gravis of more than 6 years duration, in those taking daily doses of pyridostigmine of more than 750 mg, in the presence of COPD, and in those who have a vital capacity less than 40 mL/kg.

Another muscle weakness disease encountered is the group of diseases known as the muscular dystrophies. Muscular dystrophy comprises a group of hereditary diseases of the skeletal muscles characterized by progressive weakness and degeneration of muscle. Duchenne muscular dystrophy is the most severe form, although other less severe variants exist (Table 1-55).

Duchenne muscular dystrophy is an X-linked recessive disorder occurring predominantly in males. It is typically diagnosed at 2–5 years of age, with a life expectancy of 15–20 years. The clinical findings are listed in Box 1-44.

Box 1-44 Clinical Findings in Duchenne Muscular Dystrophy

Proximal muscle weakness (gait disturbances)
Hypertrophied muscles (especially calf muscles)
Progressive kyphoscoliosis
Respiratory disease
• Inability to cough and clear secretions
• Recurrent infections
• Restrictive pulmonary defect
• Respiratory failure
• Pulmonary hypertension
Cardiomyopathy (dilated and hypertrophic)
Association with malignant hyperthermia?

Preoperative management of muscular dystrophy patients should include avoidance of depressant sedative/opioid premedicants. For major surgical procedures, especially major orthopedic, upper abdominal, and thoracic procedures, preoperative spirometry and cardiac echocardiography are appropriate.

Myotonic dystrophy is an autosomal dominant muscle disease with multisystem involvement in which muscle relaxation slows after voluntary effort or electrical stimulation. Myotonic dystrophy becomes clinically evident between the ages of 20 and 40 and progresses to an early death in the fifth or sixth decade. The myopathy has unique features including ptosis of the eyelids, sternocleidomastoid muscle atrophy, atrophy of the masseter and temporalis muscles, distal muscle group atrophy, and involvement of the pharyngeal muscles producing dysarthria and dysphagia. In the initial stages, myotonia is the predominant symptom, but as the disease progresses, increasing distal muscle weakness emerges (as apposed to the proximal muscle involvement in Duchenne muscular dystrophy). The facial, sternocleidomastoid, and pharyngeal muscles are particularly affected. Multiple organ systems are involved, as outlined in Box 1-45.

The diagnosis of myotonic dystrophy is made by the presence of typical clinical signs and symptoms and is confirmed by electromyography. Therapy is symptomatic. Drugs that have been used to help relieve the myotonia include phenytoin, quinine, mexiletine, procainamide, and beta-blockers. Mexiletine is the most effective therapy. Preoperative assessment should focus on evaluation of the cardiopulmonary system. A preoperative electrocardiogram is mandatory, taking special note of any rhythm disturbances or conduction defects. Heart failure should be excluded. The pulmonary evaluation should elicit any history of recent changes in pulmonary signs or symptoms including recent infections or changes in cough pattern or sputum production. Clinical

Table 1-55 Types of Muscular Dystrophy

Disease	Clinical Note
Duchenne muscular dystrophy	Begins early in childhood; death by late teens or early 20s; most severe form
Limb-girdle muscular dystrophy	Mostly benign clinical course
Fascioscapulohumeral muscular dystrophy	No heart involvement
Nemaline rod muscular dystrophy	
Becker's muscular dystrophy	Like Duchenne but presents later in life

---

Box 1-45   Clinical Findings in Myotonic Dystrophy

Cardiac
- Cardiomyopathy
- Atrial dysrhythmias
- Heart block

Pulmonary
- Pulmonary aspiration
- Alveolar hypoventilation
- Reduced vital capacity
- Chronic hypoxemia
- Increased sensitivity to drug-induced depression of ventilation
- Central sleep apnea and hypersomnolence

Testicular atrophy

Frontal baldness

Cataracts

Mild mental deficiency

Endocrine
- Pancreatic insufficiency
- Adrenal insufficiency
- Thyroid gland dysfunction
- Gonadal insufficiency

Gastrointestinal
- Gastrointestinal hypomotility
  - Gastric dilatation
  - Gastric regurgitation

Uterine atony

Associated with malignant hyperthermia

Prolonged contraction in response to succinylcholine

Myotonia is not relieved by anesthesia or muscle relaxants

---

evidence of thyroid, pancreatic, and adrenal hypofunction should be investigated, and this may include thyroid tests and glucose monitoring as well as perioperative steroid supplementation.

PREOPERATIVE ASSESSMENT OF PATIENTS WITH DEPRESSION

Depression afflicts about 5% of adults in the United States at any given time, with a lifetime risk of depression approaching 30%. Pharmacologic treatment of depression has been shown to be efficacious, with 65–70% of patients responding to antidepressant drug therapy, many of these experiencing complete recovery. Effective antidepressant activity has been based upon the "biogenic amine" hypothesis of depression, which holds that depression is due to a reduced functional activity of one or more of the endogenous neurotransmitter monoamines (norep-

inephrine, serotonin) at functionally important synapses in the brain. It is believed that depression is best treated by medications that stimulate neurotransmission either by (1) inhibiting the reuptake of serotonin and/or norepinephrine at the presynaptic endplate, thereby increasing synaptic amine levels and facilitating neurotransmission or (2) desensitizing inhibitory amine receptors (e.g., presynaptic serotonin or alpha-2-autoreceptors). These theories, however, do not explain why the clinical effects of antidepressant medication take 2–3 weeks to become manifest. Currently, the emphasis of research has shifted from acute reuptake effects to the slower adaptive changes in norepinephrine and serotonin receptor systems induced by chronic antidepressant therapy (e.g., "down-regulation" of the presynaptic receptors facilitating transmitter release).

Antidepressant Medications

Drugs with clinically useful antidepressant effects include the tricyclic antidepressants, selective serotonin reuptake inhibitors (SSRIs), monoamine oxidase inhibitors (MAOIs), and atypical antidepressants (bupropion, trazodone, nefazodone, and venlafaxine). An increasing number of patients are being started on SSRIs or atypical agents, as these medications have equal efficacy to the tricyclic antidepressants yet have fewer side effects and less toxicity. Tricyclic antidepressants are still being used, although they are often combined with the SSRIs in a reduced dosage. Finally, MAOIs, while still available, are usually reserved for depressive illness refractory to other therapy.

Tricyclic antidepressants

In basic terms, tricyclic antidepressant medications potentiate the actions of biogenic amines by blocking the transport or reuptake of norepinephrine into the presynaptic nerve terminals (predominantly norepinephrine reuptake). With chronic administration (>3 weeks), the presynaptic autoreceptors "downregulate", facilitating presynaptic norepinephrine release, while the postsynaptic receptors appear to remain sensitive to norepinephrine.

Selective serotonin-uptake inhibitors

Serotonin, an important chemical transmitter, is primarily synthesized from the amino acid tryptophan in the enterochromaffin cells of the gastrointestinal mucosa. In addition, a small amount is stored in platelets and the endothelial cells of the lung. Serotonin is also present in the brain, being particularly concentrated in the midbrain areas and the spinal cord, where it acts as a neurotransmitter. A very important function of serotonin is its involvement in many important psychobiological functions (including mood), which are outlined in Table 1-56.

Table 1-56 Psychobiological Function of Serotonin	
Psychobiologic Disorder	**Clinical Manifestation**
Panic disorder	Anxiety
Obsessive/compulsive disorder, post-traumatic stress disorder	Obsessionality
Behavior/personality disorders	Aggression/suicide
Schizophrenia/psychotic mood disorders	Psychosis
Major depression	Mood
Eating/sexual disorders	Appetite dysfunction

The SSRIs are a relatively new class of second-generation antidepressants that function by selectively inhibiting the presynaptic reuptake of serotonin into the presynaptic nerve terminals (rather than norepinephrine, as with the tricyclic antidepressants). With chronic administration, however, serotonin presynaptic autoreceptors become desensitized, facilitating serotonin neurotransmission, positively enhancing mood. The benefits of SSRIs over the tricyclic antidepressants are primarily related to the lack of side effects (since they have little if any effects on the H_1, muscarinic, and adrenergic receptors).

Atypical antidepressants

The medications in this class include: bupropion, venlafaxine, nefazodone, and trazodone. These agents are so classified because they possess a slightly different mechanism of action than the SSRIs; however, like SSRIs they share the beneficial properties of possessing few adverse side effects and greater safety if taken in overdose.

The preoperative assessment of patients taking tricyclic antidepressants, SSRIs, or atypical antidepressants requires nothing particularly special other than obtaining a preoperative electrocardiogram for those taking tricyclic antidepressants. All patients should continue to take their usual dose of antidepressant up to the time of surgery.

Monoamine oxidase inhibitors

Monoamine oxidase inhibitors are older agents used in the treatment of depression. Monoamine oxidase (MAO) enzymes are a group of intramitochondrial enzymes distributed widely throughout the body that are responsible for the deactivation of certain biologically active amines including norepinephrine, serotonin, and dopamine. Inhibition of MAO is thought to be effective in the treatment of endogenous depression by increasing intraneuronal neurotransmitter pools in the central nervous system. Depolarization of these cells results in an increased amount of neurotransmitter being released into the synaptic cleft, thereby increasing postsynaptic depolarization and adrenergic stimulation.

The MAO enzyme exists in two forms: MAO-A and MAO-B. Type A MAO selectively deaminates serotonin, norepinephrine, and dopamine (important neurotransmitters in affective disorders). MAOIs are divided into those agents that are nonselective and therefore inhibit both MAO-A and MAO-B enzymes and those that are selective for either the MAO-A or MAO-B enzyme. The MAOIs currently available in the United States are nonselective (inhibiting both type A and type B) and consist of two classes: hydrazine and nonhydrazine drugs. The nonhydrazine derivatives (pargyline, tranylcypromine) are reversible blockers of MAO and when discontinued have no pharmacologic effects after 24 hours. The hydrazine derivative phenelzine is an irreversible blocker of MAO, the effects lasting for at least 14–21 days after stopping therapy.

For years, the suggestion of a potential increased risk of anesthesia in association with concurrent MAOI therapy was circulated. In the past, problems associated with administering anesthesia to patients on MAOIs had included such adverse responses as hypertensive crises (especially when using indirect-acting vasopressors), arrhythmias, hypotension, prolonged narcosis or coma, and hyperpyrexia. This led to the recommendations that patients taking an MAOI should be off of the medication for at least 2 weeks before surgery (the time needed for the effects of MAOIs to dissipate). However, more recent clinical reports have shown that intraoperative adverse events are rare when appropriate monitoring techniques are used and when cardiovascular drugs and anesthesia are carefully titrated. These reports have led to the current recommendations that patients on chronic MAOI therapy may continue to take their medication up to the time of surgery as long as the potential interactions of MAOIs with specific anesthetic agents (e.g., meperidine, ephedrine) are kept in mind, as well as the importance of avoiding certain clinical scenarios that would stimulate the sympathetic nervous system (hypotension, hypovolemia, anemia, hypercarbia).

In summary, perioperative anesthetic management of patients taking MAOIs should include:

- careful monitoring of the cardiovascular system – this may include a low threshold for placing invasive monitoring devices for major surgery
- avoidance of anesthetic techniques that stimulate sympathetic responses (e.g., ketamine, pancuronium) and more emphasis on a "balanced" anesthetic technique
- maintenance of adequate arterial pressure, with particular attention to avoiding wide fluctuations in

hemodynamics; this is assured by a slow and careful anesthetic induction, meticulous titration of drug and anesthetic agents to the patient's specific needs, and careful replacement of blood and fluid losses. Should hypotension occur, it is best treated with adequate fluid volume and if needed small doses of direct-acting agents such as phenylephrine. Avoidance of indirect-acting agents (e.g., ephedrine) for the treatment of hypotension is prudent, as a rebound hypertensive crisis may occur

- careful selection of narcotics – MAOIs have been reported to adversely interact with meperidine causing agitation, excitement, restlessness, hypertension, convulsions, hyperpyrexia, prolonged narcosis, and coma. A postulated explanation for this "idiosyncratic" interaction is that it is due to meperidine-induced increases in brain serotonin (serotonin syndrome), as well as potentiation of narcotic effects secondary to MAO-induced inhibition of narcotic metabolism in the liver (cytochrome P_{450}). In addition, narcotics that induce histamine release (e.g., morphine) should probably be avoided because of the potential for hypotension that, if followed by a compensatory sympathetic-induced exaggerated release of catecholamines at the nerve terminal, may result in a hypertensive crisis and cardiac dysrhythmias.

APPENDIX: ANESTHESIA CONSENT

From Gathe-Ghermay J, Liu L. Preoperative programs in anesthesiology. Anesthesiol Clin North Am 1999; 17:335–353.

I_____authorize the administration of anesthetics under the (patient or responsible party) direction of a physician anesthesiologist member of the Department of Anesthesia at _____.
The administration of anesthesia has been explained to me and I agree to permit one or more of the following forms of anesthesia that may be appropriate for the procedure I am about to have:

- **General anesthesia** – including intravenous and/or inhaled anesthetics, which will cause unconsciousness
- **Regional anesthesia** – including needle injections near major nerves, which will temporarily cause me to lose pain sensations in certain areas of my body, and an epidural or spinal analgesia for postoperative pain relief
- **Local anesthesia** – including local anesthetic agents with or without intravenously administered sedatives.

If my regional or local anesthetic is not satisfactory, I consent to the administration of general anesthetics. I understand that, during the course of an anesthetic/operation, unforeseen changes in my condition may arise which would necessitate changes in the care being provided to me. In that case, the anesthesiologist care provider will act in my behalf with my safety as the first priority.

I am aware that no guarantees can be made concerning the results of administration of anesthetics to me. Common side effects include: nausea and vomiting, headache, backache, sore throat or hoarseness, muscle soreness, and soft tissue swelling. In addition, even minor surgery may carry with it major unforeseen anesthetic risks. These risks and complications include, but are not limited to: eye damage, damage to the mouth, teeth or vocal cords, pneumonia, numbness, dreams or recall of intraoperative events, pain or paralysis, damage to veins, arteries, liver or kidneys, adverse drug reactions, and, in rare cases, permanent brain damage, heart attack, stroke, or death. These potential risks apply to me whether I have a general, regional, or local anesthetic.

I certify that, to the best of my ability, I have told the anesthesiologist obtaining consent all of the following:

- all major illnesses I have had
- all past anesthetics I have received and any complications of these anesthetics known to me
- any drug allergies I have
- all medications I have taken in the past year
- responded truthfully to any additional questions asked by the anesthesiologist.

The nature and purpose of my anesthetic management have been explained to me. I have had the opportunity to ask questions, and my questions have been answered. I understand that I may withdraw this consent at any time prior to the administration of my anesthetic.

For the pregnant patient: I understand that anesthetics cross the placenta and may temporarily anesthetize my baby. Although fetal complications of anesthesia during pregnancy are very rare, the risks to my baby include, but are not limited to, birth defects, premature labor, permanent brain damage, and death.

Signature of patient or responsible party: _____
Date: _____
Signature of witness: _____
Date: _____
Printed name of preoperative provider: _____
Date: _____

All questions were answered and the patient consents to the anesthetic plan. The history, physical, and consent have been reviewed.

ASA Class (circle): I   II   III   IV   E

Signature of attending anesthesiologist: _____

Date: _____

SUGGESTED READING

Albright RC Jr. Acute renal failure: a practical update. *Mayo Clin Proc* 2001;76:67–74.

Braunwald E, Perloff J. Physical examination of the heart and circulation. In: Braunwald E. *Heart disease: a textbook of cardiovascular medicine*, 6th ed. Philadelphia: WB Saunders, 2001:64–75.

Brooks-Brunn JA. Predictors of postoperative pulmonary complications following abdominal surgery. *Chest* 1997;111:564–571.

Carabello BA. Clinical practice. Aortic stenosis. *N Engl J Med* 2002;346:677–682.

Clinical guideline, Part I: Guideline for assessing and managing the perioperative risk from coronary artery disease associated with major noncardiac surgery. *Ann Intern Med* 1997;127:309–312.

Dajani AS, Taubert KA, Wilson W, et al. Prevention of bacterial endocarditis: recommendations by the American Heart Association. *Circulation* 1997;96:358–366.

Detsky AS, Abrams HB, McLaughlin JR, et al. Predicting cardiac complications in patients undergoing non-cardiac surgery. *J Gen Intern Med* 1986;1:211–219.

Dierdorf SF. Anesthesia and informed consent. *Curr Opin Anesthesiol* 2002;15:349–350.

Eagle KA, Berger PB, Calkins H, et al.; American College of Cardiology; American Heart Association. ACC/AHA Guideline update for perioperative cardiovascular evaluation for noncardiac surgery – executive summary: a report of the American College of Cardiology/American Heart Association Task Force on Practice Guidelines (Committee to Update the 1996 Guidelines on Perioperative Cardiovascular Evaluation for Noncardiac Surgery). *J Am Col Cardiol* 2002;39:542–553.

Eagle KA, Coley CM, Newell JB, et al. Combining clinical and thallium data optimizes preoperative assessment of cardiac risk before major vascular surgery. *Ann Intern Med* 1989;110:859–866.

Eisenberg DM, Davis RB, Ettner SL, et al. Trends in alternative medicine use in the United States, 1990–1997: results of a follow-up national survey. *JAMA* 1998;280:1569–1579.

Fifth report of the Joint National Committee on detection, evaluation, and treatment of high blood pressure (JNC V). *Arch Intern Med* 1993;153:154–183.

Fleisher L. Preoperative evaluation. In: Barash P, Cullen B, Stoelting R, eds. *Clinical anesthesia*, 4th ed. Philadelphia: Lippincott Williams & Wilkins, 2001;473–489.

Fleisher L. Risk of anesthesia. In: Miller R. *Anesthesia*, 5th ed. New York: Churchill-Livingstone, 2000:795–823.

Frost E. Preanesthesia assessment of the patient with respiratory disease. *Anesthesiol Clin North Am* 1990;8:657–675.

Gathe-Ghermay J, Liu L. Preoperative programs in anesthesiology. *Anesthesiol Clin North Am* 1999;17:335–353.

Goldman L, Caldera DL, Nussbaum SR, et al. Multifactorial index of cardiac risk in noncardiac surgical procedures. *N Engl J Med* 1977;297:845–850.

Hayden SP, Mayer ME, Stoller JK. Postoperative pulmonary complications: risk assessment, prevention, and treatment. *Cleveland Clin J Med* 1995;62:401–407.

Lagasse RS. Anesthesia safety: model or myth? A review of the published literature and analysis of current original data. *Anesthesiology* 2002;97:1609–1617.

Lee TH, Boucher CA. Noninvasive tests in patients with stable coronary artery disease. *N Engl J Med* 2001;344:1840–1845.

Lenders JW, Keiser HR, Goldstein DS, et al. Plasma metanephrines in the diagnosis of pheochromocytoma. *Ann Intern Med* 1995;123:101–109.

Mallampati SR, Gatt SP, Gugino LD, et al. A clinical sign to predict difficult tracheal intubation: a prospective study. *Can Anaesth Soc J* 1985;32:429–434.

Mangano DT, Layug EL, Wallace A, Tateo I. Effect of atenolol on mortality and cardiovascular morbidity after noncardiac surgery. *N Engl J Med* 1996;335:1713–1720.

Mohr DN, Lavender RC. Preoperative pulmonary evaluation. *Postgrad Med* 1996;100:241–256.

Pacak K, Linehan WM, Eisenhofer G, et al. NIH Conferences: recent advances in genetics, diagnosis, localization, and treatment of pheochromocytoma. *Ann Intern Med* 2001;134:315–329.

Palda VA, Detsky AS. Clinical guideline, Part II: Perioperative assessment and management of risk from coronary artery disease. *Ann Intern Med* 1997;127:313–328.

Patel T. Surgery in the patient with liver disease. *Mayo Clin Proc* 1999;74:593–599.

Poldermans D, Boersma E, Bax JJ, et al. The effect of bisoprolol on perioperative mortality and myocardial infarction in high-risk patients undergoing vascular surgery. *N Engl J Med* 1999;341:1789–1794.

Practice advisory for preanesthesia evaluation: a report by the American Society of Anesthesiologists. *Anesthesiology* 2002;96:485–496.

Practice guidelines for preoperative fasting and the use of pharmacologic agents to reduce the risk of pulmonary aspiration: application to healthy patients undergoing elective procedures: a report by the American Society of Anesthesiologists Task Force on Preoperative Fasting. *Anesthesiology* 1999;90:896–905.

Pratt DS, Kaplan MM. Evaluation of abnormal liver-enzyme results in asymptomatic patients. *N Engl J Med* 2000;342:1266–1271.

Pugh RN, Murray-Lyon IM, Dawson JL, et al. Transection of the oesophagus for bleeding oesophageal varices. *Br J Surg* 1973;60:646–649.

Roizen M. Anesthetic implications of concurrent diseases. In: Miller R. *Anesthesia*, 5th ed. New York: Churchill-Livingstone, 2000:903–1015.

Salem M, Tainsh RE Jr, Bromberg J, *et al*. Perioperative glucocorticoid coverage: a reassessment 42 years after emergence of a problem. *Ann Surg* 1994;219:416–425.

Sheperd K, Hurford W. Pulmonary disease. In: Sweitzer BJ, ed. *Handbook of preoperative assessment and management.* Philadelphia: Lippincott Williams & Wilkins, 2000; 97–125.

Smetana GW. Preoperative pulmonary evaluation. *N Engl J Med* 1999;340:937–944.

Stone D, Gal T. Airway management. In: Miller R, ed. *Anesthesia*, 5th ed. New York: Churchill Livingstone, 2000; 1414–1451.

Thadhani R, Pascual M, Bonventre JV. Acute renal failure. *N Engl J Med* 1996;334:1448–1460.

Vanzetto G, Machecourt J, Blendea D, *et al*. Additive value of thallium single-photon emission computed tomography myocardial imaging for prediction of perioperative events in clinically selected high cardiac risk patients having abdominal aortic surgery. *Am J Cardiol* 1996;77: 143–148.

Warner DO, Warner MA, Barnes RO, *et al*. Perioperative respiratory complications in patients with asthma. *Anesthesiology* 1996;85:460–467.

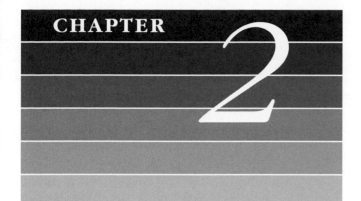

CHAPTER 2

The Operating Room

RICHARD L. APPLEGATE II

INTRODUCTION

The operating room (OR) environment is the setting for some of the most critical patient care offered by modern medicine. In many ways, the interface between the patient and the anesthesiologist is dictated by the constraints of the operating room, and the equipment we use to provide that critical care. This chapter will cover some of the basics of the operating room environment.

THE ANESTHESIA MACHINE

In its simplest form, the delivery of inhaled anesthetics requires nothing more than a soaked gauze or cloth to hold over the patient's nose and mouth. The development of more complicated surgical procedures and the development of more controlled anesthetic techniques have led to the development of more sophisticated machines. A review of the historical development of these machines is outside the scope of this chapter, but the reader should be aware that nonstandard machines may still be in existence and that thorough familiariza-

tion with the equipment available for patient care is essential for safe administration of anesthesia. The anesthesia machine allows for delivery of controlled proportions of breathing gases, addition of anesthetic vapor, and support or control of the patient's respirations.

In modern anesthesia machines, various safety systems are present that are designed to limit the harmful effects to the patient of errors or failures. The evolution of the anesthesia machine has been driven by the need for greater patient safety. Equipment malfunction, operator error and maintenance error have contributed to patient harm in the past. A series of regulations has increasingly specified the safety standards required to sell an anesthesia machine in the United States.

Gas Supply

Medical gases are supplied to the operating room through specific pipelines. The material for the pipes is specified, and the pipes should be labeled at frequent intervals to aid maintenance workers in identifying them. The outlets for medical gases are protected by safety systems. Shutoff valves are required outside the operating room and must be clearly labeled to identify the suite of rooms controlled by the valve. The connection from the supply pipe to the anesthesia machine is protected either by diameter-indexed safety system connections or by specific quick connects. Quick connects are popular because they allow rapid relocation of the anesthesia machine to different operating room sites. The quick connect depends on a specific combination of male and female connectors. These components must align correctly to allow connection of the supply hose to the wall outlet. With wear or deliberate alteration it is possible for an incorrect connection to be made, with the potential for administration of hypoxic gas mixtures to the patient. Gas is supplied to the machine at approximately 50 psi from pipeline sources (Figure 2-1).

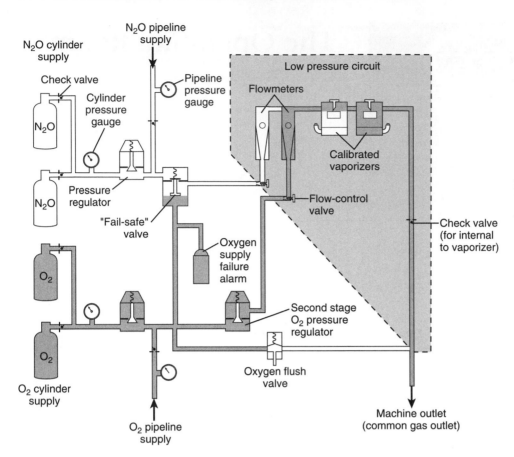

Figure 2-1 Schematic drawing of a basic anesthesia machine. The low pressure portion of the circuit is outlined (Redrawn from Andrews JJ. Inhaled anesthetic delivery systems. In: Miller R. *Anesthesia*, 5th ed. New York: Churchill-Livingstone, 2000:176.)

The anesthesia machine provides for an auxiliary or backup supply of gases with cylinders mounted on the machine. The cylinders are color-coded to assist in attaching the correct gas cylinder to the correct yoke. The cylinders have pin index safety system mounts that prevent mounting of the incorrect gas cylinder to the specific yoke on the machine. With wear or deliberate alteration, it is possible for an incorrect connection to be made with this system also, with the potential for administration of hypoxic gas mixtures to the patient. The yoke includes a check valve to prevent cross-filling or back-filling of a cylinder. A pressure gauge is present for each gas supplied by both wall and cylinder. A pressure regulator is necessary to control the gas pressure from the cylinder pressure (up to 2,200 psi for oxygen, decreasing as the tank is used) to approximately 45 psi (Figure 2-2).

The anesthesia machine has a second regulator to decrease the pressure from 45–50 psi to 12–19 psi. This lower pressure level results in less risk of barotrauma to the patient's lungs. The oxygen flush valve introduces oxygen at 45–50 psi to the fresh gas outlet and may lead to an unsafe increase in pressure in the patient breathing circuit. Flow from the oxygen flush valve may be as great as 75 L/min. If a check valve is present between the oxygen flush valve and the vaporizer, the flush valve may be used for jet ventilation. A subtle risk associated with the oxygen flush valve is the dilution of inhaled anesthetic in the circuit, which may be associated with a lightly anesthetized patient.

The delivery of safe gas mixtures to the patient is of utmost importance. A number of safety standards address this issue, and safety devices have been introduced to decrease the risk of delivering a hypoxic mixture of gases to the patient. Anesthesia machines are equipped with alarms that indicate when oxygen supply pressure falls below a limit. This audible alarm requires immediate attention. Both pneumatic and mechanical controls are employed to ensure delivery of no less than 19% inspired oxygen in compliance with standards. The first "line of defense" in prevention of delivering hypoxic gas mixtures is the oxygen failure safety valve. This device uses oxygen pressure to keep a valve controlling flow of nitrous oxide open. If oxygen pressure falls below a specific level, the valve closes, preventing delivery of nitrous oxide. It is critical to understand that this valve depends on oxygen pressure, not flow. A machine may be modified to allow delivery of 100% nitrous oxide providing oxygen pressure is above the specific lower limit (Figure 2-3).

Another approach to protecting the patient from hypoxic gas mixtures is to control the proportion of gas flow delivered to the patient. Both mechanical and pneumatic devices have been developed to accomplish this.

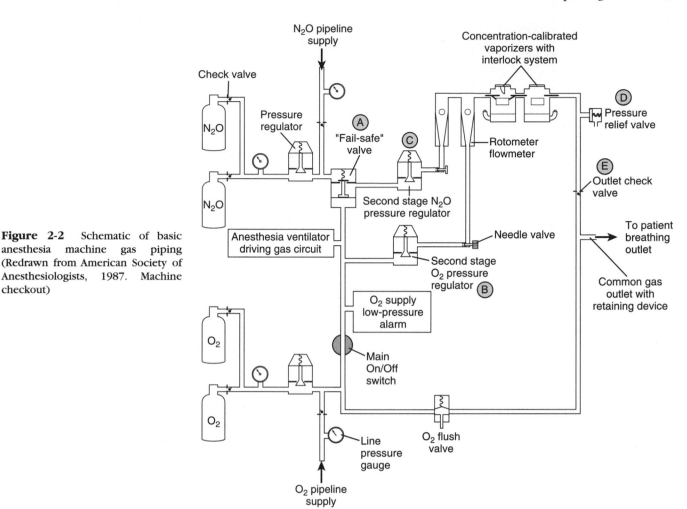

Figure 2-2 Schematic of basic anesthesia machine gas piping (Redrawn from American Society of Anesthesiologists, 1987. Machine checkout)

Figure 2-3 Schematic of oxygen failure safety valve. (Redrawn from Dorsch J, Dorsch S. *Understanding anesthesia equipment*, 2nd ed. Baltimore: Williams & Wilkins, 1984:50.)

The mechanical devices use a gear or link chain method to proportionally control oxygen flow when nitrous oxide flow is increased. The ratio of gear teeth between nitrous oxide and oxygen controls maintains an oxygen delivery above 25% if just nitrous oxide and oxygen are being delivered (Figure 2-4).

North American Drager uses a proportioning system that has both mechanical and pneumatic components. This device depends on resistors that are placed downstream of the flow valves for oxygen and nitrous oxide. The resistor in the oxygen supply path leads to generation of back pressure, which influences the position of a flow-limiting valve in the nitrous oxide outlet, which is held under tension by a spring. If oxygen flow decreases, back pressure decreases and the nitrous oxide slave control valve is closed. If oxygen flow is great enough (over 200 mL/min) the back pressure is high enough to push against the spring and open the nitrous oxide slave control valve (Figure 2-5).

Control of the amount and mixture of gases delivered to the patient depends on flowmeters. Flowmeters may be either pneumatic or electronic. The pneumatic

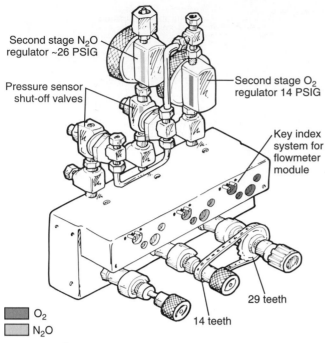

Figure 2-4 Oxygen ratio proportioning system. (Redrawn from Eisenkraft JB. Anesthesia delivery system. In: Longnecker DE, Tinker JH, Morgan, GE Jr., eds. *Principles and practices of anesthesiology*, 2nd ed. Philadelphia: Mosby, 1998: 1017, fig 48-4.)

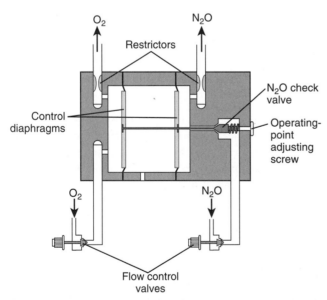

Figure 2-5 Drager Sensitive Oxygen Ratio Controller used in the Fabius GS machine. (Redrawn from Drager Fabius GS service manual.)

flowmeter depends on the relationship between the diameter of the flow tube, the characteristics of the indicator float, and the viscosity and density of the gas. The internal diameter of the flowmeter tube is tapered toward the top, with a larger effective orifice at the top. This taper requires higher gas flows to suspend the indicator float at higher levels. Flowmeters for a specific gas

may be separate for low and high flow rates. The flowmeters are color-coded and are calibrated for each specific gas. Several safety features are used on newer machines, including a different physical size and shape for the oxygen flow control valve, with a larger diameter, more prominent ridges on the outer rim, and a more prominent position out from the flowmeter compared to the other flow control knobs.

Indicator floats are of several shapes, including tapered floats and balls. The flow rate is read at the top of a tapered float or the middle of a ball float. There may be a float stop at the top of the glass flow tube. The gas from the flowmeter is gathered in a manifold at the top of the flowmeter assemblies and then piped to the vaporizers (Figure 2-6).

Electronic flowmeters are also used. These measure gas flow based on the specific heat of the gas being measured. As the gas flows through the flowmeter, the gas carries heat away. The electrical current required to maintain the temperature of the measurement chamber correlates to the gas flow through the chamber. The electrical current required is converted to a flow rate that is displayed on the anesthesia machine (Figures 2-7 and 2-8).

Glass tube flowmeters are fairly fragile and can be cracked. This can lead to delivery of a gas mixture other than desired. The location of the flowmeters on the

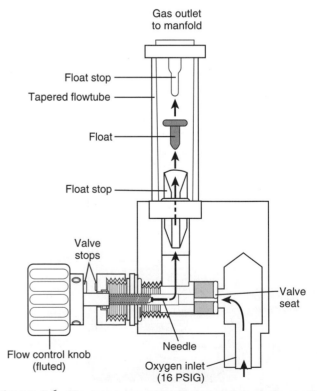

Figure 2-6 Flowmeter assembly (Redrawn from Andrews JJ. Inhaled anesthetic delivery systems. In: Miller R. *Anesthesia*, 5th ed. New York: Churchill-Livingstone, 2000:179, fig 7–6.)

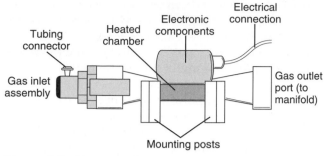

Figure 2-7 Electronic flowmeter used in Drager Fabius GS machine. (Redrawn from Drager Fabius GS service manual, page 2–34.)

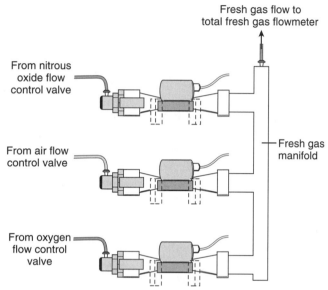

Figure 2-8 Schematic of flowmeter and manifold used in Drager Fabius GS machine. (Redrawn from Drager Fabius GS service manual, page 2–34.)

anesthesia machine is designed to decrease the risk of delivering a hypoxic gas mixture to the patient. Oxygen is the flowmeter closest to the gas manifold since this is the arrangement least likely to be associated with hypoxic gas mixtures if cracks develop in the flowmeter assemblies.

Vaporizers

Inhaled anesthetics are supplied as liquids but must be vaporized for delivery to the patient. Vaporization depends on the physical properties of the specific agent and the physical environment in which the liquid exists. For a given temperature, equilibrium exists between the liquid and vapor states of an agent that reflects the vapor pressure of the agent. As the temperature rises, the vapor pressure increases. At the boiling point, the vapor pressure equals the atmospheric pressure. In variable bypass vaporizers, gas flows through a chamber containing

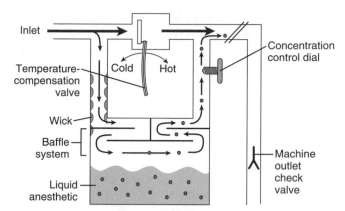

Figure 2-9 Tec 4 vaporizer showing temperature and pressure compensation systems. (Redrawn from Andrews JJ. Inhaled anesthetic delivery systems. In: Miller R. *Anesthesia*, 5th ed. New York: Churchill-Livingstone, 2000:186, fig 7–15.)

anesthetic vapor, part of which is absorbed into the gas flow and then added to the total flow going to the patient. To restate this in more obvious terms, the total flow of gas going to the patient circuit includes the fresh gas flow set at the flow meters plus the amount of anesthetic vapor entrained in the vaporizer. This amount is dependent on the temperature in the vaporizer and the vapor pressure of the agent. Modern vaporizers are calibrated for this entrainment, and have compensation systems for temperature and the effects of airway pressure on the vaporization process (Figures 2-9 and 2-10).

Factors that influence variable bypass vaporizer accuracy are related to the physics of the vaporization process and the anesthetic circuit. Among these factors are the following.

- *Flow rate*: At extremes (<250 mL/min or >15 L/min), the concentration delivered is less than the dial setting.
- *Temperature*: Nearly linear delivery of set concentration, slight increase with high temperatures.

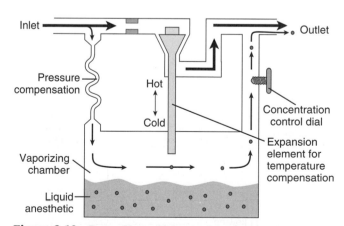

Figure 2-10 Drager Vapor 19.1 vaporizer showing temperature and pressure compensation systems. (Redrawn from Andrews JJ. Inhaled anesthetic delivery systems. In: Miller R. *Anesthesia*, 5th ed. New York: Churchill-Livingstone, 2000:186, fig 7–16.)

- *Intermittent back pressure*: A "pumping effect" caused by rapid changes in circuit pressure is seen with positive pressure ventilation. Compression of gas in the vaporizer during inspiration is rapidly released with expiration, which causes a higher concentration to be delivered than that set on the dial. This effect is more pronounced at low flow rates, low dial settings, and low liquid anesthetic levels in the vaporizer. This effect is minimal with modern vaporizers.
- *Carrier gas composition*: Probably related to viscosity and density of carrier gases and variable solubility of anesthetic agents in different gases. Generally, with these vaporizers, high nitrous oxide concentrations lead to lower delivery than that expected from the dial setting.
- *Atmospheric pressure*: Modern vaporizers deliver the same partial pressure at altitude as at sea level. This is based on the physics of these agents and the correlation between partial pressure of the anesthetic agent, not percentage of inspired gas, and the anesthetic state. Of course, partial pressure is different from percentage of a gas mixture. These vaporizers yield a mixture that has the same partial pressure of anesthetic agent whether at sea level or at higher elevations. Thus, although the percentage of anesthetic agent at the common gas outlet will be higher in Denver than in San Diego, the partial pressure of anesthetic agent will be the same. The effect at the brain correlates with partial pressure of the anesthetic agent. Although lower atmospheric pressure is associated with a greater percentage of inspired anesthetic agent, the clinical potency is relatively unchanged. Thus when using a variable bypass vaporizer at high elevation, setting the vaporizer to a desired MAC multiple will provide for the expected clinical anesthetic state.
- *Overdose* can occur if the vaporizer is tipped or overfilled. These conditions lead to liquid agent in the bypass chamber and can lead to delivery of up to 10 times the dial setting. Safe use of a vaporizer that has liquid in the bypass chamber requires the user to flush the vaporizer with high-flow gas and the vaporizer set at low output for 20–30 min before use for a patient.
- *Wrong agent in vaporizer*: The effect depends on the relative vapor pressures of agent put in compared to that of agent for which vaporizer is designed:
  - A halothane vaporizer set to 1% (1.25 minimum alveolar anesthetic concentration [MAC]) but filled with isoflurane delivers 0.96% (0.84 MAC). A halothane vaporizer filled with enflurane set at 1% delivers only 0.62% (0.37 MAC).
  - An isoflurane vaporizer set to 1.5% (1.3 MAC) but filled with halothane delivers 1.56% (1.95 MAC). An isoflurane vaporizer filled with enflurane set to 1.5% delivers only 0.97% (0.57 MAC).
  - An enflurane vaporizer set to 2% (1.19 MAC) but filled with halothane delivers 3.21% (4 MAC). If an enflurane vaporizer is set to deliver 2% but is filled with isoflurane it will deliver 3.1% (2.69 MAC).

The variable bypass vaporizer design works well for liquid anesthetic agents that have boiling points higher than room temperature. While the boiling point for isoflurane is 48.5° C, and for sevoflurane 58.5° C, the boiling point of desflurane is near 22.8° C. This boiling point reflects a vapor pressure for desflurane near 1 atmosphere. Additionally, the MAC of desflurane is much higher than the other agents, which requires a larger amount to be vaporized to achieve clinical anesthesia. The vaporization requires heat. These factors dictate that a vaporizer for desflurane must be heated and pressurized to control the administration of desflurane (Figure 2-11).

This vaporizer is essentially a gas blender, as it adds vaporized desflurane to the fresh gas flow based on the total gas flow rate. A fixed resistor is present in the fresh

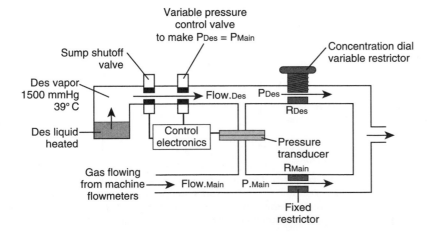

Figure 2-11 Schematic of Tec 6 vaporizer. (Redrawn from Longnecker DE, Tinker JH, Morgan GE (eds) *Principles and practices of anesthesiology*, 2nd ed. Philadelphia: Mosby, 1998:p1032, fig 48.16.)

gas flow path, which causes a back pressure proportional to the total flow rate. The back pressure is measured by the vaporizer and converted to a flow rate. The concentration dial is essentially a variable resistor, the output of which is correlated to the dial setting and the total gas flow rate. As fresh gas flow goes up, the amount of desflurane vapor blended in goes up proportionally without changing the dial setting.

Factors that influence the accuracy of the heated, pressurized vaporizer are similar to those for the variable bypass vaporizers, with important exceptions:

- *Atmospheric pressure*: Since the vaporizer works at absolute pressure, decreases in atmospheric pressure must be compensated for by manual increases in the dial setting. Similarly, using the Tec 6 under hyperbaric conditions would require decreasing the dial setting to avoid anesthetic overdose (Figure 2-12).
- *Carrier gas composition* has more impact on this type of vaporizer at low flow rates. The vaporizer is calibrated using 100% oxygen as the carrier gas. Gases with lower viscosity are associated with lower vaporizer outputs when low flow rates are used since they generate less back pressure at the primary gas flow resistor.

Safety features associated with vaporizers for desflurane include a unique filling system to limit the risk of misfilling a variable bypass vaporizer with desflurane. Additionally, the Tec 6 vaporizer has shut-off valves just downstream from the desflurane sump, which will close if major faults occur, ceasing the output of desflurane. The shut off valve will close if:

- The liquid anesthetic level falls below 20 mL
- The vaporizer is tilted
- A power failure occurs

- The pressure difference between the fresh gas circuit and the vapor circuit exceeds tolerances.

The Anesthesia Circuit

The anesthetic circuit provides for delivery of an anesthetic gas mixture to the patient from the anesthesia machine. The circle system (Figure 2-13) is the most popular breathing system in current use in the United States. The circle system has several advantages related to rebreathing. Among these are a lower use of anesthetic agent related to the lower gas flows possible with rebreathing, increases in circuit humidity with time, with a possible improvement in temperature regulation for the patient, a stable concentration of anesthetic gas in the circuit and an easier accommodation of scavenging systems to the circuit. Essential components of the circle system are:

- Fresh gas flow inlet
- Unidirectional valves in both inspiratory and expiratory limbs
- Tubes
- Y connector
- Overflow or adjustable pressure limit valve
- Reservoir bag
- Carbon dioxide absorber.

Risks associated with use of the circle system include malfunction of the valves and disconnects. The unidirectional valves may stick in either the open or the closed position. When the valve is stuck in the open position rebreathing will occur, with a resultant increase in end-tidal carbon dioxide as seen on capnometry or arterial blood gas analysis. On capnometry, rebreathing is seen as an elevated baseline. If the valve sticks in the closed position, the circuit will be occluded and the patient will not be ventilated.

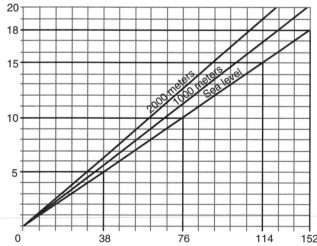

Figure 2-12 Adjustment needed with increases in elevation using Tec 6 vaporizer. (Redrawn from Datex-Ohmeda Tec 6 vaporizer brochure.)

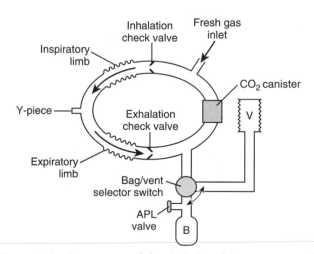

Figure 2-13 Components of the circle breathing system. B indicates reservoir bag. V indicates anesthesia machine ventilator. (Redrawn from Andrews JJ. Inhaled anesthetic delivery systems. In: Miller R. *Anesthesia*, 5th ed. New York: Churchill-Livingstone, 2000:193, fig 7.21.)

Disconnection of the breathing circuit is a significant problem. Disconnection can cause significant morbidity and even mortality. It can occur at any point between the patient and the anesthesia machine, the most common point of disconnection being at the Y connector to the endotracheal tube. Adding more connectors to a circuit increases the number of potential sites for disconnection. Disconnection is more difficult to detect and treat in patients who are positioned head away from the anesthesiologist. The significance to the practice of anesthesiology is that circuit problems are among the most common and preventable causes of anesthetic-related morbidity. Detection of disconnection requires vigilance, and should be based on a number of modalities:

- Monitoring of breath sounds – obviously, if you don't hear breath sounds during positive pressure ventilation, something is wrong.
- A hand on the bag during manual ventilation should rapidly identify changes in "compliance" when a disconnection occurs.
- In spontaneously breathing patients, light anesthesia may be the first sign of disconnection if your hand is off the bag.
- In mechanically ventilated patients, bellows that descend during exhalation may entrain room air at the point of disconnection. This would appear to show normal gas exchange at the bellows, and would lessen your ability to detect the disconnection. This event may not trigger the low-pressure alarm on your anesthesia machine. This also lessens your ability to detect the disconnection. Bellows that ascend during exhalation will not rise completely if a disconnect occurs. This should increase the ability to detect disconnection.
- Low pressure alarms:
  - An audible alarm sounds if a certain pressure is not reached during mechanical ventilation
  - Often some delay passes before the alarm sounds. On some machines this delay time can be altered
  - Some anesthesia machines allow you to alter the threshold pressure at which the alarm will sound. As a general rule, pick a pressure that is close to the peak inspired pressure of your patient
  - Pitfalls:
    - High fresh gas flows may fool the sensor
    - Inspiratory obstruction will not trigger a low pressure alarm
    - Failure of the ventilator to cycle will not trigger the low pressure alarm
    - Negative pressure via the scavenging system may trigger the alarm.

Proper function of the circle system also depends on the removal of carbon dioxide from expired gas to allow rebreathing. This is accomplished by use of chemical carbon-dioxide-absorbing agents. Currently, two agents are available for carbon dioxide absorption: soda lime and Baralyme. Reaction of either of these agents with carbon dioxide leads to the production of an inert carbonate plus water and heat. The functional status of the absorptive material is shown by color changes of an indicator substance, typically ethyl violet, which turns purple as the pH of the absorbent decreases with the reaction of carbon dioxide with the agent. The indicator dye can be deactivated, leading to the incorrect assumption that the absorbent is capable of further use. Another problem with absorbers is channeling of the gas flow, which can lead to a nonfunctional core of absorbent through which all gas is flowing. Both of these conditions will be detected by rising end-tidal carbon dioxide and a cold absorber.

The modern inhaled anesthetics can react with the absorbent material to produce unwanted substances. Sevoflurane can react with absorbents to produce compound A. The inhaled anesthetics react with desiccated absorbents to produce carbon monoxide. The concentration of carbon monoxide may be clinically significant in some settings (first case of the day on Monday, when gas was left flowing through the machine over the weekend).

Anesthesia circuits provide a mechanism for giving positive pressure ventilation to the patient. The reservoir bag is used for this purpose in addition to the function of holding gas for inspiratory flow. The pressure applied to the breathing circuit, and therefore the tidal volume given, is controlled by the adjustable pressure limit valve, also called the pop-off valve.

The anesthesia machine also allows for use of a ventilator. The ventilator may be as simple as a "bag in a box" or a more modern electronically controlled pressure- or volume-cycled ventilator. Most anesthesia ventilators are pneumatically driven bellows in a pressure chamber. Leaks in the bellows can cause dilution of the anesthetic agent in the fresh gas, and may lead to unwanted increases in tidal volume along with lighter than desired anesthetic depth. Many of these ventilators are time-cycled, and will give greater than desired tidal volumes if the fresh gas flow rate is increased. This happens because during the inspiratory phase of positive pressure ventilation with anesthesia machine ventilators, the breathing circuit receives gas from the fresh gas outlet and the bellows. This occurs because the adjustable pressure-limiting (APL, "pop-off") valve is out of circuit and the ventilator relief valve is closed during inspiration. Very high fresh gas flows will lead to larger than set or expected tidal volumes, especially with long inspiratory times. The increase will be small if the anesthesia circuit is highly compliant or leaks. Additionally, barotrauma may occur if the oxygen flush valve is triggered during the inspiratory phase. The direction the bellows move during expiration is associated with differences in safety as discussed above. Ascending bellows are associated with a greater ability to detect circuit disconnection and are the preferred type.

Waste anesthetic gases are collected and vented to outside air by a scavenging system. Scavenging systems can be associated with unwanted positive or negative pressure and should be checked during a thorough machine checkout.

Machine Checkout

The safe delivery of anesthesia to a patient depends to a great extent on a properly functioning anesthesia machine. A careful preoperative check is essential. The Food and Drug Administration has published checkout guidelines (Box 2-1).

ELECTRICAL SAFETY

The patient is exposed to numerous electrical devices in the operating room, some of which may present a threat of electrical shock to the patient. Electrical shock occurs when the patient completes the electrical circuit from the power source to ground. Electrical shock is best understood in terms of macroshock and microshock. Macroshock occurs when large amounts of current flow through and damage a patient. The damage can include burns, cardiac dysrhythmias and death. Microshock occurs when a path exists to the patient's heart, which allows very small currents to cause cardiac dysrhythmias. The path for microshock can include monitoring electrodes, central venous catheters or pacemaker wires. The current required for damage to the patient is much less for microshock (Table 2-1)

To limit the risk of microshock to the patient, monitoring equipment typically has isolation transformers in addition to the isolation transformers usually used for operating room suites. It is possible for leakage current to develop even in equipment with isolation transformers, so caution is indicated when using techniques such as intravascular electrocardiography.

Electrical equipment may also be associated with burns to the patient. Electrocautery can be associated with burns if the grounding plate is poorly applied or damaged. In such cases burns may occur at the site of the grounding pad or at other sites such as electrocardiogram pads.

ENVIRONMENTAL SAFETY

Exposure to Infection

Medical practice in the operating room exposes the anesthesiologist to several significant environmental dangers. Chief among these is the risk of infection related to needle injury. Great strides have been made in decreasing the reliance on needles for administering medications, including numerous needle-free injection systems, safety needles, and intravenous catheters. Use of safety catheters has been mandated in some areas but vascular access still depends on various needles. Care and careful practice are essential to limit the risk of needle-injury-related infection in anesthesiologists.

Anesthesiologists are also exposed to numerous bacterial and viral pathogens from their patients. Transmission of tuberculosis from patients to healthcare workers has been well documented. Concerns about transmission of the various antibiotic-resistant bacteria found in certain patients dictates careful application of infection control procedures in all operating room settings.

Latex Allergy

Another environmental concern is latex allergy. This is a significant concern for both patients and practitioners. Latex allergy is reported to be present in about 1–6% of the general population but the incidence is higher in people with a history of allergy, asthma or atopy. There may be cross-reacting antibodies to latex in patients with allergies to avocado, kiwi or bananas. Importantly, patients with no apparent risk factors may present with intraoperative anaphylaxis from latex allergy.

Treatment of intraoperative severe latex allergy or anaphylaxis from latex exposure must include pressure support with fluids and vasopressors. Epinephrine is often indicated. As the airway may be involved with bronchospasm or edema, administer 100% oxygen. Management may require postoperative mechanical ventilation. Treatment should also include antihistamines and steroids. Obviously, stopping the exposure to latex is mandatory, but it may be difficult in the setting of the solo anesthesiologist. Consider that the bellows of many ventilators on older anesthesia machines are made of a latex material, as are most reservoir bags included with anesthesia circuits. This will make ventilation of the patient difficult while you are administering various medications and intravenous fluids. It is recommended to convert to latex-free bellows, masks, endotracheal tubes, syringes, intravenous tubing, etc. and to have a latex-free cart for other items.

An American Society of Anesthesiologists taskforce developed a preoperative questionnaire to help the practitioner elicit a possibility of latex allergy. It includes a number of questions related to nonmedical exposure to latex. Even simple things like elastic bands on clothing or toy balloons may contain latex. Skin rash or wheezing after contact with any of these should raise suspicion that the patient may be latex-allergic.

What about management of a patient with known latex allergy? Meticulous avoidance of latex in the

Box 2-1   Machine Checkout Recommendations Based on the FDA Recommendations as Updated in 1997

This checkout, or a reasonable equivalent, should be conducted before administration of anesthesia. These recommendations are only valid for an anesthesia system that conforms to current and relevant standards and includes an ascending bellows ventilator and at least the following monitors: capnograph, pulse oximeter, oxygen analyzer, respiratory volume monitor (spirometer) and breathing system pressure monitor with high and low pressure alarms. This is a guideline which users are encouraged to modify to accommodate differences in equipment design and variations in local clinical practice. Such local modifications should have appropriate peer review. Users should refer to the operator's manual for the manufacturer's specific procedures and precautions, especially the manufacturer's low pressure leak test.

- **Emergency ventilation equipment**
  1. Verify backup ventilation equipment is available and functioning.
- **High-pressure system**
  2. *Check oxygen cylinder supply*: Open cylinder, verify at least half full (1,000 psi). Close cylinder.
  3. *Check central pipeline supplies*: Check that hoses are connected properly, gauges read 45–55 psi
- **Low-pressure system**
  4. *Check initial status of low-pressure system*: Close flow control valves and turn vaporizers off. Check fill level and tighten vaporizers' filler caps. Remove oxygen monitor sensor from circuit.
  5. *Perform leak check of machine low-pressure system*: Verify that the machine master switch and flow control valves are off. Attach suction bulb to common gas outlet. Squeeze bulb repeatedly until fully collapsed. Verify bulb stays fully collapsed for at least 10 seconds. Open one vaporizer at a time and repeat bulb test as above. Remove suction bulb, and reconnect fresh gas hose.
  6. Turn on machine master switch and all other necessary electrical equipment.
  7. *Test flowmeters*: adjust flow of all gases through their full range, checking for smooth operations of floats and undamaged flowtubes. Attempt to create a hypoxic oxygen/nitrous oxide mixture and verify correct changes in flow and/or alarm.
- **Breathing system**
  8. *Calibrate oxygen monitor*: Calibrate to read 21% in room air. Reinstall sensor in circuit and flush breathing system with oxygen. Verify that monitor now reads greater than 90%.
  9. *Check initial status of breathing system*: Set selector switch in "bag" mode. Check that breathing circuit is complete, undamaged and unobstructed. Verify that carbon dioxide absorbent is adequate. Install breathing circuit accessory equipment to be used during the case.
  10. *Perform leak check of the breathing system*: Set all gas flows to zero (or minimum). Close APL valve and occlude Y-piece. Pressurize breathing system to 30 cm H_2O with oxygen flush. Ensure that pressure remains at 30 cm H_2O for at least 10 seconds.
- **Scavenging system**
  11. *Check APL valve and scavenging system*: Pressurize breathing system to 50 cm H_2O and ensure its integrity. Open APL valve and ensure that pressure decreases. Ensure proper scavenging connections and waste gas vacuum. Fully open APL valve and occlude Y-piece. Ensure absorber pressure gauge reads zero when minimum oxygen is flowing, oxygen flush is activated.
- **Manual and automatic ventilation systems**
  12. *Test ventilation systems and unidirectional valves*: place a second breathing bag on Y-piece. Set appropriate ventilator parameters for next patient. Set oxygen flow to 250 mL/min and other gas flows to zero. Switch to automatic ventilation (ventilator) mode. Turn ventilator ON and fill bellows and breathing bag with oxygen flush. Verify that, during inspiration, bellows delivers correct tidal volume and that during expiration bellows fills completely. Check that volume monitor is consistent with ventilator parameters. Check for proper action of unidirectional valves. Exercise breathing circuit accessories to ensure proper function. Turn ventilator OFF and switch to manual ventilation (bag/APL) mode. Ventilate manually and ensure inflation and deflation of artificial lungs and appropriate feel of system resistance and compliance. Remove second breathing bag from Y-piece.
- **Monitors**
  13. *Check, calibrate, and/or set alarm limits of all monitors*: Capnometer, pulse oximeter, pressure monitor with high and low airway pressure alarms, oxygen analyzer, respiratory volume monitor (spirometer).
- **Final position**
  14. *Check final status of machine*: vaporizers off, APL valve open, selector switch to "bag", all flowmeters to zero (or minimum), patient suction level adequate, breathing system ready to use.

* Steps 1, 8 and 11 may be abbreviated or omitted if the same practitioner uses the same machine for following cases during the day.

Table 2-1	Comparison Between Macroshock and Microshock with 60 Hz AC Current	
Macroshock	**Microshock**
1 mA: perceptible	0.1 mA: ventricular fibrillation
Over 20 mA: can't let go	0.01 mA: recommended maximum
Around 300 mA: ventricular	leakage current
fibrillation	
About 600 mA: cardiac	
contraction/arrest	

operating room will allow management of patients with known latex allergies, without the necessity for prophylactic treatment with H_1- and H_2-blockers or steroids.

Healthcare and domestic workers are at increased risk for latex allergy, presumably because of repeated exposure to latex products. Studies of healthcare personnel have found latex sensitization in up to 15.8% of anesthesia staff, with as many as 2.4% symptomatic. There is a greater distribution in adult compared to pediatric anesthesiologists, possibly related to the more frequent use of latex gloves in adult than in pediatric anesthesiologists. For the practitioner and the patient, it is sensible to consider adopting latex-free or at least latex-minimum supplies for the operating room.

Waste Gases

Exposure to trace amounts of anesthetic agents is a reality for anesthesiologists. The long-term effects of this exposure are not clear. Governmental standards for exposure to trace amounts of these gases have been developed. As reviewed by the Occupational Safety and Health Administration (OSHA) of the United States Department of Labor, health risks of chronic exposure to trace amounts of waste gases are not entirely clear. As summarized in the OSHA report:

Despite questions about design issues or selection bias in some studies, the weight of the evidence regarding potential health risks from exposure to anesthetic agents in unscavenged environments suggests that clinicians need to be concerned. Moreover, there is biological plausibility that adds to the concern that high levels of unscavenged waste anesthetic gases present a potential for adverse neurological effects or reproductive risk to exposed workers or developmental anomalies in their offspring. While the use of prospective studies and carefully designed research protocols is encouraged to elucidate areas of controversy, a responsible approach to worker health and safety dictates that any exposure to waste and trace gases should be kept to the lowest practical level.

Workplace guidelines addressing the need for scavenging of waste gases have been put forward. The operating room should have adequate scavenging and ventilation, with evacuation of scavenged gases out of the operating room entirely. Air exchange in the operating room will also help by diluting any waste gases that are not scavenged. Additionally, several work practices may contribute to lower exposure to waste gases. Exposure to waste gases is less with the use of a circuit that allows scavenging. Stopping the flow of nitrous oxide or halogenated agents before disconnecting the circuit from the patient is prudent. The scavenging system should be adjusted to allow effective removal of waste gases without application of positive or negative pressure on the breathing circuit.

OPERATING ROOM MANAGEMENT

As the concern regarding the cost and availability of medical care has risen, the pressures surrounding practice of anesthesiology have also risen. As an anesthesiology professor once put it, the operating room is the anesthesiologist's "office" and it is essential to successful practice that the anesthesiologist understands the details of that office. This reality dictates a need to be actively involved in operating room management. Although many models have been put forward, the centralization of managerial responsibilities into a Director of Operating Room Services is reasonable. Depending on the organization, the Medical Director of the operating room may report to the Chair of the Department of Anesthesiology or Surgery, or to Hospital Administration. A close working arrangement with Hospital Administration is useful, as is a willingness to listen to varying points of view while trying to understand the different demands on operating room services. To some degree, the goals of physicians and hospital administrators will be at odds. For example, surgeons often want to have the newest equipment or adopt the latest techniques "to keep ahead of the competition," but hospital administrators may wish to have an analysis of the economics of a purchase, including a return on investment, before authorizing any purchases.

Of the various challenges facing the operating room Director, effective scheduling is often most central. Time is extremely valuable and expensive in the operating room. Much discussion occurs related to how long a process takes in the operating room. Part of this is related to differing perceptions about things such as "turnover" (Figure 2-14). For many surgeons, room turnover means the time from when they finish with a procedure until they make the next incision. For the operating room nurses, turnover is the time it takes to clean and set up an

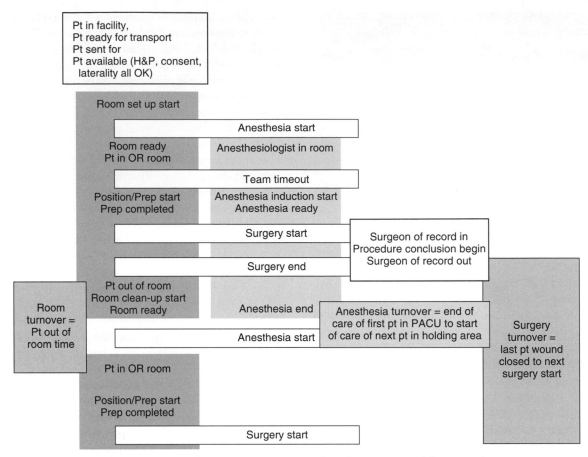

Figure 2-14   Components of operating room patient flow showing some definitions of "turnover."
Pt = patient; OR = operating room, PACU = post-anesthesia care unit.

operating room for the next case. For the anesthesiologist, turnover is the time between turning the first patient over to the care of someone else and beginning to care for the next patient. These are all a measure of turnover but will of necessity be different times. To allow focused attention on process improvement in the operating room, the various events that occur in the care of a patient through the operating room have been defined and approved by the American Society of Anesthesiologists, the Association of Operating Room Nurses, the American College of Surgeons and the American Association of Clinical Directors. Some of these times may be measured as part of improving the process of patient care in the operating room.

Effective scheduling requires measuring the use of operating room time by various surgical services and reallocating what is likely to be a limited resource to best match the actual usage patterns of surgeons using the operating room suite. Various measures of effective usage are available, including percentage block use, percentage use of time in regular hours, use of overtime resources, proportion of scheduled compared to emergency or add-on cases and cancellation rates. The optimum scheduling system has not been conclusively established to date. It seems likely that what is optimum will vary from institution to institution.

SUMMARY

The operating room is a challenging environment. The anesthesiologist must understand the various aspects of their primary place of practice, including the various aspects of the anesthesia machine, electrical safety, biological safety and operating room management.

SUGGESTED READING

Association of Anesthesia Clinical Directors. *Procedural Times Glossary of the AACD 1995*. Online at: http://www.aacdhq. org/Glossary.htm.

Berry AJ, *et al.* (ASA Committee on Occupational Health of Operating Room Personnel). *Natural rubber latex allergy: considerations for anesthesiologists*. Park Ridge, IL: American Society of Anesthesiologists, 1999.

Brown RH, Schauble JF, Hamilton RG. Prevalence of latex allergy among anesthesiologists. *Anesthesiology* 1998;89: 292–299.

Dorsch J, Dorsch S. *Understanding anesthesia equipment*, 4th ed. Baltimore: Williams & Wilkins, 1999.

Konrad C, Fieber T, Gerber H, *et al*. The prevalence of latex sensitivity among anesthesiology staff. *Anesth Analg* 1997;84: 629–633.

Occupational Safety and Health Administration, US Department of Labor. *Anesthetic gases: guidelines for workplace exposures*. 2000. Online at: http://www.osha-slc.gov/dts/osta/anesthetic-gases/index.html.

US Food and Drug Administration, Center for Devices and Radiological Health. *Anesthesia apparatus checkout recommendations, 1993, updated 1997*. Online at: http://www.fda.gov/cdrh/humfac/anesckot.html.

Positioning

THOMAS P. ENGEL

INTRODUCTION

Positioning of the patient during an anesthetic has a considerable effect on patient physiology, the ease of performing surgery and the risk of patient injury. The primary indication for a specific patient position during surgery is surgical access. This benefit should be weighed against the risks to the patient associated with the position. Nerve injuries during anesthesia are a significant cause of morbidity, accounting for about 15% of anesthesia malpractice claims (Box 3-1).

Although improper positioning may cause injury, the mechanism of injury is unclear in a large proportion of cases of nerve injury. Nerve injury may occur even when the patient position is selected and all precautions are taken to minimize the risk of injury. Responsibility for correct patient positioning lies with each member of the operating room team, including the surgeon, anesthesiologist, nurse anesthetist, nurses, and technicians caring for the patient. The patient, retractors, frames, and the operating bed frequently change during surgery. The operat-

ing room team should check the patient frequently to insure that no new risk has been created.

PHYSIOLOGIC CHANGES

Physiologic changes with patient position during general anesthesia and surgery are largely due to the effects of gravity. There is increased blood volume in the lower extremities in the vertical position and increased venous return and cardiac output in the horizontal position. Baroreceptor reflexes maintain the blood pressure. Abdominal contents are displaced inferiorly in the vertical position. The diaphragm is displaced superiorly and posteriorly in the supine position with a decrease in functional residual capacity and total lung volume. Posterior portions of the lung receive more ventilation and perfusion maintaining the ventilation/perfusion ratio with negative pressure (spontaneous) ventilation. Patients with morbid obesity, congestive heart failure or other medical problems may not be able to tolerate a horizontal position.

Additional physiologic changes occur with general anesthesia and positive pressure ventilation. Baroreceptor reflexes are attenuated. Positive pressure ventilation further reduces functional residual capacity and total lung volume. Positive pressure ventilation provides more uniform lung ventilation, impairing the ventilation/perfusion ratio. These changes result in more rapid oxygen desaturation during apnea.

Of obvious concern during a general anesthetic is the inability of the patient to signal a positioning problem. The patient may be placed in a position of undue stress or maintained in the same position for long periods of time. Tissue or nerve injury may result from direct pressure or stretching, or result from ischemia from direct pressure or stretching. Prolonged pressure on tissue may lead to ischemia and necrosis. This risk is particularly high for tissue underneath bony prominences such as the back of the head, elbows, hips, knees, ankles, and heels. Pressure to any of these areas would be painful in the awake patient and would be avoided.

Conditions such as obesity may increase risk of nerve and tissue injury because of the increased force of gravity and less space for retractors and other equipment. Patients with conditions associated with neuropathy or vasculitis such as diabetes mellitus and autoimmune syndromes may have lower tolerance of positioning problems and increased risk of injury. Hypotension or hypoperfusion states during surgery such as cardiopulmonary bypass may increase the risk of tissue ischemia and nerve injury. An extensive duration of surgery is also associated with increased risk of nerve and tissue injury.

Common patient positions during general anesthesia and surgery are supine position, lithotomy position, prone position and lateral position. Uncommon patient positions during general anesthesia and surgery include the sitting position and other positions used for specific surgeries.

COMMON POSITIONS

Supine Position

The supine position is the most common position used during surgery. This position provides surgical access to the anterior abdomen, thorax, face and extremities (Figure 3-1). The supine position generally has the lowest risk of injury for the patient when compared to other positions. The position of the arms is discussed in the section on Peripheral Nerve Injury, below. The patient's occiput and heels may be padded to reduce focal pressure and reduce the risk of alopecia or necrosis.

The patient's legs may be raised and the knees bent to increase blood volume in the thorax and reduce abdominal wall tension. Back pain after surgery in the supine position may be due to flattening of the lumbar curve, prolonged surgery and relaxation of muscles during general anesthesia. The Trendelenburg position does not always increase blood pressure in hypotensive patients. The reverse Trendelenburg position may improve pulmonary function in obese patients and may be particularly useful during emergence (Box 3-2).

Lithotomy Position

The lithotomy position is commonly used for gynecologic and urologic surgery (Figure 3-2). In the lithotomy position the patient's thighs are flexed and abducted as the legs are raised with supports attached to the bed. There is risk of injury to the common peroneal nerve if it is compressed between the support and the head of the fibula below the knee. There is risk of injury to the saphenous nerve if it is compressed between the support and the medial tibial condyle at the ankle. Obturator nerve injury at the hip may occur with flexion of the thigh and stretching of the nerve in the obturator foramen. The risk of injury to the femoral nerve in the inguinal canal may be due to tightening of the inguinal ligament with abduction of the thigh.

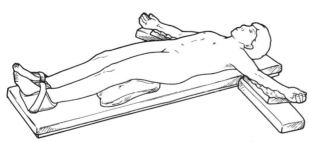

Figure 3-1   Supine position.

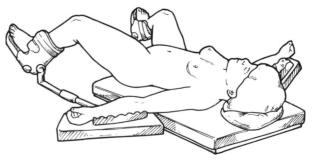

Figure 3-2   Lithotomy position.

Lower extremity compartment syndromes and deep venous thrombosis have occurred with lithotomy position. These syndromes may be related to prolonged pressure by straps or the surgeon leaning on the leg. Compartment syndromes of the hand may occur with prolonged pressure between the bed and the patient's buttocks. Fingers may be crushed in the gap between the foot and the body of the operating bed when moving the foot of the bed. The position of the hands should be checked whenever the foot of the bed is raised or lowered.

Prone Position

The prone position is used for surgery of the back and posterior aspects of the head and extremities (Figure 3-3). The weight of the patient on the chest and abdomen in the prone position results in increased intrathoracic and intra-abdominal pressure with further superior displacement of the diaphragm and further reduction in functional residual capacity and total lung volume, and may cause compression of the vena cava. Padded chest rolls are placed along the side of the chest to create space for chest and abdominal movement with ventilation.

In the prone position, the patient's arms may be placed next to the body or away from the body. One should avoid placing the arms at an angle of more than 90° to the torso, especially in patients with thoracic outlet syndrome. Direct pressure on the eye may increase intraocular pressure and reduce retinal perfusion, leading to injury. Eye injury may occur without direct pressure on the eye. The eyes should be checked frequently during surgery. Care should also be taken to avoid pressure on the lips and face from the endotracheal tube and to avoid kinking the endotracheal tube.

The jackknife position is a prone position frequently used for anal surgery. In the jackknife position, the bed is reflexed sharply in the center, elevating the buttocks. The abdominal contents are displaced superiorly in jackknife position and functional residual capacity and total lung volume are decreased.

When the prone position is selected, the patient is usually induced in the supine position on the gurney or hospital bed and moved to the prone position. Both the gurney or hospital bed and the operating bed must be locked before moving the patient to reduce the risk of the patient falling. Adequate personnel should be on hand to facilitate the move. The gurney or hospital bed should be kept nearby in case the patient must be urgently moved back to supine position.

Lateral Position

The lateral position is frequently used for thoracic and retroperitoneal surgery (Figure 3-4). Lateral positions are named for the side that is down – in the left lateral position, the patient is resting on his/her left side. Decreased ventilation and increased perfusion of the dependent lung increases ventilation/perfusion mismatch. The weight of the patient may cause ischemia or injury of dependent areas. The knees and ankles may be padded to reduce focal pressure on these areas. The arms are each usually supported to the side of the operating bed at the level of the shoulder.

Compression of the vena cava may occur with a misplaced kidney rest. The kidney rest is properly positioned under the iliac crest at the hip. Compression of the neurovascular bundle in the axilla may occur. An axillary roll should be placed under the ribs just inferior to the axilla to support the weight of the thorax and reduce pressure on the axilla. Misplacement of the roll under the axilla may displace the head of the humerus at the shoulder and increase the risk of stretch or compression injury of the brachial plexus. Proper head support may reduce the risk of neck and nondependent brachial plexus stretch injury. The head should be aligned in the neutral position.

When the lateral position is selected the patient is usually induced in the supine position on the operating bed. The patient is then moved to the lateral position.

UNCOMMON POSITIONS

Sitting Position

The sitting position is sometimes used for posterior fossa intracranial surgery. Increased venous drainage from the head may improve surgical conditions. The sitting

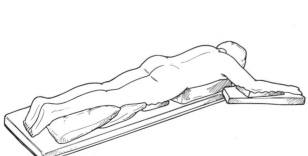

Figure 3-3   Prone position.

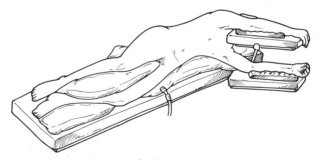

Figure 3-4   Lateral position.

Box 3-3   Use of Frames

The use of frames is becoming increasingly common in orthopedic surgery

Frames are large structures used to hold the patient in a specific position for surgical access and to create straight paths for radiography

Frames create many situations that could lead to injury, including prolonged stretching, pressure from the frame, and pressure from any straps that are used

In general, the patient's weight is supported over a smaller area when a frame is used

The frame also may allow the patient to be placed in a position that would be very uncomfortable if the patient were awake

Care must be taken to minimize the length of surgery, provide adequate padding and avoid pressure between the frame and the patient

position is also used for shoulder surgery to provide anterior and posterior access to the shoulder. The sitting position is accomplished by lowering the leg of the operating bed, flexing the bed and placing the bed in reverse Trendelenburg. Care must be taken to avoid injury to the hands and legs during manipulation of the bed.

The sitting position is similar to the reverse Trendelenburg position, with increased blood volume in the lower extremities, decreased venous return and decreased cardiac output. Abdominal contents may be displaced inferiorly, with improved functional residual capacity and ventilation/perfusion ratio compared to a horizontal position. The sitting position can place the head significantly higher than the heart, with negative venous pressures in the head.

Surgery in the sitting position includes the risk of venous air embolism if a vein is opened in the surgical field. A large venous air embolism may lead to pulmonary hypertension, hypoxia and cardiovascular collapse. Negative pressure will draw air into the vein if the vein does not collapse. Intracranial venous sinuses are held open by the dura and do not collapse when opened. Transesophageal echocardiography and transthoracic Doppler ultrasound are the most sensitive monitors for venous air embolism. Treatment of venous air embolism includes flooding the field with irrigation, lowering the head below the level of the heart and surgical occlusion of the opening (Box 3-3).

PERIPHERAL NERVE INJURY

Ulnar Nerve

Peripheral nerve injury may be an unavoidable risk of general anesthesia and surgery. The most common peripheral nerve injury during general anesthesia and surgery is injury to the ulnar nerve at the elbow. This injury accounts for one third of all nerve injuries that occur during surgery.

Current Controversies: Peripheral Nerve Injury

In many cases of peripheral nerve injury, no cause can be found

Some of these cases may represent latent disease

No screening test has been established to detect patients at highest risk

The ulnar nerve lies superficially in the groove between the medial epicondyle of the humerus and the olecranon process of the ulna in the posterior elbow. The ulnar nerve supplies sensation to the anterior and lateral portions of the fourth and fifth digits, the medial portion of the fifth digit and the anterior and lateral portions of the palm. The ulnar nerve supplies motor function for adduction and abduction of the fingers (interossei), adduction of the thumb (adductor pollicis muscle) and flexion and adduction at the wrist (interossei). Injury to the nerve may cause paresthesia, numbness, pain, and paresis or paralysis in these areas. Initial symptoms from most ulnar neuropathies are noted more than 24 hours after surgery. Patients who are male, very thin, obese, or hospitalized for prolonged periods of time are at higher risk for this injury. The injury may be transient or permanent; about half of ulnar neuropathies resolve within 1 year.

Current Controversies: Prone vs. Supine Arm Position

No consensus exists regarding whether rotation of the arm to prone position or supine position during surgery provides the lowest risk of ulnar nerve injury

The ulnar nerve is at risk whether the arms are tucked at the side, supported away from the body, held prone, or held supine. A fold of a blanket or the edge of the operating bed have been implicated in some ulnar nerve injuries. The arms and elbows should be carefully checked to insure that there is no direct pressure on the ulnar nerve.

Brachial Plexus

Brachial plexus injuries are the second most common peripheral nerve injury during general anesthesia and

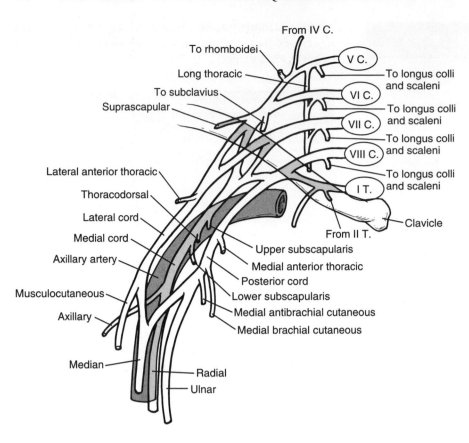

Figure 3-5   The brachial plexus.

surgery. The brachial plexus is formed from the anterior rami of the spinal nerves of C5, C6, C7, C8, and T1. These nerves form into trunks, then into divisions, and then into cords, which separate into the musculocutaneous, axillary, radial, median, ulnar, and other nerves that carry sensation from and supply motor function to the upper extremity (Figure 3-5).

Brachial plexus injury may result from stretch or compression of the plexus in the thoracic outlet or the axilla due to abduction of the arm. Brachial plexus injuries may result in paresthesia, numbness, pain, and paresis or paralysis of areas in the upper extremity. Patients undergoing cardiac surgery and sternotomy or laparoscopic surgery involving a steep Trendelenburg position may be at increased risk of brachial plexus injury. Palpation of the tendon of the pectoralis major muscle at the shoulder may suggest stretch of the brachial plexus. This should be checked whenever the arm is held away from the body.

Thoracic Outlet Syndrome

The thoracic outlet is the space between the first rib and the clavicle. The subclavian artery and the trunks of the brachial plexus pass between the anterior and middle scalene muscles and through the thoracic outlet. Compression of this space results in the thoracic outlet syndrome, with numbness, paresthesia, paresis, or coldness of the upper extremity. Symptoms may be exacerbated by abduction of the arm or raising the arm superior to the head. Patients with trauma, obesity, and poor posture are at risk for developing the syndrome. Patients with a history of thoracic outlet syndrome or brachial plexus injury should not be positioned with the arm superior to the head.

Automatic, noninvasive blood pressure measurement may be associated with peripheral nerve injury. Careful cuff placement and reduced frequency of measurement may mitigate this risk. Lower extremity peripheral nerve injuries occur most commonly when the patient is in the lithotomy position; these injuries were previously discussed in the Lithotomy Position section.

CONCLUSION

Nerve injuries are a significant cause of morbidity in patients undergoing general anesthesia and surgery. Although many of these injuries are avoidable, injuries may occur even when the patient's position during surgery is carefully selected and checked frequently to minimize risks (Box 3-4).

Box 3-4   General Strategies for Reducing the Risk of Nerve Injury

Select the safest position that facilitates the surgery
Select a position the patient is comfortable assuming
    while awake
Reduce the duration of surgery
Avoid leaning on the patient
Pad pressure points underneath bony prominences
Avoid contact between the patient and any hard surfaces
Check the patient's position frequently during surgery

SUGGESTED READING

Cheney FW, Domino KB, Caplan RA, Posner KL. Nerve injury associated with anesthesia: a closed claims analysis. *Anesthesiology* 1999;90:1062-1069.

Coppieters MW, Van de Velde M, Stappaerts KH. Positioning in anesthesiology: toward a better understanding of stretch-induced perioperative neuropathies. *Anesthesiology* 2002;97: 75-81.

Fibuch EE, Mertz J, Geller B. Postoperative onset of idiopathic brachial neuritis. *Anesthesiology* 1996;84:455-458.

Khalil IM. Bilateral compartmental syndrome after prolonged surgery in the lithotomy position. *J Vasc Surg* 1987;5: 879-881.

Partanen J, Niskanen L, Lehtinen J, *et al*. Natural history of peripheral neuropathy in patients with non-insulin-dependent diabetes mellitus. *N Engl J Med* 1995;333:89-94.

Partridge BL, Katz J, Benirschke K. Functional anatomy of the brachial plexus sheath: implications for anesthesia. *Anesthesiology* 1987;66:743-747.

Prielipp RC, Morell RC, Walker FO, *et al*. Ulnar nerve pressure: influence of arm position and relationship to somatosensory evoked potentials. *Anesthesiology* 1999;91:345-354.

Romanowski L, Reich H, McGlynn F, *et al*. Brachial plexus neuropathies after advanced laparoscopic surgery. *Fertil Steril* 1993;60:729-732.

Schaer HM. Peripheral nerve injury and automatic blood pressure measurement. *Anesthesiology* 1991;75:381.

Stoelting RK. Postoperative ulnar nerve palsy–is it a preventable complication? *Anesth Analg* 1993;76:7-9.

Stoelting RK. Brachial plexus injury after median sternotomy: an unexpected liability for anesthesiologists. *J Cardiothorac Vasc Anesth* 1994;8:2-4.

Warner MA, Warner ME, Martin JT. Ulnar neuropathy. Incidence, outcome, and risk factors in sedated or anesthetized patients. *Anesthesiology* 1994;81:1332-1340.

Warner MA, Warner DO, Harper CM, *et al*. Lower extremity neuropathies associated with lithotomy positions. *Anesthesiology* 2000;93:938-942.

Wilbourn AJ. Thoracic outlet syndromes. *Neurol Clin* 1999;17: 477-497.

CHAPTER 4

Monitoring

RIMA MATEVOSIAN
HAMID NOURMAND

INTRODUCTION

Monitoring is the essence of anesthesiology. From the earliest days of surgical anesthesia, responsible physicians realized the need to keep in contact with their patients and determine how they were doing while anesthetized. Early on, monitoring was visual observation and perhaps a finger on the pulse. Modern anesthesiologists depend on complex electronic monitors with sophisticated visual displays of complex physiologic data. Indeed, the visual image of anesthesiologists today is someone in scrubs casually looking at a display of physiologic data and removed from physical contact with the patient. Although this may seem like an improvement from the simple monitors of the early days, there are possible problems: all the complex electronic data needs to be interpreted in light of a clinical situation, which may be changing rapidly, and monitors can malfunction, giving erroneous data or even no data.

Appropriate monitoring, which can prevent hypoxia and other intraoperative or postoperative disasters, has clearly been shown to improve patient outcome and is most likely responsible for the greatly improved safety of anesthesia. Because of a rash of unfavorable anesthetic outcomes in the 1980s, the Harvard hospital system was the first to initiate standards for monitoring, on the assumption that standard monitoring would prevent such disasters as intraoperative hypoxia and subsequent brain damage. These standards were published in 1985, and the American Society of Anesthesiologists (ASA) further developed these guidelines and published their own intraoperative monitoring standards in 1986. These apply to all anesthetics and can be exceeded if indicated. Since the standards were published, anesthesia mortality has plummeted (Boxes 4-1 and 4-2).

The leaps in technology that made pulse oximetry and end-tidal (ET) CO_2 measurement easily available were essential to improving patient safety through better monitoring. Other safety efforts, such as the formation of the Anesthesia Patient Safety Foundation (APSF) in 1984 and the ASA's Difficult Airway Algorithm published in 1994, were also responsible for the improvement in anesthesia mortality. But the platform for improved intraoperative patient safety is monitoring. The specialty of anesthesiology is currently the model for patient safety efforts nationwide.

It is crucial that the anesthesiologist does a thorough preoperative evaluation. During preoperative assessment of the patient, the anesthesiologist determines what type of monitoring is necessary for the planned operation. This chapter reviews the various monitors anesthesiologists use, with focus on the standard monitors of blood pressure, electrocardiogram (ECG), pulse oximetry, capnography, and temperature. Less frequently used monitors will be briefly reviewed.

BLOOD PRESSURE MONITORING

The ultimate goal of monitoring physiologic functions under anesthesia is to attempt to maintain tissue perfusion for oxygen delivery and clearance of waste substances. Clearly, direct measurement of tissue perfusion is not easily accomplished; therefore, clinicians resort to other means to try to quantify this vital function. The most suitable single measure of the circulatory function is blood pressure.

Tissue perfusion, or flow, is dependent on the balance between the forward pressure generated by the heart and the resistance offered by the vascular bed. Many of the anesthetics commonly used influence the myocardial function and the vascular resistance, thus affecting the tissue perfusion. Blood pressure monitoring is mandated for any patient under some type of anesthesia, be it general, regional, or sedation.

Blood pressure can be measured indirectly with a cuff or directly using a transducer. It should be emphasized that the blood pressure value is only an indicator of the tissue perfusion and that other various monitors (e.g., urine output) should be employed to better gauge end-organ perfusion and function. Measured blood pressure values are affected by many factors. The site where blood

---

Box 4-1   Standards for Intraoperative Monitoring

STANDARD I

An anesthesiologist shall be responsible for determining the medical status of the patient, developing a plan of anesthesia care, and acquainting the patient or the responsible adult with the proposed plan

Qualified anesthesia personnel shall be present in the room throughout the conduct of all general anesthetics and monitored anesthesia care

STANDARD II

During all anesthetics, the patient's oxygenation, ventilation, circulation and temperature shall be continually evaluated.

a) Oxygenation
   i.   Inspired gas during general anesthesia, with an alarm for low concentrations.
   ii. Blood oxygen: Pulse oximetry continuously
b) Ventilation
   i.   Adequacy of ventilation will be continuously evaluated by qualitative clinical signs such as chest excursion, auscultation of breath sounds, and observation of the reservoir breathing bag. Continual monitoring for the presence of expired carbon dioxide (CO_2).
   ii. Correct position of an endotracheal tube or laryngeal mask airway will be verified by the presence of end-tidal CO_2.
   iii. If a ventilator is used, there will be a disconnect alarm.
   iv. During regional or monitored anesthesia care (MAC), the adequacy of ventilation shall be evaluated, by continuous observation of qualitative clinical signs.
c) Circulation
   i.   Continuous electrocardiogram (ECG) displayed
   ii. Arterial blood pressure (BP) and heart rate determined at least every 5 minutes.
   iii. Alternative monitoring of circulation
d) Temperature: When clinically significant changes in body temperature are expected.

Box 4-2   Standards for Postanesthesia Care Units

STANDARD I

All patients who have received any type of anesthesia, general, regional, or MAC shall receive appropriate postanesthesia management.

STANDARD II

A member of the anesthesia care team who is knowledgeable about the patient's condition shall accompany the patient transported to the Postanesthesia Care Unit (PACU). The patient shall be continually evaluated and treated during transport with monitoring.

STANDARD III

Upon arrival at PACU, the patient shall be re-evaluated and a verbal report given to the PACU nurse by a member of the anesthesia care team.

STANDARD IV

The patient's condition shall be evaluated continuously by the PACU.

STANDARD V

A physician is responsible for the discharge of the patient from PACU.
For complete guidelines see the ASA website: www.asahg.org/publicationsandServices/standards/02.html.

---

pressure is measured plays an important role in the accuracy of the results. Generally, upon moving away from the aorta to the smaller peripheral arteries, systolic pressure is exaggerated and the pulse pressure widens. This phenomenon is attributed to the distortion of the pressure waveform as it moves away from the heart. The accuracy of the blood pressure values also depends on the technique (noninvasive or invasive) and the type of equipment (cuff size, catheter size, etc.) used in the measurement. Anesthesiologists should be well aware of these factors and be able to use blood pressure values in conjunction with other physiologic parameters to better improve clinical judgment and decision-making.

Noninvasive Blood Pressure Monitoring

Indirect measurement of the blood pressure is a noninvasive technique using a cuff with an inflatable bladder inside. Since its invention in the late 19th century, many techniques have been proposed for blood pressure measurement using this device. All methods are based on the waves generated, and resultant sounds made, when a cuff occluding the artery is released and blood flow resumes through the artery. The most commonly used noninvasive blood pressure methods are auscultatory and oscillometric techniques.

Palpation of a pulse distal to the occluding cuff is the most basic method of determining the systolic blood pressure. When the pulse is first felt as the cuff deflates it is marked as the systolic pressure. This is a quick and easy check of the more complex methods of measuring blood pressure. Diastolic blood pressure is taken as the point when the pulse goes away as the cuff is inflated.

Auscultatory technique is the most commonly used method of blood pressure measurement outside the operating room. A stethoscope is used to listen for the appearance and subsequent loss of the Korotkoff sounds as the cuff deflates. Onset of the Korotkoff sounds marks the systolic pressure, while loss of the sounds determines the diastolic value. This approach is time-consuming, often requires long stethoscope tubing, takes the clinician's attention away from other monitors, and is difficult to use in low-flow states such as hypotension. Because of these limitations, and with the advent of the automated blood pressure machines, this method is not commonly used in the operating room.

Noninvasive automated blood pressure units are the most commonly used devices for blood pressure measurement in the operating room. Oscillometry is the most common detection technique used in these automated blood pressure devices. Upon deflating the occluding cuff, arterial pulsations result in oscillations in the cuff, which are then processed by a microprocessor, giving the systolic, diastolic, and mean blood pressure values. Automated blood pressure machines offer many advantages, with very few disadvantages. They are easy to operate, may be set to cycle intermittently, measure systolic, diastolic, and mean blood pressures, and the results are reliable and reproducible. Most importantly, they free the clinician to attend to the other physiologic monitors and patient care issues.

An important factor influencing the measurement is the size of the cuff in use. Selecting the appropriate cuff size is crucial for accuracy. The width of the cuff should be 20–50% larger than the diameter of the extremity, and the bladder inside should encircle more than half way around the limb. A cuff that is too small for the patient results in a higher blood pressure reading. In contrast, too large a cuff may result in slightly lower blood pressure values.

Complications due to the use of automated blood pressure devices are few, and these can be easily avoided. The most common problem is too-frequent cycling of the cuff, resulting in tissue edema and even compartment syndrome. Extremities with vascular abnormalities, such as arteriovenous fistulas, arterial or venous insufficiencies, and even intravenous access distal to the cuff, are best avoided. The cuff should not be applied to extremities with soft tissue or bone injuries.

Limitations of the use of this noninvasive technique include low perfusion states or during cardiopulmonary bypass, when the pulsatile arterial flow is absent. A common scenario during hypotension is frequent, rapid attempts to take the blood pressure before the cuff has finished deflating. The machine tends to jam, giving the impression that it has failed. Technically, the machine cannot start another pressure measurement until cuff deflation has finished. In this situation, the hypotension needs to be quickly confirmed by other means and treated promptly.

Invasive Arterial Blood Pressure Monitoring

Direct blood pressure measurement is an invasive technique, accomplished by cannulating a peripheral artery and displaying the pressures on a monitor continuously. The most common arterial sites used are the radial, brachial, femoral, and dorsalis pedis arteries. The radial artery is the preferred site, because of its easy accessibility and the presence of collateral flow.

Indications for the direct measurement of the blood pressure are twofold. This technique offers continuous, beat-to-beat measurement of the blood pressure and is reserved for cases where rapid fluctuations in blood pressure are anticipated or when pre-existing systemic diseases dictate tight blood pressure control. It also provides access for arterial blood sampling.

Once the artery is cannulated, the catheter is connected to a transducer via saline-filled stiff pressure tubing. The pressure transducer consists of a Wheatstone bridge circuit with a diaphragm that fluctuates with the pressure wave. This converts the mechanical energy of the blood pressure to an electrical signal that can be displayed on the monitor (Figure 4-1).

Many factors may influence the accuracy of the arterial pressure readings. The anatomic site of the measurement, as described above, affects the values. The size and length of the catheter are also important. The tubing between the catheter and transducer should be as short as possible, with very few stopcocks, filled with a saline solution, and without any air bubbles. The transducer must be zeroed at the level of the right atrium and remain at the same height throughout the case. The easiest way is to mount the transducer on the operating room table so that its relative height to the patient remains the same upon changing the height of the table. In a supine patient the transducer is placed at the mid-axillary line to be zeroed.

The normal direct blood pressure tracing consists of a steep systolic upstroke, a rather sharp peak, a dicrotic notch on the descending diastolic limb, and a slowly flattening runoff (Figure 4-2). In addition to the systolic and diastolic values, the shape and nature of the waveform

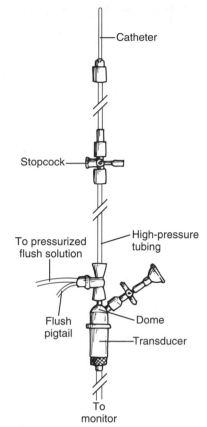

Figure 4-1   The catheter-tubing-transducer system.

could provide other valuable information. The slope of the systolic upstroke portion is an indication of the heart's contractility. A damped waveform has a smaller slope, with a rounded peak (Figure 4-3). Damping may be caused by left ventricular dysfunction or by air bubbles in the transducer tubing. The slope of the diastolic portion may become steeper with lowering of the systemic vascular resistance.

Systolic and diastolic pressures normally show variations with respiration. This variation is accentuated in mechanically ventilated patients who are also hypovolemic. This

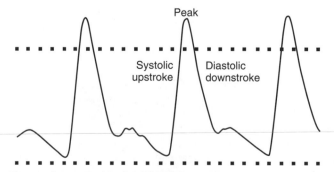

Figure 4-2   Normal arterial pressure tracing. (Redrawn from Morgan GE, Mikhail MS, Murray MJ. *Clinical anesthesiology* 3rd ed. New York: McGraw Hill, 2002.)

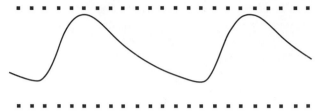

Figure 4-3   Damped arterial pressure tracing.

phenomenon is attributed to the fact that the positive pressure ventilation lowers venous return to the thorax and heart, whereas in spontaneously ventilating patients the negative intrathoracic pressure actually hastens venous return to the heart.

Direct blood pressure monitoring is an invasive technique and carries many of the potential risks and complications inherent to invasive procedures (Box 4-3). Bleeding, hematoma, infection, nerve injuries, arterial thrombosis, loss of digits, and air emboli with flushing of the system, both distal and central, are known to occur. The overall risks of invasive arterial pressure monitoring are quite low, especially in monitoring of short duration.

ELECTROCARDIOGRAM

Scientists knew of the heart's electrical activity as early as 1855; this was recorded in the laboratory on smoked drum kymographs or photographic plates. The importance of ECG monitoring intraoperatively became clear after 1936 with the introduction of cyclopropane, which often caused arrhythmias. Because the usual anesthetic agents of the time (ether and cyclopropane) were explosive, ECG machines had to be made explosion-proof before continuous ECG monitoring could be achieved in operating rooms. The first explosion-proof ECG monitor was the Cardioscope, introduced in 1954.

Monitoring of ECG is indicated during all anesthetic cases. Modern ECG monitors for the operating room are capable of displaying multiple leads, analyzing for ischemia, and detecting arrhythmias. Other information gained from intraoperative ECG monitoring includes detecting possible electrolyte abnormalities and evaluating pacemaker function.

An ECG tracing is the recording and display of the surface potential changes from the heart muscle, which, in turn, is the sum of the electrical activity of the individual myocardial cells (Box 4-4). The sinoatrial (SA) node sets the heart rate, since under normal conditions it depolarizes more rapidly than any cardiac tissue. The SA node is located on the superior right border of the heart, and the depolarization vector from the atrium follows a path downward and to the left. The ECG tracing generates an upward deflection when the depolarization vector is in the same direction as the ECG lead. By contrast, if the depolarization spreads against the direction of the ECG lead, it results in a downward deflection.

Lead Placement Techniques

Correct placement of ECG electrodes is essential for an accurate signal. Perioperative ECG monitoring may be accomplished using either a basic three-electrode or a more advanced five-electrode format. One of three bipolar limb leads (I, II, III) may be monitored continuously using the standard three electrodes (positive, negative, and ground). This format is most widely available and is simple to use. The standard electrode placement format is right arm (RA), left arm (LA), and left leg (LL). Lead II is the preferred lead to monitor since its axis is parallel to the atria, resulting in the largest P wave voltage of all the surface leads. Monitoring lead II is most useful for detection of cardiac dysrhythmias and inferior wall myocardial ischemia but offers little in way of detecting anterior wall or lateral wall ischemias; the V5 lead is best suited for this purpose.

Several modifications of the three-lead electrode placement system have been suggested to improve sensitivity for detection of anterior wall or anterolateral wall ischemias. One widely accepted variation is called "central subclavicular (CS5) lead" and is obtained when the RA electrode is placed under the right clavicle and the LA electrode is placed on the V5 position. Subsequently, modified lead I, called CS5, is monitored for ischemia and lead II is used to detect dysrhythmias.

Box 4-3   Contraindications to Invasive Blood Pressure Monitoring

Pre-existing vascular abnormalities in the extremity
Documented absence of collateral flow
Infection at the catheterization site
Coagulopathy

Box 4-4   Information Obtained from the Electrocardiogram

Heart rate
Heart rhythm
Cardiac dysrhythmia
Conduction disturbances
Myocardial ischemia
Electrolyte disturbances
Pacemaker function and/or malfunction

The newer ECG monitors offer the five-electrode format and two-lead display capabilities. The two additional electrodes are placed on the right leg (RL) and on the V5 position (in the fifth intercostal space along the anterior axillary line). Continuously monitoring leads II and V offers greater sensitivity for the detection of arrhythmias and myocardial ischemia. It should be noted that the leg electrodes (RL and LL) might be placed on the torso without compromising the ECG monitoring yield.

Detection of Myocardial Ischemia and ST Segment Analysis

Detection of myocardial ischemia is best accomplished by continuously monitoring the ST segment and comparing it to the baseline. Modern ECG monitors are capable of performing ST segment analysis electronically. The ST segment is measured from 60–80 msec after the J point (Box 4-5).

ST segment analysis for the detection of ischemia may have limited value in patients with Wolf–Parkinson–White syndrome, bundle branch block, and continuous pacemaker capture. Artifacts due to the use of electrocautery and other electrical devices and patient movement can make the ECG unreadable.

Invasive ECG monitoring:

- *Intracardiac ECG*: Monitoring intracardiac ECG is achieved by using a multipurpose pulmonary artery catheter. In addition to being superior in detecting atrial, ventricular, or atrioventricular nodal dysrhythmias and conduction blocks, this technique is also more resistant to electrocautery interference. These specialized pulmonary artery catheters may also be used to establish intracardiac atrial or atrioventricular pacing.
- *Esophageal ECG*: The ECG electrodes are incorporated into an esophageal stethoscope in order to monitor esophageal ECG. This technique offers a greater sensitivity for the detection of atrial dysrhythmias and posterior wall ischemia.
- *Endotracheal ECG*: A specialized endotracheal tube that has two electrodes implanted in it is used to monitor endotracheal ECG. This method of monitoring is most useful in pediatric patients and for the diagnosis of atrial dysrhythmias.
- *Intracoronary ECG*: During coronary angioplasty, monitoring of intracoronary ECG offers greater sensitivity for detecting acute ischemia compared to surface ECG monitoring using ST segment analysis.

PULSE OXIMETRY

Assessment of adequate oxygenation is one of the most important functions of an anesthesiologist. In the past, the color of the skin was used to evaluate the level of oxygenation and cyanosis marked the hypoxemic episodes, but it was not a reliable method. Clinical signs of hypoxemia such as altered mental status, cardiovascular instability, and cyanosis may be masked by anesthesia.

The most accurate monitor of oxygenation is direct measurement of arterial partial pressure of oxygen, but this technique is invasive and only offers intermittent readings. Pulse oximetry has revolutionized the field of anesthesiology by providing a tool for early detection and prompt intervention to prevent the catastrophic consequences of unrecognized hypoxemia. It is the most sensitive noninvasive tool for continuous monitoring of oxygenation and early detection of desaturation and impending hypoxemia. In addition to oxygen saturation, pulse oximetry provides data regarding the heart rate, heart rhythm and tissue perfusion.

Pulse oximetry uses the principle of photospectrometry. In 1939–1942, physiologist Glen Millikan developed the first practical oximeter and coined the term "oximeter." This was used to evaluate aids that might help pilots bailing out of high-altitude planes during World War II. Hypoxia at high elevation left the pilots unconscious when they fell into the sea. New flotation devices, which could maintain the airway in this situation, were evaluated using anesthetized volunteers and the Millikan oximeter.

In 1948, an oximeter was first used in the operating room to monitor hypoxemia. In 1966, the Waters Company introduced the X-350 Oximeter, based on Earl H. Wood's work in the 1950s at the Mayo Clinic. In 1971, Japanese engineer Takuo Aoyagi developed the first clinically useful pulse oximeter. This measured pulsatile light absorbance and did not need to heat the tissue. The new light-emitting diode (LED) was used as the light source. Pulsations of transmitted red and infrared light measured oxygen saturation levels.

In the 1970s, Hewlett-Packard marketed the first self-calibrating ear oximeter. It used eight wavelengths to measure oxygen saturation of the blood in the ear and used heat to "arteriolize" blood in the ear. The equipment was big, cumbersome, and quite expensive. In 1983,

---

Box 4-5   Established Criteria for Detection of Myocardial Ischemia Using ECG

Upsloping ST segment depression of 0.2 mV (2 mm)
Flat or downsloping ST segment depression of 0.1 mV (1 mm)
ST segment elevation
T-wave inversion

William New, an anesthesiologist at Stanford, co-founded the Nellcor company, the first manufacturer of pulse oximeters. It was this Nellcor pulse oximeter that first associated the pitch of the pulse-tone with the level of oxygen saturation. In 1990, as its clinical usefulness became clear, pulse oximetry became an ASA standard for intraoperative monitoring. In 1992, this ASA standard was also applied to postanesthesia care unit (PACU) patients. Since then, pulse oximetry has become an essential tool in patient care and has saved many lives.

It is important to understand how pulse oximeters work, so accurate data can be obtained. Pulse oximetry uses the concepts of spectrophotometry and plethysmography. The spectrophotometric technique of measurement involves shining light through a sample and measuring the amount of light absorbed. The pulse oximeter probe contains an LED that generates two different wavelengths of light: red light at 660 nm and infrared light at 940 nm. These two wavelengths are absorbed differently by oxyhemoglobin and deoxyhemoglobin. Oxyhemoglobin absorbs more infrared light at 940 nm, while deoxyhemoglobin absorbs more red light at 660 nm. The difference in absorption is picked up by the probe's photodetector. The difference between light emitted and light detected is converted to the percentage oxygen saturation.

Lambert-Beer's law explains the absorption of light as it passes through a sample compound. This law defines the linear relationship between the absorbance and the concentration of the absorber of light. When light is shone through a solution containing an absorber (in this case hemoglobin), a portion of light is absorbed and provides an indirect measurement of the absorber concentration. The light absorbed by blood depends on the concentration of oxyhemoglobin and deoxyhemoglobin present and the wavelength of the light. This change in light absorption during arterial pulsations is the fundamental basis of oximetry. The ratio of absorbance at red and infrared wavelengths is analyzed by the microprocessor, which, based on an algorithm, calculates the oxygen saturation of the arterial pulsations (S_pO_2).

Other substances besides oxygenated hemoglobin absorb light from the LED, such as deoxygenated hemoglobin, bone, tissues, and other blood solutes. To account for this, plethysmography is utilized to identify the arterial pulsations, allowing corrections for nonpulsatile venous blood. Arteries expand during systole and relax during diastole, but tissue and veins stay relatively unchanged. Therefore, these pulsatile changes in the arterioles were used to create two different measurements. The two phases characterized as nonpulsatile include absorption during diastole from tissues, venous blood, capillary blood, and nonpulsatile arterial blood. In the pulsatile phase, absorbance occurs during systole, which includes absorption by pulsatile arterial blood. By obtaining absorbances of each

wavelength during the two phases, saturation can be calculated from a specific algorithm. These algorithms are proprietary and vary by manufacturer, so each type of pulse oximeter technology is slightly different in its characteristics and accuracy (Box 4-6).

Technically, all pulse oximeters have inherent limitations because of the method used to measure S_pO_2. Algorithms used to calculate the S_pO_2 values are derived experimentally by correlating the measured S_pO_2 with the arterial oxygen saturation (S_aO_2) values. In general, there is a 98% correlation ($\pm2\%$ error) when S_aO_2 is greater than 70%. Oxygen saturations of less than 70% are not as accurate because of the lack of experimental values (it would be unethical to allow the experimental subjects to desaturate below 70%). Because of variations in readings by different oximeters, hospitals should standardize to one model of pulse oximeters.

Pulse oximetry depends on pulsatile blood flow to an extremity. Hypotension, hypovolemia, vasoconstriction, congestive heart failure, hypothermia, and nonpulsatile flow states (such as cardiopulmonary bypass or cardiac arrest) may fail to produce enough arterial pulsation to produce an adequate signal. These devices may then seem to "fail" at a time when they are most needed. Numerous instances of presumed pulse oximeter failure due to low-flow states have occurred. A common response is for the anesthesiologist to call for a replacement pulse oximeter, because the one in the room "isn't working." By the time the replacement monitor comes, valuable time has been lost to possibly rescue a deteriorating situation. When a pulse oximeter seems to "fail," clinical signs (e.g., skin color, a central pulse if the abdomen is open, or heart sounds) should be quickly checked before presuming that the pulse oximeter has failed and needs replacing. The problem must be presumed to be the patient, and not the machine, until proven otherwise.

Box 4-6   Advantages of Pulse Oximetry

Early detection of hypoxemia allows prompt intervention to prevent serious injury
Noninvasive and continuous monitoring
Provides data on heart rate, heart rhythm and tissue perfusion
Reduces need for blood gas analysis
Provides reliable and reproducible results
Low cost comparable to the invaluable information that it gives
Portable and fast start time
Simple to use
Assesses viability of limbs
Helpful in limiting O_2 toxicity in neonates by allowing quick O_2 titration

There is a lag factor in measuring S_pO_2 that should be taken into consideration. This delay averages 5–20 seconds and varies by probe location. The farther away from the central circulation the probe is, the longer the delay. Delay averages 10 seconds for probes on the earlobe, 30 seconds for finger probes, and more than 30 seconds for probes on the toe.

Motion artifacts have been a major source of error. As the patient moves while awakening, for example, movement may be picked up by the probe as a "flow" signal. This confuses the detector and often results in an alarm. This is an area of current intense work by manufacturers. Finally, overhead lights can affect the amount of light measured by the sensor; opaque covering of the probe can reduce inaccuracies due to ambient light.

Abnormal hemoglobins, such as carboxyhemoglobin (COHb), methemoglobin (MeHb), and sulfhemoglobin (SuHb), can give false pulse oximeter readings. Carboxyhemoglobin and oxyhemoglobin (HbO_2) absorb light at 660 nm identically. Pulse oximeters that only compare two wavelengths of light will register a falsely high reading in patients suffering from carbon monoxide poisoning. Methemoglobin has the same absorption coefficient at both red and infrared wavelengths. The absorption ratio is 1:1 and corresponds to a saturation reading of 85%. Methemoglobinemia then causes a falsely low saturation reading when the S_aO_2 is actually greater than 85%, and *vice versa*, a falsely high reading when saturation is less than 85%. Sulfhemoglobinemia secondary to drug or chemical exposure can give false readings. Other issues to consider are as follows.

- High concentrations of hemoglobin do not affect the S_pO_2. In anemia (2.3–8.7 g/dL), the S_pO_2 accurately correlates with S_aO_2.
- Skin pigmentation, for example melanin, can result in slightly low S_pO_2 readings while high bilirubin levels have little or no effect on S_pO_2.
- Fingernail polish (especially blue or black) can decrease S_pO_2 by 3–5%.
- Dyes commonly used in the operating room (e.g. methylene blue, indocyanine green, and isosulfan blue) can falsely lower the S_pO_2 readings, as a result of increased absorbance of light.

CAPNOGRAPHY

Another monitor that has revolutionized anesthesia care and has resulted in increased anesthesia safety is capnography. It can detect unrecognized esophageal intubations and prevent subsequent hypoxia, identify inadequate or abnormal ventilation such as bronchospasm or respiratory obstruction, and also detect circuit disconnects. "Capno" is derived from the Greek *kapno*s, which means "smoke." Capnometry is measuring

ET-CO_2; capnography is visual display of the exhaled CO_2 tracing on a monitor. Capnography is now the gold standard for verification of endotracheal tube placement. The presence of ET-CO_2 for six consecutive breaths, or after 1 minute of ventilation, indicates that the endotracheal tube is in the trachea and not in the esophagus. In some rare situations, such as difficult mask ventilation before intubation, the tube may be in the esophagus and CO_2 may be present, but the waveform is abnormal. The waveform should always be checked for accuracy after intubation; it should show a square wave pattern with a plateau. Capnography cannot be used to detect endobronchial intubations. Bilateral auscultation of the chest still has to be done to assure correct placement of the endotracheal tube. Methods to measure CO_2 include mass spectrometry, Raman scattering, electrochemical, and infrared analysis. The CO_2 level may be reported as either partial pressure or volume percent. It may be displayed continuously or as a peak end-tidal value.

Most capnometers use the principles of Lambert–Beer's law and spectrophotometry as they apply to gases. A special frequency of infrared light is readily absorbed by carbon dioxide. This infrared light is passed through a sample gas and also through a known reference gas. The difference in the amount of light that passes through a sample gas and that of the reference gas is measured. Calculation of ET-CO_2 becomes possible by utilizing the rate of gas aspiration from the breathing circuit, the diameter of the sample tubing, the length of the sampling tubing, and the amount of the unknown gas.

The two common types of capnographs acquire their samples differently, either by "flow-through" or by aspiration of a sample from the anesthetic gases.

Flow-through

Flow-through, or mainstream, capnographs measure CO_2 passing through an adapter placed in the breathing circuit. Infrared light transmission through the sample gas is measured, and the concentration of CO_2 is calculated by the monitor (Boxes 4-7 and 4-8).

Box 4-7   Advantages of Mainstream Capnography

Fast response because there is no delay getting the sample

No scavenging is necessary because no gas is removed from the breathing system

Water and secretions are not a problem

Uses fewer disposable items than aspiration capnographs

A standard gas is not required for calibration

Box 4-8   Limitations/Disadvantages of Mainstream Capnography

The adapter between the patient and the breathing system increases the circuit dead space slightly – this could be significant in pediatric patients

They are difficult to use with spontaneously breathing patients

The sensors are bulky and can cause traction on an endotracheal tube, possibly resulting in dislodging of the endotracheal tube

The circuit adapter must be cleaned and disinfected between the cases

---

Aspiration

A continuous side-stream suction pump aspirates gas from the breathing circuit into a sample cell within the monitor. The amount of CO_2 is determined by infrared absorption through the sample cell in a CO_2-free chamber. Sample aspiration rates of 250 mL/min and low dead-space sample tubing increase the sensitivity and decrease the lag time for measurement (Boxes 4-9 and 4-10).

One of the tremendous advantages of capnography is the ability to view continuous waveforms of CO_2. These give extremely important information about the patient's respiratory status, circulation and ventilation as well as the anesthesia circuit. The waves have been analyzed and divided into four parts (Figure 4-4):

- *First phase (A–B)* shows the initial stage of expiration. This is gas sampled during the phase that occupies the anatomic dead space. Therefore it does not contain CO_2.
- *Second phase (B–C)* shows the beginning of expiration, when CO_2-containing gas is presented to the sample site, followed by a sharp upstroke. The slope of this upstroke is a function of uniformity of ventilation and alveolar emptying. This phase is a mixture of dead space and alveolar gas.
- *Third phase (C-D)* is the alveolar or expiratory gas plateau. Normally, this part of the waveform is horizontal with slight upstroke at D, which is the ET-CO_2.

Box 4-9   Advantages of Sidestream Capnography

Easy sampling from spontaneously breathing patients

Fast warm-up

Calibration and zeroing is usually automatic

Light weight

Minimal dead space

Less potential for cross contamination between patients

Box 4-10   Limitations/Disadvantages of Sidestream Capnography

Aspiration units are prone to water precipitation in the sample cell, as well as in the sample tubing – this can result in inaccurate readings and damage analyzers

Disposable items are needed

Low aspiration rates, less than 50 mL/min, can slow the end-tidal CO_2 measurement and underestimate it during rapid ventilation

Contamination of the operating room with anesthetic gases can result from a leak during the continuous sample aspiration

In pediatric patients, the small tidal volumes combined with a high rate of aspiration may lead to fresh gas being entrained from the circuit and diluting the sample, falsely lowering the CO_2 reading

---

The highest concentration of CO_2 is reached at the end of expiration, which is why it is called ET-CO_2. Point D is the best reflection of alveolar CO_2. In patients with severe chronic obstructive pulmonary disease (COPD), the plateau may not be reached before the next inspiration. In this situation, the gradient between ET-CO_2 and arterial CO_2 is increased. Depression during this phase shows recovery of spontaneous breathing.

- *Fourth phase (D-E)* demonstrates the beginning of inspiration. Fresh gas is entrained and there is a sharp down stroke to baseline. The baseline should reach zero unless rebreathing of CO_2 is taking place, either from incompetent valves or exhausted CO_2 absorbent.

The relationship between ET-CO_2, arterial CO_2 (P_aCO_2), and alveolar CO_2 (P_ACO_2) is dependent on several factors.

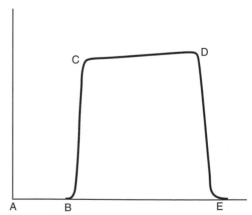

Figure 4-4   Normal CO_2 waveform. The capnogram is divided into four phases: AB is the exhalation of CO_2-free gas at the beginning of expiration contained in dead space. BC is the expiratory upstroke. CD shows the expiratory, or alveolar plateau. Because of the uneven emptying of alveoli, the slope has a slight upstroke. Point D is the best end-expiration. DE is the inspiratory downstroke.

Table 4-1	Factors that Alter ET-CO$_2$ During Anesthesia

Increased ET-CO$_2$	Decreased ET-CO$_2$
Altered CO$_2$ Production	
Conditions with increased metabolic rate	Conditions with decreased metabolic rate
Hyperthermia	Hypothermia
Malignant hyperthermia	Hypothyroidism
Hyperthyroidism	
Sepsis	
Shivering	
Altered CO$_2$ Elimination	
Hypoventilation	Hypoperfusion
Re-breathing	Hyperventilation
	Embolic phenomenon

In an ideal situation, with no ventilation/perfusion mismatch and no sampling errors during measurement:

$$ET\text{-}CO_2 = \text{arterial } CO_2 \ (P_aCO_2) = \text{alveolar } CO_2 \ (P_ACO_2).$$

(This is because CO$_2$ is a highly soluble gas.) There is normally a 5–10 mmHg gradient between ET-CO$_2$ and P_aCO_2. The maldistribution of ventilation and perfusion that occurs in many diseases and the induction of general anesthesia can increase this gradient. Conditions with increased dead space ventilation, $\dot{V}_D$ (wasted ventilation with no perfusion) decrease ET-CO$_2$. Common clinical scenarios with increased dead space resulting in increased gradient between P_aCO_2 and ET-CO$_2$ include embolic conditions, for example air, fat, thrombus and amniotic fluid. Hypoperfusion states with decreased pulmonary blood flow and chronic obstructive pulmonary disease can also result in increased $\dot{V}_D$ and lower than expected ET-CO$_2$ (Table 4-1).

INSPIRED OXYGEN ANALYZER

Inspired oxygen monitoring is used to measure the oxygen concentration that is delivered to the patient from the anesthesia circuit (F_iO_2). It is the most important machine monitor and is used to avoid delivery of hypoxic mixtures. Historically, hypoxic gas mixture delivery to the patient posed a significant problem in anesthesia. Usually, hypoxic gas incidents were due to gas mix-ups in the days when tanks were used as gas sources, or due to errors made during machine maintenance, when nitrous oxide (N$_2$O) and oxygen (O$_2$) lines might be crossed. The integrity of the circuit can also be measured with these monitors. Advances in electrode technology made this monitor possible.

All modern anesthesia machines now come with self-contained inspired oxygen analyzers. The analyzer's electrode is placed in the circuit between the patient and the anesthesia machine. Inspired O$_2$ analyzers are of two types, paramagnetic and electrochemical.

Paramagnetic Oxygen Analyzers

Oxygen is a highly paramagnetic gas and is attracted into a magnetic field. This paramagnetic property of oxygen is the result of its molecular structure, which has unpaired electrons in the outer shell. In contrast, nitrogen (N$_2$) is repelled from a magnetic field. A gas-tight chamber containing two glass spheres is connected in an arrangement and placed in a nonuniform magnetic field. Oxygen and nitrogen are added to the chamber. A magnet is switched on and off rapidly. Signal changes during electromagnetic switching correlate with the oxygen concentration within the sample line. This difference is detected by a pressure transducer and is converted into an electrical signal displayed as partial pressure, or is converted to volume percent on the monitor. The main disadvantage of the paramagnetic oxygen analyzers is that the gas from the analyzer is returned to the breathing circuit. The air that is used as a reference will dilute the other gases and cause an increase in nitrogen (N$_2$).

Electrochemical Oxygen Analyzers

This analyzer has a sensor that measures F_iO_2 in the inspiratory limb of the anesthesia breathing circuit. The sensor contains an anode and a cathode surrounded by an electrolyte gel. A gas-permeable membrane holds the gel. Oxygen molecules in the delivered anesthetic gases diffuse through this membrane located at the tip of the electrode into the electrolyte solution. Oxygen molecules are then reduced within the electrolyte solution, resulting in current flow between the electrodes. The magnitude of current flow is proportional to oxygen concentration within the electrolyte solution, which, in turn, is proportional to the partial pressure of oxygen in the delivered gas. The monitor then converts this current into a percentage of oxygen in the inspiratory limb. The rate of oxygen entry into the cell and the current generated is proportional to partial pressure outside the membrane. These analyzers can be subdivided by type of electrode into polarographic or galvanic.

Polarographic (Clark) Electrode

Developed by Leland Clark, this was the first oxygen analyzer used clinically in 1954. The electrode of the analyzer is placed in the anesthesia circuit between the patient and the ventilator in the inspiratory limb. Oxygen molecules diffuse through a Teflon or polyethylene membrane at the tip of the electrode, and then enter an electrolyte (KCl) solution in the form of a gel. Here, oxygen molecules are reduced to hydroxide ions and a current flow is produced, which is proportional to the oxygen concentration in the sample. After temperature compensation, the current is measured and converted to millimeters of mercury or percentage of oxygen in the gas sample and displayed on the monitor.

Galvanic (Fuel Cell) Electrodes

These were introduced in 1975. Oxygen molecules diffuse through an oxygen-permeable membrane located at the tip of the electrode and enter a KOH electrolyte solution. The hydroxide ion made at the gold cathode reacts with the lead anode to make lead oxide, which is gradually consumed. An electron flow between the anode and the cathode is generated that is proportional to the partial pressure of oxygen in the sample. This is an electrolytic reaction; no battery is needed. This type of electrode needs less maintenance than paramagnetic ones and has a guaranteed life span. The life of these electrodes may be prolonged by removing them from the circuit and leaving them exposed to room air when not in use.

ANESTHETIC GAS ANALYZERS

Only recently have we been able to analyze anesthetic gases continuously. The common techniques for analyzing multiple anesthetic gases include mass spectrometry, Raman spectrometry and infrared analysis.

Mass Spectrometry

Mass spectrometry provides the ability to analyze multiple gases within a mixture continuously. It offers measurement of O_2, CO_2, N_2, N_2O, and the inhalation agents of halothane, enflurane, isoflurane, and sevoflurane.

From a side port in an anesthesia breathing circuit, a vacuum pump within the mass spectrometer draws a continuous gas sample. The sample is passed through a magnetic field, where an electron beam ionizes the gas sample. The ions are sorted according to their mass-to-charge ratios. The mass spectrometer provides output signals that are proportional to the concentration of each gas within the gas mixture. Two types of mass spectrometry systems are available:

- A shared system where the mass spectrometer is located outside of the anesthetizing sites, but within the operating room suite. There are multiple sites from which gases are sampled and to which data is returned, resulting in delays.
- Dedicated mass spectrometers are used in only one location. A cable connects the analyzer and the display unit. Short tubing carries the gas sample from the sampling site to the analyzer. It uses a lower sampling flow rate than a shared spectrometer (Boxes 4-11 and 4-12).

Box 4-11   Advantages of Mass Spectrometry

Ability to detect multiple agents and mixtures of volatile anesthetics
Reliable

Box 4-12   Limitations/Disadvantages of Mass Spectrometry

Costly installation
Measures only preprogrammed gases
Scavenging needed
Long warm-up time

Infrared Analysis

Infrared analyzers are based on the fact that gases like N_2O, CO_2, and halogenated anesthetic agents have two or more dissimilar atoms in the molecule. These agents have specific and unique absorption of infrared light. The amount of light absorbed is proportional to the concentration of the absorbing molecules; thus concentration can be calculated by comparing the absorbance with that of a known standard.

Diverting (Side-stream)

The sample gas is transported from the airway to a remote analyzer. These analyzers use one wavelength to measure inhalation agents and therefore are unable to distinguish between agents and mixture of agents. Usual sampling rates are 150 mL/min.

Nondiverting (Main-stream)

Mainstream analyzers monitor the respiratory gas stream through a chamber with two windows. A cuvette is placed between the patient and the breathing system. Gas is aspirated through the cuvette and is analyzed by the sensor.

Photoacoustic

This method is based on the fact that absorption of infrared light by molecules causes the gases to expand and causes the pressure of the gas to increase. It has better long-term durability than other infrared analyzers because it measures the gases directly rather than indirectly (Boxes 4-13 and 4-14).

Raman Spectrometry

Raman spectrometry takes the sample gas mixture and illuminates it with an intense laser beam. Gas sample molecules are scattered by the intense laser beam, causing a

Box 4-13 Advantages of the Infrared Analyzers

Multi gas capability, it measures N_2O, CO_2, and all the volatile agents

No need to scavenge gases since they can be returned to the breathing system

Response time is fast enough to measure both inspired and expired concentrations – response time for anesthetic agents and N_2O is longer than for CO_2

Short warm-up time

Needs only periodic calibration with standard gas mixture

Box 4-14 Limitations/Disadvantages of the Infrared Analyzers

Oxygen and nitrogen concentrations cannot be measured

Water vapor absorbs infrared light and can cause increased CO_2 and volatile agent readings

Slow response time if rapid respiratory rates are present

Addition of air to the breathing system from the returned agent monitor can increase nitrogen levels because of air added to the sample gas after it has passed through the analyzing chamber

Interference from radio frequencies – hand-held radios, pagers and cell phones may increase CO_2 readings.

shift in the light's frequency (wavelength). The amount of frequency shift is dependent on the type of molecules present in the gas sample. The intensity of the scattered light at that frequency depends on the concentration of the gas in the sample mixture.

CARDIAC PRESSURES

Cardiac pressures are monitored to estimate cardiac filling volume, which in turn determines the stroke volume of the right and left ventricles. According to the Frank–Starling principal, the contraction force of cardiac muscle is directly proportional to end-diastolic muscle fiber length at any given contractility. The muscle fiber length, or preload, is proportional to end-diastolic volume. This section will examine central venous pressure (CVP) for evaluation of right heart function and pulmonary artery catheterization for evaluation of the left heart.

Central Venous Pressure Monitoring

Indirect assessment of CVP by visual inspection of neck veins is a basic tool of cardiovascular assessment by physical exam. This is not a useful technique in the operating room. Since its introduction into clinical practice, percutaneous venipuncture of a central vein and pressure measurement is the most reliable method for right heart monitoring in anesthetized patients.

Central venous pressure is the hydrostatic pressure generated by the blood within the right atrium and/or the great veins of the thorax near the right atrium. This pressure is a function of the volume of blood returning to the heart from the systemic circulation and also of the ability of the right ventricle to pump blood through the pulmonary circulation. CVP, by consensus, is the pressure at the junction of the vena cava and the right atrium. Multiple factors such as vascular tone of the venous capacitance vessels as well as intravascular blood volume can influence this function and change the CVP.

Cannulation of a large neck vein, usually the right internal jugular, is the standard clinical method for monitoring CVP. The catheter is inserted into the venous circulation and advanced until the tip of the catheter is within the superior vena cava parallel to the vessel wall and just above the right atrium. In the past, CVP was measured using a fluid-filled manometer attached to the CVP catheter. Today, pressure transducers are used to measure CVP. They are accurate and have rapid response. The transducer converts the pressure generated at the distal orifice of the catheter into an electrical signal, which is then displayed in torrs or millimeters of mercury. Reliable, disposable transducers have made CVP monitoring much more convenient, and continuous monitoring of the CVP waveform display is possible. CVP reflects right ventricular preload, which is an indirect measurement of right ventricular end-diastolic volume. In the absence of cardiac or pulmonary disease, CVP can, but does not always, correlate with left ventricular preload. Normal CVP varies between 1 and 10 mmHg.

Central Pressure Waveform

Display of the CVP waveform provides additional information. The normal CVP waveform consists of three upstrokes (a, c, v) and two descents (x, y) that correspond to events in the cardiac cycle (Figure 4-5). By observing the waveform, anesthesiologists may be able to diagnose pathophysiologic events affecting the right heart function. For example, in atrial fibrillation no a wave is present and, in tricuspid regurgitation there is a giant "V" wave that replaces the normal c, x, and v waves.

- The *a wave* represents atrial contraction, the "atrial kick", which coincides with the end-diastole phase of the cardiac cycle.
- The *c wave* represents decline in atrial pressure and bulging of tricuspid valve into the atrium, which

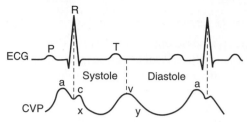

Figure 4-5   The normal central venous pressure (CVP) waveform consists of three upstrokes (a, c, v) and two descents (x, y), which correspond to events in the cardiac cycle. (Redrawn from Mark JB. *Atlas of cardiovascular monitoring*. New York: Churchill Livingstone, 1998.)

coincides with early systole (early phase of right ventricular contraction).

- The *v wave* represents the increase in atrial pressure that occurs when the atrium fills against a closed tricuspid valve. This coincides with late systole.
- The *x descent* follows the c wave and it represents downward movement of the ventricle and tricuspid valve during the later stages of ventricular contraction. This coincides with midsystole.
- The *y descent* represents a decline in ventricular pressure as the ventricle relaxes, the tricuspid valve opens and blood enters the ventricle from the right atrium. This coincides with early diastole.

Technique

There are several approaches to central vein cannulation (Box 4-15). Central veins can be cannulated via the internal jugular vein, subclavian vein, external jugular vein, femoral vein, and axillary vein. A peripheral approach through an antecubital vein was used in the past. This has been abandoned because of the difficulty

---

Box 4-15   Indications for Central Venous Pressure Monitoring

As a guide for fluid management, in operations with large blood loss or fluid shifts
When a pulmonary artery catheter will be needed
When transvenous cardiac pacing is needed
Temporary hemodialysis
Drug administration
- Chemotherapy
- Agents irritating to peripheral veins
- Prolonged antibiotic administration
- Hyperalimentation
- Vasoactive agent
Rapid infusion of fluids or blood
Aspiration of air emboli during neurosurgical procedures
Inadequate peripheral intravenous access
Sampling site needed for repeated blood testing

---

of making the turn into the central circulation at the shoulder.

The patient is placed in the Trendelenburg position to decrease the risk of air embolism and to distend the veins. Central venous catheterization requires full aseptic technique, including sterile gloves, mask, gown (not standard but recommended), and drapes. The skin should be prepared with iodophor solution or another antiseptic. In awake patients, local anesthesia should be used to infiltrate the area in order to minimize patient discomfort.

The two most common techniques for CVP catheterization are:

- *Passing a catheter through a needle*: A 14 gauge needle is introduced into a vessel, then the catheter is threaded through the needle and into the vein. The needle is then removed.
- *Passing the catheter over a guide wire*: This is the most common method and is referred to as the Seldinger technique since Seldinger first described it in 1953. An 18 or 20 gauge needle is introduced into a central vein; a J-shaped tip or a soft flexible straight-ended guide wire is then threaded through the needle and into the vein. The needle is removed, leaving the guide wire in the vessel. Arrhythmias are relatively common at this point, so the ECG should be observed for arrhythmias. Typical treatment is pulling the wire back. If normal rhythm doesn't resume promptly, intravenous lidocaine (1 mg/kg) should be given. The puncture site is enlarged, using a No. 11 scalpel blade, to the desired size, depending on the type of intended catheter. A firm, tapered-tip catheter is used as a dilator to make room for smooth placement of a larger catheter. The dilator is then removed, leaving the wire still in place, and the catheter is advanced over the wire to an appropriate depth, usually 15–18 cm. The guide wire is withdrawn, and the catheter is sutured in place. Finally, the air in the catheter lumen(s) is aspirated, it is flushed with a saline solution, and the catheter is then attached by a Luer lock connector to the monitoring or infusion tubing. A sterile gauze or transparent dressing is applied.

Several different styles of catheter are available for central venous catheterization. Catheters are chosen based on the size of the patient, the site, and the purpose of the catheterization. Catheters come in a variety of lengths, gauge, composition, and lumens. Single-lumen catheters are available with single-port and multiple-port tips. Multilumen catheters are especially popular. These allow simultaneous continuous pressure monitoring and drug and fluid infusion, but they are associated with a higher rate of infection. Large-bore catheter introducer sheaths (8.5 Fr) with a side port extension are popular for CVP monitoring as well as for access availability for pulmonary artery catheter placement.

A follow-up chest radiograph is required for verification of correct placement of the catheter, as well as for diagnosis of possible complications. Before monitoring or infusion begins, aspiration of blood (to confirm correct intravenous placement) as well as aspiration of any air from the tubing system should take place. Ultrasound-guided insertion techniques are becoming more popular and offer many advantages, including increased success rate, reduced procedure time and decreased complication rates.

Sites for Central Venous Cannulation
Right Internal Jugular Vein

Anesthesiologists prefer the right internal jugular vein approach to central venous cannulation. There are reliable anatomic landmarks, the vein has a short, straight course to the superior vena cava and the location is easily accessible for anesthesiologists. There are several approaches to internal jugular vein cannulation:

- *Low anterior*: The needle is introduced at an angle of 30° where the sternal and clavicular heads of the sternocleidomastoid muscle join. It is then advanced toward the ipsilateral nipple until the internal jugular vein is entered and blood is aspirated.
- *High anterior*: The carotid artery pulse is palpated at the level of cricothyroid membrane. The needle is introduced lateral to the carotid pulsation at an angle of 30° and is advanced toward the ipsilateral nipple until the internal jugular vein is entered.
- *Posterior*: The needle is introduced posterior to the junction of the external jugular vein and the posterior border of the sternocleidomastoid muscle. It is advanced until the internal jugular vein is entered and blood can be easily aspirated.

Left Internal Jugular Vein

Left internal jugular vein cannulation is associated with more difficulties and more complications. The cupola of the pleura is higher on the left than on the right; therefore there is a higher chance of pneumothorax. The thoracic duct may be injured on the left side approach since it enters the venous system at the junction of the left internal jugular and subclavian veins. In the majority of patients, the left internal jugular vein is smaller than the right and has more overlap with the carotid artery when the head is rotated. Catheters inserted on the left side must cross the innominate vein and enter the superior vena cava perpendicularly, so the distal tip of the catheter may impinge on the wall of the superior vena cava and cause injury.

Subclavian Vein

This vein is popular with surgeons, who use this route for long-term use and for emergency volume resuscitation. The advantages are lower risk of infection than other sites, ease of insertion in trauma patients with cervical injury and increased patient comfort for long-term

therapy such as hyperalimentation. The subclavicular approach is usual. The needle is aimed along the posterior border of the clavicle in the direction of the sternal notch until the subclavian vein is entered and blood is aspirated. The incidence of pneumothorax and subclavian arterial puncture is higher with this approach. These complications are directly related to the number of attempts made for access.

External Jugular Vein

The right and left external jugular veins are safe alternatives for central access, but technically more difficult than a "straight shot" directly to an internal jugular vein. The external jugular vein can be visualized crossing the sternocleidomastoid muscle when the patient is in the Trendelenburg position. The needle is advanced in a parallel direction to the vessel. There may be difficulty advancing the guide wire or the catheter into the central circulation because the patient's anatomy often directs the catheter into the subclavian vein. If difficulty is encountered advancing the catheter, abducting the ipsilateral shoulder 90° prior to advancing the guide wire may help. Since the external jugular vein is superficial, the incidence of pneumothorax or unintentional arterial puncture is extremely low.

Femoral Vein

In burns and trauma patients and surgical procedures that involve the neck, the femoral approach may be useful. Femoral venipuncture is made below the inguinal ligament, medial to the femoral artery. Either a long (40–70 cm) or a short (15–20 cm) catheter can be used. The catheter is inserted from the femoral vein into the common iliac vein. Both techniques provide intra-abdominal venous pressure measurements that agree closely with superior vena cava CVP. This technique avoids the complications of pneumothorax. Disadvantages with this route are thromboembolic and infectious complications. Femoral arterial or venous injury may lead to intra-abdominal hemorrhage.

Axillary and Peripherally Inserted Central Venous Catheters

The axillary route is reserved for patients with extensive burns. Venipuncture is made 1 cm medial to the palpated axillary artery. Peripherally inserted central venous catheters have the advantages of extremely low complication rates and ease of insertion. Access is obtained through an antecubital vein. The basilic vein approach is more successful than the cephalic vein, because the course of the cephalic vein is more tortuous.

Complications of Central Venous Catheters

Multiple complications are associated with placement and use of central venous catheters. Some complications are higher in frequency depending on the site of cannulation. These complications may be categorized as follows:

- Complications associated with insertion of CVP catheters (Box 4-16)
- Catheter-related complications (Box 4-17)
- Late complications
- Miscellaneous complications.

Late complications associated with central venous catheterization include infection, vascular damage, hematoma formation, extravascular migration of the catheter and dysrhythmias (Box 4-18).

Other miscellaneous complications include misinterpretation and misguided use of data.

Pulmonary Artery Pressure Monitoring

Cardiologists Swan, Ganz and colleagues introduced pulmonary artery catheterization into clinical practice in 1970 as a way to measure left heart pressures. Right-sided heart pressures may not reflect left-sided pressures since the right heart acts as a low-pressure, highly distensible conduit. Their balloon-tipped, flow-directed catheter has become an important tool in critical care medicine; it allows better assessment of left-sided filling pressures

---

Box 4-16 Complications Associated with Insertion of Central Venous Catheters

Hematoma from arterial puncture or vascular injury
Hemomediastinum from arterial puncture or vascular injury
Hemothorax from arterial puncture or vascular injury
Arterial thromboembolism
Airway compromise
Pneumothorax
Subcutaneous, mediastinal emphysema
Brachial plexus nerve injury
Phrenic nerve injury
Vocal cord paralysis
Stellate ganglion injury
Tracheal puncture with or without endotracheal tube cuff perforation
Chylothorax if left neck site is used

Box 4-17 Catheter-related Complications

Air embolism
Catheter shearing and embolism
Guide wire embolization
Arterial cannulation
Venous injury, right facial vein avulsion
Guide-wire-induced arrhythmias
Guide-wire-induced heart block

Box 4-18 Late Complications Associated with Central Venous Catheterization

Phlebitis
Cellulitis
Bacteremia, sepsis, fungemia
Aortoatrial fistula
Venobrachial fistula
Pseudoaneurysm
Right atrial, ventricular, or superior vena cava perforation
Cardiac tamponade
Venous thrombosis
Pulmonary embolism
Impaired venous drainage
Superior vena cava syndrome
Hydrothorax
Hydromediastinum
Catheter fracture and embolism
Catheter migration, malposition, arrhythmias

---

and calculations of cardiac work. After many years of acceptance, there is now controversy about its usefulness in improving patient outcome.

Pulmonary artery catheters allow measurement of intracardiac pressures, thermodilution cardiac output, and mixed venous oxygen saturation. The most frequently directly measured hemodynamic parameters are right atrial pressure or CVP, pulmonary arterial pressure, and intermittent measurement of pulmonary capillary wedge pressure (PCWP). PCWP is used to indirectly assess left ventricular end-diastolic pressure (LVEDP) or left ventricular end-diastolic volume (LVEDV). The preload of the left ventricle, which correlates with LVEDP, is also measured. Because increases in left ventricular volume should result in an increase in left ventricular pressure, there should be some correlation between LVEDP and LVEDV. In normal hearts, an increase in LVEDV will result in an increase in LVEDP. This correlation is not necessarily found in the failing heart. Factors, such as myocardial ischemia, that cause decreases in left ventricular compliance will result in large changes in left ventricular pressures, with small changes in left ventricular volumes.

The clinical picture cannot be defined with just pressure data. Calculations can be made to determine the state of systemic vascular resistance, pulmonary vascular resistance, cardiac output and cardiac work (Table 4-2). The accuracy of these calculations depend entirely on the accuracy of the pressure numbers. Small slips in technique, such as air bubbles in the transducer tubing, can lead to erroneous pressure numbers and then incorrect hemodynamic calculations and possibly inappropriate and harmful therapy.

Table 4-2   Calculations of Hemodynamic Variables

Measurement	Formula	Normal	Units
Cardiac index	$\dfrac{CO\ (L/min)}{BSA\ (m^2)}$	2.2–4.2	$L/min/m^2$
Total peripheral resistance	$\dfrac{(MAP-CVP) \times 80}{CO\ (L/min)}$	1,200–1,500	dynes/sec
Pulmonary vascular resistance	$\dfrac{(MAP - PAOP) \times 80}{CO\ (L/min)}$	100–300	dynes/sec
Stroke volume (SV)	$\dfrac{CO\ (L/min) - 1,000}{Heart\ rate\ (beats/min)}$	60–90	mL/beat
Stroke index (SI)	$\dfrac{SV\ (mL/beat)}{BSA\ (m^2)}$	20–65	$mL/beat/m^2$
RVSWI	$0.0136\ (MPAP - CVP) \times SI$	5–10	$g\text{-}m/beat/m^2$
LVSWI	$0.0136\ (MPAP - PCWP) \times SI$	45–60	$g\text{-}m/beat/m^2$

BSA, body surface area; CO, cardiac output; CVP, central venous pressure; g-m, gram meter; LVSWI, left ventricular stroke work index; MAP, mean arterial pressure; MPAP, mean pulmonary arterial pressure; PAOP, pulmonary artery occlusion pressure; PCWP, pulmonary capillary wedge pressure; RVSWI, right ventricular stroke work index.

Indications for Pulmonary Artery Pressure Monitoring

These are listed in Box 4-19.

Contraindications

There are no absolute contraindications for pulmonary artery catheter placement. Relative contraindications are listed in Box 4-20.

Technique

Pulmonary artery catheters can be placed from any of the central venous cannulation sites described in CVP monitoring. The catheter has a 7–8 French circumference and is 110 cm in length, with 10 cm interval markings. It is a multilumen catheter, with one lumen leading to the distal port at the catheter tip, which is used for pulmonary artery pressure (PAP) monitoring. The second lumen leads to a proximal port, about 30 cm from the catheter tip. This is used to measure CVP as well as for intravenous fluid and drug administration. The third lumen leads to a balloon near the tip of the catheter. The fourth lumen contains fine wires leading to a temperature thermistor proximal to the balloon that monitors pulmonary artery blood temperature, which is needed for cardiac output (CO) determination. Some catheters have a fiberoptic channel incorporated for continuously measuring mixed venous oxygen saturation. Other Swan–Ganz catheters allow pacing of the heart, and some are capable of measuring right ventricular ejection fraction. There are also catheters that contain an additional proximal infusion port (PIP) lumen, which is used for infusion of vasoactive medications. Newer technology allows catheters with continuous cardiac output monitoring capabilities.

The pulmonary artery catheter is inserted through a sterile plastic sheath, which covers the length of the catheter, and is threaded into a large introducer, typically a Cordis. This sterile sheath allows minor manipulations

Box 4-19   Indications for Placement of a Pulmonary Artery Catheter

Severe ischemic heart disease, valvular, or congenital heart disease

Major organ system disease in patients undergoing major surgery with large fluid shifts

Recent myocardial infarction (less than 6 months old)

Patient with poor left ventricular function, ejection fraction less than 40%

Severe left ventricular wall motion abnormality

Shock states

Adult respiratory distress syndrome

Pulmonary hypertension with right ventricular failure

Sepsis

Acute renal failure

Acute burns

High-risk obstetrics, e.g. severe toxemia, placental abruption

Surgery that will involve aortic cross-clamping

Severe valvular disease

Patients undergoing cardiac surgery, cardiac transplantation, lung transplantation, and liver transplantation

Resuscitation of major trauma victims

Box 4-20   Relative Contraindications to Pulmonary Artery Catheter Insertion

Coagulopathies
Severe thrombocytopenia
Endocardial pacemaker leads
Prosthetic right heart valve
Complete left bundle branch block

Box 4-21   Complications of Placing a Pulmonary Artery Catheter

Complications associated with venipuncture itself are the same as described for central venous catheter placement
Complications associated with pulmonary artery catheterization:
- Supraventricular arrhythmias, atrial fibrillation.
- Ventricular arrhythmias, ventricular tachycardia, ventricular fibrillation
- Right bundle branch block may occur from distortion of the intraventricular septum close to the right ventricular outflow tract, causing disruption of the ventricular conducting pathway
- Complete heart block may occur in patients with pre-existing left bundle branch block
- Catheter tip misplacement
- Air embolism
- Mechanical problems from catheter coiling, entrapment, knotting and migration
- Introducer sheath problems
- Balloon rupture from hyperinflation of the balloon
- Thrombosis, pulmonary embolism
- Thrombocytopenia
- Pulmonary infarction can occur when pulmonary artery blood flow is occluded; this can happen with prolonged balloon inflation times
- Infection, sepsis, endocarditis
- Pulmonary artery rupture is the most serious complication of pulmonary artery catheter placement. Rapid hypotension and hemoptysis result. If the patient survives, pseudoaneurysm can occur
- Structural damage to the endocardium and perforation of cardiac chambers may occur, resulting in shock, cardiac tamponade, hemothorax, and hemoptysis
- Tricuspid and pulmonic valve damage
- Dislodgment of pacing wires.
Inaccurate and misguided use of data

---

of the catheter, while maintaining sterility. The distal and proximal ports of the catheter are attached to a pressure transducing system, which allows the waveforms to be displayed on a monitor. These ports are flushed with heparinized saline solution, to flush the air from the catheters and also to make certain that they are not obstructed. To make sure there are no leaks in the balloon, it is inflated with air using the volume-limited 1.5 mL syringe packaged with the pulmonary artery catheter. The inflated balloon helps to "float" the catheter along with the blood flow towards its final position in the pulmonary artery. With the distal (PA) port transducing, the catheter is inserted through the hemostasis valve of the introducer to a depth of 20 cm. At this point, a CVP waveform should be seen, which would indicate that the tip of the catheter is in the superior vena cava or right atrium.

The balloon is inflated and the catheter is advanced into the right atrium, carried forward by the inflated balloon acting as a "sail" in the ongoing blood. It then goes through the tricuspid valve into the right ventricle. After passing through the pulmonic valve into the pulmonary artery, it finally reaches the "wedge position" in a small pulmonary arteriole. Characteristic waveforms and pressure changes during passage of the catheter confirm its route until it reaches its final destination in a distal pulmonary vessel. After pulmonary artery wedge pressure (PAWP) is measured, the balloon is deflated, allowing reappearance of the PAP waveform (PAWP is also called pulmonary artery occlusion pressure, PAOP). The balloon should always stay deflated except when taking PCWP measurement. The catheter should not be aggressively forced forward but should be allowed to "float" into position, to avoid vascular trauma or possibly fatal complications. As the catheter moves through the right ventricle, dysrhythmias can occur. These should disappear once the catheter tip is advanced beyond the right ventricle into the pulmonary artery. Otherwise, catheter advancement should stop and it should be pulled back out of the right ventricle. Intravenous lidocaine may be needed to advance through the right ventricle without dysrhythmias.

Possible complications are listed in Box 4-21.

Pulmonary Artery Pressure Waveforms

As the catheter enters the central vein, a typical CVP waveform appears, as was described before. The right ventricular diastolic pressure characteristically has the same value, but systolic levels are much higher than for the CVP. Then, after the catheter goes through the pulmonic valve into the main pulmonary artery, the pulmonary artery waveform is seen. Pulmonary artery and right ventricular systolic pressures have the same value, but pulmonary artery diastolic pressure is higher than right ventricular systolic ("diastolic step up"). With continued advancement, the balloon wedges into a small branch of a pulmonary artery, with its typical waveform (Figure 4-6).

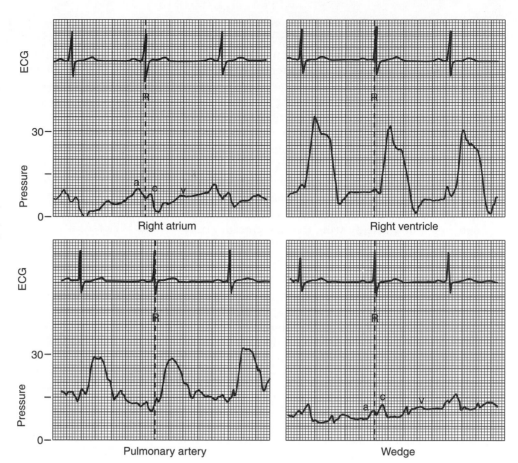

Figure 4-6 Pulmonary artery pressure waveforms. (Redrawn from Mark JB. *Atlas of cardiovascular monitoring*. New York: Churchill Livingstone, 1998.)

Cardiac Output Measurement

Cardiac output measurement is essential for assessment of the circulatory system. Using PAP and PCWP measurements to manage a patient without knowing the cardiac output is risky. Not enough information is available. For example, someone with a normal PCWP and blood pressure may have a low cardiac output. Pharmacologic interventions to manipulate preload, afterload, and contractility can be effective only if cardiac output is known. Cardiac output is most commonly measured by the thermodilution technique.

Thermodilution Technique

This consists of injection of 5–10 mL of fluid below body temperature (room or iced temperature) into the right atrium. The change in temperature of the blood is sensed by the thermistor at the tip of the pulmonary artery catheter. The cold or room temperature injectate is injected at the proximal port of the Swan–Ganz catheter. The temperature of the diluted injectate is measured at the proximal port and cardiac output is calculated using an algorithm. The amount of temperature change is inversely proportional to cardiac output. The temperature change is small if cardiac output is high, but great if cardiac output is low in low-flow states. By plotting the temperature change versus time, a thermodilution curve can be produced. The area under this curve is then calculated by a microprocessor, and the cardiac output is estimated. Accurate measurements depend on knowing the volume and temperature of the injectate and smooth, rapid injection of the solution. In patients with tricuspid regurgitation and cardiac shunts, this measurement technique does not accurately reflect cardiac output, since only right ventricular output is being measured.

Other Techniques

Other methods of measuring cardiac output are as follows.

• *The Fick principle* states that amount of oxygen consumed $\dot{V}O_2$) by an individual equals the difference between arterial and venous (a − v) oxygen content (*C*) multiplied by cardiac output. Mixed venous oxygen content can be determined if a pulmonary artery catheter and an arterial line are in place. Oxygen consumption can be calculated from the difference between the oxygen content in inspired and expired gas.

$$CO = \frac{\text{Oxygen consumption}}{\text{Difference in a} - \text{vO}_2 \text{ content}} = \frac{\dot{V}O_2}{C_aO_2 - C_vO_2}$$

- *The dye dilution technique* for measurement of cardiac output consists of injecting an indicator (green dye) through a central venous catheter. Then, with an appropriate detector (a densitometer for green dye) the arterial circulation level can be measured. The area under the dye indicator curve is the cardiac output. The problems with this technique are recirculation of the dye and buildup of the indicator.
- *The ultrasonography technique* utilizes the Doppler principle. When ultrasound waves strike moving objects, the way they are reflected back to their source depends on the velocity of the moving objects and the angle at which the beams of the ultrasound strike them. Red blood cells flowing through a major artery serve as the moving objects.
  - Transesophageal echocardiography (TEE) assesses left ventricular filling, ejection fraction, wall motion abnormalities and contractility.
  - Transtracheal Doppler measures cardiac output from the diameter of the ascending aorta and the blood velocity. The Doppler transducer is attached to the distal end of the endotracheal tube.
  - Pulsed Doppler measures the velocity of aortic blood flow.
  - Transesophageal Doppler color flow mapping assesses valvular function and presence of intracardiac shunting. Blood flow is measured by color indicating flow direction and velocity.

Mixed Venous Oximetry

Some pulmonary artery catheters have fiberoptic bundles in the catheter tip to determine the oxygenation of pulmonary blood. A computer connected to the pulmonary artery catheter displays the mixed venous oxygen saturation continuously and enables thermodilution cardiac output measurements. The catheter needs to be calibrated for accuracy, and the tip of the catheter must be in the correct position for best results. Mixed venous oximetry catheters are used to measure cardiac output via thermodilution, arterial and mixed venous oxygen content, and oxygen consumption using the Fick equation.

TEMPERATURE MONITORING

Thermoregulation

To maintain core body temperature, humans balance heat production from metabolism and the heat loss to the environment. The hypothalamus maintains core body temperature within a very narrow range, referred to as the *interthreshold range*. This is accomplished when regional temperature information from sites like skin, muscle, body cavities, spinal cord, and brain are integrated and processed by the central nervous system. Deviations in the body temperature by a fraction of a degree beyond the set point trigger temperature dissipating, temperature conserving, or heat producing mechanisms. Thus, increases in temperature induce sweating and vasodilation while lowering the temperature induces vasoconstriction and shivering.

In adults, thermoregulation involves control of the basal metabolic rate, muscular activity, sympathetic arousal, vascular tone increase, and hormonal activation.

Shivering is modulated by the hypothalamus and consists of spontaneous, asynchronous, random contraction of skeletal muscles in an effort to increase the basal metabolic rate. Infants younger than 3 months of age cannot shiver and rely on nonshivering thermogenesis to mount a caloric response. Brown fat, which is only present in infants, is a unique type of fat capable of high-energy production.

Temperature monitoring is a standard of anesthesia care. The risks of accidental heat loss and malignant hyperthermia require constant monitoring of temperature during anesthesia. Body temperature may vary markedly during anesthesia. This is especially significant during general anesthesia when body cavities are open and thermoregulatory functions are depressed by inhalation anesthetics. The cold operating room environment also facilitates heat loss. General and regional anesthetics inhibit afferent and efferent control of thermoregulation. Regional procedures of short duration (i.e. less than 15 minutes) may not require temperature monitoring. Blood and fluids given to patients at room temperature, as well as the cool air in the operating room, can lead to a significant drop in core body temperature. The fact is that anesthetized patients reflect the temperature of the external environment. Thus, the role of the anesthesiologist should be to attempt to maintain central core temperature at near-normal levels in all patients undergoing anesthesia.

The four mechanisms of heat loss are radiation, conduction, convection, and evaporation. Radiation involves the infrared rays emanated from all objects to cooler surroundings. It accounts for up to 60% of total heat loss, depending on factors such as cutaneous blood flow and the area exposed. Conduction is the transfer of heat to a cooler adjacent object and is dependent on the temperature gradient and thermal conductivity. It contributes to 5% of the total heat loss. Evaporation comprises up to 20% of the total heat loss through the latent heat of vaporization (the energy required to vaporize water from the serosal and mucosal surfaces). For every gram of water that evaporates, 0.58 kcal of heat is lost. The amount lost depends on the exposed surface area and the relative humidity of the air. Convection results in loss of heat by the airflow on the exposed surfaces and accounts for 15% of heat loss.

Hypothermia

Hypothermia is the clinical state of subnormal body temperature in which there is not enough production of heat to provide energy for body functions. Hypothermia is defined as body temperature below 36° C, and occurs frequently during anesthesia and surgery. Below this level, shivering and autonomic responses are unable to compensate completely without assisted warming.

In the operating room, the cold ambient air, prep solutions, and exposure of the patient are the major causes of hypothermia. One unit of refrigerated blood or 1 L of room-temperature crystalloid solution decreases body temperature about 0.25° C. Cutaneous heat loss accounts for 90% of intraoperative net heat loss.

The first drop in the temperature during general anesthesia occurs during the first hour of anesthesia (phase I). It is followed by a gradual decrease during the next 3–4 hours (phase II) until it reaches an equilibrium point (phase III). The redistribution of heat from the warm central compartments (abdomen, thorax) to cooler peripheral tissues (arms and legs) caused by anesthetic-induced vasodilation accounts for the initial drop in the temperature. During this phase, actual heat loss plays a minor role in the temperature drop. After this period, continuous heat loss is responsible for the slower subsequent decline in body temperature. Once steady-state equilibrium is reached, heat loss equals metabolic heat production and there is no net change in body temperature.

Elderly patients, infants, patients with reduced autonomic vascular control, burns patients, patients with hypothalamic lesions, and spinal cord injuries that involve autonomic dysfunction are especially at risk for hypothermia. Endocrine abnormalities such as hypothyroidism also increase this risk. Of interest, the basal metabolic rate decreases by 1% per year after age 30.

The normal central thermoregulation of core body temperature and shivering are inhibited by the use of anesthetics. Inhalation anesthetics produce vasodilation, which leads to increasing heat loss. Additionally, these agents cause impairment of the hypothalamic function and its thermoregulatory role. Isoflurane, for example, produces a dose-dependent decrease in the vasoconstrictive threshold (3° C for each 1% of isoflurane). Opioids have a sympatholytic property that prevents vasoconstrictive mechanisms. Barbiturates also cause peripheral vasodilation. Muscle relaxants prevent shivering thermogenesis by decreasing muscle tone. Regional anesthesia may induce sympathetic block, muscle relaxation, and sensory block of the thermoreceptors, preventing adjusting responses. Spinal and epidural anesthesia cause vasodilation and subsequent redistribution of the heat (phase I), leading to hypothermia. Rather than a central effect, regional anesthesia appears to alter the perception of temperature in the blocked dermatomes by the hypothalamus, thus increasing the interthreshold range. Nonshivering thermogenesis is carried out in brown fat, a high-energy tissue capable of rapidly producing heat. (Adults do not have brown fat.)

Management of hypothermia consists of passive or active rewarming. Passive rewarming entails covering exposed areas to minimize losses due to radiation and convection. This relies on intact hypothalamic mechanisms and shivering thermogenesis and adequate glycogen stores, to allow the body to produce the necessary heat. Active rewarming uses methods available in the operating room such as administration of warmed intravenous fluids, use of radiant warmers or heat lamps in pediatric patients, warming blankets for conductive transfer of heat (mainly those that blow warm air on the surfaces), and heated humidifiers in the anesthetic circuit to decrease evaporative losses and warm compressed gases. It is important to maintain closed or low-flow semiclosed circuits to minimize evaporative losses. Also included in this class is the use of heated irrigation fluids for peritoneal lavage or bladder instillation and extracorporeal rewarming with cardiopulmonary bypass.

A secondary drop in body core temperature can occur with rewarming because of the return of cold blood from the periphery. Prevention of phase I can be accomplished by prewarming for a minimum of 30 minutes with convective forced-air warming blankets in order to eliminate the central–peripheral temperature gradient. There are many methods of minimizing heat loss during phase II, such as the use of forced-air warming blankets, heated humidification of inspired gases, warm-water blankets, warming of intravenous fluids, and raising operating room temperature. Unless most of the body is covered, passive insulators such as heated cotton blankets have little utility. Humidification of inspiratory gases is important to prevent airway drying and maintain ciliary function.

Perioperative hypothermia is associated with increased morbidity and mortality, depending on the degree of the temperature depression. Box 4-22 lists these adverse events. With mild hypothermia (32–35° C) there is a decrease in metabolic rate, the central nervous system is depressed, and tachycardia and shivering may occur. The patient can present with dysarthria, amnesia, ataxia, and apathy. In moderate hypothermia (27–32° C) there is a further decrease in level of consciousness, a mild depression of vital signs, arrhythmias, and cold diuresis. Severe hypothermia (<27° C) is characterized by coma, areflexia, and depressed vital signs. At about 33° C sedation occurs and at 30° C cold narcosis ensues.

The increase in metabolic heat production by shivering increases the oxygen consumption as much as 300%. This is undesirable in patients with coronary artery

---

Box 4-22   Physiologic Effects of Hypothermia

Decreased basal metabolic rate
Vasoconstriction and decreased tissue perfusion
Metabolic acidosis
Increased vascular resistance and central venous pressure
Increase in oxygen consumption and myocardial oxygen demand
Ventricular arrhythmias and myocardial depression
Increased pulmonary vascular resistance
Decreased hypoxic pulmonary vasoconstriction
Hypoxemia and ventilation/perfusion mismatch
Decreased ventilatory drive and bronchomotor tone
Decreased renal blood flow and glomerular filtration rate
Increased diuresis and protein catabolism
Decreased sodium reabsorption and hypovolemia
Decreased ability to concentrate or dilute urine
Decreased hepatic blood flow
Decreased cerebral blood flow
Increased cerebral vascular resistance
Decrease in drug metabolism
Left shift of the hemoglobin dissociation curve
Platelet dysfunction and aggregation and visceral sequestration
Thrombocytopenia
Increased blood solubility
Reduced activity of clotting factors
Impaired coagulation
Increased fibrinolysis
Decreased cutaneous blood flow (increased peripheral vascular resistance)
Poor wound healing
Postoperative protein catabolism and stress response
Decreased aqueous humor production

---

disease or pulmonary insufficiency. The arterial oxygen saturation is decreased, predisposing these patients to myocardial ischemia and angina. Postoperative shivering can be successfully treated with intravenous meperidine (12.5–25 mg). Prevention, however, continues to be the best solution.

As hypothermia worsens, a decrease in heart rate, cardiac output, and oxygen consumption is noted. The carbon dioxide content of blood drops by 50% for each 8° C decrease in temperature, leaving little respiratory stimulus to breathing and diminishing respiratory drive. The pH of arterial blood rises by 0.015 units for each 1° C decrease in temperature. The minimal alveolar concentration (MAC) of volatile agents is decreased, causing delayed emergence, drowsiness, and confusion. The MAC of inhalational agents is decreased by 5–7% for each 1° C decrease in core body temperature, but the speed of inhalational induction is unchanged.

Hepatic and renal blood flow is decreased, leading to slower metabolism and clearance of drugs and their prolonged effect. An example is the prolonged duration of neuromuscular blocking agents. Hypothermia also causes an increase in protein binding.

Cerebral metabolic oxygen consumption is reduced by 7% for each 1° C drop in temperature. Motor and somatosensory evoked potential (EP) latencies are increased in hypothermia.

Hypothermia can lead to wound infection and delayed wound healing. This is due to impairment of the immune system and the decrease in oxygen delivery to the wound caused by thermoregulatory vasoconstriction.

The clinical signs of hypothermia are summarized in Table 4-3.

The ECG manifestations of hypothermia vary depending on the degree of temperature depression, summarized in Table 4-4.

A prolonged Q-T interval may be observed. An elevation of the J point or ST segment, known as the hypothermic hump, may be observed in temperatures lower than 32° C. It is seen in leads II and V6 and may spread to leads V3 and V4. Nodal rhythms are common below 30° C. Ventricular fibrillation and asystole are relatively unresponsive to countershock, atropine, or pacing at body temperatures below 28° C; therefore, resuscitative efforts should be carried on until the patient is rewarmed.

Infants are particularly susceptible to hypothermia because of their large body surface area to body mass ratio. Hypothermia in pediatric patients should be avoided because of the serious problems that can occur postoperatively. Because anesthetic blood solubility is greater at lower temperatures, these patients take longer to recover from anesthesia and their $P_a\mathrm{CO_2}$ is higher. The higher $P_a\mathrm{CO_2}$ can also be explained by the hypoventilation caused by hypothermia.

Several measures can be taken to avoid hypothermia in this age group. The operating room should be warmed to 37–39° C. The smaller the patient, the higher the temperature should be. The infant should be put under an infrared heater for operation and the head should be protected with a thermal cap. An attempt should be made to cover the body as much as possible and for as long as feasible. The legs should be wrapped with sheet wadding. Placement of a heating pad under the patient, set at

---

Table 4-3   Clinical Signs of Hypothermia

Early Signs	Late Signs
Shivering	Altered mental status
Decreased sweating	Muscle weakness
Vasoconstriction	Decreased motor activity

Table 4-4 **Electrocardiographic Changes with Hypothermia**		
Mild	**Moderate**	**Severe**

Sinus bradycardia	Prolonged P–R interval
	Widened QRS complexes
	Prolonged Q–T Interval
		Premature ventricular
		  contractions
		Atrioventricular blocks
		Spontaneous atrial/ventricular
		  fibrillation
		Asystole

36–37° C, reduces conductive heat loss during anesthesia. Solutions should be warmed to body temperature, and inspired gases should be warmed and humidified at 32–37° C to reduce the heat loss and prevent tracheal mucosal damage.

Hypothermia may offer one advantage. Since hypothermia results in decreased metabolic rate and oxygen requirement, it may have some brain protective effects during periods of central nervous system hypoperfusion.

Hyperthermia

Hyperthermia is an increase in temperature of 2° C per hour. It is uncommon in anesthetized patients, and its cause must be investigated. It can occur with the use of thermal insulation (sterile drapes) or the use of anticholinergic drugs and inhalation anesthetics, which can affect the thermoregulatory function. Hypermetabolic states such as sepsis or fever (endogenous pyrogens) are the usual causes. In this situation, the temperature should be lowered before the induction of anesthesia. Bacteremia during surgery and vigorous warming techniques are some of the other causes. Hypothalamic lesions secondary to trauma, anoxia or tumor, hyperthyroidism (thyroid storm), and pheochromocytoma are less common. Neuroleptic malignant syndrome, transfusion reactions and medications such as sympathomimetics, monoamine oxidase inhibitors, cocaine, amphetamines, and tricyclic antidepressants, which increase basal metabolic rate, can also cause hyperthermia. Anticholinergics and antihistamines suppress sweating, elevating the temperature.

Hyperthermia increases the basal metabolic rate and hepatic metabolism and decreases the half-life of anesthetics, increasing their requirement. This hypermetabolic state increases oxygen consumption and minute ventilation, sweating, and vasodilation. Intravascular volume and venous return are reduced. Heart rate increases by 10 beats per minute (BPM) per 1° C increase in temperature.

Malignant hyperthermia is a relatively rare genetic condition in which body temperature rises rapidly, but tachycardia, increased ET-CO$_2$, and hypertension precede the fever. Malignant hyperthermia is a true medical emergency and must be recognized and treated promptly.

Clinical manifestations of hyperthermia in awake patients include general malaise, nausea, lightheadedness, tachycardia, sweating, and vasodilatation. In prolonged cases, the patient may present with symptoms of heat exhaustion or heat stroke. In the anesthetized patient, the signs and symptoms include tachycardia, hypertension, increased ET-CO$_2$, increased drug metabolism, and possibly dehydration.

Treatment of hyperthermia includes exposing skin surfaces to a cool environment, cooling blankets, cool intravenous fluids, and administration of antipyretics. The etiology of the hyperthermia should be investigated and corrected.

Temperature Monitors

Routine intraoperative measurement of the body temperature is usually carried out with electronic thermometers such as thermistors or thermocouples. Thermistors are tiny beads of semiconductor material whose electrical resistance decreases predictably with warming. An example is the circuit incorporated into an esophageal probe producing a voltage that varies linearly with temperature, thus not needing calibration. Thermistor circuits form the basis of most digital electronic thermometers. Analog thermistor thermometers comprise of a single thermistor and use a nonlinear scale for temperature reading. A thermocouple is a circuit of two dissimilar metals joined at the point of temperature measurement so that a potential difference or voltage is generated and measured when the metals are at different temperatures at this junction. Thermocouple temperature probes maintain one junction at a known temperature and place the second junction on the temperature probe tip. Skin temperature may be monitored using a liquid crystal thermometer. Temperature strips, however, do not correlate well with core temperature measurements.

Surface temperature monitoring with a sensor applied to the forehead is noninvasive and convenient. However, it is not considered accurate enough for use in major cases and is not the standard of care. Liquid crystal technology is used for this purpose. The appropriate liquid compound is laminated into a thin plastic sheet. As the temperature varies, the liquid changes structure and color. By geometric arrangement of various chemical mixtures, an interpretation through an overlying numerical display is possible. This is used for forehead temperature monitoring when information on temperature trend is desired, as changes in temperature are well tracked. Mercury thermometers are not useful during anesthesia because they fail to respond to decreases in temperature and are breakable.

Disposable probes are available for monitoring temperature at various sites. The site for monitoring temperature during anesthesia depends on the surgical procedure, type of anesthesia, and reason for temperature monitoring. There are no absolute contraindications for temperature monitoring, although a particular site may not be suitable in certain patients or certain cases. During endotracheal anesthesia, central core temperature is usually monitored in the distal esophagus. Temperature probes for monitoring may also be placed into the bladder, external ear canal, axilla, trachea, nasopharynx, or rectum.

The skin does not accurately reflect the mean core body temperature because it is 3-4° C cooler than the core temperature. Axillary temperature monitored over the brachial artery with the arm adducted is approximately 1° C below core temperature, and depends on skin perfusion. The rectum does not reflect rapid changes of core temperature in central organs, and rectal perforation is a rare complication. It is also more difficult to insert a rectal probe since the rectum is not easily accessible.

A probe in the lower third of the esophagus accurately reflects core and blood temperature. Combined with an esophageal stethoscope, it is also useful for auscultation of the heart and breath sounds, since it is placed behind the heart to avoid measurement of the temperature of tracheal gases. It provides early detection of early changes in core temperature by recording the average temperature of the blood returning to the heart. It can be unreliable if influenced by pulmonary ventilation or local cooling of the heart.

Nasopharyngeal temperature reflects the brain temperature because of its proximity to the internal carotid artery. The complications include epistaxis, especially in pregnancy, and coagulopathy. Nasopharyngeal temperature monitoring is contraindicated in head trauma with evidence of cerebrospinal fluid rhinorrhea.

The temperature at the external auditory meatus correlates well with the core temperature because of its proximity to the internal carotid artery, and it approximates that of the regulatory centers of the brain. Tympanic membrane perforation, especially in patients unresponsive to pain, is a possible complication. Cerumen insulation can prevent accurate measurements.

A pulmonary artery catheter gives an accurate estimate of the core temperature.

Box 4-23   Advantages and Disadvantages of Transcutaneous Oxygen Measurement

ADVANTAGES

Noninvasive
Continuous

DISADVANTAGES

Less accurate than analysis of blood samples
If cardiac output falls, readings are unreliable because of low skin perfusion
Increased inaccuracy when there is a shift in oxygen dissociation curve with high or low temperatures
Reduction in skin perfusion because of edema from high temperature of the electrode
Risk of skin burns

Transcutaneous Oxygen Measurement

This is a noninvasive continuous technique of assessing oxygenation at the skin level. It is most commonly used in neonates and pediatric patients.

The skin is warmed to 43-44° C, to arterialize skin blood flow and liquefy the stratum corneum. A thermistor controls skin temperature. A polarographic electrode placed on the skin senses the oxygen that diffuses from the capillaries through the skin to the electrode. Electrode position should be changed every 3-6 hours, to avoid skin damage from heat.

This technique is used in infants and neonates and is most successful in this group because of their thin skin layer. It also avoids the need to have an arterial line or do arterial sampling in this technically difficult age group (Box 4-23).

Transcutaneous Carbon Dioxide Measurement

This is a noninvasive continuous technique of assessing ventilation. It is most commonly used in the neonatal and pediatric patient populations.

A sensor containing a CO_2 electrode with a heating device is attached to the skin. CO_2 electrodes measure changes in pH and this is converted to a P_{CO_2} reading. The heating device vasodilates capillary vessels and increases gas diffusion by liquefying the stratum corneum (Box 4-24).

NEUROMUSCULAR MONITORING

During general anesthesia, muscle relaxants are used to achieve muscular paralysis. Muscle relaxants are agents that interfere with the transmission of nerve impulses at the neuromuscular junction. Perioperative muscular paralysis is desirable to facilitate tracheal intubation, improve surgical exposure, and increase the efficacy of the mechanical ventilation.

For normal muscular contraction to occur, a nerve action potential is generated and reaches the nerve terminal. This causes the release of acetylcholine into the synaptic cleft. The released acetylcholine diffuses across the synaptic cleft and binds to the nicotinic receptors on the muscle membrane, leading to the contraction of the muscle fiber. Generally, muscle relaxants interfere with and interrupt this transmission of motor nerve impulses across the synaptic cleft.

Muscle relaxants are divided into two groups: depolarizing muscle relaxants and nondepolarizing muscle relaxants (NDMRs). Succinylcholine is the only depolarizing muscle relaxant used in clinical practice. Once succinylcholine is administered, it gains access to the neuromuscular junction. It then binds and activates the nicotinic cholinergic receptors and leads to the depolarization of the muscle membrane, and then the muscle fasciculates. Because succinylcholine is not degraded by the cholinesterase present in the synaptic cleft, the depolarization is prolonged and causes the muscle membrane to become inexcitable. Termination of the action of succinylcholine is achieved when it diffuses out of the synaptic cleft, and it is then hydrolyzed by plasma cholinesterase (pseudocholinesterase).

The typical dose of succinylcholine administered for endotracheal intubation is about 1.0–1.5 mg/kg. The neuromuscular blockade caused by this dose range is termed phase I block. Phase II block may happen when larger doses of succinylcholine are administered, and it mimics the type of neuromuscular blockade achieved by NDMRs.

Nondepolarizing muscle relaxants are divided into two major groups based on their chemical structure. Steroid derivatives include vecuronium, pancuronium, rocuronium, and pipecuronium. The other group, benzylisoquinolines, includes atracurium, cis-atracurium, mivacurium, tubocurarine, and doxacurium. If agents of two different groups (e.g., vecuronium and atracurium) are combined, they act synergistically. NDMRs are more commonly categorized based on their duration of action: short-acting (mivacurium), intermediate-acting (vecuronium, atracurium, rocuronium, and cis-atracurium) and long-acting (pancuronium, pipecuronium, and doxacurium).

Nondepolarizing muscle relaxants exert their action by binding the nicotinic cholinergic receptors on the muscle end-plate, resulting in the competitive inhibition of the receptors. Unlike succinylcholine, the paralysis caused by the nondepolarizers may be reversed if the concentration of the acetylcholine in the synaptic cleft is raised sufficiently.

Assessment of Neuromuscular Function

Assessment of neuromuscular function, or muscle strength, can be accomplished clinically or by using a peripheral nerve stimulator. Clinical evaluation relies on such factors as handgrip, head lift, negative inspiratory pressure, tidal volume, and vital capacity. However, under anesthesia estimation of muscle strength based on these clinical factors is inaccurate and not easily reproducible. During surgery a peripheral nerve stimulator is used for the purpose of neuromuscular monitoring. Two types of nerve stimulator are used in clinical practice. The most common type, the mechanomyelograph, assesses the contractile response to nerve stimulations. In contrast, electromyelographs measure the electrical response to stimulations. The nerve stimulators used commonly in the operating room rely on mechanomyelography to evaluate neuromuscular function and assess the visual or tactile muscle response to the stimulus.

For the nerve stimulator to function properly, a rather superficial nerve should be used. The most common site for this purpose is the ulnar nerve. It is close to the surface at two sites: at the elbow, and at the wrist. Stimulations of the ulnar nerve cause contraction of the adductor pollicis muscle, resulting in the adduction of the thumb at the metacarpophalangeal joint. Other alternative sites include:
- Ophthalmic branch of the facial nerve – contraction of the orbicularis oculi muscle
- Posterior tibialis nerve – plantar flexion of the foot
- Peroneal nerve – dorsiflexion of the foot.

It is crucial to place the electrodes on the nerve, and not directly on the muscle, to avoid direct stimulation of the muscle. Additionally, different muscle groups have different sensitivities to the effects of muscle relaxants. For example, the diaphragm and vocal cords are more resistant to the paralytic effects of the muscle relaxants, which are more closely paralleled by that of the orbicularis oculi muscle. Therefore, monitoring of the ulnar nerve may underestimate the strength and function of the diaphragm or vocal cords.

The peripheral nerve stimulators used in clinical practice are capable of delivering stimuli of different frequency and amplitude. The impulses are monophasic, and of constant duration of 0.2 msec. The stimuli are said to be supramaximal, meaning that current output is 20% above that of maximal stimulation, typically set at 50–60 mA. Various patterns of stimulation are employed: single twitch, train of four (TOF), tetanus, post-tetanic facilitation, post-tetanic count, and double-burst stimulation (DBS).

Single Twitch

The simplest mode of a nerve stimulator delivers a single twitch. This is a supramaximal stimulus of 0.2 msec duration, at a frequency of 0.15–0.1 Hz (one every 6–10 sec). Twitch height begins to decrease once 75% of the receptors are blocked and disappears at 90–95% blockade. A 95% depression corresponds to intubating conditions and surgical relaxation. This mode is mostly reserved for establishing the baseline response.

Train of Four

This mode was introduced into clinical practice in the 1970s and today is most commonly used to evaluate neuromuscular function. Four supramaximal stimuli at 2 Hz are delivered at 10–12 sec intervals. Depending on the type of the blockade, depolarizing versus nondepolarizing, the responses to the TOF differ. TOF mode offers many advantages: it gives a good measure of relaxation, it is also very useful in assessing recovery, and it causes only moderate discomfort in the awake patients. But TOF is not very useful in quantifying the degree of depolarizing blockade.

Train of four is the most commonly used mode to evaluate nondepolarizing blockade. Upon disappearance of the fourth response, 75–80% of the receptors are blocked, which corresponds to 75% of depression of the single twitch (Table 4-5). All four responses disappear when 90–95% of the receptors are occupied. Presence of one or two twitches of the TOF corresponds to surgical relaxation.

Clinical recovery from muscle relaxants is assessed based on the TOF ratio (T4:T1). This is described as the ratio of the height of the fourth TOF response to the first. At a TOF ratio of greater than 0.7, the height of the single twitch has returned to control, and there would be no fade during a 50 Hz tetanus. This corresponds to adequate clinical recovery, with normal vital capacity, inspiratory force, and protective airway reflexes.

It should be noted that with phase I blockade, the TOF ratio remains 1, but the height of all four responses decreases in relation to the degree of the neuromuscular blockade. Phase II blockade, in contrast, mimics the characteristics of NDMR blockade (Figure 4-7).

Tetanus

Tetanic nerve stimulation is used to evaluate fade and post-tetanic facilitation. During this mode, a tetanic stimulus at a frequency of 50 Hz and a duration of 5 seconds is delivered to the peripheral nerve. All muscle relaxants cause a reduced response to tetanic stimulation, although phase I blockades do not exhibit fade with tetanus, whereas phase II and NDMR blockade reveal fade in this mode. A major disadvantage of tetanus is that it is very uncomfortable in awake patients. In addition, tetanic stimulation may accelerate recovery in the stimulated muscle and lead to confusion and underestimation of the level of neuromuscular blockade.

Post-tetanic Facilitation

Post-tetanic potentiation is enhancement of the height of a single twitch delivered shortly of the tetanic stimulation. It is observed with phase II and NDMR blockade, but not with phase I blockade.

Post-tetanic Count

During intense NDMR blockade, the time to recovery may be assessed using this mode. A 50 Hz tetanic stimulus of 5 seconds duration is delivered, followed by single-twitch stimulation. The number of observed twitches corresponds to the time to twitch recovery.

Double-Burst Stimulation

One of the disadvantages of the TOF and tetanic stimulation is that the evaluation of fade is unreliable. This has led to the development of a newer mode, DBS. In this mode, two tetanic stimuli of 50 Hz are delivered, separated by 750 msec. Residual NDMR causes a decrease in the response of the second stimulus. The awake patient more easily tolerates DBS than tetanic stimulation.

Clinical Factors

Although evaluation of neuromuscular transmission based on clinical factors is not reliable, some parameters may be used more successfully than others. While an adequate tidal volume may be achieved with 80% receptor blockade, a negative inspiratory pressure of 50 cmH_2O is thought to mean that 80% of receptors are unblocked.

Complications

Very few complications are associated with the use of peripheral nerve stimulators. Occasionally, skin erythema or mild abrasions caused by the electrodes may be encountered. Needle electrodes, on the other hand, may cause skin blisters or bruises.

Table 4-5 Relationship Between Train of Four Count and Level of Receptor Blockade					
TOF Count	4	3	2	1	0
Receptor blockade (%)	<75	75–80	85	85–90	95
Depression of single twitch height (%)	75	80	90	100	

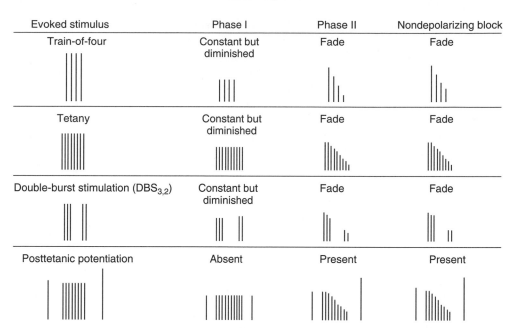

Evoked stimulus	Depolarizing block		Nondepolarizing block
	Phase I	Phase II	
Train-of-four	Constant but diminished	Fade	Fade
Tetany	Constant but diminished	Fade	Fade
Double-burst stimulation (DBS$_{3,2}$)	Constant but diminished	Fade	Fade
Posttetanic potentiation	Absent	Present	Present

Figure 4-7 Evoked responses during depolarizing (phase I and phase II) and nondepolarizing block. (Redrawn from Morgan GE, Mikhail MS, Murray MJ. *Clinical anesthesiology* 3rd ed. New York: McGraw Hill, 2002)

Less frequently, skin burns have been reported, possibly due to frequent use of high-output tetanic stimulations.

URINE OUTPUT

Perioperative monitoring of the urine output provides valuable information about renal function, which is a great indicator of overall tissue perfusion. Identifying patients with increased risk for renal dysfunction is crucial. Perioperative renal failure has a poor prognosis, with potential for life-threatening complications. It also accounts for half of all patients requiring acute dialysis. Urine output monitoring requires an in-depth understanding of the physiology of urine formation, the influence of anesthetic drugs, and the effects that intraoperative events have on the normal physiology of renal function. General anesthesia decreases renal function by decreases in urine output, glomerular filtration rate (GFR), renal blood flow and electrolyte excretion. This effect is reversible and temporary. Spinal and epidural analgesia may depress renal function to a lesser extent.

Direct monitors of renal function are still very rudimentary, and indirect measures (CVP, MAP, CO) are frequently used as the most reliable renal protective measures to preserve renal function in high-risk patients. Urine volume is used intraoperatively as the only true indicator of renal function and kidney perfusion.

Urine output is measured by transurethral insertion of a Foley catheter connected to a urinometer, a calibrated collection reservoir. Urine output is then measured and recorded periodically, typically every 30–60 minutes.

Specialized Foley catheters also allow measurement of the bladder temperature. Computerized urine output measurements allow more frequent recording of data, for example every 10 minutes. An alternative technique to the transurethral approach is suprapubic bladder catheterization.

Adequate urine output is between 0.5 and 1.0 mL/kg/hr. Oliguria is defined as urine output less than 0.5 mL/kg/hr. Generally, the possible etiologies of oliguria are categorized as prerenal, renal, or postrenal. The most common intraoperative cause of oliguria is intravascular volume depletion.

Catheterization of the urinary bladder is the only reliable method of monitoring urine output. Urine output monitoring is indicated in patients with significant preexisting systemic diseases, such as cardiovascular, renal, or hepatic abnormalities, as well as burns or trauma patients. Patients with pre-existing renal disease are at risk of deterioration of their renal function and acute tubular necrosis when subjected to surgery and anesthesia. The type and extent of the surgery is another important factor to consider for this monitor. Patients undergoing cardiac, major vascular, liver, or bowel surgery, among others, and procedures involving major fluid shifts require urine output monitoring. Lengthy operations may be yet another indication. Catheterization of the urinary bladder prevents overdistension of the bladder and subsequent increase in sympathetic output.

In patients with abnormal urethral anatomy or when catheter insertion is found to be difficult, a urologist should be consulted. In such instances, insertion of a suprapubic catheter may be required as the last resort for urine output monitoring.

The most common risks associated with the insertion of Foley catheters include urethral trauma and urinary tract infections. Interestingly, the most common nosocomial infection in the United States is urinary tract infection. The incidence of bacteriuria in catheterized patients is directly related to the duration of catheterization. Among these patients, 10–25% will develop symptoms of infection and 3% will develop bacteremia, a serious and life-threatening complication

Urine output is only an indicator of the kidney perfusion and renal function, and not a direct parameter. Various nonrenal factors can affect urinary flow, including intravascular volume, cardiac output, systemic vascular resistance, and medications such as diuretics. Some studies have shown that there is no correlation between urine volume and GFR, creatinine clearance, or histological evidence of acute tubular necrosis in patients with burns, trauma, shock states, or cardiovascular surgery. Moreover, normal urine output may not definitively rule out renal failure since perioperative nonoliguric renal failure has been documented. Finally, the data does not even prove that oliguria is a reliable sign of renal dysfunction.

NEUROLOGIC MONITORING

The fundamental principles of neurological assessment should always include a thorough physical examination with special focus on evaluation of the nervous system. This is obviously not possible during general anesthesia (Box 4-25).

The driving force that allows blood flow through the brain tissues is the cerebral perfusion pressure (CPP).

CPP is dependent on MAP and intracranial pressure (ICP):

$$CPP = MAP - ICP.$$

Normal ICP is about 10–13 mmHg. The cranium has a fixed volume; therefore, an increase in volume of any of the intracranial components (brain tissue, cerebral blood volume, cerebrospinal fluid [CSF]) will increase the ICP, unless it is offset by a decrease in volume of another component. Brain tissue makes up 80–85% of the intracranial volume. It consists of intracellular water, extracellular water, and solid matter. Cerebral blood volume is about 7 mL/100 g of brain. It makes up 5–8% of the intracranial volume. It is contained within the venous, arterial, and capillary beds of the intracranial space. CSF is formed at a rate of 400–600 mL/day, mostly by the choroidal plexuses of the ventricles and some by nonchoroidal surfaces of the ventricles. CSF accounts for 7–10% of the intracranial volume.

A pressure–volume compliance curve (Figure 4-8) illustrates the relationship between intracranial volume and ICP. At the end of the compliance curve, even a small increase in volume will result in a large increase in ICP.

Increases in intracranial volume can be caused by increased brain tissue volume due to space occupying diseases or brain edema, increased cerebral blood volume from hematoma or intravascular causes such as vasodilation, and CSF volume increases due to blockage of CSF circulation. Intracranial volume increase from any of these causes can lead to increased ICP and a decrease in CPP, with resultant cerebral ischemia. If increased ICP is not treated and CPP falls even further, brain herniation may ensue and death can occur. ICP monitoring and management may help decrease the morbidity and mortality associated with elevated ICP.

Methods of Monitoring Intracranial Pressure

External Transducers
Intracranial placement of transducer implantation is done utilizing fluid-coupled external transducers.

Box 4-25   Signs and Symptoms of Increased Intracranial Pressure

Headache
Vomiting
Papilledema
Drowsiness
Decerebrate rigidity
Oculomotor palsy
Abnormal respiration
Arterial hypertension
Absent brain-stem reflexes
Unconsciousness
Bilateral, fixed, dilated pupils
Apnea

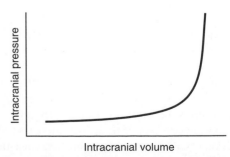

Figure 4-8   Intracranial pressure versus intracranial volume.

Advantage
- Easily calibrated, recalibrated and zeroed

Subdural Bolt (Richmond Bolt)

The bolt is threaded into the skull via a drill hole through a small dural opening. The tip lies 1 mm below the surface of the dura and the head of the bolt is connected to a transducer via saline-filled tubing.

Advantage
- No need to puncture the brain tissue

Disadvantages
- Malfunction of the bolt from loose connection or malposition
- Infection
- Occlusion from wound debris, the dura or blood
- May underread at higher ICPs

Ventriculostomy

The most commonly used method of monitoring ICP. A catheter is introduced through a burr hole into the anterior horn of one of the lateral ventricles.

Advantages
- Accurate measurement of ICP
- Allows therapeutic drainage of the CSF

Disadvantages
- Technical difficulties in catheter placement when the brain is swollen and normal anatomy is distorted
- Possibility of brain damage during placement of the catheter
- Obstruction of the catheter
- Infection
- Accidental venting of the CSF

Intracranial Placement of an Electronic Transducer

A miniature fiberoptic catheter with a transducer tip is placed into the:
- Ventricular system
- Epidural space
- Subdural space or
- Brain parenchyma.

Advantages
- Self-enclosed electronic system, therefore decreased incidence of infection and catheter drift
- Simple, noninvasive, and accurate, so it may gain widespread use
- The transducer is at the tip of the catheter; therefore, the level of the transducer is of no concern

Disadvantages
- Inability to calibrate and re-zero following placement into the cranial cavity
- Unstable for use for prolonged period of time

Transcranial Doppler

Transcranial Doppler (TCD) is a noninvasive method of evaluating cerebral hemodynamics. It is used to assess regional cerebral perfusion. TCD measures the blood velocity in the basal arteries. It does not measure flow, and therefore the cerebral blood flow is only estimated if the diameter remains constant. Technically, the middle cerebral artery (MCA) is the easiest vessel to insonate, and it is also the most important artery since about 80% of the cerebral blood flows through the MCA. Thus, it has a high sensitivity for detecting vasospasm in the MCA, but to a lesser extent with the anterior cerebral artery.

Since TCD only measures flow velocities, it would be difficult to differentiate between hyperemia and vasospasm when high flow velocities are detected; therefore, a second modality is desirable. In contrast, a decreased TCD reading is a good indicator of diminished cerebral blood flow.

Low frequency ultrasound penetrates areas of the cranium and allows estimation of the velocity of the blood flow by detection of the reflected signal. A computer is used to calculate and display systolic, diastolic, and mean blood velocity transformed from the Doppler signals. Mean blood velocity serves as an index of cerebral blood flow in a region. Three regions are described. The temporal bone is used to determine the mean blood velocity of the anterior, posterior and middle cerebral arteries (Box 4-26).

Electroencephalogram

The electroencephalogram (EEG) is a record of the electrical activity from the superficial cerebral cortex. This represents the small electrical signals (0.010–0.100 mV) from the postsynaptic excitatory and inhibitory potentials of the neurons. The standard EEG electrode placement, termed *montage*, is the 10–20 system – 20

Box 4-26   Advantages and Disadvantages of Transcranial Doppler Monitoring

ADVANTAGES

Detects intracranial air or particulate embolism
Beat-to-beat changes in mean blood velocity correlates with changes in regional cerebral blood flow
Early warning for detection of critical reduction in cerebral blood flow

DISADVANTAGES/LIMITATIONS

Subjective measure requiring technical expertise
Values are unpredictably influenced by intracranial pressure and cerebral perfusion pressure
P_aCO_2 values affect the accuracy of measurements
Occasional false-positive results
Measures velocity at a certain point, not the cerebral blood flow

electrodes are placed symmetrically on the scalp and a 16-channel EEG recording is obtained. A normal EEG tracing is symmetrical across the two hemispheres.

The raw EEG tracing may only be read and interpreted by trained personnel. This EEG recording contains three parameters: amplitude, frequency, and time. The height of the EEG wave is its amplitude, measured in volts (V). Frequency is the number of cycles, or basically the number of times the wave crosses the zero line, per unit of time, and is reported in hertz (Hz). The raw EEG recording is continuous in time but for the purpose of processing the EEG a sample *epoch* is selected.

Four EEG frequency bands have been described: alpha (8–13 Hz), beta (>13 Hz), theta (4–7 Hz) and delta (<4 Hz). The predominant rhythm in awake patients is in the beta range, which is a high-frequency, low-amplitude waveform. Under deep anesthesia, lower-frequency rhythms predominate.

Interpretation of the raw EEG essentially entails correlating the tracing with the described clinical states. This correlation is derived experimentally, and requires training and experience. With the advent of more sophisticated modern microprocessors, computerized interpretation of the raw EEG has gained popularity. Through computerized analysis, the data contained in the EEG is converted into a format that is more easily comprehensible. (One such algorithm has been developed for use in a device called the bispectral index (BIS) monitor, described later.) Typical clinical states identified by EEG are consciousness, unconsciousness, sleep, epilepsy, and coma.

Intraoperatively, clinicians may desire to use the EEG for: adjustment of anesthetic doses to prevent recall and avoid overdose; diagnosis and prevention of acute cerebral ischemia; and achievement of electrocerebral silence.

Indeed, anesthesiologists have long tried to use the EEG, in conjunction with hemodynamic data, to monitor the depth of anesthesia. This has not been very successful, for two major reasons:

- The drugs used in modern anesthesiology practice do not produce the same effect on the EEG signal. This is compounded by the fact that anesthesiologists commonly use a combination of medications in their regimen.
- Other factors may influence the EEG signal, including hypoxia, hypotension, and hypothermia.

The EEG effects produced by isoflurane, sevoflurane, and desflurane are very similar. With increasing dose, there is initial slowing, progressing to burst suppression and, ultimately, total suppression of the EEG at high doses. This same pattern is seen with increasing doses of barbiturates, propofol, and etomidate. Other drugs, such as opiates and benzodiazepines, even other inhalational anesthetics, produce different effects on the EEG signal.

Early diagnosis and prevention of acute cerebral ischemia relies on detecting the changes in the EEG tracing

---

Box 4-27   Indications for Intraoperative Electroencephalographic Monitoring

Intraoperative monitoring is indicated for the prevention of cerebral ischemia, including:
Cerebrovascular surgery: carotid endarterectomy
Cardiopulmonary bypass and/or deep hypothermia
Controlled hypotension
Epilepsy surgery

Box 4-28   Limitations of Intraoperative Electroencephalographic Monitoring

Need for trained personnel for interpretation
Expensive and bulky equipment
Electrical interferences
Polypharmacy in the clinical practice of anesthesiology
Individual variability

---

indicative of cellular dysfunction due to hypoxemia. At this stage, the neurons are still alive and salvageable by restoring perfusion to the ischemic areas. It is estimated that 50% of the brain oxygen consumption is directed toward the generation of the EEG signal. Administration of barbiturates leads to dose-related slowing of the EEG. Higher doses result in burst suppression, eventually progressing to electrical silence. Although controversial, barbiturate-induced electrocerebral silence has been suggested as a modality to reduce cerebral oxygen demand as a method of brain protection (Boxes 4-27 and 4-28).

Bispectral Index

The bispectral index monitors and processes the EEG to yield a single number ranging from 0 to 100. The sensor used is for a frontotemporal electrode montage. It is a single patch containing three electrodes. The monitor itself displays the raw EEG, the electromyelographic strength, the BIS number, and the BIS trend. The lower the BIS number the deeper the hypnotic state. The BIS is a single number derived from the information obtained from the EEG. A sample epoch of 30 seconds is analyzed for EEG power and frequency, and additional data is computed through a mathematical technique called *bispectral analysis*. The BIS is an empirical, statistically-derived number based on a large pool of EEG readings. This number correlates with the level of sedation or hypnosis, regardless of what agent was used to produce this clinical state.

Table 4-6   Bispectral Index Monitoring

Bispectral Index Number	Clinical State
100	Awake
70–90	Light to moderate sedation
60–70	Light hypnotic state (low probability of recall)
45–60	Moderate hypnotic state
<40	Deep hypnotic state
0	Isoelectric electroencephalogram

Bispectral index monitoring uses an algorithm to analyze the raw EEG patterns and translate them into a number that correlates with the hypnotic level (Table 4-6).

It is widely accepted that a BIS value between 45 and 60 is associated with the hypnotic level needed for general anesthesia. This range correlates well with the loss of consciousness and lack of recall.

Intraoperative monitoring with the BIS may offer many potential benefits, including reduced risk of awareness and recall, and anesthetic dose adjustment to the individual patient's requirements, minimizing underdosing or overdosing and leading to a faster recovery.

The bispectral index value is highly predictive of the hypnotic level and probability of recall. It is not greatly valuable as a predictor of movement and hemodynamic response to surgical stimulation. These are mostly dependent on the anesthetic technique. Movement in response to surgical stimulation is a spinal cord reflex. A patient who is anesthetized by isoflurane alone with a BIS value indicative of adequate hypnosis may still react to surgical stimulation. Indeed, the concentration of isoflurane required to prevent movement or hemodynamic response to stimulation is higher than that needed to achieve hypnosis. However, when opioid analgesics are administered as adjuncts during general anesthesia, the BIS value does not correlate with the patient's response to surgical stimulation.

In addition, other factors may affect the reliability of the derived BIS value. They include cerebral ischemia with subsequent EEG slowing, hypothermia resulting in EEG suppression, and artifact interfering with accurate data collection and analysis.

Finally, the potential for cost savings promised by the BIS technology is, at least partially, offset by the cost of the equipment and its sensors.

Evoked Potentials

Evoked potentials are electrical signals generated in the neural pathways in response to external stimuli. These small evoked responses are then recorded at various points along the neural pathway to examine the functional integrity of the tested structures. EPs generated in the cortex and subcortex have a much smaller amplitude (0.1–20 μV) than the background EEG; therefore the EP signal has to be extracted from the EEG.

Evoked potentials are represented by a plot of voltage versus time. An evoked response is commonly described by the latency and the peak amplitude of each of the waveforms. *Latency* is the time from the stimulation to the time the response is recorded, and *amplitude* is the strength of the recorded signal. The overall purpose of monitoring EP is to detect any injury to the nervous system in the early stages before it is irreversible. It is crucial to determine the baseline latency and peak amplitude prior to any manipulations. Any change from the baseline, such as increased latency, decreased amplitude, change in waveform morphology, or total loss of the signal, is significant and has to be investigated for the possible cause.

Evoked potentials are subcategorized into two groups: sensory evoked potentials (SEPs), and motor evoked potentials (MEPs). Three sensory pathways are used for intraoperative monitoring: somatosensory, brain-stem auditory, and visual. SEPs are recorded using scalp electrodes positioned according to the international 10–20 montage. MEPs assess the descending motor pathways. Many factors affect the EP signals, including inhalational and intravenous anesthetics and physiologic factors such as hypothermia and hypotension (see Box 4-22).

Somatosensory Evoked Potentials

The SSEP is the most common type of EP monitored in the operating room. Generation of the SSEP involves stimulating a sensory nerve, at a rate of 1–2 Hz, and measuring the electrical response rostrally along the nervous system tract activated. The electrical stimulus is delivered to the nerve by a skin-surface electrode or a subcutaneous fine-needle electrode. If the integrity of the neural pathway is intact, the electrical signal is transmitted from the periphery to the contralateral sensory cortex. The most commonly used peripheral nerves are median, ulnar, peroneal, and posterior tibial nerves. Other possible sites are trigeminal and pudendal nerves and the tongue.

Multiple recording sites are usually employed along the stimulated nerve, over the spinal cord, brain stem, and cerebral cortex. This allows for evaluation of the response, after traversing the surgical site, allows for some redundancy in case of technical problems, and helps point to the site of insult with better accuracy. SSEP monitoring allows for continuous evaluation of the spinal cord function throughout the surgical procedure as opposed to the wake-up test. The neuronal activities from the upper extremity primarily represent proprioception and vibration and ascend in the spinal cord via the ipsilateral dorsal column. In contrast, neuronal activities from the lower extremity have additional components that pass in the spinocerebellar pathways. The posterior columns are supplied completely by the posterior spinal artery, whereas the anterior spinal artery, which also supplies the motor tracts, supplies the spinocerebellar tract. Therefore, ischemic injury to the spinocerebellar tract would be expected to affect the motor tracts as well.

The correlation of SSEP monitoring and neurologic injury is not exact, and there are reports of neural injury without intraoperative changes in SSEP. The spinal cord can tolerate ischemia for about 20 minutes, and continuous loss of the SSEP waveform for less than 15 minutes is not associated with permanent neurologic deficit. In contrast, persistent loss of the waveform for longer periods would probably result in neurologic injury.

Many nonpathologic factors may influence the SSEP signal, including the anesthetic agents and technique used, and some physiologic factors, such as hypothermia and hypotension. In general, intravenous anesthetics have a much less depressant effect on the SSEP than inhalational agents. A generally acceptable technique for SSEP monitoring would constitute a 0.7 MAC of inhalational agents supplemented with an intravenous infusion of an opiate.

Somatosensory EP monitoring is indicated during spinal fusion with Harrington rod instrumentation or spinal stabilization, resection of spinal tumors, repair of aortic aneurysms, and brachial plexus exploration.

A major limitation of SSEP monitoring is that the region at risk may not be amenable to monitoring.

Brain-Stem Auditory Evoked Potentials

The auditory pathway is the most metabolically active part of the conscious brain and is the last sense suppressed by anesthesia. Brain-stem auditory evoked potentials (BAEPs) are recorded by stimulation of the cochlea using pulse sound waves delivered into the ear canal. The evoked responses are transmitted along the auditory pathway. The recording electrodes are placed on the lobe of the ipsilateral ear and on top of the head. BAEP monitoring is indicated for acoustic neuroma resection, posterior fossa exploration, basilar artery aneurysm clipping, and procedures involving cranial nerves V, VIII, and IX. Volatile anesthetics increase the latency of the BAEP, while the amplitude is not affected. BAEP are relatively resistant to the effects of hypotension.

Visual Evoked Potentials

Visual evoked potentials (VEPs) are cortical EPs recorded after stimulation of the retina by flashing lights by recording electrodes placed on the scalp. VEP monitoring is indicated during surgery around the optic nerve and tract, such as pituitary surgery and craniopharyngioma resection, and surgery on the anterior cranial fossa.

The use of VEP monitoring is limited by technical difficulties due to the site of the surgery (anterior fossa), closed eyelids, and size of the pupil. In addition, VEPs are

the modality most sensitive to the effects of inhalational anesthetics.

Motor Evoked Potentials

Whereas SSEP monitors the dorsolateral tracts, motor evoked potentials (MEPs) monitor the functional integrity of the descending motor pathways in the anterior spinal cord. The motor cortex is stimulated, either electrically or by a magnetic field, and the evoked responses are recorded along the spinal cord, a peripheral nerve, or the innervated muscle. Alternatively, the spinal cord may be directly stimulated at levels above the surgical field and the responses are then registered along the cord but beyond the surgical field, or over the nerve and the muscle itself. Simultaneous monitoring with MEP and SSEP may offer the opportunity to monitor both the anterior and posterior pathways during surgical procedures. Indeed, loss of motor function without recorded changes in SSEP has been reported. MEPs are profoundly depressed by inhalational anesthetics, even at relatively low concentrations. The management of muscle relaxants while monitoring MEP is complex. It is safest to avoid these agents but they may be used if the EPs are recorded along the spinal cord and over the nerve, and not on the muscle. The efficacy of MEP monitoring as a predictor of surgical outcome has not been tested by large studies, and is mostly based on anecdotal reports.

Motor evoked potential monitoring is indicated during procedures where the structural integrity or blood supply to the spinal cord, especially the ventral pathways, may be at risk, including neurosurgical, orthopedic, or vascular surgery.

Electromyelogram

The electromyelogram is recorded from fine wires inserted into muscle innervated by a nerve that is stimulated by surgical irritation or instrumentation, and represents the muscle's spontaneous electrical activity. Its most common application is for intraoperative monitoring of the facial nerve, and it is best to avoid the associated use of muscle relaxants.

Other Considerations

Evoked potentials are affected by many factors other than neurologic damage. General anesthesia can influence the synaptic transmissions and neuronal activity, either directly or by altering tissue perfusion. Volatile anesthetics influence the evoked responses by increasing the latency and decreasing the amplitude. In general, intravenous anesthetics are safer to use, especially when monitoring SEP. Etomidate is a unique agent. It has minimal effect on the MEP, while increasing both latency and amplitude of the SEP.

Various physiologic factors affect EPs, including hypothermia, hypotension, hypocarbia, hypercarbia, and anemia. Finally, the structures at risk of injury during the surgical procedure may not be amenable to monitoring.

No contraindications to EP monitoring have been reported. Potential risks and complications are mostly related to the electrodes, including electrical shock or burn, skin irritation, and possible breakage of the fine-needle electrodes.

Brain Tissue Oxygen Partial Pressure

Brain tissue oxygen partial pressure ($P_{bti}O_2$) monitoring is an invasive technique for continuous measurement and evaluation of brain tissue oxygenation. The monitor consists of a sensor that is inserted into the brain parenchyma through a small hole in the skull. Whereas jugular venous oxygen saturation ($S_{jv}O_2$) monitors global cerebral oxygenation, $P_{bti}O_2$ monitoring provides direct measurement of brain tissue PO_2.

The type of tissue into which the sensor is to be placed remains controversial. There is good reason not to place the probe in the infarcted tissue. Probably, the sensor must be placed in the "penumbra zone" or even the undamaged brain tissue, because then the therapy can be better directed.

Studies have shown a good correlation between different CPP values and both $S_{jv}O_2$ and $P_{bti}O_2$. Additionally, as compared to $S_{jv}O_2$, $P_{bti}O_2$ yields better quality measurements when both monitors are inserted simultaneously.

In summary, $P_{bti}O_2$ measurement gives good-quality information about brain tissue oxygenation, and its measure is complementary to that given with jugular bulb oxygen determinations, providing the opportunity for better patient management (Box 4-29).

Jugular Venous Oxygen Saturation

Jugular venous oxygen saturation is the result of the difference between cerebral oxygen delivery and cerebral metabolic rate for oxygen ($CMRO_2$). Cerebral oxygen delivery is affected by such factors as cerebral blood flow (CBF), arterial oxygen saturation (S_aO_2), hemoglobin concentration (Hb), and the hemoglobin dissociation curve. The Fick equation relates these variables:

$$CMRO_2 = CBF \times a - vDO_2,$$

where $a - vDO_2$ is the arteriovenous O_2 difference, which is the difference in content of oxygen (C_aO_2), and:

$$C_aO_2 = ([Hb] \times \% \text{ saturation} \times 1.34) + (\text{arterial or venous } O_2 \text{ tension} \times 0.003).$$

Thus, it is apparent that $S_{jv}O_2$ is a function of arterial saturation, $CMRO_2$, and cerebral blood flow. The normal range of $S_{jv}O_2$ is 55–75%, although this range remains controversial. Low $S_{jv}O_2$ readings may indicate inadequate cerebral perfusion, while elevated $S_{jv}O_2$ readings could be due to cerebral hyperemia. In general, assessment of $S_{jv}O_2$ may indirectly indicate whether cerebral blood flow is coupled with the brain's energy requirements.

Jugular venous oxygen saturation can be obtained by intermittent sampling of the internal jugular venous blood, or continuously monitored by inserting a fiberoptic catheter into the jugular bulb. The catheter is placed similarly to an internal jugular approach for CVP monitoring. Once the internal jugular vein is cannulated percutaneously, a 5 French introducer or 4.5 French peel-away introducer is placed into the vein using a Seldinger technique. The fiberoptic catheter is inserted over the introducer into the vein until the tip is felt to be at the base of the skull. The catheter tip placement is then confirmed radiologically.

It is also crucial to choose the correct side to insert the catheter. The flow rate in the right and left jugular veins may not be the same from individual to individual. Indeed, cranial venous drainage is asymmetric, and usually greater on the right (in 55–65% of individuals). In general, the side most affected by the pathology should be selected. For bilateral global monitoring, the dominant side may be identified by using ultrasound imaging, and cannulated.

Indications for intraoperative monitoring of $S_{jv}O_2$ include neurosurgical cases, management of acute brain injuries, and cardiac surgery with cardiopulmonary bypass and hypothermia. Complications include carotid artery puncture, hematoma formation, thrombosis, and, rarely, raised ICP (Box 4-30).

Box 4-29   Advantages and Disadvantages of Brain Tissue Oxygen Partial Pressure Measurement

ADVANTAGES

Provides data for oxygenation at the tissue level
Complements the data regarding the global oxygenation from $S_{jv}O_2$

DISADVANTAGES/LIMITATIONS

An invasive monitor with potential risks and complications similar to those of ICP
Provides focal oxygenation data and may not adequately represent other cerebral regions
Clinical reliability not yet proven

Transcranial Cerebral Oximetry

Transcranial cerebral oximetry (TCCO) is a continuous, direct, noninvasive method of monitoring cerebral oxygen saturation. It continuously measures the cerebral concentrations of oxyhemoglobin and deoxyhemoglobin by detecting the absorption of near infrared light;

Box 4-30   Advantages and Disadvantages of Jugular Venous Oxygen Saturation Monitoring

ADVANTAGES

Reflects the overall balance between cerebral oxygen supply and demand

Provides an early warning of cerebral ischemia and augments the knowledge of what happens with cerebral blood flow and autoregulation. May be a valuable tool for detecting and treating insufficient cerebral oxygenation in patients after intracranial hemorrhage

Plays a significant role in the management of neurologically critically ill patients, to optimize therapy and for outcome prediction

DISADVANTAGES/LIMITATIONS

Unilateral $S_{jv}O_2$ measurement may not be representative of truly mixed bihemispheric cerebral venous blood

A global measurement of cerebral oxygenation and metabolism and as such may not detect small regions of ischemia. A normal or elevated $S_{jv}O_2$ does not exclude the presence of cerebral ischemia

$S_{jv}O_2$ values are indicative of the adequacy of cerebral blood flow relative to $CMRO_2$. Changes in $S_{jv}O_2$ reflect changes in cerebral blood flow *only* if $CMRO_2$ remains constant. $CMRO_2$ values range from 0.72 to 4.85 mL O_2/100 g/min

Other variables such as S_aO_2, Hb, and the Hb dissociation curve affect the value of the $S_{jv}O_2$

Readings are not sensitive for cerebellum/brain-stem blood flow and/or ischemia

Technical limitations such as need for frequent calibration and inaccuracies due to the catheter tip resting against the vessel wall

---

Box 4-31   Advantages and Disadvantages of Transcranial Cerebral Oximetry

ADVANTAGES

Noninvasive

Allows frequent readings

Easy to use and may be readily accessible

DISADVANTAGES/LIMITATIONS

Accuracy is affected by extracranial blood flow

Has a high rate of false-positive readings

In patients with severe head injury, readings do not correlate well with $S_{jv}O_2$ values because TCCO does not reflect changes in blood pressure or in P_aCO_2

Clinical reliability, sensitivity, and specificity for detecting brain ischemia are not yet determined

---

therefore it is also referred to as transcranial near-infrared spectroscopy (NIRS). Although its reliability in clinical practice is yet to be proved, studies have shown that TCCO is at least as sensitive to cerebral hypoxia as the EEG, and that it reliably detects changes in cerebral oxygenation during carotid endarterectomy.

A commercial model, INVOS 3100 (Somanetics Corp., Troy, MI), uses two wavelengths (750 and 850 nm) and displays a percentage value of regional cerebral oxygenation, calculated from the ratio between oxygenated hemoglobin and total hemoglobin in brain tissue. It is capable of detecting tissue hypoxia deep to the scalp. INVOS uses two detectors: the close one measures saturation of the superficial structures (scalp and skull), and the far detector samples both superficial and deep structures (scalp, skull, and brain). By subtracting the value of close detector sample from the far one, the oxygen saturation of the deep structures (brain) is calculated (Box 4-31).

Neuromonitoring: A Summary

The proper management of CNS injury consists of early prevention, detection, and correction of ischemia. In patients undergoing CNS surgery, without pre-existing CNS injury, perioperative monitoring with EEG and EP may be sufficient. On the other hand, if prior CNS injury, such as head injury or intracranial hemorrhage, is a concern, then other modalities may be employed to better guide the therapeutic management. ICP and CPP monitoring give an indication of cerebral blood flow. Monitoring TCCO could be an adjunct to CPP management to better guide cerebral perfusion. In turn, combined $S_{jv}O_2$ and $P_{bti}O_2$ measurements help determine whether cerebral blood flow is coupled with the brain's energy requirements. TCD ultrasonography may give additional information about cerebral hemodynamic status. Concomitant monitoring with TCD and TCCO may be a reliable method for detecting reduced cerebral circulation in clinical practice. Table 4-7 is a summary of various clinical settings and the neuromonitors that may be most appropriate for the setting.

SUMMARY

Basic and more advanced monitors have become an essential part of intraoperative patient care. The benefits of these monitoring modalities can only be realized by integrating the information obtained from the monitors with those obtained from the history and physical examination. When considering the potential applications of these monitors, the following are necessary conditions before deciding on the need for a particular monitor.

Table 4-7 Value of Different Neuromonitors in Various Clinical Settings

	Exam	EEG	SSEP	BAEP	VEP	MEP	ICP	TCD	$S_{jv}O_2$	TCCO	CNM
Head trauma	++++	+	+	+	0	0	++++	++	++	++	0
Carotid endarterectomy	++++	++++	+++	0	0	0	0	+++	++	+	0
Cardiopulmonary bypass	0	++	+	0	0	0	0	+++	++	++	0
Supratentorial tumor	0	+	+	0	0	0	+-++++	0	+	+	0
Brain-stem surgery	0	0	++	+++	0	0	0	0-+	0	0	+++
Cerebral aneurysm	++++	++	+++	0-++	0-++	0	0-+++	+++	++	++	0
Acoustic neuroma	++++	0	0-+	++++	0	0	0	0	0	0	++++
Cranial nerve surgery	++++	0	+	0-+++	0	0	0	0	0	0	++++
Pituitary surgery	0	0-+	0-+	0	+++	0	0	0	0	0	0
Spinal surgery	++++	0	++++	0	0	+++	0	0	0	0	0

0, none; +, minimal; ++, moderate; +++, considerable; ++++, might be considered a standard of care. BAEP, brain-stem auditory evoked potential; CNM, cranial nerve monitoring; EEG, electroencephalogram; ICP, intracranial pressure; MEP, motor evoked potential; $S_{jv}O_2$, jugular venous oxygen saturation; SSEP, somatosensory evoked potential; TCCO, transcranial cerebral oximetry; TCD, transcranial Doppler; VEP, visual evoked potential.

- Thorough preoperative evaluation is a key factor in deciding what additional intraoperative monitoring is necessary.
- The monitor must have a reasonable sensitivity and specificity for early detection of pathologic conditions.
- The intraoperative team must be able to interpret changes and distinguish injury from benign variations, anesthetic effect, or technical failure.
- The intraoperative team must have the latitude and therapeutic options to respond appropriately to these pathologic conditions.

Even the most sophisticated monitors cannot and will not replace the role of a vigilant anesthesiologist, to care for the anesthetized patient, to monitor the physiologic parameters, and to integrate the data to optimize care and safety.

Acknowledgments

We would like to extend our gratitude to Dr Selma Calmes for her mentoring and guidance, and to Dr Rachel Micelli for her valuable assistance with this project.

CHAPTER 5

Anesthetics and Anesthetic Adjuvants

RANDALL M. SCHELL

EDWIN A. BOWE

INTRODUCTION

The choice of anesthetic agents used and anesthetic technique (e.g., regional, general, local, sedation) performed vary by patient and procedure. The goals of general anesthesia, including hypnosis, amnesia, analgesia, and possibly immobility and blockade of autonomic responses, can be provided by multiple combinations of intravenous and inhaled anesthetics. There is a paucity of data to prescribe one technique over another with regard to important measures of outcome. Therefore, the choice of anesthetic agents and adjuvants administered during the perioperative period is often based on anesthesiologist preference, associated side effects, and economics.

Although clinical perceptions and theoretical considerations suggest that regional anesthesia should be safer than general anesthesia, current outcome studies suggest there is no difference in mortality and major morbidity between the two in most populations, including the elderly.

The concept of preinjury analgesic administration (pre-emptive analgesia) in an attempt to reduce postoperative pain remains controversial.

Current Controversies: Pre-emptive Analgesia

Concept: To reduce the magnitude and duration of postoperative pain by the pre-injury administration of various medications

Pre-emptive analgesia may be attempted by intravenous and oral premedicants (e.g., non steroidal anti-inflammatory drugs [NSAIDs], acetaminophen, opioids, ketamine), regional anesthesia techniques, and local anesthetic presurgical wound infiltration

The benefit from pre-injury analgesic administration has been demonstrated experimentally in animals but at present there is minimal support for the belief that pre-emptive techniques aid recovery in humans

A recent meta-analysis did not support the potential beneficial effect of pre-emptive analgesia on postoperative pain

Future studies are likely to focus on "protective analgesia" strategies aimed at the prevention of pain hypersensitivity or pathologic pain

LOCAL ANESTHETIC AGENTS

Local anesthetic action can occur on any electrically excitable cell in the central or peripheral nervous system and cardiac muscle, producing conduction blockade of neural impulses and insensitivity to stimuli by reversibly blocking sodium channels. With progressive increases in concentrations of local anesthetics, the transmission of autonomic, sensory, and motor impulses is interrupted. Local anesthetics are applied cutaneously, subcutaneously, adjacent to peripheral nerves, and in the subarachnoid and epidural space to produce anesthesia. Lidocaine is also administered intravenously to deepen general anesthesia, reduce the pain associated with intravenous injection of induction agents such as propofol and etomidate, and treat ventricular dysrhythmias. The major factors distinguishing the various local anesthetics include the class (ester versus amide), onset time, duration of action, and risk of systemic toxicity when absorbed.

Chemistry

The local anesthetic molecule consists of (1) a lipophilic group (aromatic ring), connected by (2) an intermediate side chain (ester or amide) to (3) a hydrophilic ionizable group (usually a tertiary amine). The prototypical ester local anesthetic is procaine and the prototypical amide local anesthetic is lidocaine (Figure 5-1). The intermediate chain bond, ester or amide, determines local anesthetic class and mode of metabolism (Table 5-1). The ester linkage is hydrolyzed very rapidly in the blood by plasma esterases and the amide linkage more slowly by liver microsomal oxygenases. The tertiary amine group of the local anesthetic can accept a proton and become a charged quaternary amine. Local anesthetics are there-

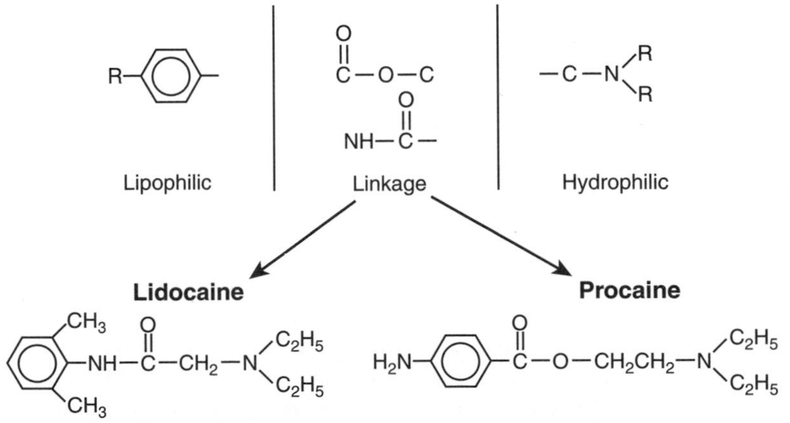

Figure 5-1 The prototypical ester local anesthetic procaine and amide local anesthetic lidocaine.

Table 5-1	Local Anesthetic Classes
Esters	**Amides**
Cocaine	Lidocaine (Xylocaine)
Procaine (Novocain)	Bupivacaine (Marcaine, Sensorcaine)
Tetracaine (Pontocaine)	Levobupivacaine (Chirocaine)
Chloroprocaine (Nesacaine)	Etidocaine (Duranest)
Benzocaine (Americaine)	Prilocaine (Citanest)
	Ropivacaine (Naropin)
	Mepivacaine (Carbocaine, Isocaine)
	Dibucaine (Nupercaine)

As a general rule, esters have only one "i" in their generic name (procaine) while amides have two (lidocaine).

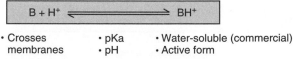

Figure 5-2   The pH of tissues and pKa of the local anesthetic determines the relative amount in the ionized or non-ionized state.

fore weak bases. The non-ionized lipophilic form (B) crosses membranes and enters nerve cells while the ionized cationic form (BH+) is thought to be the active form at the sodium channel. The pH of tissues and pKa ($\approx$7.6–9.1) of the local anesthetic determines the relative amount in each state. They are marketed as hydrochloride salts at a low pH which are then highly ionized and water-soluble (Figure 5-2).

Action

The un-ionized lipid soluble form (B) of the ester or amide local anesthetic crosses the lipid barriers of the epineurium and the cell wall. The molecule exists as both the ionized and un-ionized form in an equilibrium dependent on the surrounding pH and the pKa of the local anesthetic. The ionized form (BH+) enters the internal portion of the sodium channel during the open depolarized state and disrupts sodium conductance. The membrane expansion theory, a less recognized explanation of local anesthetic action, hypothesizes that lipophilic local anesthetics such as benzocaine become incorporated into the cell membrane, expanding it and

preventing the opening of pores like the sodium channel. The rate of depolarization of the nerve action potential is slowed such that the threshold potential is not reached and an action potential cannot be propagated. Local anesthetics do not change the threshold potential or resting membrane potential (Figure 5-3).

Susceptibility to Blockade

Different types of nerve fibers differ significantly in their susceptibility to local anesthetic blockade on the basis of size and myelination (Figure 5-4). The preganglionic autonomic fibers (B fibers) are the class of nerve fibers most easily blocked by local anesthetics, as evidenced by hypotension soon after administration of spinal anesthesia. Large myelinated fibers (A-alpha) are the most resistant to block, which explains why motor blockade occurs last.

Some generalizations can be made about susceptibility to blockade. The thicker the fiber the less readily it is blocked (e.g., A-alpha/motor fibers). Myelinated fibers are more readily blocked because of the need to produce blockade only at the nodes of Ranvier. The thicker the nerve fiber, the farther apart the nodes tend to be, which explains, in part, the greater resistance to blockade of larger myelinated fibers than smaller myelinated fibers. For myelinated nerves, three successive nodes of Ranvier must be blocked by the local anesthetic to halt impulse propagation and this has been termed *critical length*. Local anesthetics gain access to receptors only when sodium channels are in the activated-open state. Therefore, a resting nerve is less sensitive to local-anesthetic-induced conduction blockade

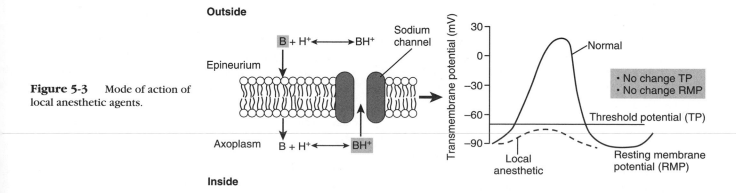

Figure 5-3   Mode of action of local anesthetic agents.

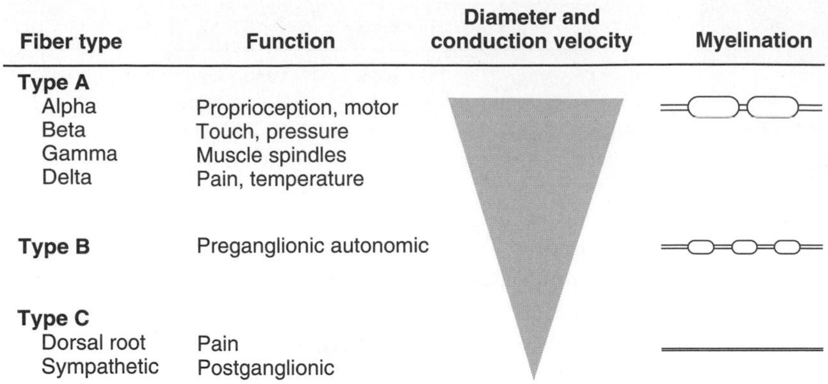

Fiber type	Function	Diameter and conduction velocity	Myelination
Type A			
Alpha	Proprioception, motor		
Beta	Touch, pressure		
Gamma	Muscle spindles		
Delta	Pain, temperature		
Type B	Preganglionic autonomic		
Type C			
Dorsal root	Pain		
Sympathetic	Postganglionic		

Figure 5-4   Different nerve fiber types differ in their function, size, and conduction velocity (A < B < C), and presence or absence of myelination.

than is a nerve that is repeatedly stimulated. This has been termed *frequency-dependent blockade*. Since thick nerve fibers are less readily blocked by local anesthetic agents than thin ones, it is possible to block pain completely (A-delta and C fibers) without significantly affecting motor function (A-alpha fibers), termed *differential blockade*. When local anesthetic is placed in the subarachnoid space, blockade usually progresses in the following order; sympathetic block with peripheral vasodilation (B fibers), loss of pain and temperature sensation, loss of proprioception, loss of touch and pressure sensation, and then motor paralysis.

In summary, other things being equal, the minimum concentration (C_m) of local anesthetic necessary to produce conduction blockade of nerve impulses is less for smaller-diameter fibers, myelinated fibers, increased tissue pH, high frequency of nerve stimulation, and sensory fibers. Conversely, the C_m is increased for larger-diameter fibers, decreased tissue pH, and motor fibers.

Pharmacokinetics

Clinically, local anesthetics are injected as close to the targeted nerves as possible. The un-ionized form (B) crosses the membranes and penetrates the nerve sheath and diffuses through the epineural connective tissues before entering the nerve bundles, the final and major barrier being the perilemma. The ionized form (BH^+) binds to sodium channels. Eventually, equilibrium is reached between the nerve membrane and surrounding medium, and the block begins to regress from the outer portion of the nerve first, and then the core.

Absorption

Local anesthetics rapidly diffuse through tissue and are absorbed into the systemic circulation via surrounding capillaries and lymphatics. The rate of systemic absorption is proportionate to the vascularity of the site of injection; intravenous > tracheal > intercostal > caudal >

remainder of the epidural space > brachial plexus > lower extremity nerve blocks > subcutaneous tissue. In general, local anesthetics (excluding cocaine) relax vascular smooth muscle, resulting in vasodilation. If a vasoconstrictor such as epinephrine (concentration 1:200,000 = 5 μg/mL) is added to a local anesthetic, systemic absorption can be slowed, minimizing peak blood levels of the local anesthetic and clinically prolonging the block by up to 50%, especially for the short- and intermediate-duration local anesthetics. Epinephrine should not be added to local anesthetics for peripheral nerve block anesthesia in areas that may lack collateral blood flow such as the ears, nose, fingers, penis, and toes. The addition of epinephrine to local anesthetics is also not recommended in patients with unstable angina pectoris, cardiac dysrhythmias, a history of hypertension, and uteroplacental insufficiency, and for intravenous regional anesthesia (e.g., Bier block). The maximum dose of epinephrine should not exceed 10 μg/kg in pediatric patients or 200–250 μg in adults.

Physiochemical Properties

Lipid Solubility

The most important property determining the potency of a local anesthetic is lipid solubility. Potency is also increased by increasing the length of the intermediate chain and amino groups.

Duration of Action

The duration of action of local anesthetics is related to their affinity for protein compounds (e.g., protein binding) such as the sodium channel, itself a protein structure. In general, the potent, long-acting, highly lipophilic agents such as tetracaine, etidocaine, and bupivacaine are highly protein-bound. In the near future, local anesthetics with liposomes and polymer microspheres will likely provide extended duration of analgesia of days following a single injection, without the need for catheters, pumps, or infusion systems.

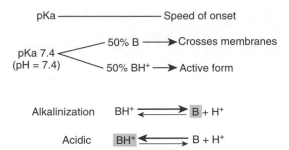

Figure 5-5   The pH of the surrounding environment and pKa of the local anesthetic determine the relative amount in the ionized or non-ionized state. Alkalinization of the local anesthetic speeds the onset and acidification slows the onset of local anesthetic action.

Drug Interactions: Local Anesthetics

Succinylcholine and ester local anesthetics depend on pseudocholinesterase for metabolism – possible potentiation of effects when administered concomitantly

Pseudocholinesterase inhibitors (e.g., echothiophate, neostigmine, phenelzine, cyclophosphamide, and trimethaphan) can potentiate ester local anesthetic effects and duration of action.

Nondepolarizing muscle relaxant blockade is potentiated by local anesthetics

Medications that decrease hepatic blood flow (cimetidine, propranolol) may decrease amide local anesthetic (lidocaine) clearance.

pKa

The pKa determines speed of onset of neural blockade (Figure 5-5). The pKa of commonly used local anesthetics ranges from 7.6–8.9. The amine group of the weak base local anesthetic exists both in the uncharged base form (B) and as a positively charged cation (BH$^+$). The pKa is the pH at which 50% of the local anesthetic is in the charged form and 50% uncharged. Agents with a lower pKa value, such as mepivacaine (pKa 7.6) and lidocaine (pKa 7.8), will have a faster onset because a greater fraction of the molecules will exist in the uncharged form and thus will more easily diffuse across nerve membranes. However, the pKa of local anesthetics is greater than 7.4, the normal pH of the body. Therefore, more of the local exists as BH$^+$ at normal tissue pH, the form that doesn't cross membranes as well. Commercially prepared solutions containing epinephrine are more acidic, which prevents spontaneous hydrolysis of the solution. The greater acidity leads to more immediately available ionized drug (BH$^+$) and slows the onset of action of local anesthetic. Addition of bicarbonate (e.g., 1 mL bicarbonate to 9 mL lidocaine, 0.1 mL bicarbonate for each 9.9 mL bupivacaine) to a local anesthetic before injection increases the un-ionized form, the form that easily crosses lipid membranes and speeds the onset of neural blockade. Local anesthetics are not very effective when injected into infected tissue such as an abscess, which has a low pH, causing more of the drug to be in the ionized (BH$^+$) form and less in the non-ionized form (B).

Metabolism

The amide local anesthetics undergo slow metabolism by hepatic microsomal enzymes. Hepatic insufficiency and drugs such as cimetidine decrease hepatic clearance. Ester local anesthetics are rapidly hydrolyzed in the blood by plasma cholinesterase, which prevents accumulation of ester local anesthetics in the plasma and decreases the risk of systemic toxicity. The duration of action may be prolonged in patients with pseudocholinesterase deficiency.

Clinical Pharmacology

Most local anesthetics are poorly soluble in oil and therefore do not cross lipid membranes such as the skin very well. However the local anesthetics used for topical anesthesia may be placed on mucous membranes of areas such as the nose, mouth, tracheobronchial tree or anus to produce topical anesthesia of the most superficial layers of skin and mucosa. Cocaine is used for topical anesthesia and vasoconstriction in nasal surgery. Lidocaine, tetracaine, and benzocaine provide topical anesthesia of the mouth and tracheobronchial tree. Eutectic mixture of local anesthetics (EMLA) is a cream composed of a mixture of two amide local anesthetics, lidocaine (2.5%) and prilocaine (2.5%), placed on the skin to provide analgesia for superficial surgical procedures and for the placement of intravenous catheters. Local infiltration is designed to produce sensory anesthesia in the injected area without any attempt to block specific nerves. Lidocaine (0.5-2.0%) is frequently used for infiltration to provide anesthesia for suturing wounds. Longer-acting agents such as bupivacaine (0.25-0.5%) are infiltrated into surgical wounds for postoperative pain management. Local anesthetics may be injected into the tissues surrounding individual peripheral nerves or nerve plexuses such as the brachial plexus (e.g., ≈30-40 mL) to provide anesthesia and skeletal muscle paralysis of the area supplied by that nerve. Bupivacaine (0.25-0.5%), ropivacaine (0.25-0.5%), lidocaine (0.5-1.5%), mepivacaine (0.5-1.5%), and 2-chloroprocaine (1-2%) are the most frequently used. Local anesthetics placed into the lumbar epidural space provide analgesia for labor and delivery, and for abdominal and lower extremity surgery. By increasing the volume administered, the dermatomal level may be raised, and by increasing the concentration both sensory and motor blockade may be produced. Bupivacaine, lidocaine, chloroprocaine, and ropivacaine are most commonly used. Spinal anesthesia is produced by injection of the local anesthetics lidocaine, bupivacaine, or tetracaine into the lumbar subarachnoid space, blocking sensory, motor, and sympathetic fibers resulting in loss of sensation, inability to move muscles, and decreased blood pressure.

Side Effects

Allergic Reactions

The overall incidence of true allergic reactions to local anesthetics is very low, the majority of those being related to ester local anesthetics. Ester local anesthetics are metabolized to para-aminobenzoic acid (PABA) derivatives responsible for allergic reactions evidenced by dermatitis, bronchospasm, or anaphylaxis in a small percentage of the population sensitized by prior exposure to chemical environs. Allergic reactions to amides are extremely rare. The preservatives methylparaben and metabisulfite, present in multi-dose vials, can provoke an allergic response. Intravascular injection in the dentist's office after attempted oral block with local anesthetics containing high concentrations of epinephrine can result in tachycardia, palpitations, and tinnitus, which may be reported as an "allergy" to local anesthetics.

Systemic Toxicity

The adverse systemic effects of local anesthetics result from absorption of toxic amounts of these agents into the bloodstream. The magnitude of this systemic absorption and toxicity depends on the local anesthetic agent (e.g., ester << amide), dose and speed of injection, inclusion of a vasoconstrictor in the local anesthetic solution, and site of injection (e.g., intercostal nerve block). Mixtures of local anesthetics such as lidocaine and bupivacaine should be considered to have roughly additive toxic effects. Ester local anesthetics are rapidly hydrolyzed by cholinesterase enzyme, principally in the plasma but also in the liver. 2-chloroprocaine is rapidly metabolized with a plasma half-life less than 30 seconds, greatly reducing the risk of systemic toxicity following accidental intravascular injection and decreasing the risk of neonatal local anesthetic toxicity in the parturient. The initial sign of systemic toxicity is often circumoral or tongue numbness and lightheadedness. The cardiovascular system is more resistant than the central nervous system to toxic effects. Hypoxia, acidosis, hypercarbia, and pregnancy potentiate systemic toxicity. Treatment of local anesthetic systemic toxicity is with supplemental oxygen, assisted ventilation and protection of the airway as required, possibly anticonvulsant therapy (e.g., midazolam, thiopental), and cardiovascular resuscitation.

Clinical Controversy: Lidocaine Toxicity and Tumescent Liposuction

Tumescent liposuction involves infiltrating fatty tissue with large volumes of dilute lidocaine and epinephrine to facilitate anesthesia and decrease blood loss

The doses of lidocaine used and recommended from small case series or uncontrolled trials in tumescent liposuction are up to eight times (55 mg/kg) the classic recommended maximum dose for lidocaine with epinephrine of 7 mg/kg

Why don't all patients have toxicity from lidocaine?
- Relatively low blood flow to adipose tissue
- Vasoconstriction from epinephrine that retards absorption
- Decreased vascularity of adipose tissue
- Increased lipophilicity of lidocaine with potential sequestration in adipose tissue

No well-designed studies have examined the pharmacokinetic and pharmacodynamic effects of tumescent lidocaine/epinephrine, although practical experience suggests that larger doses of lidocaine than classically recommended can be used in many patients without toxicity

Patients have died following tumescent liposuction, with extremely high lidocaine metabolite levels.

Central Nervous System

Initially, local anesthetics block inhibitory pathways in the brain, producing excitation demonstrated clinically by muscle twitching, and seizures. Higher doses cause blockade of both inhibitory and facilitatory pathways producing central nervous system (CNS) depression clinically manifested by coma and respiratory arrest.

Cardiovascular System

Local anesthetics in high concentrations block sodium channels in the heart. Toxicity is manifested by hypotension secondary to decreased ventricular contractility, decreased electrical conduction with block of the sinoatrial and atrioventricular node, and vasodilation that may lead to cardiovascular collapse. If cardiac arrest occurs with bupivacaine, prolonged resuscitation is indicated as it is highly protein-bound and washout from the sodium channels in the heart is slow. For persistent or recurrent ventricular fibrillation or ventricular tachycardia (VF/VT), defibrillation, epinephrine or vasopressin, and amiodarone (per Advanced Cardiac Life Support [ACLS] protocol) may be used. Bretylium was recommended in the past as the antiarrhythmic drug of choice in this scenario but is not currently available. Two newer local anesthetics, ropivacaine and levobupivacaine, contain only the S-isomer rather than the more cardiotoxic R-isomer. Standard bupivacaine is a racemic mixture of R- and S-isomers. Cocaine blocks reuptake of norepinephrine, and toxicity is known to cause hypertension, tachycardia, myocardial ischemia and infarction, and ventricular dysrhythmias. Nitroglycerin is recommended to manage coronary vasoconstriction and myocardial ischemia associated with cocaine toxicity. Although beta-blockers such as esmolol have been recommended to treat associated tachycardia, they may accentuate cocaine-induced coronary artery vasospasm.

Methemoglobinemia

Prilocaine administered in high doses (>600 mg) may result in accumulation of a metabolite (*O*-toluidine) that oxidizes hemoglobin (Fe^{2+}) to methemoglobin (Fe^{3+}), potentially resulting in cyanosis. The reduction in oxygen-carrying capacity is rarely symptomatic but may be treated after confirmation of the diagnosis (e.g., arterial blood/gas with high methemoglobin level), with oxygen supplementation and methylene blue (1–2 mg/kg intravenously). Large doses of benzocaine contained in EMLA cream and in over-the-counter sunburn treatments on disrupted skin or over large areas of the body (i.e. infant) have the potential of causing methemoglobinemia.

Neurologic/Neurotoxicity

Permanent neurologic injury after regional anesthesia is extremely rare. However, transient neurologic symptoms in the distribution of the lumbosacral nerves after "single-shot" intrathecal injection of local anesthetic and following 5% lidocaine administered through previously available spinal microcatheters has been described. Chloroprocaine has been associated with severe back pain following epidural administration. The mechanism may involve the preservative ethylenediaminetetraacetic acid (EDTA) chelating calcium in the paravertebral muscle with resultant muscle spasm. Chloroprocaine is available in a preservative-free formulation, which should be used for epidural blockade.

Clinical Caveat: Transient Neurologic Symptoms after Spinal Anesthesia

Characterized by transient neurologic symptoms or transient radicular irritation of the lumbosacral nerves manifested as moderate to severe pain in the lower back, buttocks, and posterior thighs that appears within 24 hours after complete recovery from spinal anesthesia with full recovery typical within 7 days

The delayed onset of pain reflects the time required for the neural inflammatory reaction to develop. However, pathogenesis is unclear – neurotoxicity versus inflammation?

Pain may be erroneously attributed to surgical positioning

More commonly associated with hyperbaric lidocaine for spinal anesthesia, with incidence up to 12%, and less common with tetracaine (1.6%) or bupivacaine (1.3%). Other local anesthetics (ropivacaine, mepivacaine, prilocaine, procaine) have also been associated with transient neurologic symptoms but much less than lidocaine

Incidence is highest among outpatients after surgery in the lithotomy position and lowest in inpatients and surgical positions other than lithotomy

The use of spinal lidocaine has been questioned

Clinical Calculations

A 1% solution of local anesthetic has 10 mg/mL. Therefore, a 10% solution is 100 mg/mL, and a 0.5% solution 5 mg/mL. A local anesthetic containing epinephrine at 1:200,000 concentration contains 5 μg/mL of epinephrine and 1:400,000 contains 2.5 μg/mL epinephrine. Each local anesthetic has a maximal recommended dose per weight in kilograms. The maximal dose of

Table 5-2 Local Anesthetics – Summary Points	
Amides	
Lidocaine	Maximum dose 3–4 mg/kg without epinephrine, 7 mg/kg with epinephrine (based on subcutaneous administration), transient radicular irritation with spinal use
Mepivacaine	Low pKa, fast onset
Bupivacaine	Mixture $R(+)$ and $S(-)$ isomer, cardiac toxicity, 0.75% for epidural not available, good differential block, maximum dose 2 mg/kg
Levobupivacaine	$S(-)$ isomer of bupivacaine with lower cardiovascular toxicity than racemic bupivacaine, otherwise similar pharmacology
Ropivacaine	Compared to bupivacaine, ropivacaine is the pure $S(-)$ isomer, has a different chemical structure, is less lipid-soluble, has a higher therapeutic index (less cardiotoxic), and induces greater sensory than motor blockade
Prilocaine	Component of EMLA along with lidocaine. In toxic doses may cause methemoglobinemia
Esters	
Chloroprocaine	Toxicity low, back pain/spasm after epidural (?EDTA), not for intrathecal use
Cocaine	Topical use (maximum dose 3 mg/kg), vasoconstriction, blocks reuptake of norepinephrine, causing hypertension and ventricular ectopy. Treat cocaine toxicity with nitroglycerin
Tetracaine	Potent, spinal and topical use

lidocaine without epinephrine for subcutaneous injection (infiltration) is 3-4 mg/kg and with epinephrine 7 mg/kg. A summary of local anesthetic points of clinical interest is given in Table 5-2.

PHARMACOLOGY OF PREMEDICATION

The goals of premedication may include anxiolysis, sedation, amnesia, the alleviation of preoperative pain, reduction of gastric fluid volume, increase in gastric fluid pH, reduction of the incidence of postoperative nausea and vomiting (PONV), drying of excessive secretions, prevention of autonomic reflex responses, or prophylaxis against allergic reactions. Pharmacologic premedication is typically administered 1-2 hours before induction of anesthesia, often intravenously and occasionally by the intramuscular, oral, or nasal route. The anxiolysis and amnesia provided by intravenous midazolam (0.5-2.0 mg intravenous incremental doses) make it a popular premedicant.

Benzodiazepines

Benzodiazepines (midazolam, lorazepam, and diazepam), usually administered intravenously or orally, can produce anxiolysis, anterograde amnesia, and sedation at lower doses with progression to stupor and unconsciousness at higher doses. Benzodiazepines have anticonvulsant and muscle relaxant (i.e., mediated at the spinal cord, not the neuromuscular junction) properties but lack significant analgesic effects. Diazepam and lorazepam are not water-soluble and their intravenous use necessitates nonaqueous vehicles (e.g., propylene glycol, polyethylene glycol, benzyl alcohol), which may cause local irritation and thrombophlebitis of veins, and pain on intramuscular injection. Midazolam formulations are water-soluble and less irritating and undergo a unique chemical change at physiologic pH, making the drug lipid-soluble, which allows it to readily cross the blood-brain barrier. Lorazepam is the least lipid-soluble of the benzodiazepines and midazolam the most. Lorazepam is more potent than midazolam, which is more potent than diazepam. All three undergo hepatic metabolism, with diazepam having clinically significant active metabolites. The elimination half-life of diazepam is long (diazepam > lorazepam > midazolam) and can result in excessive and prolonged sedation. The benzodiazepine antagonist flumazenil can reverse excessive sedation.

Brain sensitivity to midazolam is increased, clearance decreased, and recovery dramatically prolonged in the elderly. The net effect is a nearly 75% reduction in the dose of midazolam needed for elderly patients. Premedication with only 2 mg intravenous midazolam in elderly patients is associated with a high incidence of oxygen desaturation to less than 94% on pulse oximetry and with increased time to postanesthesia care unit discharge after short surgical procedures.

Anticholinergics

Anticholinergic medications such as atropine, scopolamine, and glycopyrrolate compete with acetylcholine at multiple effector sites in the nervous system. They are not routinely given as pharmacologic premedicants but may be used to decrease secretions, block vagal reflexes, and provide sedation and amnesia (e.g., scopolamine). Atropine and scopolamine are tertiary amines that cross the blood-brain barrier and can cause confusion and somnolence in the postoperative period. This is termed anticholinergic syndrome and can be reversed by the centrally acting anticholinesterase physostigmine (0.5-2.0 mg intravenously), which inhibits acetylcholine breakdown and therefore increases acetylcholine in the CNS. Glycopyrrolate is a quaternary amine charged molecule that does not cross the blood-brain barrier to produce CNS effects. Glycopyrrolate is commonly used for its antisialagogue effect and lack of CNS side effects, atropine for desired vagal blockade, and rarely scopolamine for amnesia and sedation. Side effects of anticholinergics include CNS toxicity (e.g., confusion), tachycardia, dilated pupils and blurred vision (e.g., mydriasis and cycloplegia), increased body temperature from suppression of sweating, lower esophageal sphincter relaxation, and increased physiologic dead space.

Opioids

Advantages of opioids for pharmacologic premedication include the absence of direct myocardial depression and the production of analgesia in patients who are experiencing pain preoperatively or who will undergo painful procedures prior to the induction of anesthesia. Morphine sulfate and meperidine are the most commonly administered opioid premedicants. In equianalgesic doses all opioids cause respiratory depression to a similar extent. Opioids stimulate the chemoreceptor trigger zone in the medulla, which in turn activates the nearby vomiting center. All opioids are capable of releasing histamine (meperidine > morphine), although the newer synthetic opioids (fentanyl, sufentanil) do not do so in clinically significant amounts. If an opioid that releases histamine is injected rapidly, hypotension may result. Opioids that do not release histamine have little or no effect on the human myocardium. Almost all commonly used opioids are not pure mu-1-receptor site agonists. Therefore, along with analgesia, they may cause drowsiness, euphoria, or dysphoria.

Increase Gastric pH and/or Decrease Gastric Volume

A major risk of anesthesia is aspiration of gastric contents into the lungs. If aspiration occurs with larger volume of gastric contents of an acidic pH (classically pH <2.5), severe pneumonitis can result. Although routine prophylaxis in all patients is not recommended, histamine receptor (H_2) blockers such as cimetidine and ranitidine, which increase gastric pH, may be administered the night before surgery and prior to anesthesia in patients at high risk (e.g., parturients, morbid obesity, symptoms of esophageal reflux, anticipated difficult airway management) for aspiration. Histamine receptor antagonists will not facilitate gastric emptying or alter the pH of gastric fluid that is present before administration of the drug.

Metoclopramide, with an onset of 1–3 minutes after intravenous injection, speeds gastric emptying by selectively increasing the motility of the upper gastrointestinal tract and relaxing the pyloric sphincter. Metoclopramide should be avoided in patients with Parkinson's disease (e.g., dopamine receptor blockade) and in the presence of gastrointestinal obstruction. Oral antacids such as sodium citrate can be administered 15–30 minutes before induction of anesthesia to immediately raise the pH of gastric contents but will also increase the gastric volume. Proton pump inhibitors (e.g., omeprazole), which inhibit secretion of hydrogen ions, effectively raise the gastric pH. Anticholinergics are not predictably effective in increasing gastric fluid pH or decreasing gastric fluid volume.

Prophylaxis Against Postoperative Nausea and Vomiting (PONV)

Factors associated with increased risk of PONV include use of inhaled volatile anesthetics and opioids, certain types of surgical procedure (e.g., laparoscopic, ear, nose and throat, plastic, and ophthalmologic procedures), younger age, female gender, inadequate hydration, nonsmokers, and history of motion sickness or postoperative nausea, pain, and anxiety.

The use of combinations of antiemetic agents may be more cost-effective than a single agent for routine prophylaxis. Combining low-dose droperidol (0.625 mg intravenously) and the 5-HT_3 (serotonin) antagonists (ondansetron 4 mg or dolasetron 12.5 mg intravenously) with dexamethasone (4–10 mg intravenously) may be the "optimal" combination for prophylaxis in the very-high-risk patient population. Notwithstanding the Food and Drug Administration's concerns regarding possible adverse cardiovascular side effects of droperidol (0.625–1.25 mg), it remains an extremely useful antiemetic, especially when combined with other antiemetic therapies.

Drug Interactions: Droperidol

Droperidol in low doses (0.625–1.25 mg intravenously) was widely accepted as first-line therapy for the prophylaxis and treatment of postoperative nausea and vomiting, with approximately 25 million unit doses in year 2000

December 2001: FDA Black Box Warning of possible death, cardiac dysrhythmias, and *torsade de pointes*

FDA: 100 "unique" reports of cardiovascular events and 20 reports of QT/QTc interval prolongation or *torsade de pointes* – 74% of reports are from outside the United States, with confounding factors often associated

However, not a single case report in the literature during its more than 30 years of clinical use in the perioperative period documented that droperidol caused a cardiac arrhythmia

There is no apparent safety or efficacy advantages of ondansetron (4 mg IV) over droperidol (0.625 or 1.25 mg IV)

If droperidol is used, pretreatment screening 12-lead electrocardiography (ECG) must be performed – droperidol should not be administered if QTc is increased in duration (male >440 msec, female >450 msec) – and continuous ECG monitoring for up to 3 hr

Medications and clinical scenarios associated with increased QT and potential adverse interaction with droperidol include: atrioventricular block, sinus bradycardia, hypokalemia, some cardiac antiarrhythmic medications (classes I and III), many antidepressants, monoamine oxidase inhibitors, antibiotics (erythromycin), and even the 5-HT_3 antagonists (ondansetron)

The efficacy of prophylactic antiemetics is affected by the timing of their administration. Ondansetron has been shown to be more effective when administered at the end of surgery rather than after induction. Droperidol and dexamethasone are usually administered at the time of induction of general anesthesia or shortly thereafter, to avoid the possible dysphoric effects of droperidol and occasional perineal pain associated with intravenous dexamethasone.

Prophylaxis Against Allergic Reactions

Antihistamines and steroids are used as pharmacologic premedication to provide prophylaxis against intraoperative allergic reactions in patients with a history of chronic atopy, latex allergy, or undergoing procedures (e.g., radiographic dye studies) known to be associated with allergic reactions. Although controversial, pretreating latex allergic patients with H_1- and H_2-blockers and steroids is not recommended, since avoidance of latex exposure is the most important aspect of preparation. Histamine antagonists such as diphenhydramine and cimetidine do not decrease histamine blood levels but block histamine's action.

Perioperative Beta-blockade

Initiation of beta-blockade should be considered in patients at risk for perioperative myocardial ischemia and beta-blockers should be continued in those already taking them preoperatively. Ideally, beta-blockade should be started before surgery in patients deemed appropriate for beta-blockade therapy and continued postoperatively for days to weeks. Contraindications to beta-blockade include symptomatic bradycardia, or symptomatic hypotension, severe heart failure requiring diuretics or inotropes, cardiogenic shock, asthma or reactive airway disease requiring bronchodilators and/or steroids, and second- or third-degree atrioventricular block.

Clinical Caveat: Perioperative Prophylactic Beta-blockade

Appropriately administered beta-blockers reduce perioperative ischemia and may reduce the risk of myocardial infarction and death in high-risk patients

Two randomized, placebo-controlled trials have been performed; one demonstrated reduced perioperative cardiac events and the other improved 6-month survival

Class I indication ("evidence and/or general agreement that a given procedure/therapy is useful and effective"): When required in the recent past to control symptoms of angina or patients with symptomatic arrhythmias or hypertension and patients at high cardiac risk owing to the finding of ischemia on preoperative testing who are undergoing vascular surgery

Class IIa indication ("conflicting evidence but weight of evidence/opinion is in favor of usefulness/efficacy"): When preoperative assessment identifies untreated hypertension, known coronary disease, or major risk factors for coronary disease

When indicated and possible, beta-blockers (e.g., atenolol) should be started days or weeks before elective surgery, with the dose titrated to achieve a resting heart rate between 50 and 60 beats/min

Whether initiation of beta-blockade with longer acting beta-blockers such as atenolol or metoprolol at the time of induction and without postoperative continuance has benefit is unknown

INTRAVENOUS ANESTHETIC AGENTS

Propofol and thiopental are the most frequently used intravenous agents to induce general anesthesia, with etomidate and ketamine usually reserved for patients with cardiovascular instability. Occasionally, benzodiazepines and opioids are used, alone or in combination to induce general anesthesia.

Mode of Action

Barbiturates, benzodiazepines, and probably propofol and etomidate, decrease neuronal excitability by augmenting the inhibitory action of gamma-amino butyric acid (GABA) in the central nervous system (Figure 5-6). GABA decreases the excitability of neurons by its action at the postsynaptic GABA receptor complex. When GABA occupies the binding site of the complex, it allows inward flux of chloride ions, resulting in hyperpolarization of the cell and therefore the subsequent resistance of the neuron to stimulation by excitatory neurotransmitters.

The action of ketamine is at least partly explained by its antagonism at the N-methyl-D-aspartate (NMDA) receptor, although it has action at opioid receptors, and muscarinic receptors among others. Glutamate, or its analog NMDA, is excitatory. When glutamate occupies the binding site on its receptor, the channel opens and allows ions to either enter or leave the cell. Flux of these ions leads to depolarization of the postsynaptic neuron and initiation of an action potential and activation of other pathways. Ketamine blocks this open channel and prevents further ion flux, thus inhibiting the excitatory response to glutamate and causing dissociation between limbic and thalamocortical systems (e.g., dissociative anesthesia). Ketamine does not interact with GABA receptors.

Opioids act as agonists at the opioid receptors mu (mu-1 and mu-2), kappa, and delta, and at presynaptic and postsynaptic sites in the CNS. The commonly used opioids bind and activate the mu or "morphine-preferring" receptor, resulting in profound analgesia, respiratory depression, and euphoria.

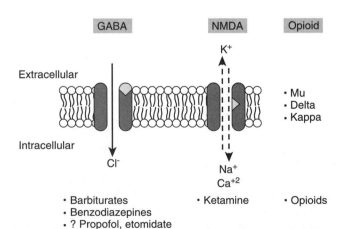

Figure 5-6 Proposed major mode of action of intravenous anesthetic agents include augmentation of the inhibitory tone of gamma-amino butyric acid (GABA) in the central nervous system by most intravenous anesthetic agents, antagonism at the N-methyl-D-aspartate (NMDA) receptor by ketamine, and opioid receptor binding.

Propofol

Propofol is prepared as a 1% (10 mg/mL) lipid emulsion containing egg:lecithin, glycerol, and soybean oil to which either sulfite or EDTA may be added as preservative. Propofol may be used for induction (2-2.5 mg/kg intravenous bolus), sedation (25-75 μg/kg/min, titrated to effect) and maintenance of general anesthesia (100-150 μg/kg/min intravenously, titrated to effect). It is associated with a rapid recovery, reduced incidence of PONV, a high incidence (50-75%) of pain on injection, which may be reduced by addition of local anesthetic or prior administration of an opioid, and hypotension with induction. Induction doses and maintenance infusion rates tend to be higher in pediatric patients but should be reduced in the elderly. Propofol should be used cautiously or not at all in patients with hemodynamic compromise or disorders of lipid metabolism (e.g., hyperlipidemia).

Drug Interactions: Propofol and Propofol Infusions

Two brands: Diprivan (Zeneca Pharmaceuticals) and Propofol (Baxter Pharmaceuticals). One preparation contains sulfite preservative which may pose a risk of allergic reactions in susceptible patients, and bronchospasm in asthmatics

Lipid emulsion preparation can support bacterial growth (e.g., discard unused open propofol after 6 hours) and cause pain with injection

Prolonged sedation of children in the intensive care unit with propofol has been associated with unexplained metabolic and lactic acidosis and cardiovascular collapse and is no longer recommended

Barbiturates (Thiopental, Thiamylal, Methohexital)

Intravenous administration of the thiobarbiturates, thiopental, or thiamylal (3-5 mg/kg intravenously), or the more potent oxybarbiturate, methohexital (1-1.5 mg/kg intravenously), produces induction of hypnosis in less than 30 seconds and recovery within 5-10 minutes. Recovery is the result of redistribution of drug away from the brain to the lean tissues (peak ≈15-30 min) and fat (peak ≈300 minutes) followed by slow hepatic clearance of 10-15% per hour. Barbiturates are very alkaline (pH >10) and are usually prepared as dilute solutions (1-2.5% [10-25 mg/mL]). Solutions of thiopental may be incompatible with and cause precipitate with drugs or

fluids in more acidic solution such as lactated Ringer's, muscle relaxants (e.g., rocuronium, pancuronium, vecuronium), sufentanil, alfentanil, and midazolam.

Venous thrombosis, a complication after intravenous administration, presumably reflects deposition of barbiturate crystals in the vein. The pathogenesis of arterial occlusion and ischemia that occurs following accidental intra-arterial injection is not due to the alkalinity of the solution but more probably a chemical endarteritis. Treatment of an involved upper extremity after intra-arterial injection includes anticoagulation and possibly thrombolytics, sympathectomy (e.g., stellate ganglion block or brachial plexus block), administration of intra-arterial vasodilators, and dilution of the drug with saline through the needle or catheter that still remains in the artery.

Undesirable effects of barbiturates include hypotension resulting from myocardial depression and venodilation, hyperalgesia, histamine release, and rare (1:30,000 patients) anaphylactic or anaphylactoid response. Hepatic enzyme induction and acute tolerance can develop with sustained drug administration over days. Induction of delta-aminolevulinic acid synthetase with increased porphyrin production and possible paralysis and death may occur in patients with some forms of porphyria.

The calculated barbiturate dose based on weight should be decreased or another induction agent used:

- When protein binding is reduced and therefore more free drug is present (e.g., neonates, cirrhosis, renal failure, malnutrition, burns, malignancy)
- When hypovolemia or shock are present
- In the presence of acidosis, when more non-ionized drug is available to cross the blood–brain barrier
- Where minimum anesthetic alveolar concentration (MAC) is already decreased (e.g., acute alcohol intoxication, hypothermia).

The increased sensitivity of the elderly is more likely to be caused by a pharmacokinetic (e.g., early distribution of drug) than a pharmacodynamic (e.g., increased brain sensitivity) mechanism.

Methohexital is often used to provide general anesthesia for cardioversion, electroconvulsive therapy, and outpatient procedures. The most important advantage of methohexital over thiopental is a more rapid recovery of consciousness resulting from a high rate of hepatic clearance. Disadvantages include an increased incidence of excitatory phenomena such as skeletal muscle movement (e.g., myoclonus), and pain on injection.

Etomidate

Etomidate is a hypnotic agent used to induce general anesthesia (0.2-0.3 mg/kg intravenously) and is supplied as a 0.2% (2 mg/mL) solution in propylene glycol that, like midazolam, is water-soluble in acidic solutions and lipid-soluble in physiologic solutions. Etomidate is frequently chosen to induce anesthesia in patients with cardiovascular instability, poor cardiac function, or intracranial hypertension.

Adverse effects include pain on injection and delayed thrombophlebitis of the vein used due to the propylene glycol vehicle myoclonic movements (e.g., >50% of patients) that in approximately 20% of patients are associated with spikes on the electroencephalogram; and a 30–40% incidence of PONV. Prolonged sedation with etomidate is not recommended secondary to a dose-dependent, reversible inhibition of the enzyme 11-β-hydroxylase and adrenal steroid production. A single induction dose of etomidate may slightly decrease cortisol levels but for less than 24 hours and without clinical consequences. However, etomidate should probably be avoided in the hypoadrenal patient because of the potential for further adrenal suppression. Etomidate should be used with caution in patients with a history of seizure disorder and probably not at all in those with acute intermittent porphyria.

Ketamine

Ketamine is a structural analogue of phencyclidine with hypnotic, amnestic, and analgesic properties but with psychotomimetic side effects that limit its usefulness. Ketamine is often used for induction of anesthesia in hemodynamically compromised patients and those with severe reactive airway disease. Ketamine may be administered intravenously (1–2 mg/kg) and intramuscularly (5–10 mg/kg), producing unconsciousness in 30–60 seconds and approximately 5 minutes respectively. It is supplied as a water-soluble 1% or 10% solution that is a racemic mixture, the S^+ isomer having increased anesthetic potency and decreased psychotomimetic side effects.

Adverse effects include increased muscle tone, myoclonic movements, increased intracranial pressure, eye movements with increased intraocular pressure, increased oral secretions, and emergence delirium. There is an increased incidence of hallucinations and unpleasant dreams when ketamine is used in higher doses (>2 mg/kg), in female patients and the elderly, and when benzodiazepines or propofol are not used concomitantly.

Ketamine–propofol total intravenous anesthesia (TIVA) has gained some popularity in outpatient surgical settings in an attempt to reduce opioid use and the incidence of PONV. Monitoring the depth of ketamine anesthesia remains a challenging problem. The established range of bispectral index (BIS) is not applicable in patients under ketamine anesthesia.

Comparative Pharmacokinetics

Thiopental, propofol, etomidate, and ketamine are lipid-soluble and have a large volume of distribution (e.g., V_d 100–500 L). Rapid awakening after a single intravenous bolus results from redistribution of drug away from vessel-rich groups. The clinical effect after prolonged infusion is terminated by hepatic metabolism. Thiopental has a rather low hepatic extraction ratio and an elimination half-life of approximately 10 hours compared to 1.5–2.5 hours for propofol, etomidate, and ketamine. Methohexital has a similar pharmacokinetic profile to thiopental with regard to lipid solubility, ionization, and protein binding, and therefore the onset time of clinical effect is similar. However, methohexital has a shorter half-life ($\approx$3 hr) because of its high rate of clearance. The clearance of propofol actually exceeds hepatic blood flow implying extrahepatic metabolism. Thiopental, propofol, and etomidate are all relatively highly protein-bound while ketamine is not.

Comparative Pharmacodynamics

Cardiovascular System

Propofol and thiopental produce a dose-dependent decrease in mean arterial pressure. Barbiturates produce direct venodilation, depression of myocardial contractility, and reduced cardiac output despite a reflex increase in heart rate. Hypertensive patients exhibit greater hypotension for a given dose than normotensive patients. Propofol produces a greater reduction in mean arterial blood pressure than thiopental, the result of decreased systemic vascular resistance and venodilation, direct myocardial depression, reduced sympathetic activity, lack of reflex increase in heart rate, and significant blunting of baroreflexes. Etomidate has minimal affects on the cardiovascular system with observed decreases in mean arterial pressure and cardiac output (e.g., decrease $\approx$10%) similar to the nonanesthetized natural sleep state. Ketamine causes release of endogenous catecholamines with associated increases in heart rate, systemic blood pressure, and pulmonary artery pressure that may be undesirable in patients with coronary artery disease, heart failure, or pulmonary artery hypertension. The direct effect of ketamine, however, is myocardial depression, which may be unmasked in patients with autonomic nervous system blockade (e.g., spinal cord transection) or depleted catecholamine stores (e.g., end-stage shock).

Central Nervous System

Cerebral blood flow, cerebral metabolic rate of oxygen consumption (CMR_{O_2}), and intracranial pressure are decreased by thiopental, propofol, and etomidate. Cerebral perfusion pressure is best preserved by etomidate and thiopental. Ketamine is a cerebrovasodilator that increases cerebral blood flow, intracranial pressure, and CMR_{O_2}.

Barbiturates provide some protection of the brain from adverse effects produced by regional or focal cerebral ischemia but not global cerebral ischemia (e.g., cardiac arrest).

Somatosensory Evoked Potentials/ Electroencephalogram

Thiopental and propofol increase the time for the electrical signal to go from stimulus site to recording site (e.g., latency) and decrease the amplitude of the recording in a dose-dependent manner. Etomidate and ketamine may actually increase the amplitude and enhance SSEP recordings when reproducible responses are difficult to obtain.

Thiopental and propofol can be used to produce an isoelectric electroencephalogram (EEG). Methohexital and etomidate may activate seizure foci. Methohexital is often used to provide general anesthesia for electroconvulsive therapy where a seizure is desirable, and etomidate during intraoperative mapping and resection of seizure foci.

Respiratory System

Propofol, thiopental, and, to a much lesser extent, etomidate produce dose-dependent respiratory depression with decreased tidal volume, decreased minute ventilation, a right shift of the CO_2 response curve, and ultimately apnea at higher doses. Blunting of laryngeal reflexes is better accomplished with propofol than with equivalent doses of thiopental or etomidate. Bronchospasm and laryngospasm may occur in response to stimulation of the patient's airway in the presence of inadequate drug-induced depression of laryngeal reflexes but this is not unique to thiopental as was initially believed. Thiopental can be safely used for induction of anesthesia in asthmatic patients.

Ketamine has a minimal effect on respiratory drive, with maintenance of spontaneous ventilation, although rarely apnea may occur with high doses or when combined with other respiratory depressant medications. Ketamine increases salivation (sympathetic cholinergic activity), frequently necessitating co-administration of an anticholinergic agent such as glycopyrrolate; it has bronchodilatory effects secondary to release of endogenous catecholamines with beta-2-agonist action; and it maintains upper airway reflexes, although aspiration of gastric contents in the absence of a cuffed endotracheal tube is still a possibility.

Benzodiazepines

Midazolam (0.15-0.3 mg/kg intravenously) and, less commonly, diazepam (0.3-0.5 mg/kg) are occasionally used to induce general anesthesia when myocardial depression and decreased systemic vascular resistance are especially undesirable (e.g., in aortic stenosis).

Benzodiazepine receptor binding facilitates GABA receptor binding, which increases the membrane conductance of chloride (Cl^-), reducing neuronal membrane firing and inhibiting neuronal function. Benzodiazepines have minimal cardiovascular affects and cause a mild decrease in systemic vascular resistance and mean arterial pressure with a slight reflex tachycardia. When given with opioids, a synergistic decrease in mean arterial blood pressure and systemic vascular resistance is often observed. Benzodiazepines decrease the minute ventilation response for a given P_aCO_2, which is usually insignificant unless administered with other respiratory depressants but on occasion can cause apnea. They reduce cerebral blood flow and $CMRO_2$ (although not to the extent that barbiturates do), decrease volatile anesthetic MAC by up to 30%, and have centrally mediated muscle relaxant properties. Benzodiazepine-mediated unconsciousness can be reversed with flumazenil (0.2-1.0 mg intravenously).

Opioids

The synthetic opioids fentanyl, sufentanil, alfentanil, and remifentanil, as intravenous bolus or continuous infusion, are useful adjuncts to general anesthesia and in higher doses provide surgical anesthesia. Opioids bind to their specific receptors, which are heavily concentrated in the periaqueductal gray area of the brain and the substantia gelatinosa of the spinal cord. Activation of the mu-1 receptor is speculated to produce supraspinal and spinal analgesia while the more undesirable effects, such as respiratory depression and bradycardia, are mediated via the mu-2 receptor. Opioid receptor activation causes a decrease in neurotransmission that is due largely to presynaptic inhibition of neurotransmitter release. The MAC of volatile anesthetics is reduced by concomitant administration of opioids but with a ceiling effect. Higher doses provide hypnosis but are not reliably amnestic. The opioids are mainly differentiated by potency, onset, mode of metabolism, and duration of action.

Potency

Sufentanil > fentanyl ≈ remifentanil > alfentanil. In general, the more lipid soluble the more potent the opioid.

Onset

Alfentanil and remifentanil have a rapid onset secondary to an effect site equilibration of just over 1 minute as compared to approximately 6 minutes for fentanyl and sufentanil following intravenous administration. At physiologic pH, opioids (pKa ≈8) exist mainly in the ionized and less lipid soluble form. An exception is alfentanil, which has a pKa of 6.5 such that nearly 90% of the drug exists in the lipid-soluble, non-ionized form at physiologic pH, which readily crosses the blood–brain barrier.

Metabolism

All opioids except remifentanil are dependent on hepatic metabolism. Remifentanil is hydrolyzed by nonspecific plasma and tissue esterases to inactive metabolites. Remifentanil metabolism is independent of hepatic or renal function and is unaffected by pseudo-cholinesterase deficiency.

Duration of Action

Remifentanil has a short elimination half-time (≈6 min) and does not accumulate, relatively independently of the duration of infusion. This makes high-dose remifentanil anesthetic techniques associated with a rapid recovery and less risk of postoperative respiratory depression than similar techniques with other opioids. The shorter duration of action of alfentanil versus fentanyl is explained by the very small V_d and lower lipid solubility of alfentanil which keeps more of the drug in the blood and available for metabolism. Alfentanil actually has a lower hepatic clearance (mg/kg/min) than fentanyl.

Context-sensitive half-time describes the time necessary for the plasma drug concentration to be decreased by half after discontinuing a continuous infusion of a specific duration (Figure 5-7). The context-sensitive half-time of remifentanil is independent of the duration of infusion and is estimated to be only approximately 4 minutes. For infusions of up to 8 hours duration, sufentanil actually has a shorter context-sensitive half-time than does alfentanil. After termination of a continuous infusion of fentanyl for even a relatively short time, fentanyl drug levels decrease more slowly than sufentanil, alfentanil, or remifentanil. The clinical implication is that awakening following prolonged infusion of remifentanil should be more predictable and of shorter duration than from sufentanil and alfentanil, with fentanyl having the least favorable characteristics in this regard. Opioid-induced unconsciousness

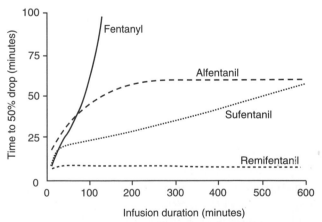

Figure 5-7   Context sensitive half-time describes the time necessary for the plasma drug concentration to be decreased in half after discontinuing a continuous infusion of a specific duration. Note that the context-sensitive half-time of remifentanil is independent of the duration of infusion. (Redrawn from Egan TD, Lemmens HJM, Riset P, *et al.* The pharmacokinetics of the new short-acting opioid remifentanil (G187084B) in healthy adult male volunteers. *Anesthesiology* 1993;79:881–892.)

and apnea can be reversed with naloxone in incremental doses of 10–40 μg intravenously every 1–2 minutes.

Physiologic Effects of Opioids
Cardiovascular

In general, opioids exert their cardiovascular effects by reducing sympathetic output via vasomotor centers in the medulla and increasing parasympathetic tone via vagal pathways. Although opioids do not cause significant myocardial depression and provide relative hemodynamic stability, hypotension secondary to dose-dependent central vagally-mediated bradycardia and arterial and venous vasodilation can occur. An exception is meperidine, which can cause tachycardia (its chemical structure is similar to atropine) and direct myocardial depression. Meperidine and morphine (meperidine > morphine), but not sufentanil, fentanyl, remifentanil, or alfentanil, can cause clinically significant release of histamine and vasodilation.

Central Nervous System

In the absence of hypoventilation, opioids produce a modest decrease (10–25%) in cerebral blood flow, $CMRO_2$ and intracranial pressure. The effect of most opioids on the EEG is minimal, without seizure activity and with slower delta-wave predominance at higher doses. Myoclonus, without EEG evidence of seizure, is occasionally observed. Bispectral analysis (BIS) correlates well with the clinical dose-response of hypnotic drugs but not with opioids. Opioid analgesics confound the use of BIS as a measure of anesthetic adequacy.

Stimulation of the medullary chemoreceptor trigger zone is responsible for a high incidence of PONV, the Edinger–Wesphal nucleus of the oculomotor nerve with miosis. Interaction with dopamine and GABA receptors a likely explanation for the thoracoabdominal muscle stiffness ("stiff chest syndrome") and vocal cord closure that may make ventilation difficult after rapid intravenous administration of an opioid.

Respiratory

Opioid administration decreases minute ventilation mainly by decreasing the respiratory rate but, at higher doses, the tidal volume also decreases. Opioids have a direct effect on the respiratory centers in the medulla producing a dose-dependent depression of ventilatory response to carbon dioxide (shift CO_2 response curve to the right), blunt the normal increase in ventilation that occurs in response to hypoxia (hypoxic drive) and increase the highest P_aCO_2 at which a patient remains apneic (apneic threshold). Maximal respiratory depression occurs approximately 5–7 minutes after intravenous administration of fentanyl as compared to 20–30 minutes after intravenous morphine. Opioids do not interfere with hypoxic pulmonary vasoconstriction and are useful anesthetics during one-lung ventilation techniques.

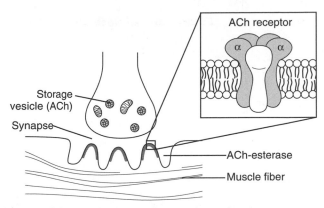

Figure 5-8   Both depolarizing and nondepolarizing neuromuscular blocking agents bind to the alpha subunits of the postjunctional nicotinic cholinergic (acetylcholine, ACh) receptor. Acetylcholinesterase (ACh-esterase) is present in the junctional folds and rapidly hydrolyzes acetylcholine but not succinylcholine.

Clinical Caveat: Remifentanil in Clinical Practice

Remifentanil has a faster onset of clinical effect than fentanyl or sufentanil, potency similar to fentanyl, and an extremely short elimination half-time ($\approx$6 min). In

Remifentanil is metabolized by *nonspecific* tissue and plasma esterases to inactive metabolites

Clearance is independent of liver or renal function, pseudocholinesterase deficiency or cholinesterase inhibitors

Very short context-sensitive half time ($\approx$4 min). In contrast to other opioids, there is a lack of drug accumulation following repeated boluses and the rate of decline of the remifentanil plasma concentration on discontinuance is essentially independent of the infusion duration

The bispectral index is relatively insensitive to the addition of an opioid such as remifentanil

Need to supplement with another longer-acting opioid if remifentanil infusion is discontinued and postoperative analgesia is desirable

NEUROMUSCULAR BLOCKADE

Neuromuscular blocking agents (NMBs) lack amnestic or analgesic properties but facilitate endotracheal intubation and improve surgical conditions thereby decreasing the concentration of inhalation anesthesia required. Clinically, the choice of NMB is based on onset time, duration of action, mode of metabolism/clearance, associated side effects, and cost.

Basic Neuromuscular Junction and Receptor Physiology

With arrival of a nerve action potential at the presynaptic nerve terminal and with extra-cellular influx of calcium, synaptic vesicles release acetylcholine into the synaptic cleft to bind to postjunctional receptors. Each postjunctional nicotinic cholinergic receptor is composed of protein subunits; two alpha (the site of acetylcholine and NMB binding), and one each of beta, delta, and epsilon. When acetylcholine binds to the active site of both alpha subunits, a central channel is formed by a protein conformational change through which ions can flow, leading to depolarization of the cell membrane and muscle contraction. Both nondepolarizing and depolarizing (succinylcholine) NMBs act on this receptor (Figure 5-8). Acetylcholinesterase is present in the junctional folds to facilitate rapid hydrolysis of acetylcholine.

Cholinergic Receptors: Postjunctional versus Extrajunctional

Postjunctional Nicotinic Cholinergic Receptors

The depolarizing muscle relaxant succinylcholine binds to postsynaptic nicotinic receptors at the alpha subunit similar to acetylcholine. If two alpha subunits are occupied simultaneously, the ion channel opens, producing ion flow and muscle contractions (fasciculations). Because succinylcholine is not hydrolyzed by acetylcholinesterase, the channel remains open for a longer period of time, causing persistent depolarization, prevention of propagation of an action potential, and short-term flaccid paralysis. When a nondepolarizing NMB occupies one or more of the alpha subunits of the postsynaptic nicotinic receptor, it competitively antagonizes acetylcholine but lacks intrinsic activity and the ion channel remains closed. If enough channels are closed, neuromuscular transmission is prevented.

Extrajunctional Receptors

Extrajunctional receptors proliferate beyond the neuromuscular junction and over the postjunctional muscle membrane whenever there is deficient stimulation of the skeletal muscle membrane by the nerve following trauma or denervation (Figure 5-9). Conditions associated with increased extrajunctional receptors include upper (e.g., stroke, spinal cord injury) and lower motor neuron disease, muscular disease (e.g., disuse/ immobilization, muscular dystrophies), and burns.

These extrajunctional receptors are similar to their postjunctional counterparts but a gamma subunit is substituted for the epsilon subunit. Interestingly, this receptor pattern and type is similar to that found in the fetus. The extrajunctional receptors are as responsive

Extrajunctional Receptors

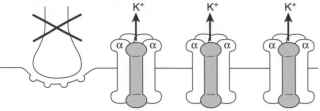

- UMN
- LMN
- Muscle disease
- Burns

- ↑ Numbers and proliferate beyond NMJ
- Stay open longer
- Responsive to ACh and SCh
- Short half-lives
- One subunit different

Figure 5-9 Extrajunctional receptors proliferate beyond the neuromuscular junction (NMJ) with upper motor and lower motor neuron (UMN, LMN) disease, muscle disease, and after burn injury. Potassium (K$^+$) release may occur with succinylcholine (SCh) administration.

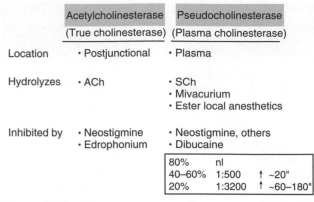

	Acetylcholinesterase (True cholinesterase)	Pseudocholinesterase (Plasma cholinesterase)
Location	• Postjunctional	• Plasma
Hydrolyzes	• ACh	• SCh • Mivacurium • Ester local anesthetics
Inhibited by	• Neostigmine • Edrophonium	• Neostigmine, others • Dibucaine

80%	nl	
40–60%	1:500	↑ ~20"
20%	1:3200	↑ ~60–180"

Figure 5-10 Esterase enzymes and neuromuscular blockade physiology. Dibucaine inhibits normal (nl) pseudocholinesterase activity by 80%, heterozygous atypical by 40–60% and homozygous atypical by 20%, which occurs in 1 case out of 3,200 and results in prolongation of the clinical effect of succinylcholine (SCh) to 60–180 minutes duration. ACh, acetylcholine.

to acetylcholine and succinylcholine as junctional receptors but remain open approximately four times longer. This change in subunit type and the greatly increased number of receptors present results in agonist-triggered potassium release with succinylcholine. Extrajunctional receptors have short half-lives of less than a day as opposed to longer than a week for the usual junctional receptor.

Esterase Enzymes and Neuromuscular Blocking Agents (Figure 5-10)

Pseudocholinesterase (e.g., plasma cholinesterase, butyrylcholinesterase, nonspecific cholinesterase) hydrolyzes succinylcholine, mivacurium, and ester local anesthetics and is located in the plasma and liver but not at the motor endplate. Pseudocholinesterase concentration is decreased by cirrhosis and pregnancy, and enzyme activity is inhibited by anticholinesterases, echothiophate, trimethaphan, cyclophosphamide, and phenelzine. There are genetic variants of pseudocholinesterase with varying degrees of activity. Plasma activity is increased in obese patients and succinylcholine dose requirements may be higher.

Acetylcholinesterase (i.e., true cholinesterase) hydrolyzes acetylcholine but not succinylcholine, and is located at the motor endplate near the postjunctional cholinergic receptor. It is inhibited by the anticholinesterase reversal agents such as neostigmine.

Nonspecific plasma esterases hydrolyze atracurium, which is also broken down by spontaneous nonenzymatic degradation at body temperature and pH (Hoffman elimination).

Succinylcholine

Succinylcholine binds to the postjunctional receptor and precipitates prolonged depolarization, causing it to become unresponsive to subsequent stimuli. A depolarizing blockade is also referred to as phase I blockade. However, when the dose of succinylcholine exceeds ≈3–5 mg/kg intravenously, a phase II block (desensitization neuromuscular blockade – mechanism unknown), which resembles blockade by a nondepolarizing muscle relaxant, can occur (Table 5-3).

Termination of Succinylcholine Effect

Intravenously administered succinylcholine is rapidly hydrolyzed by plasma cholinesterase (pseudocholinesterase) to succinylmonocholine and then to succinic acid and choline, causing only a small fraction of the administered dose to reach the neuromuscular junction. Diffusion of succinylcholine away from the neuromuscular junction into the extracellular fluid rather than hydrolysis within the folds of the postjunctional membrane

Table 5-3	Characteristics of Phase I and Phase II Neuromuscular Block	
	Phase I Block	**Phase II Block**
Type of relaxant	Succinylcholine	Nondepolarizer Succinylcholine (≈>3–5 mg/kg)
Train-of-four	>70%	<30%
Tetanic fade	No	Yes
Post-tetanic potentiation	No	Yes
Response to neostigmine	Prolong block	Reversal of block
Administration of nondepolarizer	Antagonize	Augment

terminates its effect. This explains why even pseudo-cholinesterase-deficient patients eventually recover neuromuscular function after administration of succinylcholine. Dibucaine, an amide local anesthetic, normally inhibits pseudocholinesterase activity by 80% (i.e., dibucaine number) and is used to detect genetic variants of this enzyme. The duration of succinylcholine blockade may be increased to approximately 20 minutes in the heterozygous variant (incidence ≈1:500) of this enzyme, which is inhibited 40–60% by dibucaine and prolonged to 60–180 minutes in the homozygous variant (incidence ≈1:3,200) with a dibucaine number of 20%. Side effects of succinylcholine are summarized in Table 5-4.

Nondepolarizing Neuromuscular Blocking Agents

The nondepolarizing NMBs can be separated according to their molecular class (benzoisoquinolones or aminosteroid) and their duration of action (long, intermediate, or short). Note that the names of the currently used benzoisoquinolones end in "-ium" (atracurium, cisatracurium, mivacurium) while the names of the steroidals end in "-onium" (pancuronium, vecuronium, rocuronium, rapacuronium). Table 5-5 is a summary of the pharmacology of nondepolarizing muscle relaxants. The aminosteroids may increase heart rate by their vagolytic action (pancuronium > rocuronium > vecuronium) while the benzylisoquinolines are associated with histamine release at higher doses (atracurium > mivacurium) and do not have organ-dependent elimination

(atracurium, cisatracurium, mivacurium). The standard intubating dose is about two to three times the ED_{95} (i.e., the dose needed to produce 95% suppression of the single twitch response). The time to return to 25% twitch height or more is ≈60–90 minutes for pancuronium, ≈20–35 minutes for the intermediate-duration NMBs, and ≈12–20 minutes for the short-acting NMB mivacurium.

Pharmacokinetics and Pharmacodynamics
Chemistry

Muscle relaxants mimic acetylcholine in their chemical structure and they may have action not only at postjunctional cholinergic receptors on muscle but also at pre- and postganglionic sites in the autonomic nervous system (Figure 5-11). The cardiovascular effects of succinylcholine (e.g., bradycardia in infants, tachycardia in adults with first dose) and the nondepolarizing muscle relaxant pancuronium can be explained accordingly. NMBs are charged molecules containing at least one quaternary ammonium. This may be an antigenic site associated with allergic reactions for both succinylcholine and nondepolarizers and suggests that if a patient is allergic to one NMB they may be allergic to others. They are highly ionized, water-soluble compounds at physiologic pH with a low V_d. Low lipid solubility and high ionization limits their passage through lipid barriers such as the gastrointestinal tract, the blood–brain barrier, and the placenta. Therefore, they are not absorbed orally, they do not produce CNS effects, and maternal administration does not affect the fetus. Unlike the intravenous induction agents, they have low protein binding.

Table 5-4 Side Effects of Succinylcholine	
Hyperkalemia	• 0.5–10 mEq/L increase in $[K^+]$ • Massive release with conditions associated with extrajunctional receptor proliferation (upper and lower motor neuron disease, burns, crush injury, muscular dystrophy)
Dysrhythmias	• Bradyarrhythmias most common, especially in children and after second dose of succinylcholine (SCh). Give atropine before second dose of SCh, although it does not always prevent heart rate slowing • Ganglionic stimulation may cause increase in heart rate and blood pressure
Muscle pains	• From fasciculations – may be associated with myoglobinemia and increased creatine kinase • Lower incidence in children (less fasciculations) • Defasciculating dose of nondepolarizer before SCh (SCh dose should then be increased) prevents fasciculations but does not reliably decrease myalgias
Malignant hyperthermia	• Trigger for malignant hyperthermia in patients at risk (muscular dystrophy, myotonic dystrophy, osteogenesis imperfecta)
Phase II block	• From prolonged infusion and increased dose (≈3–5 mg/kg) of SCh
Prolonged paralysis	• If decreased pseudocholinesterase activity or quantity
↑ Intracranial pressure	• Although intracranial pressure can be increased by SCh, it has been an inconsistent observation and SCh is not contraindicated when needed for rapid securing of the airway, even in patients with head injury • Increase appears to be secondary to arousal phenomenon caused by increased afferent traffic from muscle spindles. • Attenuated by defasciculation
↑ Intraocular pressure	• Mild transient increase (5–10 min) in intraocular pressure (IOP), mechanism unknown; *theoretical* risk of extrusion of global contents; acceptable rapid sequence in penetrating eye injury with defasciculation, adequate anesthesia, and prevention of coughing/bucking, which increases IOP significantly more than SCh
↑ Intragastric pressure	• Increased intragastric pressure is an inconsistent finding. Does not increase in infants and children.

Table 5-5 Summary Pharmacology of Nondepolarizing Neuromuscular Blocking Agents

	Intubating Dose (mg/kg)	Primary Route of Elimination	Histamine Release	Vagal Blockade	Comments
Long-acting					
Pancuronium	0.1	Kidney > liver*	0	++	Inexpensive
Intermediate-acting					
Vecuronium	0.1	Liver > kidney	0	0	Hemodynamic stability
Rocuronium	0.6–1.2	Liver > kidney	0	+	Rapid onset. Precipitates with thiopental
Atracurium	0.4–0.5	Ester hydrolysis + spontaneous degradation	+	0	Laudanosine (CNS stimulant) a metabolite
Cisatracurium	0.1–0.15	Spontaneous degradation	0	0	No histamine release
Short-acting					
Mivacurium	0.15–0.2	Plasma cholinesterase	+	0	Prolonged with atypical pseudocholinesterase
Rapacuronium	1.5–2.0	Liver > kidney	+	↑ HR	**No longer available** Bronchospasm >3%

*Liver elimination may refer to hepatic degradation and/or biliary excretion.
HR, heart rate.

Relationship of Low Potency and Fast Onset

The discovery that low-potency NMBs tend to have a faster onset led to the development of rocuronium. This low-potency (intubating dose ≈0.6–1.2 mg/kg intravenously) steroidal muscle relaxant has a faster onset than the more potent drugs such as pancuronium and vecuronium (intubating dose 0.1 mg/kg intravenously).

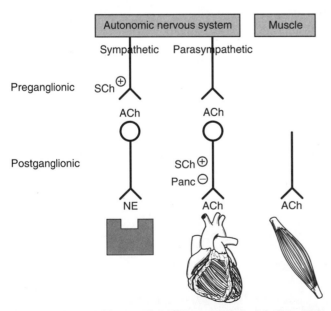

Figure 5-11 Cardiovascular effects of succinylcholine (SCh) and pancuronium (Panc). +, stimulatory; –, inhibitory; ACh, acetylcholine; NE, norepinephrine.

Pharmacodynamic Response – Clinical Factors Altering Normal Response

Both nondepolarizers and succinylcholine are potentiated by anesthetics (isoflurane, desflurane, sevoflurane > halothane > nitrous/opioid), hypermagnesemia, some antibiotics (e.g., aminoglycosides, tetracyclines, clindamycin, bacitracin – not penicillins or cephalosporins) and lithium. Local anesthetics, diuretics, and hypothermia can potentiate NMBs. An acute decrease in extracellular [K^+], making the cell membranes farther from the firing threshold, causes resistance to succinylcholine and increased sensitivity to nondepolarizers.

Pattern of Neuromuscular Blockade and Recovery

Different muscles vary in their sensitivity to NMBs (Figure 5-12). Speed of onset is characterized by larynx > diaphragm > orbicularis oculi > adductor pollicis. Orbicularis oculi is a better indicator of laryngeal blockade than adductor pollicis. When profound surgical relaxation is required, absence of the train of four at the adductor pollicis cannot be relied upon to avoid hiccups, cough, or extrusion of the abdominal contents. Diaphragmatic paralysis correlates better with response at the orbicularis oculi than at the adductor pollicis. Speed of recovery is characterized by larynx > orbicularis oculi = diaphragm > adductor pollicis. Therefore, monitoring adductor pollicis for adequacy of recovery is suggested, since recovery at the adductor pollicis insures that laryngeal reflexes are recovered.

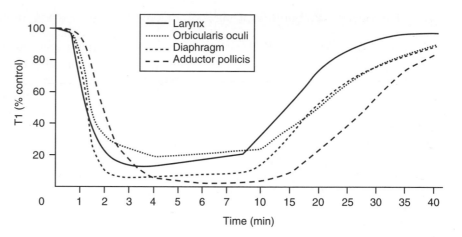

Figure 5-12   Different muscles differ in the speed of onset and recovery from neuromuscular blockade. (Redrawn from Donati F, *et al*. Vecuronium neuromuscular blockade at the adductor muscles of the larynx and adductor pollicis. *Anesthesiology* 1991;74:833-837.)

Disease States and Special Populations with Altered Response to NMB

Age Differences

Pediatric Population

Functional maturation of the neuromuscular junction is not complete until approximately 2 months of age and, in general, neonates and infants are more sensitive to nondepolarizing muscle relaxants than adults (i.e., neuromuscular blockade occurs at a lower blood concentration) and their response varies more. However, the initial dosage calculated on the basis of the infant's body weight should not be decreased because infants have a larger V_d. The increased V_d and slower clearance increases the duration of action - the exceptions being cisatracurium, atracurium, and mivacurium. For example, the duration of vecuronium is prolonged in the newborn, making it similar to pancuronium in this regard. The intubating dose of succinylcholine is increased to 1.5-2 mg/kg intravenously and reliable muscle relaxation may occur within 3-4 minutes after 4-5 mg/kg intramuscular succinylcholine administration. Rocuronium may also be administered intramuscularly, with more dependable relaxation when administered in the deltoid rather than the quadriceps muscle. While important in the armamentraium of children requiring rapid sequence induction (e.g. pyloric stenosis), routine use of succinylcholine in healthy children is contraindicated. Intractable cardiac arrest with hyperkalemia, rhabdomyolysis, and acidosis may develop following succinylcholine, particularly in patients with undiagnosed muscular dystrophy of the Duchenne type (i.e., male, 2-5 years old).

Elderly Population

Acetylcholine receptor sensitivity to nondepolarizing muscle relaxants is not altered by advanced age. Physiologic changes, including decreased hepatic and renal function, are responsible for the prolonged duration of action of many nondepolarizing muscle relaxants.

Organ Dysfunction

Renal Failure

Succinylcholine is not contraindicated in renal failure. However, since succinylcholine will transiently increase the serum potassium level by 0.5-1.0 mEq/L, it is best avoided if serum potassium levels are high. Pseudocholinesterase may be decreased after hemodialysis. The duration of action of most nondepolarizing muscle relaxants is increased in renal failure while atracurium, cisatracurium, and mivacurium are the least altered. The elimination half-life of laudanosine, the principal metabolite of atracurium associated with CNS stimulation and an increase in MAC in animals, is increased in renal failure but with little clinical consequence. The plasma clearance of anticholinesterase reversal drugs will be delayed for as long as, if not longer than, the nondepolarizing muscle relaxants and return of muscle paralysis after reversal (i.e., recurarization) is unlikely.

Hepatobiliary Disease

The effect of hepatic disease on NMBs is complex. Succinylcholine is not contraindicated. However, plasma cholinesterase may be decreased when liver disease is severe and this may modestly prolong the duration of action of succinylcholine and mivacurium. Cirrhosis is associated with an increased volume of distribution and a need for a larger initial dose of nondepolarizing neuromuscular relaxant to produce the required plasma concentration; but if the agent is dependent on hepatic metabolism, prolongation of action is expected. Atracurium and cisatracurium clearance is affected to a minor degree.

Burns

A hyperkalemic response to succinylcholine may occur in burn patients, especially if administered more than 48 hours after the injury and less than 1-2 years after complete healing. Proliferation of extrajunctional receptors or altered affinity of cholinergic receptors has been used to explain the marked resistance to nondepolarizing NMBs observed in patients with burns involving 30% or more of their body.

Neuromuscular Disease

The response to succinylcholine and nondepolarizers is summarized in Table 5-6. Note that proliferation of extrajunctional receptors results in a risk of a hyperkalemic response to succinylcholine and resistance to nondepolarizing NMBs.

Prolonged Paralysis Following Long-term Use of Muscle Relaxants in the Intensive Care Unit

Approximately 20% of patients who receive muscle relaxants for more than 6 days will have prolonged paralysis upon discontinuing neuromuscular blockade. Persistent weakness has several pathologic forms:

- Pharmacologic neuromuscular blockade secondary to metabolites with muscle relaxant properties
- A myopathy associated with elevations in creatine kinase that was initially believed to only occur with the steroidal NMBs and is now believed to be independent of structure, and with the incidence increased in asthmatic patients receiving NMBs and concomitant high-dose steroids
- A motor neuropathy without myopathy
- A persistent motor weakness without sensory involvement.

Reversal Issues: Anticholinesterase Drugs

Edrophonium (0.5–1.0 mg/kg intravenously), neostigmine (0.03–0.06 mg/kg intravenously up to 5 mg total dose), and pyridostigmine (0.25 mg/kg intravenously) inhibit acetylcholinesterase. They increase the length of time acetylcholine can spend at the motor endplate on nicotinic cholinergic receptors, reversing nondepolarizing neuromuscular blockade, and at muscarinic receptors, causing muscarinic side effects such as bradycardia if an anticholinergic is not administered concomitantly. Edrophonium has a more rapid onset of action (i.e., administer with atropine rather than glycopyrrolate) and a shorter duration of action than neostigmine and pyridostigmine. However, neostigmine is more effective than edrophonium or pyridostigmine at antagonizing intense (>90% twitch depression) neuromuscular blockade. Physostigmine is the only reversal agent that crosses the blood–brain barrier, and is used to treat central anticholinergic syndrome characterized by excitation, delirium, and hyperpyrexia following atropine or scopolamine administration.

- *Reversal of mivacurium*: Since neostigmine decreases not only true cholinesterase (acetylcholinesterase) activity but also plasma cholinesterase (pseudocholinesterase), which metabolizes mivacurium, reversal agents could interfere with the usual rapid spontaneous recovery of neuromuscular function (Figure 5-13). However, moderate levels of mivacurium NMB are antagonizable with anticholinesterases.
- *Anticholinesterase–succinylcholine interaction*: Neostigmine administration immediately followed by

Table 5-6   Summary of the Effects of Neuromuscular Diseases on Neuromuscular Blocking Agent Pharmacology

	SCh	Nondepolarizers	Comments
Neuromuscular Junction Disease			
Myasthenia gravis	↓	↑	↓ Postjunctional receptors, Rx pyridostigmine; prolong SCh
Myasthenic syndrome	↑	↑	Oat cell cancer of lung ↓ presynaptic release of ACh
Nerve Injury/CNS Injury			
Stroke/hemiplegia	K^+	↓ (affected side)	Monitor blockade on unaffected side
Muscular denervation	K^+	↓	Proliferation of extrajunctional receptors
Peripheral Neuropathy			
Guillain-Barré syndrome	K^+	↑ or ↓	
Myelopathy			
Multiple sclerosis	K^+	↓	? Proliferation of extrajunctional receptors
Amyotrophic lateral sclerosis	K^+/contractures	↑	
Dystrophinopathies			
Duchenne muscular dystrophy	K^+	↑	Avoid routine use of SCh in children
Myotonias			
Myotonic dystrophy	Contractures	Normal or ↑	SCh induced contractures may make ventilation difficult Nondepolarizers will not attenuate intraoperative myotonia
Familial periodic paralysis	K^+/Myotonia	? Normal	Hypokalemic form of disease more common than hyperkalemic
Cerebral palsy	–	↓	SCh is not contraindicated in stable neurologic disease

↑, increased sensitivity or hypersensitivity; ↓, decreased sensitivity or resistance; K^+, hyperkalemic response. ACh, acetylcholine; SCh, succinylcholine.

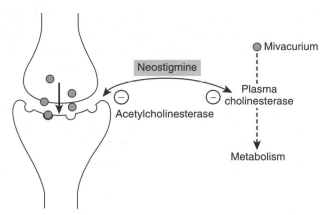

Figure 5-13 Neostigmine decreases not only acetylcholinesterase activity but also plasma cholinesterase (pseudocholinesterase) activity, potentially interfering with the usual rapid spontaneous recovery of neuromuscular function after mivacurium administration.

administration of succinylcholine may result in unpredictable prolongation of succinylcholine duration. This can be partly explained by inhibition of pseudocholinesterase by anticholinesterase agent.

- *Postoperative weakness*: The incidence of weakness in the postoperative period despite drug-assisted antagonism is more frequent in patients who have received pancuronium compared with an intermediate- or short-acting NMB. Once the maximum effect of the antagonist is achieved (≈10 minutes), recovery from profound blockade is dependent on clearance of the relaxant, and recovery from the long-acting NMB is slower.

- *Reversal administration prior to return of first twitch*: The administration of reversal agent only 5 minutes after neuromuscular blockade with rocuronium or at time of return of twitch height to 1%, 10%, or 25%, does not increase the time (≈25 min) from relaxant administration to a train of four ratio or more

than 0.7. These results suggest that reversal of intense rocuronium neuromuscular blockade need not be delayed until return of appreciable neuromuscular function has been demonstrated.

INHALED ANESTHETICS

Chemical and Physical Characteristics

The inhaled volatile anesthetics sevoflurane and desflurane were developed because their low blood solubilities predicted fast onset/recovery profiles and an ability to control anesthetic depth more rapidly and precisely. The chemical and physical characteristics of the inhaled anesthetics are summarized in Figure 5-14. Halogenation with only fluorine distinguishes sevoflurane and desflurane from isoflurane and halothane. The substitution of fluorine for chlorine and bromine increases chemical stability (i.e., decreased metabolism), decreases anesthetic potency, decreases blood solubility, and increases vapor pressure at room temperature. Unlike the alkane halothane, desflurane, sevoflurane, and isoflurane are ethers that do not sensitize the heart to exogenous catecholamines.

Desflurane Vaporizer (Tech 6)

The boiling point of 22.8° C at 1 atmosphere and high vapor pressure of desflurane requires it to be in sealed bottles with a valve that only opens when it is inserted into the filler port of a desflurane vaporizer. Controlled vaporization requires an electrically heated and pressurized vaporizer. Liquid desflurane is heated to 39° C within a sealed chamber forming gaseous desflurane at approximately 2 atmospheres (1,500 mmHg). Desflurane delivery via a conventional vaporizer would result in initial high, uncontrollable concentrations.

	Desflurane	Sevoflurane	Isoflurane	Halothane	Xenon
V_p (20°C, mmHg)	664	157	238	243	–
MAC (%)	6.0	1.4–3.3	1.28	0.75	71
MAC-awake	0.33 MAC	0.33 MAC	0.38 MAC	0.52 MAC	–
MAC (pp, mmHg)	45.6	10.6–25.1	9.7	5.7	–
Solubility (B/G)	0.42	0.69	1.4	2.3	0.14
Metabolites (%)	<<0.2	2–5	0.2	20	0

Figure 5-14 Chemical and physical characteristics of the inhaled volatile anesthetics. B/G, blood/gas; MAC, minimal alveolar concentration; V_p, vapour pressure

Potency

In general, the greater the oil:gas solubility, the more potent the inhaled agent. MAC is the minimum alveolar concentration (%) of anesthetic at 1 atmosphere pressure required to eliminate movement in response to skin incision in 50% of patients (MAC-skin incision). However, the partial pressure is a more fundamental measure of anesthetic concentration and MAC can be expressed as such. The MAC of desflurane is 6% at 1 atmosphere but is 45.6 mmHg as a partial pressure (i.e., 0.06×760 mmHg). Variations on the MAC concept may be used to estimate the potency of other anesthetic endpoints (e.g., MAC-awake < MAC-skin incision < MAC-intubation < MAC BAR).

MAC-awake is the concentration permitting voluntary response to command (eye opening) in 50% of patients emerging from anesthesia. MAC-awake is approximately 0.33 MAC for desflurane and sevoflurane but 0.52 MAC for halothane and 0.67 MAC for N_2O, implying that less anesthetic must be eliminated to reach wakefulness after N_2O and halothane anesthesia. *MAC-intubation* is the MAC that would inhibit movement and coughing during endotracheal intubation. *MAC-BAR* is the MAC necessary to prevent adrenergic response to skin incision as measured by the concentration of catecholamines in venous blood ($\approx 1.5 \times$ MAC). MAC-BAR desflurane is $1.66 \times$ MAC skin incision or approximately 10%. The anesthetic dose at which 95% rather than 50% of patients have no response to skin incision (AD_{95}) is approximately $1.3 \times$ MAC. MAC is highest in infants at approximately 6 months of age with a steady decline throughout life ($\approx 6\%$ decrease per decade) except for a slight increase at adolescence. Factors that increase, decrease, or have no effect on MAC are summarized in Table 5-7.

Table 5-7 Factors that Increase, Decrease or Have No Effect on Minimal Alveolar Concentration

"No" Effect	Decrease MAC	Increase MAC
Gender	Hypoxia	Young age
Duration of anesthesia	Hypothermia	Hyperthermia
Ethnicity	Other anesthetics	Chronic ETOH
P_aCO_2 15–95 mmHg	Severe anemia	Acute amphetamine use
P_aO_2 >38 mmHg	Pregnancy	
Blood pressure >40 mmHg	Elderly	Hypernatremia
Thyroid dysfunction	Acute ETOH	MAO inhibitors
Decerebration (animals)	Chronic amphetamine use	Cocaine
	Hyponatremia	
	Clonidine	
	Lithium	

ETOH, alcohol; MAO, monamine oxidase.

Electroencephalographic parameters such as the BIS have not correlated well with predicting movement to incision but have correlated quite well with hypnotic clinical endpoints such as sedation and loss of consciousness.

Clinical Caveat: Cerebral Electrophysiologic Signals and Anesthetic Depth

The bispectral index (BIS, Aspect Medical System Inc.), PSA 4000 (Physiometrix), and A-line (Alaris Medical Systems, Inc.) attempt to use cerebral electrophysiologic signals to track anesthetic depth

The BIS uses several variables from the electroencephalogram, combining them with various weightings in a prediction rule to render a measure of hypnosis on a linearized BIS scale from 0 to100

The algorithm for determining this number is continuously being changed and refined. A BIS number of 50–60 suggests an adequate hypnotic component of an anesthetic

Similar BIS values are found in the young as in the elderly (excluding Alzheimer's dementia).

The BIS is a monitor of hypnosis (sleep) and is not a credible monitor of movement, awareness, or hemodynamic response to incision

The contention that BIS monitoring reduces the risk of awareness is unproven

Various anesthetic regimens may impact the BIS differently

Physiologic Effects

Cardiovascular

Halothane, isoflurane, desflurane, and sevoflurane produce a similar and dose-dependent decrease in mean arterial pressure when administered to healthy volunteers, but by different mechanisms. Sevoflurane, desflurane and isoflurane decrease blood pressure mainly by decreasing peripheral vascular resistance and, although they depress myocardial contractility (Enflurane [E], halothane [H] > isoflurane [I], desflurane [D], sevoflurane [S]), the heart rate increases (I, E, D, S > H) and cardiac output is maintained. Halothane decreases blood pressure, mainly by decreases in myocardial contractility and cardiac output. Coronary artery vascular resistance is decreased (I > H > E). Isoflurane has been associated with coronary steal in animals but the clinical significance of this is debatable. Desflurane and sevoflurane do not produce coronary steal syndrome. Sympathetic nervous system activation with increased heart rate and blood pressure can occur transiently (e.g., 4–6 min) when the inspired concentration of desflurane, and less so isoflurane, is rapidly increased. This may result from stimulation of medullary centers via irritant receptors in the airway. However, a similar response is observed when the desflurane concentration is rapidly increased during cardiopulmonary bypass (CPB) where it is administered via the CPB circuit bypassing endotracheal administration. This neurocirculatory response is attenuated by pretreatment with beta-blockers and fentanyl or a slow increase in desflurane concentration.

Clinical Controversy: Desflurane and Coronary Artery Disease

The transient sympathetic stimulation associated with desflurane may be limited or minimized by:
- Not exceeding 6% desflurane
- Increasing the desflurane concentration slowly
- Prior administration of opioids
- Clonidine or beta-blocking drugs such as esmolol

The receptors mediating this rapidly adapt to the increase in desflurane concentration

Desflurane (and other potent inhaled anesthetics) does not cause clinically relevant degrees of coronary steal

Desflurane (and other potent inhaled anesthetics) has protective actions in animal models of coronary artery occlusion and reperfusion

Desflurane (and other inhaled anesthetics) and various intravenous approaches to anesthesia have similar safety records in patients with coronary artery or peripheral vascular disease

Desflurane is *not* contraindicated in patients with coronary artery disease

Respiratory

All inhaled volatile anesthetics produce alveolar hypoventilation and arterial hypercarbia in a dose-dependent manner when administered with spontaneous respiration. The characteristic respiratory pattern is a decrease in tidal volume and an increase in respiratory rate (I < S, D, E, H). However, the increase in respiratory rate does not match the decrease in tidal volume and minute ventilation decreases, alveolar ventilation decreases (i.e., increased dead space/tidal volume ratio), and hypercarbia ensues. All agents cause a dose-dependent depression of the ventilatory response to hypercarbia and raise the apneic threshold. The ventilatory response to hypoxia is even more affected than the response to carbon dioxide. The ventilatory response to hypoxia is profoundly decreased even by subanesthetic concentrations (0.1 MAC [D < S, E, I, H]) of inhaled anesthetics and totally abolished by anesthetic concentrations greater than 1.0 MAC. This can be particularly important in patients with severe chronic lung disease, who normally

retain CO_2 and depend on hypoxic drive to increase minute ventilation.

All potent inhaled anesthetics cause an increase in the alveolar–arterial oxygen gradient. All diminish bronchomotor tone and can be used efficaciously in asthmatic patients. All produce airway irritation (D > I > E > H > S) and during light anesthesia may produce coughing, laryngospasm, or bronchospasm. Pulmonary compliance and functional residual capacity are decreased and hypoxic pulmonary vasoconstriction is mildly impaired. Tracheal ciliary activity is decreased.

Central Nervous System

All potent inhaled agents decrease $CMRO_2$, decrease cerebrovascular resistance, increase cerebral blood flow (H > I, S, D), and can potentially increase intracranial pressure. Desflurane, isoflurane, and sevoflurane depress the EEG in a dose-related manner. Enflurane, especially when associated with hypocapnia, and sevoflurane (rarely) can cause convulsive activity on the EEG, particularly with rapid increases in concentration. Somatosensory evoked potentials (SSEP) are decreased in amplitude and the time for the signal to reach the receiving electrode is increased (latency). Intraocular pressure is decreased.

Neuromuscular/Uterine Smooth Muscle

Volatile anesthetics cause a dose-dependent decrease in muscle tone and enhance the effects of muscle relaxants (I, D, S, E > H). Volatile anesthetics, including desflurane and sevoflurane, may trigger malignant hyperthermia in a genetically susceptible individual, although halothane is the most potent trigger. They produce similar and dose-dependent decreases in uterine smooth muscle tone and blood flow that are modest at 0.5 MAC and become substantial at concentrations above 1 MAC.

Uptake and Distribution

Diffusion of anesthetics across the alveolar membrane is generally very efficient. The anesthetic concentration in arterial blood is close to that of the alveolar gas and, because the brain is a well perfused organ, the anesthetic concentration in the brain equilibrates rapidly with the concentration in arterial blood. Therefore, the rate of rise of partial pressure of the anesthetic agent in the alveolus correlates with the rate of onset of the anesthetic state. The partial pressure of agent in the alveolus depends on the balance between delivery of the agent to the alveolus and removal of the agent from the alveolus (partial pressure = delivery − removal). End-tidal concentration after equilibration ($F_A \simeq F_I$) is used to estimate the concentration in the brain. Blood/gas solubility, ventilation, and circulation affect uptake and distribution (Table 5-8).

The various factors involved in uptake of inhalational anesthetics are studied by means of F_A/F_I curves, where F_A is the alveolar concentration of the

Table 5-8	Factors that Alter the Rise of Partial Pressure of Inhaled Volatile Anesthetic in the Lung
↑ **Rate of Rise of Partial Pressure**	↓ **Rate of Rise of Partial Pressure**
Increased alveolar ventilation (S > I)	Increased cardiac output (S > I)
Increased inspired concentration (F_I)	Increased solubility of agent in blood
Second gas effect	
↓ FRC, ↓ circuit dead space	Large arteriovenous differences in partial pressure of agent

FRC, functional residual capacity; I = insoluble agents (lower blood/gas solubility); S = soluble agents (higher blood/gas solubility).

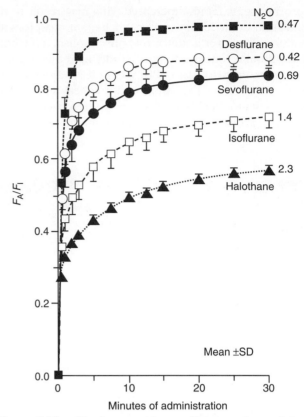

Figure 5-15 Blood:gas partition coefficients and rate of rise of alveolar (F_A) to the inspired anesthetic (F_I) concentration demonstrating that F_A/F_I increases more rapidly with the less soluble agents. (Redrawn from Yasuda N *et al.* Comparison of the kinetics of sevoflurane and isoflurane in humans. *Anesth Analg* 1991;72:316–324.)

anesthetic agent and F_I is the inspired concentration of the anesthetic agent. These curves represent the time over which the alveolar concentration of the anesthetic agent approaches the inspired concentration of the agent. The low blood/gas solubility of the newer inhaled agents results in a faster rise in F_A/F_I, less alteration of F_A/F_I with changes in cardiac output or alveolar ventilation, but greater changes with alterations in $\dot{V}/\dot{Q}$ (mismatch). Of note, the faster rise in F_A/F_I of nitrous oxide, despite it being more soluble than desflurane, is secondary to the "concentration effect" or the effect of increased F_I (nitrous oxide ≈70% versus desflurane 7-10%) on the rate of onset of inhalational anesthesia (e.g. 70% nitrous oxide reaches a higher F_A/F_I faster than 10% nitrous oxide [Figure 5-15]).

Uptake in Infants and Children

Anesthetic uptake in infants and children is more rapid than in adults. The reasons include:

- Infants and children have a higher alveolar ventilation
- Smaller functional residual capacity
- There is a greater proportion of cardiac output going to vessel-rich groups such as the brain
- The inhaled anesthetics are less soluble in children (i.e., higher water content of children).

Recovery Profile

Recovery is a mirror image of uptake except that there is no concentration effect and, although the lungs are the major route of elimination, metabolism may be important in the elimination of halothane (20% metabolized). The low blood/gas solubility of desflurane and sevoflurane provides a more rapid decline in the arterial partial pressure after termination of anesthesia than with the older, more soluble agents. With increasing duration of anesthesia these differences are magnified. Time to awakening is decreased in most studies of adults and children when insoluble agents are used, while time to discharge may or may not be shortened.

Biodegradation, Degradation, Toxicity

There is little toxicity from metabolism of modern inhaled anesthetics. Major pathways of volatile anesthetic metabolism are oxidative. A reductive pathway exists for halothane. Dehalogenation results in liberation of halogens (F^-, Br^-). Enzyme induction may be associated with increased metabolism of inhaled anesthetics. Desflurane is extremely resistant to degradation. However, toxicity may result from degradation of inhaled anesthetics by CO_2 absorbents. A dry absorbent can degrade desflurane to carbon monoxide. A dry or normal (moist) absorbent can degrade sevoflurane to compound A. Future CO_2 absorber compounds may not degrade anesthetics independent of absorber wetness.

Carbon Monoxide Formation

Carbon monoxide generation, with increased carboxyhemoglobin and falsely increased pulse oximeter readings (Figure 5-16), may occur from degradation of

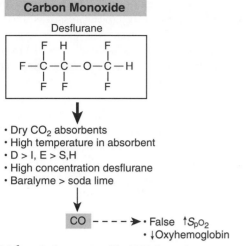

Figure 5-16 Carbon monoxide (CO) formation can occur from degradation of desflurane (D), isoflurane (I), enflurane (E), and much less from sevoflurane (S) and halothane (H). S_pO_2, pulse oximetry oxygen saturation.

inhalational anesthetics ($D \geq E > I >> S$, H) by desiccated CO_2 absorbents. Factors associated with increased CO production include dry absorbent, higher temperatures in absorbent, choice of anesthetic, concentration of anesthetic, and type of CO_2 absorber (e.g., Baralyme > soda lime).

Compound A (Vinyl Halide Toxicity)

Compound A, a dose-dependent nephrotoxin in rodents, is a product of sevoflurane degradation in the CO_2 absorber. Accumulation of compound A increases with increased respiratory gas temperature (e.g., low flows), increased CO_2 production, barium hydroxide absorber (e.g., Baralyme), high sevoflurane concentration, and long duration of anesthesia. Fresh gas flow rates below 1 L/min are not recommended. Nevertheless, the amount of compound A produced under clinical conditions has consistently been far below concentrations associated with nephrotoxicity in animals. Moreover, comparisons of the renal effects of sevoflurane and isoflurane using fresh gas flows of 1 L/min have not demonstrated any difference in indices of renal function.

Fluoride Ion

Metabolism of fluorinated volatile anesthetics to F^- ($S? > E >> I$, D) with high serum fluoride levels (historically >50 μmol/L) may result in fluoride-induced nephrotoxicity characterized by polyuria, hypernatremia, hyperosmolarity, and inability to concentrate urine (i.e., vasopressin-resistant high-output renal failure [nephrogenic diabetes insipidus]). Although both enflurane and sevoflurane are appreciably defluorinated metabolically, sevoflurane has little potential to produce F^- nephrotoxicity.

Immune-mediated Hepatic Injury

Acetylated liver proteins (neoantigens) capable of evoking an antibody response may be produced after exposure to the inhaled anesthetics other than sevoflurane (H ["halothane hepatitis"] $>E > I > D \neq S$). Enflurane, isoflurane, and desflurane could produce hepatotoxicity by a mechanism similar to that of halothane but at a lower incidence since they are metabolized to a lesser extent to the trifluoroacetylated adduct that binds to liver proteins (Figure 5-17). Volatile anesthetic degradation and toxicity issues are summarized in Figure 5-18.

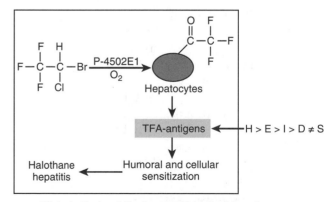

- Clinical: Eosinophilia, fever, rash, arthralgia, prior exposure
- Risk: Female, obesity, multiple exposure, not children

Figure 5-17 Immune-mediated hepatic injury. Inhaled anesthetics – halothane (H) and, less probably, enflurane (E), isoflurane (I), or desflurane (D), not sevoflurane (S) – may be metabolized to the trifluoroacetylated adduct (TFA), which binds to liver proteins creating a neoantigen capable of evoking an antibody response. (Redrawn from Njoku D, Laster MJ, Gong DH, *et al*. Biotransformation of halothane, enflurane, isoflurane, and desflurane to trifluoroacetylated liver proteins: association between protein acylation and hepatic injury. *Anesth Analg* 1997;84:173–178.)

Volatile Anesthetic Degradation and Toxicity

Summary

• Metabolism	H>S, E>I>D
• Carbon monoxide	D (I, E>>S, H)
• Compound A	S
• Fluoride	S (E)
• Immune-mediated hepatic injury	H (E>I>D≠S)

Figure 5-18 Summary of volatile anesthetic degradation and toxicity issues.

Topics of Interest in Anesthetic Delivery

Volatile Anesthetic Delivery at Altitude

To understand the effect of changes in atmospheric pressure on anesthetic delivery, one must understand (1) vapor pressure, (2) MAC as a partial pressure, and (3) vaporizer function. The vapor pressure of a liquid is a measure of its affinity for transition into the gaseous state or, more simply put, how easily it will vaporize. Vapor pressure is dependent on the physical characteristics of a liquid and also varies directly with temperature. It is independent of atmospheric pressure. However, changes in altitude (atmospheric pressure) can be an important factor in the delivery of volatile anesthetics. The desflurane vaporizer is a heated and pressure-regulated unit. As such, its internal environment does not vary with changes in altitude and its delivery of anesthetic in percentage concentration is constant. However, at higher elevations, this percentage concentration represents a lower partial pressure of anesthetic (6% of 760 mmHg $\simeq$ 46 mmHg [$\simeq$ 1 MAC as a partial pressure]; 6% of 600 mmHg = 36 mmHg [<1 MAC]). It is the partial pressure of an anesthetic agent and not its relative percentage concentration that correlates with MAC levels. Thus for desflurane delivery at 7,000 feet elevation (ambient pressure ≈600 mmHg) the vaporizer dial would have to be increased to approximately 7.6% ($0.76 \times 600 = 46$ mmHg) to deliver the same partial pressure as 6% at sea level. Contemporary variable bypass vaporizers deliver a constant partial pressure and therefore do not need adjustment at different elevations. At higher elevations these vaporizers (S, I, E, H) will actually deliver higher percentage concentrations than the corresponding dial setting, yet the partial pressure delivered will remain the same.

Vaporizer Filling Error

It is difficult to put an inappropriate liquid anesthetic in the sevoflurane or desflurane vaporizer because of the agent-specific, keyed filling devices that are used. However, a potential for misfilling exists for vaporizers not equipped with keyed fillers (I, H, E). A mass spectrometer and some newer gas monitors are able to detect the mixture of gases that may result from this mistake. Vaporizers are agent-specific and misfilling may result in anesthetic under- or overdosing.

To predict the consequences of a vaporizer filling error, one must know the vapor pressures and MAC of each anesthetic. Note that the vapor pressure of halothane and isoflurane is similar at ≈240 mmHg and enflurane and sevoflurane vapor pressure is similar at ≈170 mmHg.

What if halothane was placed in an isoflurane vaporizer? If you dialed 1.5%, believing it was isoflurane, you would deliver approximately 1.5% gas (similar vapor pressures) but it would be halothane. This dose of halothane is ≈2.0 MAC and not the ≈1.0 MAC isoflurane that you thought you were giving, therefore an overdose. If you unintentionally filled an enflurane-specific vaporizer with halothane it could lead to an anesthetic overdose: First, halothane's vapor pressure (≈240 mmHg versus ≈170 mmHg) will cause approximately 40% more anesthetic vapor to be released. Second, halothane is more than twice as potent as enflurane. Conversely, filling a halothane vaporizer with enflurane will cause an anesthetic underdose.

Desflurane has a very high vapor pressure; as it vaporizes, it cools rapidly and therefore requires a heated and pressurized vaporizer to maintain a constant output. In a nonheated vaporizer there would be an initial very high uncontrollable delivery of anesthetic. The vaporization of desflurane would eventually cool the vaporizer to the point where little or no output would occur.

Nitrous Oxide

Nitrous oxide (N_2O) is a colorless, odorless inorganic gas with a low blood solubility (blood:gas partition coefficient of 0.47) and low potency (MAC 104%) that is usually administered with inhaled volatile anesthetics or opioids in concentrations of 50–70% to produce general anesthesia. The addition of N_2O decreases the requirements of the volatile inhaled anesthetics, attenuating their potentially adverse circulatory and respiratory effects. Nitrous oxide has analgesic properties; it may produce amnesia at higher concentrations but, unlike the volatile anesthetics, causes minimal skeletal muscle relaxation. It is nonflammable but will support combustion.

When N_2O is one of the carrier gases used to vaporize the volatile agent in a variable bypass vaporizer it can effect vaporizer output. When the carrier gas is changed from air/oxygen to oxygen and nitrous oxide, the N_2O dissolves in the liquid volatile agents, initially decreasing vapor concentration output. Once the output concentration is stable and when the carrier gas is changed back to air/oxygen from N_2O/oxygen, there is a transient (≈15 min) increase in vapor concentration delivered. As with the inhaled volatile anesthetics, the mechanism of how nitrous oxide produces general anesthesia is unclear.

Physiologic Effects

Although the direct effect of nitrous oxide on myocardial contractility is depression, the *in vivo* effect is little change or slight increase in heart rate, arterial blood pressure, or cardiac output because of its tendency to stimulate the sympathetic nervous system. Nitrous oxide can increase pulmonary vascular resistance and right atrial pressure in adults and is usually avoided in patients with pulmonary hypertension. It is a mild respiratory depressant but causes minimal change in minute ventilation and resting arterial CO_2 levels. Nitrous oxide is a cerebrovasodilator, although much less than the other volatile anesthetics. It is not contraindicated for neurosurgical procedures but when intracranial pressure is persistently elevated or the brain is "tight" it should be discontinued. The addition of nitrous oxide to a given concentration of a potent inhaled anesthetic may decrease cortical sensory evoked potentials and make initial low amplitude signals even harder to interpret.

Potential Adverse Effects

Nitrous oxide can expand closed air spaces. In noncompliant spaces (e.g., middle ear, brain after pneumoencephalography, eye within 4 weeks following use of sulfur hexafluoride for retinal detachment surgery) it causes a rapid increase in pressure and, in compliant spaces (e.g., pneumothorax, pneumoperitoneum, bowel gas, air embolus, cuff of endotracheal tube), a rapid increase in volume. If nitrous oxide is used during carotid endarterectomy surgery, it should be discontinued prior to release of the carotid clamp for fear of increasing the size of air emboli that can occur with reperfusion. Nitrous oxide should not be used following cadiopulmonary bypass.

Nitrous oxide inactivates vitamin B_{12} and methionine synthetase, both essential for the production of methionine, a precursor for maintenance of the myelin sheath. Subacute combined degeneration, a myeloneuropathy characterized by progressive demyelination of the posterior columns with associated symptoms, has been described weeks following a single, otherwise uncomplicated nitrous oxide anesthetic in patients with vitamin B_{12} deficiency. Early treatment with vitamin B_{12} or cyanocobalamin injections stops progression of the disease.

The association of nitrous oxide with increased PONV has not been a consistent link, particularly in children. However, meta-analysis of published studies does suggest an association and therefore nitrous oxide is usually avoided in those patients at high risk for PONV. Concerns regarding the safety of nitrous oxide have led to continued interest in alternatives such as inhaled xenon.

Inhaled Xenon

The noble gas xenon has a MAC of ≈65%, is extremely insoluble in blood, with a blood-gas partition coefficient less than one-third that of N_2O, is chemically stable, provides rapid induction and emergence, exerts analgesic effects, and has minimal systemic and pulmonary hemodynamic effects. However, its expense has limited its use. Low fresh gas flows and development of a xenon-recycling system may offset this disadvantage in the future.

Clinical Controversy: Does the Anesthetic Profile of Xenon Warrant its Cost?

Environmental advantages of xenon:
- Does not affect the ozone layer, unlike nitrous oxide and volatile anesthetics
- Is not a greenhouse gas

Medical advantages of xenon:
- Rapid induction and emergence
- Lacks teratogenicity
- Has analgesic properties and suppresses hemodynamic and catecholamine responses to surgical stimulation
- Potent hypnotic agent
- Lack of cardiac depression
- Does not trigger malignant hyperthermia.

Potential disadvantages:
- Cost - xenon currently costs approximately $10.00/L and at 1 MAC for 240 minutes under closed circuit conditions costs an estimated $167.00
- Potency is relatively low - MAC ≈ 63% (50-70%)
- Xenon has been demonstrated to be effective and safe with rapid recovery but it is unknown if it improves outcome by providing more optimal hemodynamics

---

PHARMACOLOGY OF POSTOPERATIVE PAIN MANAGEMENT

Although intravenous opioids or peridural opioids are the mainstay of pain management in the postoperative period, concern about side effects, including respiratory depression and PONV, can result in administration of an inadequate dose for pain relief. The nonopioid analgesics ketorolac and acetaminophen, and the new cyclooxygenase (COX)-2 inhibitors, alone or more commonly in combination with opioids, have a useful role in the management of acute postoperative pain.

Opioids

Intermittent titration of small intravenous doses of fentanyl (25–50 μg), morphine (2–4 mg), meperidine (12.5–25 mg), hydromorphone (0.25–0.5 mg), and, rarely, continuous low-dose infusion of remifentanil (0.05–0.2 μg/kg/min) is employed to manage moderate to severe immediate postoperative pain.

The analgesic effects of these intravenously administered opioids usually peak within 4–5 minutes, with the exception of morphine. The relatively low lipid solubility and high degree of ionization of morphine explains the slow onset of peak analgesia (15–30 min) as compared to the more lipid-soluble meperidine and fentanyl.

All opioids produce a similar amount of PONV and respiratory depression when administered at equianalgesic doses. However, peak onset of respiratory depression after an analgesic dose of morphine (≈15–30 min) is slower than that after comparable doses of fentanyl (≈5–10 min). Opioids should not be administered immediately prior to discharge from the recovery room in patients who will not have intensive respiratory monitoring.

Meperidine is unique in that it rarely causes bradycardia, causes more histamine release than the other opioids, and has antishivering properties that are most likely due to stimulation of kappa receptors and a decrease in the shivering threshold. Meperidine should not be administered to patients taking monamine oxidase inhibitors because of its association with the neuroleptic malignant syndrome.

Renal failure alters morphine and meperidine pharmacokinetics significantly but has much less effect on fentanyl metabolism and excretion. Morphine is the opioid most likely to accumulate active metabolites (morphine 6-glucuronide) in the presence of renal failure. Normeperidine is the chief metabolite of meperidine that accumulates in patients with renal failure. Normeperidine has analgesic and CNS excitatory effects and may elicit seizure activity.

Nonsteroidal Anti-inflammatory Drugs – Ketorolac

Ketorolac, a nonsteroidal anti-inflammatory drug (NSAID), reversibly inhibits prostaglandin synthesis by inhibiting both cyclooxygenase-1 (COX-1) and cyclooxygenase-2 (COX-2). It exhibits moderate anti-inflammatory activity, is antipyretic, has potent analgesic effects, and, unlike aspirin, inhibits platelet function in a reversible manner.

Ketorolac may be administered orally, intramuscularly, or intravenously. Peak plasma concentrations occur 45–60 minutes after intramuscular injection and the elimination half-life is approximately 5 hours. Ketorolac is metabolized in the liver and excreted by the kidneys. Clearance is decreased in the elderly and the dose should be less (e.g., 15 mg) than for younger patients. Ketoralac 30 mg intramuscularly is approximately equipotent to morphine 10 mg or meperidine 100 mg.

Ketorolac is useful for providing postoperative analgesia for less painful procedures when administered as the sole analgesic and as a useful adjunct for severe pain when used to supplement parenteral or epidural opioids. The maximum daily dose should not exceed 150 mg on the first day and 120 mg on subsequent days for a maximum of 5 days.

There is no ventilatory or cardiovascular depression and little or no effect on the biliary tract. Ketorolac may be most beneficial and cost-effective by allowing reduced opioid use in patients at increased risk for postoperative respiratory depression or emesis. Contraindications to NSAIDs, such as ketorolac, in the postoperative period include coagulopathy or abnormal platelet function, peptic ulceration, gastrointestinal bleeding, renal impairment, allergy to aspirin or NSAIDs, aspirin-induced asthma, labor, and breast feeding.

Clinical Caveat: Perioperative Use of Ketorolac

Most of the published literature suggests that the overall risk of gastrointestinal or operative site bleeding related to ketorolac therapy is only slightly higher than with opioids

Some recent reports have associated an increased incidence of bleeding after tonsillectomy with the perioperative us of ketorolac; however, a recent (2003) meta-analysis was equivocal

Some practitioners will avoid ketorolac with its anti-inflammatory effects for orthopedic surgery when fusion is performed secondary to the theoretical possibility of inhibition of osteoblastic activity

The risk of adverse events increases with high doses, with prolonged therapy (>5 days) or in vulnerable patients (e.g., elderly, pre-existing renal insufficiency, hypovolemic patients)

Cyclooxygenase-2 Inhibitors

Cyclooxygenase-2-selective inhibitors (coxibs) are attractive opioid-sparing analgesic options in the perioperative setting. NSAIDs such as ketorolac have a role in postoperative pain management but concerns about increased bleeding (COX-1 effects) and inhibited wound healing and bone fusion, gastrointestinal effects (ulcers, bleeding), and renal dysfunction have limited their use.

Celecoxib and rofecoxib are two of the most commonly used COX-2 inhibitors for treatment of acute pain. Valdecoxib and parecoxib (an injectable pro-drug of valdecoxib) may be used more in the future. A single intravenous dose of parecoxib appears to be as effective as intravenous ketorolac, and superior to intravenous morphine 4 mg. Interestingly, results of premarketing and post-marketing trials have raised doubts about the cardiovascular safety of COX-2 inhibitors, including worsening of stable treated hypertension and potentially increased stroke and myocardial infarction risk. The role of COX-2 inhibitors in perioperative pain management has yet to be defined.

Acetaminophen

Acetaminophen (paracetamol) is a useful adjuvant during the perioperative period and compares favorably to the NSAIDs in children. Acetaminophen is an analgesic and antipyretic drug without significant anti-inflammatory effects. Unlike aspirin or NSAIDs, acetaminophen does not produce gastric irritation or adversely effect platelet function. The opioid-sparing effect of acetaminophen is dose related. Acetaminophen is usually given in doses of 10–15 mg/kg by mouth or up to 20 mg/kg per rectum. However, there is more recent evidence to suggest that larger doses may be more effective. Doses of 25–30 mg/kg by mouth or 40 mg/kg per rectum are found to achieve more effective blood levels. A maintenance dose of 20 mg/kg every 6–8 hours is used during the early postoperative period. The total dose should not exceed 90 mg/kg per 24 hours for fear of hepatic injury.

Dexmedetomidine

Dexmedetomidine (Precedex™) is a more selective alpha-2-adrenoceptor agonist than clonidine and is indicated for sedation of intubated and mechanically ventilated patients during treatment in an intensive care setting. It stimulates the alpha-2 receptors in the locus ceruleus to provide sedation and in the spinal cord to enhance analgesia. It also causes sympatholysis via central and peripheral mechanisms (Figure 5-19). Dexmedetomidine also has analgesia-sparing properties

Precedex™ (dexmedetomidine)

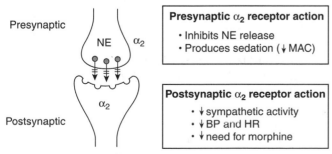

Figure 5-19   Dexmedetomidine is a selective α_2 adrenoreceptor agonist. (NE, norepinephrine; MAC, minimal alveolar concentration; BP, blood pressure; HR, heart rate.)

and, at therapeutic doses, is not associated with respiratory depression despite profound levels of sedation. It is not necessary to discontinue infusions prior to extubation. Dexmedetomidine decreases MAC, intraoperatively, and is most frequently used for sedation for less than 24 hours duration in mechanically ventilated patients in the intensive care unit.

For adult patients, dexmedetomidine is generally initiated with a loading infusion of 1.0 µg/kg over 10 minutes, followed by a maintenance infusion of 0.2–0.7 µg/kg/hr. The rate of the maintenance infusion should be adjusted to achieve the desired level of sedation but the infusion time should not exceed 24 hours. Bradycardia and hypotension may result from administration of dexmedetomidine and caution should be exercised when administering it to patients with advanced heart block or severe ventricular dysfunction.

A summary of the current understanding of dexmedetomidine in clinical practice includes the following caveats:

- Dexmedetomidine can blunt the perioperative stress response and has a possible beneficial role as a perioperative anti-ischemic agent
- Despite intubation and ventilation, patients are usually easily arousable and able to cooperate with procedures and evaluations
- Reproducible evoked potentials can be obtained and BIS monitoring employed
- Postoperative shivering is reduced
- Dexmedetomidine does not inhibit adrenal steroidogenesis
- Dexmedetomidine decreases cerebral blood flow in healthy volunteers.

The appropriate use of dexmedetomidine in patients or procedures with the potential for cerebral ischemia (e.g., cerebrovascular surgery) has yet to be determined.

PHARMACOLOGIC MANAGEMENT OF POSTOPERATIVE NAUSEA AND VOMITING

Patients are stratified preoperatively with regard to their risk of PONV. Those with minimal risk of PONV are not prophylactically treated while those with moderate to severe risk (female, gynecologic surgery, laparoscopic procedures, previous history of PONV) may be treated with multimodal therapy including a 5-HT$_3$ antagonist such as ondansetron and the steroid dexamethasone. Currently, the best prophylaxis against PONV is achieved with the fewest side effects by the combination of dexamethasone and a 5-HT$_3$ antagonist.

Nausea and vomiting occurring in the postoperative period are treated pharmacologically after evaluating and treating any underlying causes of PONV such as hypoxia, hypotension, hypoglycemia, or pain. Medications that have antagonist action at the serotonin (ondansetron), histamine (promethazine), muscarinic (atropine, scopolamine), and dopamine (droperidol) receptors may be beneficial.

Until recently, droperidol (0.625–1.25 mg intravenously) was considered first-line therapy. Although controversial, concerns about Q-T prolongation and cardiac dysrhythmias has now limited the use of droperidol to patients failing other antiemetic therapies who do not have Q-T prolongation and will be monitored for dysrhythmias for 2–3 hours after treatment.

Ondansetron or dolasetron is costly but does not alter dopamine, histamine, adrenergic, or cholinergic receptor activity, and the most commonly reported side effects are headache, diarrhea, and transient increases in the plasma concentrations of liver transaminase enzymes. Ondansetron is also available in tablet, liquid, melt (dissolves sublingually), and suppository form.

Dexamethasone 4–10 mg intravenously is additive in the treatment of PONV and has late efficacy. Promethazine 12.5–25 mg intravenously or prochlorperazine suppository (25 mg per rectum) may be added to dexamethasone and a 5-HT$_3$ antagonist but are usually reserved for recalcitrant cases of PONV. Antiemetics with dopamine antagonist activity (e.g., metoclopramide, phenothiazines, droperidol) should be avoided in patients with Parkinson's disease. The role of scopolamine administered transdermally in the prevention and treatment of PONV is unclear. Side effects, including visual disturbances and dry mouth, may limit its usefulness.

ANESTHETIC REVERSAL PHARMACOLOGY

A relative overdose with opioids or benzodiazepines may necessitate pharmacologic reversal in the perioperative period. If a patient is confused or delirious following the administration of scopolamine or atropine, the diagnosis of central anticholinergic syndrome should be considered.

Naloxone

Naloxone is a pure competitive antagonist at opioid receptors in the brain and spinal cord and is used to reverse undesired opioid-induced depression of the respiratory or central nervous system. Naloxone (1–4 μg/kg intravenously) reverses opioid-induced analgesia and depression of ventilation within 1–2 minutes but has a short duration of action of only 30–60 minutes, which is less than that of fentanyl, morphine, and meperidine. Supplemental doses or continuous infusion (5 μg/kg/hr)

of naloxone may be required for sustained antagonism of these opioid agonists.

Adverse effects of naloxone administration include reversal of analgesia, nausea and vomiting, sudden perception of pain with cardiovascular stimulation evidenced by tachycardia, hypertension, cardiac dysrhythmias (including ventricular fibrillation), pulmonary hypertension, and pulmonary edema. Naloxone crosses the placenta and can precipitate withdrawal in the neonate of an opioid-dependent parturient.

Flumazenil

Flumazenil is a specific and competitive antagonist of benzodiazepines at benzodiazepine receptors. Titration of flumazenil in low doses (0.2 mg intravenously) allows reversal of hypnotic effects and patient awakening from benzodiazepine overdose without reversing the anxiolytic effects. The recommended initial dose of 0.2 mg intravenously typically reverses the CNS effects of benzodiazepine agonists within 1–2 minutes. Repeat doses of 0.1 mg intravenously administered at 60 second intervals to a total dose of 0.3–0.6 mg will usually allow adequate evaluation of a patient who is relatively oversedated or anesthetized by a previously administered benzodiazepine. The dose required for desired clinical effect varies. The lowest doses reverse hypnosis followed by muscle relaxation, amnesia, sedation, anticonvulsant effects, and then anxiolysis with increasing dose.

Flumazenil may precipitate withdrawal in benzodiazepine-dependent patients and, because the elimination half-life (60 minutes) is less than that of the longer-acting benzodiazepines (diazepam), re-sedation may occur necessitating repeat doses. Flumazenil lacks intrinsic agonist effects on the cardiovascular, respiratory, or central nervous systems and does not affect the MAC of inhalational anesthetics.

Physostigmine

Physostigmine (0.5–2.0 mg intravenously) is effective in the treatment of central anticholinergic syndrome characterized by restlessness and confusion and due to the central anticholinergic action of administered atropine or scopolamine. It is a tertiary amine that readily crosses the blood–brain barrier, inhibiting cholinesterase both centrally and peripherally. Possible consequences of peripheral inhibition of cholinesterase and increased acetylcholine include bradycardia, asystole, hypotension, and bronchospasm. The duration of action of physostigmine is shorter than that of scopolamine and atropine and repeat administration may be necessary.

SUMMARY

The introduction of extremely insoluble and easily titratable inhaled anesthetics such as desflurane, less toxic local anesthetics, opioids that can be turned "on and off" in minutes like remifentanil, and intravenous anesthetic induction agents with near ideal characteristics, such as propofol, have been big advances in the practice of anesthesiology.

Although there remains a paucity of prospective, randomized trials to definitively recommend one anesthetic technique over another with regard to outcome measures, a detailed understanding of the pharmacologic and physiologic characteristics of the anesthetic agents and adjuvants allows a more rationale approach to perioperative anesthetic care.

SUGGESTED READING

Conzen PF, Kharasch ED, Czerner SFA, *et al*. Low-flow sevoflurane compared with low flow isoflurane anesthesia in patients with stable renal insufficiency. *Anesthesiology* 2002; 97:578-584.

Eagel KA, Berger PB, Calkins H, *et al*. ACC/AHA Guideline for perioperative cardiovascular evaluation for noncardiac surgery — executive summary. *Anesth Analg* 2002;94:1052-1064.

Henzi I, Walder B, Tramer MR. Dexamethasone for the prevention of postoperative nausea and vomiting: a quantitative systematic review. *Anesth Analg* 2000;90:186-194.

Mangano DT, Layug B, Tateo I, *et al*. Effect of atenolol on mortality and cardiovascular morbidity after noncardiac surgery. *N Engl J Med* 1996;335:1713-1720.

Moiniche S, Kehlet H, Dahl JB. A qualitative and quantitative systematic review of preemptive analgesia for postoperative pain relief. *Anesthesiology* 2002;96:725-741.

Moiniche S, Romsing J, Dahl JB, Tramer MR. Nonsteroidal anti-inflammatory drugs and the risk of operative site bleeding after tonsillectomy: a quantitative systematic review. *Anesth Analg* 2003; 96:68-77.

Muzi M, Lopatka CW, Ebert TJ. Desflurane-mediated neurocirculatory activation in humans. Effects of concentration and rate of change on responses. *Anesthesiology* 1996;84:1035-1042.

Prielipp RC, Wall MH, Tobin JR, *et al*. Dexmedetomidine-induced sedation in volunteers decreases regional and global cerebral blood flow. *Anesth Analg* 2002;95:1052-1059.

Romsing J, Moiniche S, Dahl JB. Rectal and parenteral paracetamol, and paracetamol in combination with NSAIDs, for postoperative analgesia. *Br J Anaesth* 2002;88:215-226.

Rosow C, Manberg PJ. Bispectral index monitoring. *Anesthesiol Clin North Am* 2001;19:947-966.

Rossaint R, Reyle-Hahn M, Schulte am Esch J, *et al*. Multicenter randomized comparison of the efficacy and safety of xenon and isoflurane in patients undergoing elective surgery. *Anesthesiology* 2003;98:6-13.

Tang J, Li S, White PF, *et al*. Effect of parecoxib, a novel intravenous cyclooxygenase type-2 inhibitor, on the postoperative opioid requirement and quality of pain control. *Anesthesiology* 2002;96:1305-1309.

Tong D, Wong J, Chung F, *et al*. Prospective study on incidence and functional impact of transient neurologic symptoms associated with 1% versus 5% hyperbaric lidocaine in short urologic procedures. *Anesthesiology* 2003;98:485-494.

White PF. The role of non-opioid analgesic technique in the management of pain after ambulatory surgery. *Anesth Analg* 2002;94:577-585.

White, PF. Droperidol: A cost-effective antiemetic for over thirty years. *Anesth Analg* 2002;95:789-90.

Wissing H, Kuhn I, Warnken U, Dudziak R. Carbon monoxide production from desflurane, enflurane, halothane, isoflurane, and sevoflurane with dry soda lime. *Anesthesiology* 2001;95: 1205-1212.

Airway Management

RICHARD L. APPLEGATE II

INTRODUCTION

The importance of safe management of the airway cannot be overstated. Anesthesiologists rightly consider themselves experts at airway management. Our worse nightmares often involve cases in which the airway cannot be secured, with the patient suffering physiologic insult. While managing patients with normal airway anatomy is a key component of safe practice, management of patients with difficult airway anatomy is critically important. Various studies report that between 1% and 18% of patients have difficult airway anatomy. Of these, 0.05–0.35% are not intubated successfully and a significant portion may be difficult to ventilate by mask. Put in the perspective of the average practice, it is likely that the practitioner will encounter between one and 10 patients per year in whom intubation of the trachea will be difficult or impossible. The impact of the resultant respiratory compromise varies but can include signifi-

cant brain injury and death. The risks related to inadequate management of the patient's airway are reflected in the malpractice claims analyzed in the American Society of Anesthesiologists Closed Claims Project, in which adverse respiratory events represent the largest single source of settled claims, with a high incidence of death and brain damage occurring in patients in whom a claim related to respiratory complications has been closed. The goals of this chapter are to discuss the basics of airway anatomy and normal airway management, and to highlight some of the factors that contribute to the safe management of the patient with a difficult airway.

AIRWAY ANATOMY

Taken as a system, the airway begins at the external openings of the mouth and nose and ends in the alveolar units. An understanding of the anatomic relationships in the airway is helpful in managing patients in the perioperative setting. A review of basic airway anatomy with an emphasis on functional concerns follows. For convenience, airway anatomy will be discussed in terms of the supraglottic airway, the larynx, and the subglottic airway.

The Supraglottic Airway

The Nose
The nose serves to warm and humidify air as it enters the body. The nasal passage may be limited by the size of the turbinates, which are highly vascular. Passage of endotracheal tubes or bronchoscopes through the nose may be associated with profuse bleeding. The nasal septum is often deviated, giving a smaller passage on one side than the other. The nasopharynx opens into the oropharynx. Branches of the fifth cranial nerve provide sensory innervation to the nose.

The Pharynx

The space in the posterior portion of the oral cavity is divided into the nasopharynx, oropharynx, and hypopharynx. Lymphoid tissue around the pharynx may hinder passage of an endotracheal tube. The internal muscles of the pharynx serve to elevate the palate during swallowing. The external muscles of the pharynx are constrictors and serve to push food into the esophagus, but may impair passage of an endotracheal tube or bronchoscope in awake or lightly anesthetized patients. The innervation of the pharynx is from the ninth cranial nerve for somatic sensory and motor function with the exception of the levator veli palatini, which is innervated by the fifth cranial nerve.

Obstruction of the airway may occur at the pharyngeal level. In this event, the soft tissues of the pharynx are apposed, limiting airflow. This blockage of airflow can occur at the soft palate, which can come into contact with the nasopharyngeal wall. Similarly, the tongue may move posteriorly in the pharynx and obstruct the airway by contacting the posterior wall of the oropharynx. This condition occurs in anesthetized and sedated patients but may also occur in sleeping patients. The obstruction occurs as muscle tone decreases and a decrease in the functional lumen of the pharynx ensues. With spontaneously breathing patients, a decrease in functional airway lumen may be associated with an increased respiratory effort and resultant greater negative pressure below the level of obstruction. This can lead to a worsening of the obstruction as the negative pressure pulls more soft tissue into the area of collapse. A significant form of this problem is obstructive sleep apnea.

The Larynx

The larynx is a complicated structure that serves to protect the lower airway, as the organ of phonation and as the conduit for respiration. These functions depend on the interaction of the cartilaginous, bony and soft tissue components of the larynx and pharynx. There are 9 cartilages of the larynx including the midline epiglottis, thyroid and cricoid cartilages and the paired arytenoids, cuneiform and corniculate cartilages. The muscles of the larynx are both extrinsic and extrinsic. Innervation of the upper airway is rich, with both sensory and motor supply.

Structures of the Larynx

The structures of the larynx are illustrated in Figure 6-1. The *hyoid bone* suspends the larynx, and is attached to the temporal bone by the stylohyoid ligament.

Cartilages of the Larynx

- *Thyroid cartilage*: The largest cartilage of the larynx, this has a more acute angle in males, which gives a more prominent appearance and longer, lower-pitched vocal cords. It is attached by membranes to the hyoid

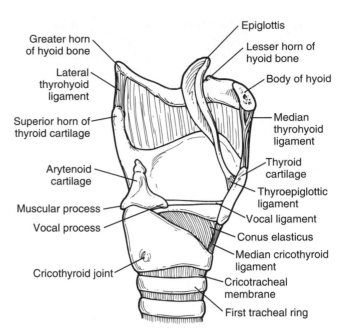

Figure 6-1   Lateral view of the larynx with the right half of the thyroid cartilage removed. (Redrawn from Black SM, Chambers WA. *Essential anatomy for anesthesia.* New York: Churchill Livingstone, 1997:21.)

bone above and articulates with the cricoid cartilage below. The stem of the epiglottis and the vocal and vestibular ligaments attach to the inner surface.

- *Cricoid cartilage*: A complete ring with a broader posterior portion that attaches to the esophagus. The anterior arch attaches to the thyroid cartilage by the cricothyroid membrane. The cricothyroid membrane is relatively avascular and may provide for emergency access to the airway via a midline incision or needle insertion.

- *Arytenoid cartilages*: Pyramidal in shape, the arytenoids are the anchor points for several of the internal muscles of the larynx and of the vocal cords. The cuneiform and corniculate cartilages are found in ligaments attached to the arytenoid cartilages.

- *Epiglottis*: A relatively large cartilaginous structure that has been described as shaped like a tear or a leaf, or even as a bicycle seat. It is flexible and variably sized, and is positioned vertically behind the hyoid bone, to which it is attached by the hyoepiglottic ligament. The base of the epiglottis attaches to the arytenoids via the aryepiglottic folds. The mucosa of the epiglottis sweeps forward and laterally forming a space between the pharyngoepiglottic folds called the vallecula. This space is a site for impaction of foreign material such as food, and is the proper place to place the tip of a Macintosh laryngoscope blade.

Interior of the Larynx

The interior of the larynx is also a complicated structure. The inlet to the larynx from the pharynx is almost vertical. The laryngeal cavity can be divided into segments. The vestibule extends from the inlet to the vestibular folds, which are also known as the false cords. The ventricle of the larynx extends from the false cords to the true cords. The area between the vocal cords when closed and the arytenoid cartilages is called the rima glottidis. This is the narrowest portion of the upper airway in adults. The infraglottic portion of the larynx extends from the vocal cords to the upper portion of the trachea. It is bounded by the cricothyroid membrane and the cricoid cartilage, and is the narrowest portion of the airway in the child (Figure 6-2, Box 6-1).

Muscles of the Larynx

The extrinsic muscles of the larynx move the larynx in relationship to other structures in the neck and play a role in swallowing. These muscles include the sternohyoid, sternothyroid, thyrohyoid, thyroepiglottic, stylopharyngeus, and inferior pharyngeal constrictor muscles.

The intrinsic muscles of the larynx work in concert to adduct the vocal cords to close the laryngeal opening during swallowing, abduct the vocal cords during inspiration, and alter the tension of the vocal cords during phonation. The muscles of the larynx are:

- *Oblique arytenoid*: Closes rima glottidis
- *Transverse arytenoid*: Adducts arytenoids, closes rima glottidis
- *Lateral cricoarytenoid*: Adducts vocal cords
- *Posterior cricoarytenoid*: Abducts vocal cords
- *Cricothyroid*: Tenses vocal cords
- *Thyroarytenoid*: Relaxes tension on vocal cords
- *Vocalis*: Relaxes vocal cords.

Closure of the laryngeal opening is an important function. The larynx can be closed at three levels: the aryepiglottic folds, the false vocal cords and the true vocal cords. The larynx is closed during swallowing, which occurs in three phases. In the first, the voluntary phase of swallowing, food is pushed to the posterior pharynx by the tongue. In the second phase of swallowing, respiration is halted, the

---

Box 6-1 Differences in Airway Anatomy in the Pediatric Patient

The differences between adult and pediatric airway anatomy (Figure 6-3) are most pronounced in neonates and young children, with growth leading to adult anatomy by about 6 years of age. The major differences in pediatric airway anatomy compared to adult airway anatomy can be summarized as follows:

- Smaller nares
- Relatively large tongue
- Smaller larynx compared to the rest of the airway
- More cephalad location of larynx: C3–C4 in neonate, C5 by age 6
- Softer epiglottis, described as being "floppy", angled in the direction of the glottis
- Arytenoids larger compared to the glottic opening
- Cricoid cartilage in continuity with the larynx, narrowest part of larynx in infants
- Trachea shorter
- Head and occiput larger compared to rest of body
- Relatively short neck

---

palatoglossal muscles contract, and the oropharynx is cut off from the nasopharynx and larynx by the combined action of several of the strap muscles effectively pulling the larynx superiorly to allow the epiglottis to block the opening to the larynx. The third phase of swallowing carries the food into and down the esophagus.

Innervation of the Larynx

The laryngeal structures have both sensory and motor innervation (Table 6-1). The motor functions are adduc-

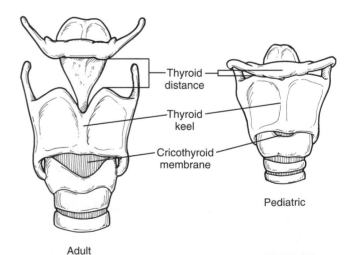

Figure 6-3   Anterior view of larynx in an adult and an infant. Note overlapping of hyoid, thyroid, and cricoid in the infant. (Redrawn from Reynolds P. Pediatric difficult airways. In: Norton ML, ed. *Atlas of the difficult airway*. St Louis: Mosby/Year Book, 1996:247.)

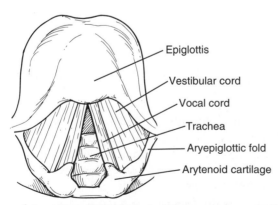

Figure 6-2   View of the larynx at laryngoscopy. (Redrawn from Black SM, Chambers WA. *Essential anatomy for anesthesia*. New York: Churchill Livingstone, 1997.)

Table 6-1   Innervation of the Larynx

Nerve	Function Sensory	Function Motor
Superior laryngeal, interior division	Epiglottis, base of tongue, supraglottic mucosa, thyroepiglottic joint, cricothyroid joint	None
Superior laryngeal, external division	Anterior subglottic mucosa	Cricothyroid: vocal cord tension
Recurrent laryngeal	Subglottic mucosa, muscle spindles	Thyroarytenoid: adduction, glottic sphincter
		Lateral cricoarytenoid: adduction
		Interarytenoid: adduction
		Posterior cricoarytenoid: abduction

tion (closing vocal cords), abduction (opening vocal cords), and tension (tightening vocal cords to produce higher-pitched sounds). All motor and sensory innervation to the intrinsic laryngeal structures comes from branches of the vagus nerve. The superior laryngeal nerve is a branch of the vagus nerve that passes deep to the carotid artery before dividing into internal and external branches. The larger internal branch pierces the thyrohyoid membrane between the greater cornu of the thyroid cartilage and the hyoid bone. This branch then supplies the sensory innervation to the larynx. The external branch of the superior laryngeal nerve carries motor fibers from the spinal accessory nerve. This branch travels along the thyroid cartilage to supply the cricothyroid muscle. The recurrent laryngeal nerve leaves the vagus in the chest and then runs superiorly to the larynx in the tracheoesophageal groove. The recurrent laryngeal nerve supplies motor innervation to all the intrinsic muscles of the larynx except the cricothyroid muscle.

Laryngeal reflexes may be stimulated at the larynx or at supraglottic levels and may lead to closure of the vocal cords up to the point of laryngospasm. Sensory block of the mucosa of the larynx requires block of the superior laryngeal nerve for the mucosa down to the vocal cords plus a recurrent laryngeal nerve block or topical application of local anesthetic, for example by transtracheal injection or spray for the mucosa below the vocal cords. Complete motor block, to facilitate intubation for example, requires a block of the recurrent laryngeal nerve, since this nerve supplies motor function to all intrinsic nerves of the larynx except the cricothyroid muscle. This block is usually carried out by transtracheal or cricothyroid injection or spray of local anesthetic.

Stimulation of the supraglottic structures can lead to glottic closure or laryngospasm. These structures respond briskly to touch, heat and chemical stimuli. This response is usually brief. Laryngospasm is a state in which glottic closure persists after removal of the stimulus. It is initiated in response to repeated stimulation of the nerves in the supraglottic region and may persist to the point of hypoxia and hypercapnia, at which point it usually ceases.

Subglottic Airway

The subglottic airway extends from the cricoid cartilage to the alveolar units. A complete review of this anatomy is outside the scope of this chapter; however, a brief discussion of the anatomy of the major bronchi is included.

Trachea

The trachea begins at the cricoid cartilage and extends approximately to the T5 level (about 10–20 cm in length). The tracheal cartilage forms incomplete rings, with the posterior portion thus flattened and unsupported by cartilage. The tracheal bifurcation into the left and right main stem bronchi is such that the angle is less acute to the right bronchus in adults. Thus unintended single-lung intubation is more likely to occur in the right main bronchus.

Lobar Bronchi

The right and left lungs have different lobar anatomy (Table 6-2). The right lung has three lobes – upper, middle, and lower – while the left lung has just upper and lower.

Table 6-2   Lobes and Segments of the Lungs

	Lobes	Segments
Right lung	Upper	Apical, anterior and posterior
	Middle	Lateral and medial
	Lower	Superior, medial basal, anterior basal, lateral basal, posterior basal
Left lung	Upper	Apical, posterior, anterior, superior lingual, inferior lingual
	Lower	Superior, medial basal, anterior basal, lateral basal, posterior basal

The origin of the right upper lobe bronchus is quite proximal compared to the origin of the left upper lobe bronchus. This difference may be useful in distinguishing left from right during bronchoscopy. The lobes are further divided into segments.

MANAGEMENT OF PATIENTS WITH NORMAL AIRWAY ANATOMY

Mastering ventilation by bag and mask is critical for safe practice. The basic maneuvers used to facilitate air exchange in spontaneously breathing or paralyzed patients are directed to opening the airway above the glottis. Motions that move the tongue and other soft tissues of the supraglottic airway anteriorly will generally improve air exchange. These maneuvers include chin lift, jaw thrust, head tilt, and introduction of oral or nasal airways (Figure 6-4).

Difficulty with mask ventilation may be predicted in some patients. Factors reported to correlate to difficult mask ventilation include:
- Presence of a beard
- Body mass index greater than 26
- Lack of teeth
- Age over 55 years
- History of snoring.

Motions required for intubation in the normal patient are performed to allow visualization of the larynx from the opening of the mouth. In patients with normal airway anatomy, the major components of this positioning are flexion of the neck, particularly in the lower cervical spine, and extension of the head at the atlantooccipital

joint. This position is referred to as the "sniffing position" and is best understood in terms of the major axes of three parts of the airway. In the adult airway, the long axis of the mouth is horizontal, roughly parallel to the floor when standing. The long axis of the pharynx is nearly vertical. The long axis of the larynx is off vertical with a posterior to anterior course. Alignment of these three axes allows visualization of the vocal cords from the mouth (Figure 6-5).

Patients in whom cervical spine motion is limited will appear to have an "anterior" position of the larynx, which may make intubation difficult.

Use of laryngeal mask airway (LMAs) can be considered to be an intermediate type of airway management. In many patients, the LMA can be used safely in place of endotracheal intubation. There is a clear role for LMA use in managing patients with difficult airway anatomy, as will be discussed later. Finally, there may be a role for the LMA in emergency or trauma settings, perhaps even by paramedical personnel.

MANAGEMENT OF THE DIFFICULT AIRWAY

Ideally, all patients would have normal airway anatomy, so any patient requiring a controlled airway would have no additional risk above that of the surgical procedure. Since this is not realistic, the anesthesiologist must have a way to identify and care for patients with abnormal airway anatomy. Simplistically, safe management of patients with a difficult airway comes down to three "P"s:
- Prediction
- Preparation
- Practice.

Prediction

Identification of patients at risk for abnormal airway anatomy allows the anesthesiologist to consider options for management in a non-emergency setting. This is important, as some of the techniques to be discussed later are difficult if airway bleeding occurs, and as some patients will become apneic and potentially hypoxic following induction of anesthesia. There are several popular methods of predicting ease or difficulty of intubation using a physical examination. Prior to evaluating the predictive tests, some clarification is needed.

Difficulty in intubating the trachea can be said to occur when an experienced practitioner is unable to pass an endotracheal tube in the normal time and fashion. It may be defined as an intubation that requires more than one attempt. However, more difficult intubations can be related

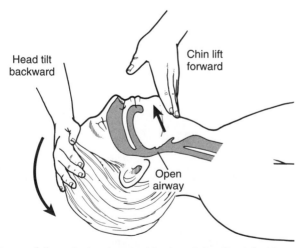

Figure 6-4   The head is tilted back and the chin lifted forward, both of which contribute to opening the airway. (Redrawn from Benumof JL. *Airway management: principles and practice*, St Louis: Mosby, 1996:233.)

Head and neck position and the axis of the head and neck and upper airway

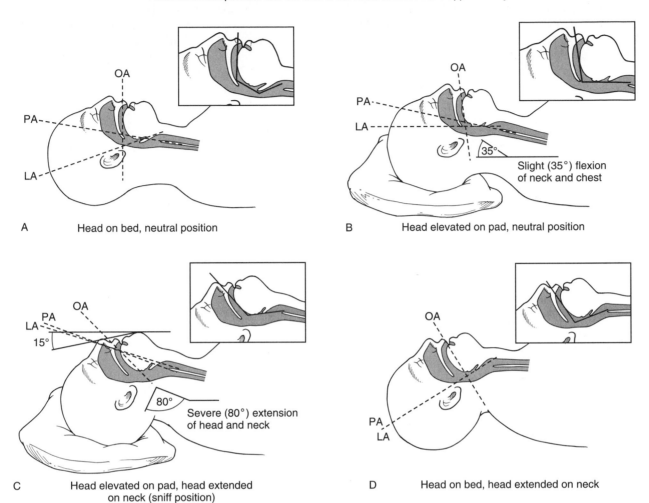

A   Head on bed, neutral position

B   Head elevated on pad, neutral position

C   Head elevated on pad, head extended on neck (sniff position)

D   Head on bed, head extended on neck

Figure 6-5   **The alignment of the oral axis (OA), pharyngeal axis (PA), and laryngeal axis (LA) in four different head positions**. Each head position is accompanied by an inset that magnifies the upper airway (the oral cavity, pharynx, and larynx) and superimposes, as a variously bent bold line, the continuity of these three axes within the upper airway. **A**, The head is in a neutral position with a marked degree of nonalignment of LA, PA, and OA. **B**, The head is resting on a large pad that flexes the neck on the chest and aligns the LA with the PA. **C**, The head is resting on a pad (which flexes the neck on the chest); concomitant extension of the head on the neck, which brings all three axes into alignment (sniff position), is shown. **D**, Extension of the head on the neck without concomitant elevation of the head on a pad, which results in nonalignment of the PA and LA with the OA. (Redrawn from Benumof JL. *Airway management: principles and practice*, St Louis: Mosby, 1996:Fig. 14-1.)

to the grade of laryngoscopic view (Figure 6-6). Difficulty during intubation is likely with a grade III or IV view.
- Grade I: Vocal cords are visible
- Grade II: Vocal cords are only partly visible
- Grade III: Only the epiglottis is seen
- Grade IV: Not even the epiglottis is seen.

Recent investigations have compared various predictive tests in an attempt to determine the best way to predict difficult intubation. There are various factors to evaluate when assessing a patient for endotracheal intubation.

- *History*: Most patients will not relate any significant history about prior intubation if no problems were encountered. However, patients who give a history of prior difficult intubation have a very high incidence of difficult intubation. The presence of conditions associated with difficult intubation should be ascertained. These conditions include:
  - Congenital syndromes, including Down, Goldenhar, Treacher Collins, Pierre Robin, and mucopolysaccharidoses, among others

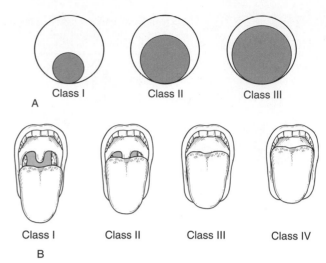

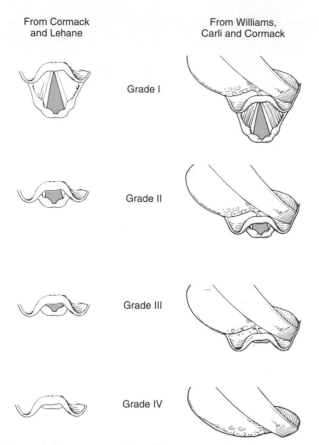

From Cormack and Lehane — From Williams, Carli and Cormack

Grade I

Grade II

Grade III

Grade IV

Figure 6-6   Four grades of laryngoscopic view. Grade I is visualization of entire laryngeal aperture; grade II is visualization of just the posterior portion of laryngeal aperture; grade III is visualization of just the epiglottis; and grade IV is visualization of just the soft palate. It is assumed that care has been taken to get the best possible view of the vocal cords. (Redrawn from Benumof JL. *Airway management: principles and practice*, St Louis: Mosby, 1996:Fig. 6-3.)

Class I Class II Class III

A

Class I Class II Class III Class IV

B

Figure 6-7   A, The conceptual basis of the Mallampati Airway Classification is determining the size of the tongue (shaded area) relative to size of the pharyngeal cavity (open circle). **B,** Samsoon and Young modification of the Mallampati Airway Classification. (Redrawn from Benumof JL. *Airway management: principles and practice*, St Louis: Mosby, 1996:Figs 7-2, 7-3.)

- Bony diseases, including rheumatoid arthritis, ankylosing spondylitis, mandibular fracture or fixation, ankylosis of the temporomandibular joint
- Soft tissue abnormalities, including obesity, tumors, hemangiomas, abscesses, airway infections such as epiglottitis, bleeding
- Trauma to face or neck, burns, postoperative changes including scarring, radiation-induced changes.
- *Dentition*: Prominent upper central incisors can limit the ability to see the larynx during intubation. Be especially wary of patients with chipped teeth in a pattern that would fit a laryngoscope blade.
- *Temporomandibular joint mobility* is assessed by mouth opening as measured by the interincisor distance and by the ability to prognath. Interincisor distance must at least allow passage of a standard laryngoscope blade.
- *Oropharyngeal class*: This is commonly called Mallampati class; the opening in the pharynx is evalu-

ated. Scores of 3 or 4 are associated with a greater chance of difficult intubation (Figure 6-7).
- *Width of the palate*: Patients with long narrow palates are more likely to have difficult airway anatomy.
- *The thyromental distance* is the distance from the inner aspect of the most anterior portion of the mandible to the top of the thyroid cartilage. The smaller this distance the more anterior the larynx will appear.
- *Compliance of the mandibular space* is an important factor to evaluate. During normal intubation, the tongue and other soft tissues of the floor of the mouth are pushed anteriorly into the mandibular space, allowing visualization of the larynx. Patients whose mandibular space is poorly compliant, as in postradiation conditions, significant obesity or infection, will have a limited view of the larynx.
- *Body habitus*, especially length and thickness of the neck, and the presence of any anatomic factors that will limit motion of the head such as fat pads between the scapulae should be evaluated.
- *Neck mobility* is assessed for flexion and extension. Movement of the head at the atlanto-occipital junction is assessed. Limited motion at the atlanto-occipital junction will make the larynx appear anterior.

The value of these tests has been demonstrated in the literature. The more factors evaluated, the greater the likelihood of accurately predicting patients with difficult airway anatomy. Significantly, the negative predictive value of a multifactorial examination of the patient for difficult airway anatomy is very high. If all factors in the multifactorial airway examination indicate normal airway

Table 6-3   Nonreassuring Findings of the Airway Examination

Airway Examination Component	Nonreassuring Finding
Length of upper incisors	Relatively long
Relationship of maxillary and mandibular incisors during normal jaw closure	Prominent "overbite" (maxillary incisors anterior to mandibular incisors)
Relationship of maxillary and mandibular incisors during voluntary protrusion of mandible	Patient cannot bring mandibular incisors anterior to (in front of) maxillary incisors
Interincisor distance	Less than 3 cm
Visibility of uvula	Not visible when tongue is protruded with patient in sitting position (e.g., Mallampati class greater than II)
Shape of palate	Highly arched or very narrow
Compliance of mandibular space	Stiff, indurated, occupied by mass, or non-resilient
Thyromental distance	Less than 3 ordinary finger-breadths
Length of neck	Short
Thickness of neck	Thick
Range of motion of head and neck	Patient cannot touch tip of chin to chest, or cannot extend neck

anatomy, the likelihood of a difficult intubation is very small.

Examination of the airway may be performed several ways. The American Society of Anesthesiologists (ASA) Task Force on Difficult Airway Management has published an extensive examination with findings that are "nonreassuring." Nonreassuring findings (Table 6-3) are more likely to be associated with difficult intubation.

One set of maneuvers that seems to work well and allows evaluation of the significant factors is outlined below. With the patient in a sitting or semi-sitting position evaluate:

- *Body habitus*, especially the distribution of body fat around the head and neck
- *Thyromental distance, mandibular compliance*: "I'm going to put my hand under your chin"
- *Teeth, mouth opening and oral–pharyngeal space*: "Open your mouth as wide as you can;" if the Mallampati score is not 1 or 2, ask for phonation
- *Temporomandibular joint mobility*: "Relax. Now stick your chin out to put your lower teeth in front of your upper teeth"
- *Neck flexion*: "Pick your head up and try to touch your chin to your chest"
- *Head extension*: "I'm going to hold my hand behind your neck. Tip your head back as far as you can, like you are trying to look at the ceiling."

This examination puts the patient in an exaggerated sniffing position. If there are no nonreassuring findings and the patient can do the maneuver with little or no limitation or pain, intubation is likely to be easy. If a portion of the examination is abnormal, be suspicious of a difficult intubation. For example, if the patient can flex the neck but cannot extend the head, the larynx will seem anterior.

This is often seen in patients with degenerative joint disease, rheumatoid arthritis, or obesity. Several significant points are clear from the literature:

- In a busy anesthesiology practice, you are likely to encounter a significant number of patients each year with difficult airways. A portion of these will be difficult or impossible to ventilate.
- Prediction of difficulty intubating is more accurate with more factors evaluated.
- A positive history of previous difficult intubation is very significant and should be treated as true. At least some practitioners believe that these patients should be registered with Medic Alert or a similar organization.
- If all the measures you use to evaluate a patient's airway indicate that the patient has normal airway anatomy, you will probably be able to intubate the airway easily. Some patients in whom you predict a difficult intubation will be easy to intubate.
- Importantly, in some patients with expected normal airway anatomy, difficulty may be encountered. Because of this, the anesthesia care provider must always be prepared to care for patients with difficult airway anatomy.

Preparation

Adequate preparation to care for patients with difficult airway anatomy requires acquisition of knowledge and equipment. The knowledge necessary for safe management of these patients is an extension of the knowledge needed to provide care for any patient but with additional points. The ASA addressed these additional knowledge points and developed and published an algorithm for difficult airway management. The algorithm suggests the following steps:

1. Assess the likelihood and clinical impact of basic management problems:
   a. Difficult ventilation
   b. Difficult intubation
   c. Difficulty with patient cooperation or consent
   d. Difficult tracheostomy.
2. Actively pursue opportunities to deliver supplemental oxygen throughout the process of difficult airway management.
3. Consider the relative merits and feasibility of basic management choices:

   A. Awake intubation   versus   Intubation attempts after induction of general anesthesia

   B. Non-invasive technique for initial approach to intubation   versus   Invasive technique for initial approach to intubation

   C. Preservation of spontaneous ventilation   versus   Ablation of spontaneous ventilation

4. Develop primary and alternative strategies (Figure 6-8). Successful application of the algorithm is dependent on identifying patients at risk for difficult airway anatomy, ventilation, and cooperation. The practitioner needs to consider the various methods of management (awake or asleep? surgical or nonsurgical airway?). Safe management depends on providing adequate oxygenation and ventilation during the time needed to control the airway. It is clear from the algorithm that identification of the patient at high risk allows you to alter the management technique chosen to promote ventilation and oxygenation. A number of the tools available can help to turn a difficult intubation into a successful intubation (fiberoptic, retrograde, etc.) or unable-to-ventilate patients into able-to-ventilate patients (transtracheal jet, possibly LMA). The equipment you choose to add to your practice will depend on your own skills and preferences. The range of choices is wide, and some of the options will be discussed.

Tools for Management of the Difficult Airway

Airways

Oral or nasal, these may turn a "can't ventilate" into a "can ventilate" scenario.

Stylets, Intubation Guides and Bougies

These are available as standard wires that provide added stiffness to the endotracheal tube, thus allowing better "steering" into the larynx. They are especially useful in the setting of an anterior larynx. Stylets are available as lighted devices that can be used to facilitate blind intubation by transillumination of the larynx. Intubating stylets may also be "ventilation" designs with a small central port to allow jet ventilation or verification of carbon dioxide return once the stylet is placed in the airway.

Airway Exchange Catheter

This allows administration of oxygen during endotracheal tube exchange and monitoring of carbon dioxide during the endotracheal tube change. It may be used with jet ventilation to improve oxygenation during endotracheal tube change.

Specialized Forceps

These are available to assist in guiding the endotracheal tube into the larynx or to facilitate retraction of the tongue during fiberoptic intubation.

Laryngoscopy

Laryngoscopy is done with a variety of tools. Rigid, direct-vision laryngoscopes are available in a wide assortment of blade shapes and sizes. Some patients have anatomy that is more suited to one type of blade than another. For example, patients with a long, "floppy" epiglottis are often easier to intubate using a straight blade than a Macintosh blade. Rigid, semi-direct laryngoscopes have a prism on the blade to allow vision of the laryngeal structures when the patient's anatomy doesn't allow direct vision. Rigid fiberoptic laryngoscopes such as the Bullard™ and Upsher™ scopes allow visualization of laryngeal structures via fiberoptics. These scopes may be very useful in patients with an anterior larynx. Advantages of the rigid fiberoptic intubating scopes include:
- Rigid scope more similar to usual laryngoscopes
- Possibly shorter learning curve
- Possibly more durable than flexible fiberoptic scopes.

Disadvantages of the rigid fiberoptic intubating scopes include:
- The endotracheal tube is passed into the larynx while watching through the fiberoptic eyepiece, not directly over the scope
- Technique may be difficult or awkward
- Patient size limits related to the relatively large blade size.

Fiberoptic Bronchoscopic Intubation

Fiberoptic bronchoscopic intubation (FBI) uses flexible bronchoscopes to intubate the trachea. Many manufacturers have developed scopes specifically for intubation that are typically longer and of smaller diameter than standard diagnostic bronchoscopes. The advantages of FBI include:
- The endotracheal tube is passed into the trachea directly over the scope
- Acceptable range of patient sizes, since different-sized scopes are available

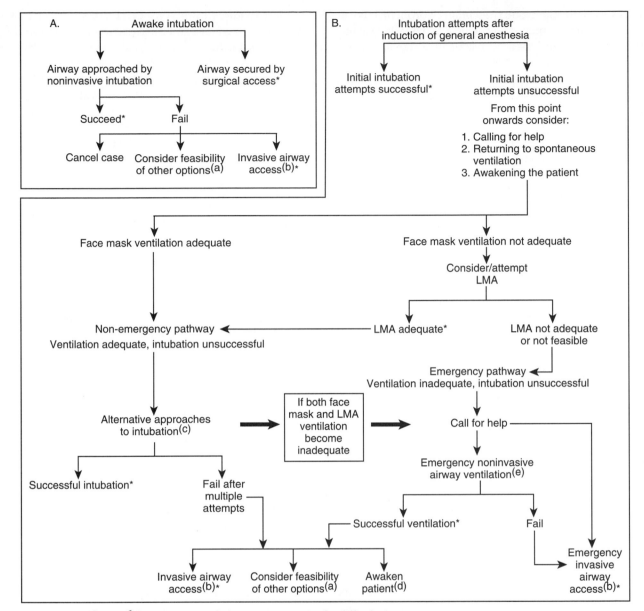

Figure 6-8 Primary and alternative strategies for difficult airway management.
* Confirm tracheal intubation or LMA placement with exhaled CO_2.
Difficult airway algorithm:
a. Other options include (but are not limited to): surgery utilizing face mask or LMA anesthesia infiltration or regional nerve blockade. Pursuit of these options usually implies that mask ventilation will not be problematic. Therefore, these options may be of limited value if this step in the algorithm has been reached via the Emergency Pathway.
b. Invasive airway access includes surgical or percutaneous tracheostomy or cricothyrotomy.
c. Alternative non-invasive approaches to difficult intubation include (but are not limited to): use of different laryngoscope blades, LMA as an intubation conduit (with or without fiberoptic guidance), fiberoptic intubation, intubating stylet or tube changer, light wand, retrograde intubation, and blind oral or nasal intubation.
d. Consider re-preparation of the patient for awake intubation or canceling surgery.
e. Options for emergency non-invasive airway ventilation include (but are not limited to): rigid bronchoscope, esophageal–tracheal combitube ventilation, or transtracheal jet ventilation.

- Therapeutic uses include placement of bronchial blockers and double-lumen endotracheal tubes. Additionally, the bronchoscope may be useful in removing secretions from the bronchi.

Disadvantages of FBI include:
- The technique can be difficult to learn
- The cost and fragility of the equipment are of concern.

Pitfalls of FBI include:
- Blood/secretions may obscure view
- Easy to "get lost" in airway, especially off midline
- Distorted anatomy
- Special problems with FBI:
  - Endotracheal tube may "hang up" on laryngeal structures
  - Scope may loop in pharynx
  - Lens may fog.

Fiberoptic Intubation Tips

- How many? Generally, it takes about 10 tries to learn how to reliably operate the bronchoscope, about 25 to reliably intubate normal patients and more to reliably intubate abnormal patients.
- How to learn? Get acquainted with the scope. Learn how to hold it and how to make the tip move the way you want it to: do this the same way every time. Keep the scope straight between your hands to ensure that the tip moves the way you think it will when you twist the scope. Introduce the scope into the pharynx, taking care to stay in the midline. Nasal intubations are easier at first because the nose is a midline structure and will help to keep the scope in the midline. It helps to keep a finger on the patient's nose or lip for oral intubations. As you advance the scope use an "inching" technique with thumb and first finger to gradually work the scope into the airway. Identify the structures of the upper airway; advance 8–10 cm. You must flex the tip of the scope upward/anteriorly to see the larynx, and then rotate the distal end of the scope as needed to get to the midline position at the vocal cords. To pass the vocal cords, return the tip of the scope to the neutral position, or even posterior, to advance into the trachea. Position the scope above the carina but be aware that touching the carina may induce bronchospasm or coughing. Thread the endotracheal tube into the trachea while keeping the carina in view. If endotracheal tube won't pass easily, try the maneuver described below. Remember that using brute force is usually the wrong thing to do and may damage the airway or scope.
- *Anesthetic techniques*: Start with normal patients, asleep, paralyzed and ventilated by mask by an assistant. Progress to asleep, breathing patients, with or without airway regional anesthesia. Master this before attempting FBI in awake, sedated, breathing patients. Regional anesthesia of the airway will facilitate intubation in awake/sedated patients. Adequate anesthesia for intubation requires both sensory and motor block of the laryngeal surfaces and musculature. This requires block of both the superior laryngeal and recurrent laryngeal nerves to provide both sensory and motor block. There are risks related to regional anesthesia of the airway. Superior laryngeal nerve block provides sensory block to the base of the tongue and epiglottis and may leave the patient at risk for aspiration as refluxed material may not trigger the normal laryngeal closure reflex when sensory block is present. Additionally, recurrent laryngeal nerve block will provide motor block to the laryngeal adductors and will prevent the normal closure reflex to refluxed material, further worsening the risk for aspiration of gastric contents when regional anesthesia of the airway has been performed. For these reasons, regional anesthesia of the airway is relatively contraindicated if the patient has a full stomach or significant gastroesophageal reflux disease.
- *Aids to intubation*: There are several adjuncts available. Intubating airways allow you to pass the scope via a channel while holding the oropharyngeal space open. Intubating masks are available, allowing the patient to be ventilated by a colleague while you do the intubation. The cuffed oropharyngeal airway (COPA) can be used, and again the patient can be ventilated while intubation is performed. However, you must push the tip of the scope past the cuff of the COPA to visualize the cords, then intubate. You may intubate via a LMA. The best adjunct may be a good assistant to hold either jaw thrust or tongue traction as you perform endoscopy.
- *Potential problems*: Some patients may require a different approach to intubation. The most common problems happen after getting the tip of the scope in the trachea: "the endotracheal tube won't pass." Causes include: the tip of the endotracheal tube catching on cartilage, or the scope looping in posterior pharynx. Force will generally not cure this and may damage the airway. Retract the scope slightly, keeping the trachea in view, and corkscrew the tube in. Realize that just because you can clearly view the main carina you are not done with the intubation. The endotracheal tube may not pass during nasal intubation and may cause bleeding that prevents successful fiberoptic endoscopy. The endotracheal tube may be too large for the patient; or the patient may be closing the vocal cords, blocking passage of the tube.
- *Small patients*: If the endotracheal tube is too small to fit over the scope, under direct vision you may pass a guidewire (from a ureteral stent or a retrograde intubation kit) through the suction port of the bronchoscope into the trachea. Remove the bronchoscope and leave the wire in the trachea. Pass the endotracheal tube over the wire while visualizing the larynx with the bronchoscope.

Learn to use the bronchoscope by intubating asleep, paralyzed patients. For most, it takes 10–20 intubations to successfully intubate normal patients. When some degree of proficiency is attained, the technique is applied to asleep, breathing patients. With some additional practice (approximately 40 intubations total) the practitioner is usually able to successfully intubate the trachea in patients with abnormal airway anatomy, even with the patient awake.

Role of the Laryngeal Mask Airway in Difficult Airway Management

The LMA can be used to change a "can't ventilate" to a "can ventilate" situation. This allows you to continue the anesthetic with the LMA as your airway device or awaken the patient to allow a safe alternative intubation or tracheostomy. However, once ventilation is assured through the LMA, other techniques may be used to secure the airway. The intubating LMA (ILMA) adds another tool for management of patients with difficult airway anatomy. Successful placement of the endotracheal tube is possible in nearly all patients, often on the first attempt. The ILMA should be considered early in management of patients with unsuspected difficult airway anatomy as it may allow rapid conversion of a difficult airway to a controlled airway. If an ILMA is not available, the LMA may still be used as a conduit to intubation, as a blind technique or with airway exchange catheters or fiberoptic bronchoscopes (Table 6-4).

Blind Endotracheal Tube Intubation via Laryngeal Mask Airway
- Place LMA and verify ventilation via LMA
- Pass a well-lubricated endotracheal tube down the LMA, rotated 90° from normal to ease passage through bars on LMA; at 20 cm, rotate endotracheal tube into normal position
- Pass the endotracheal tube into trachea, inflate cuff, verify ventilation
- Secure the endotracheal tube and LMA in place or cut and split LMA to allow for securing of the endotracheal tube alone

Fiberoptic Intubation via Laryngeal Mask Airway
- Place LMA and verify ventilation via LMA
- Lubricate endotracheal tube well, position on bronchoscope
- Pass bronchoscope down LMA, into trachea, advance endotracheal tube along bronchoscope
- Verify position of endotracheal tube visually, withdraw bronchoscope
- Secure endotracheal tube and LMA in place or cut and split LMA to allow for securing of the endotracheal tube alone

Passage of Intubating Guide via Laryngeal Mask Airway
- Place LMA and verify ventilation via LMA
- Pass ventilating or nonventilating intubation guide via LMA – ventilating guide allows verification of position of guide by capnometry before endotracheal tube passage
- Remove LMA, pass appropriate-sized endotracheal tube over guide, remove intubating guide
- Verify position of endotracheal tube in trachea by bronchoscopy, capnometry and ventilation
- Secure endotracheal tube

Laryngeal Mask Airways Allow Ventilation of Patient During Other Airway Management Techniques
- Tracheostomy
- Retrograde wire-guided intubation

Pitfalls of Laryngeal Mask Airway in Difficult Airway Management
- Epiglottis may fold down during insertion of the airway and limit the ability to pass other devices into the trachea – this may happen even though some ventilation is possible
- Bars on LMA may limit passage of other devices
- The endotracheal tube may be too short to completely enter the trachea via LMA
- The LMA/endotracheal tube combination may be difficult to secure and may slip out of trachea
- Risk of aspiration of gastric contents – Proseal may decrease this risk

---

Table 6-4   Laryngeal Mask Airway Sizes and Corresponding Endotracheal Tube (ETT)

Size	Weight	Maximum Air in Cuff	ETT Size that will Pass
1	<5 kg	4 mL	3.0 uncuffed
1.5	5–10 kg	7 mL	
2	10–20 kg	10 mL	4.5 uncuffed
2.5	20–30 kg	14 mL	
3	30 kg to small adult	20 mL	6.0 uncuffed
4	Adult	30 mL	6.0 cuffed
5	Large adult/poor seal with 4	40 mL	7.5 cuffed

ADVANCED AIRWAY TECHNIQUES

- *Retrograde intubation*: Passage of an endotracheal tube can be facilitated by a guide wire passed through the cricothyroid membrane into the upper airway in a retrograde fashion. This technique is facilitated by use of one of the commercial prepackaged kits available. With practice, this technique can be done in a relatively short time.
- *Transtracheal jet* ventilation: In the presence of a patent upper airway, jet ventilation via a catheter passed into the trachea through the cricothyroid membrane will entrain enough gas to adequately ventilate a patient in whom intubation is not possible. Jet ventilation requires a high-pressure gas source to be effective, such as from the gas flush on the anesthesia machine or from a separate control valve connected to the wall oxygen source. Transtracheal jet ventilation can be life-saving but should be seen as a bridge to a more definitive method of airway management, as there are significant risks associated with the technique, including barotrauma of the airway and subcutaneous emphysema.
- *Cricothyroidotomy*: The airway may be entered through the cricothyroid membrane by a scalpel incision or using a needle and guide wire combination. An endotracheal tube can then be passed into the trachea and ventilation assured. Several commercially available kits provide all the components needed to rapidly secure the airway using this technique.
- *Tracheostomy*: There are patients in whom the appropriate airway management choice is tracheostomy, sometimes with the patient awake. This surgical approach to airway management provides a secure way to ventilate the patient.

DIFFICULT AIRWAY CART

The equipment needed to safely manage patients with difficult airway anatomy must be tailored to the practitioner. Many institutions have standardized this equipment to some degree. For example, each operating room may have an oxygen regulator/jet ventilator setup hanging by the anesthesia machine. These are connected to the oxygen supply and ready for immediate use. Further standardization includes a "difficult airway" cart. These carts may be located centrally in the main operating rooms and in the obstetric suite. They contain a selection of the equipment used for managing patients with difficult airways. Custom-made holders may be mounted on the back of the cart to protect the fiberoptic bronchoscopes. An oxygen cylinder with a regulator attached may be mounted on the side of the cart. Equipment used for airway management may be in the drawers of the cart, as follows:

- *Drawer 1*: Yankauer suction catheters; laryngoscope handles (small and large) and blades (Mac 3, 4, Miller 2, 3); tape; tube clamp; Magill forceps
- *Drawer 2*: Medications; syringes; prep solutions; lubricant; antifog solution
- *Drawer 3*: Miscellaneous equipment such as swivel adapters, stylets, etc.
- *Drawer 4*: Rigid fiberoptic laryngoscope
- *Drawer 5*: Oxygen masks, guide wires (0.035), endotracheal tubes (sizes 2–9); cricothyrotomy set; retrograde intubation kit
- *Drawer 6*: LMA (sizes 1–5); disposable Ambu bag; oral airways; nasal trumpets; oral airways for fiberoptic intubation; gum elastic bougie.

To state the obvious, the time to collect and organize the equipment you need for managing patients with a difficult airway anatomy is before you really need it. However, having the equipment is not enough. The anesthesia care provider must also be able to use the equipment successfully when needed. This requires practice.

Case Study: Unanticipated Difficult Airway

A 65-year-old male patient is brought to the operating room for exploratory laparotomy following trauma. The patient is inebriated but quite cooperative. The airway examination appears normal. Following preoxygenation and induction of anesthesia, direct laryngoscopy attempts show only a grade 4 view. Attempts at mask ventilation are unsuccessful and the patient's oxygen saturation begins to decrease.

Clinical need : Rapid intervention to prevent hypoxic brain damage and to ensure adequate ventilation.

Response: A LMA is inserted but ventilation is still unsuccessful. A call for help goes out and the difficult airway cart is brought to the operation room. Management options at this point are very limited because of the patient's progressive hypoxia, and a choice must be made between transtracheal jet ventilation as a bridge to securing an airway and a surgical technique such as cricothyroidotomy or tracheostomy. Jet ventilation is initiated using a 14-gauge catheter and a manually controlled high-pressure oxygen source. Jet ventilation is continued while intubation of the trachea is successfully performed by fiberoptic bronchoscopy.

Conclusion: In the emergency setting, management choices may be limited and must be anticipated in advance. The time to prepare the necessary equipment and learn appropriate management techniques is before they are needed in the operating room. Collecting equipment in a portable difficult airway cart may be very helpful.

APPROACHES TO AIRWAY ANESTHESIA

- *None*: Really only appropriate for the comatose patient or the occasional very cooperative patient. Most patients will require some type of anesthetic to tolerate instrumentation of the airway.
- *General anesthesia*: May be either intravenous or inhalational, if carefully administered. Spontaneous ventilation allows the practitioner to follow air/bubbles to larynx. Additionally, spontaneous ventilation may preserve airway patency better than paralysis. Controlled ventilation with or without relaxant may be appropriate for some patients. This approach may give more time for procedure because of better ventilation and oxygenation.
- *Topical anesthesia* may be appropriate in a wide range of patients. There are several tools you may use to anesthetize the airway with local anesthesia. One collection includes self-grabbing forceps, atomizer, medicine cup, bent needle for depositing local anesthetic solution on the vocal cords, tongue retractor, and mirror. To do an adequate job of anesthetizing the airway, you must understand the innervation of the airway. Complete airway anesthesia entails blocking portions of three nerves – the trigeminal nerve for the nasopharynx, the glossopharyngeal nerve for the oropharynx, and the laryngeal branches of the vagus nerve for the epiglottis and larynx. These blocks can be achieved either by topical application of local anesthetic solution or by injection into the nerves. Topical application may be carried out using pledgets soaked in local anesthetic solution, by nebulizing the airway, by atomizing, or by direct instillation of local anesthetic into the airway. Of the various local anesthetics available, only a few have widespread use for this application:
  - Cocaine, 2–4% solutions. Provides good local anesthesia and vasoconstriction but is a controlled substance. Duration 30–60 minutes.
  - Lidocaine, 2–4% solutions, doses up to 200 mg in adults. Provides good local anesthesia, and vasoconstriction if epinephrine or phenylephrine is added. Duration 60–180 minutes.
  - Benzocaine, spray or lozenges. Provides rapid onset, relatively good local anesthesia. Duration 30–60 minutes. Be aware of the risk of methemoglobinemia with large doses of benzocaine.

Administration Options

- *Local anesthetic solution administered by nebulizer*: 4% lidocaine, 2 mL in med nebulizer device while the patient is awake, preferably in the preoperative holding area. This may provide very good airway anesthesia, if the patient will perform the deep inspirations necessary for entrainment of anesthetic all the way down the trachea.
- *Direct application by atomizer*, usually done with the patient in the operating room. If the local anesthetic solution is administered by atomizer, the vocal cords can be sprayed by withdrawing the patient's tongue and angling the tip of the atomizer down. Alternatively, the vocal cords may be anesthetized by direct application of local anesthetic solution using the suction port of the fiberoptic bronchoscope or a special needle. This method will lead to fairly rapid abduction of the vocal cords.
- *Direct application of local anesthetic using a pledget*: Local-anesthetic-soaked gauzes or cotton swabs can be pressed against the tonsillar pillars to block the glossopharyngeal nerve or, with use of a special self-holding forceps, the epiglottis and vocal cords.
- *Glossopharyngeal nerve block* can also be performed by nebulizer or atomizer or by direct injection with an angled needle.
- *Transtracheal instillation of local anesthetic solution into the airway*: This is done by inserting a needle or intravenous catheter through the anterior wall of the trachea, generally through the cricothyroid membrane. Angulation of the needle in a caudad direction helps limit the risk of direct vocal cord trauma from the needle. After aspiration of air to prove intratracheal position of the needle tip, 2–4 mL of local anesthetic solution is rapidly injected. This will generally stimulate a cough, which helps spread the local anesthetic up to the vocal cords and epiglottis.
- *Superior laryngeal nerve block*: Laryngeal structures have sensory and motor innervation. The motor functions are adduction (closing vocal cords), abduction (opening vocal cords) and tension (tightening vocal cords: produces higher-pitch sounds). All motor and sensory innervation to laryngeal structures is from branches of the vagus nerve (see Table 6-1).

Laryngeal reflexes may be stimulated at the larynx or at supraglottic levels and may lead to closure of the vocal cords up to the point of laryngospasm. Sensory block of the mucosa of the larynx requires a superior laryngeal nerve block for the mucosa down to the vocal cords plus recurrent laryngeal nerve block for the mucosa below vocal cords. Laryngeal nerve block may be performed by midline or lateral approaches. Pushing the hyoid bone toward the side you wish to block facilitates the lateral approach. Local anesthetic solution is injected in a fan pattern, with slight insertion and withdrawal of the needle to bathe the nerve as it pierces the cricothyroid membrane. Complete motor block (to facilitate intubation for example) requires block of the recurrent laryngeal nerve, since this nerve supplies motor function to all intrinsic nerves of the larynx except the cricothyroid muscle, and is usually done by transtracheal or cricothyroid spray of local anesthetic.

Case Study: Recognized Difficult Airway

A 14-year-old patient with significant temporomandibular joint ankylosis presents for elective temporomandibular joint replacement surgery. Preoperative assessment demonstrates a maximum interincisor distance of only 7 mm.

Clinical need: Controlled airway to allow surgical procedure under general anesthesia.

Response: A choice must be made between awake and asleep intubation. In the patient who is both highly motivated and cooperative, an awake intubation may be performed, with or without fiberoptic bronchoscopic intubation. In the noncooperative patient, asleep intubation during spontaneous/assisted ventilation may be the most practical choice. Alternatives for anesthesia include inhalational agents or carefully titrated intravenous agents such as propofol. With the patient spontaneously breathing during propofol infusion, regional anesthesia of the airway is provided by transtracheal injection of lidocaine and superior laryngeal nerve blocks. Fiberoptic bronchoscopic intubation is performed and the endotracheal tube is successfully passed on the first attempt. Surgery proceeds without complication and the patient is extubated in the recovery area after complete return of consciousness, verification of no postoperative bleeding, and assessment for possible airway edema.

Conclusion: Identification of difficult airway anatomy allows the greatest number of management choices for successful intubation.

PRACTICE

Using the various pieces of equipment available is the only way to attain the proficiency needed to ensure success when a technique is used to manage a patient with difficult airway anatomy. While practitioners can and should take advantage of workshops designed to teach the use of this equipment, they can also practice the techniques in normal patients. We have found that using the equipment in asleep, paralyzed patients allows the beginner to gain enough proficiency to use the equipment when needed. As an example, flexible fiberoptic bronchoscopes may be used to intubate the trachea in patients with normal airway anatomy as a method of gaining mastery of the technique. With a careful approach, the patient is subject to no additional risk related to the intubation. This same approach can be used with the other techniques you choose for your practice. It adds only a little time to your cases and, when you are faced with a patient with an abnormal airway, you will have the proficiency needed to succeed.

SUMMARY

Successful management of patients with abnormal airway anatomy depends on prediction, preparation, and practice. The best way to ensure successful management of the patient with a difficult airway is to recognize the airway difficulty prior to the induction of anesthesia. Accurate prediction is essential to allow you time to plan and perform safe techniques of intubation. Preparation includes having and using alternate plans if your first choice for management is not successful. This is the benefit of practice guidelines such as the ASA difficult airway algorithm. You must know when to switch to a different technique if the technique you choose first is not successful. Preparation for patients with difficult airways includes gathering all the equipment desired into a location that is accessible, for example a difficult airway cart. Preparation also includes practice, since all the devices designed to assist the practitioner in intubating the trachea in patients with difficult airways require mastery of the associated technique to improve the success rate. This practice should be in non-emergency situations to allow mastery of the techniques you choose to add to direct laryngoscopy. Adequate practice to allow mastery in emergency settings is essential.

There will be patients in whom one technique may be more successful than another. Thus the practitioner must have more than one option available for managing the difficult airway. Practical tips – airway management is easier if the patient is still oxygenated, accurate prediction allows more options, and have more than one option. Select the adjunctive techniques you prefer, and then practice in normal patients in an elective setting to gain mastery. Finally, don't be afraid to call for help.

SUGGESTED READING

ASA Task Force on Management of the Difficult Airway. Practice guidelines for management of the difficult airway. *Anesthesiology* 1993;78:597-602.

Benumof JL. Laryngeal mask airway and the ASA difficult airway algorithm. *Anesthesiology* 1996;84:686-699.

Domino KB, Posner KL, Caplan RA, Cheney FW. Airway injury during anesthesia: a closed claims analysis. *Anesthesiology* 1999;91:1703-1711.

Langeron O, Masso E, Huraux C, *et al*. Prediction of difficult mask ventilation. *Anesthesiology* 2000;92:1229-1236.

Langeron O, Semjen F, Bourgain JL, *et al*. Comparison of the intubating laryngeal mask airway with the fiberoptic intubation in anticipated difficult airway management. *Anesthesiology* 2001;94:968-972.

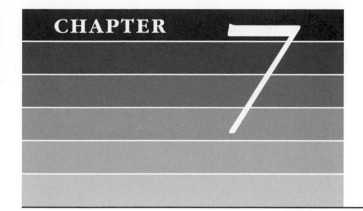

CHAPTER 7

Acid–Base Balance

MICHELLE S. KIM

INTRODUCTION

The process for regulation of hydrogen ion (H^+) and bicarbonate ion (HCO_3^-), or acid–base balance, is of prime importance to the anesthesiologists. It is vital to understand the physiologic derangements that can occur with acid-base disturbances and factors that can be manipulated, such as ventilation and perfusion, that can rapidly alter acid-base disturbances. Maintenance of H^+ over a narrow range is necessary for optimal enzyme function, oxygen saturation of hemoglobin, electrolyte balance, and organ function. In order to maintain acid-base balance, it is necessary to interpret blood gases, be familiar with acid-base chemistry, and have knowledge of the differential diagnosis for acid-base disturbances and treatment during anesthetic management.

Acid–Base Chemistry

In order to sustain life, there is a narrow range of pH that the body must maintain for optimal cell function. The body has buffering systems and compensatory mechanisms to regulate the pH between 7.36 and 7.44 in adults. To understand how the pH is calculated, one must be familiar with the Henderson-Hasselbach equation:

$$pH = 6.1 + \log \frac{HCO_3^-}{0.03 \times P_a\text{co}_2}$$

To maintain a physiologic pH, the optimal ratio of HCO_3^- to arterial partial pressure of carbon dioxide ($P_a\text{co}_2$) is 20:1. This ratio of 20:1 is regulated by the lungs ($P_a\text{co}_2$) and kidneys (plasma HCO_3^-). An acid-base disturbance with a decrease in HCO_3^- will increase alveolar ventilation to maintain a proportional ratio. Any change in the acid-base balance is therefore corrected by the buffering system and renal compensation.

Buffer System

All body fluids contain a buffer system to maintain pH near 7.4. An acid is a proton donor, which increases H^+ concentration, and a base, a proton acceptor, which decreases the H^+ concentration. The buffering system is dependent on the hydration of carbon dioxide (CO_2) to carbonic acid (H_2CO_3) in the plasma and erythrocytes. Carbon dioxide is a product of aerobic metabolism and the balance of production and elimination determines the amount of carbon dioxide in the body. The major extracellular buffering system is composed of bicarbonate (HCO_3^-) and carbonic acid (H_2CO_3).

The process of carbonic acid conversion is slower in the plasma than erythrocytes which is accelerated by the presence of carbonic anhydrase. The carbonic acid will then spontaneously dissociate to hydrogen and bicarbonate. The H^+ is then buffered by the reduced hemoglobin, and the bicarbonate ion is absorbed in the plasma, to function as a buffer. Electrical neutrality is maintained by absorbing chloride ions in the erythrocyte.

Protein is the most potent buffering system in the intracellular space. It accounts for about 75% of the buffering system based on the high intracellular concentration. Further compensation to maintain acid–base balance includes alveolar ventilation changes, reabsorption of HCO_3^- or secretion of hydrogen (H^+) by the renal tubules, or increased ammonia production. Renal compensation is the most powerful tool to correct acid–base disturbances; however, the process requires 12–24 hours and, in contrast, respiratory changes and buffering systems take place within minutes.

ACID–BASE DISTURBANCES

The specific acid-base disturbances are respiratory acidosis, respiratory alkalosis, metabolic acidosis, and metabolic alkalosis. Each category is determined by the direct measure of pH, P_aCO_2, along with plasma concentration of HCO_3^-. Acidosis is defined as pH less than 7.36 and alkalosis as pH greater than 7.44. Respiratory acidosis or hypoventilation involves a P_aCO_2 greater than 44 mmHg, and alkalosis or hyperventilation a P_aCO_2 less than 36 mmHg. Respiratory disturbance can be determined by using the rule of thumb "for every 10 mmHg change in P_aCO_2, the pH will change 0.08 units in the opposite direction." Metabolic disturbances are characterized by deviation above or below a HCO_3^- concentration of 24 mEq/L (Table 7-1).

Primary or simple disorders and compensated or mixed acid–base disorders can be determined by the severity of deviation from the range of normal values of P_aCO_2 and HCO_3^- to pH values. It is essential to differentiate the causes of the acid–base disturbance in order to select a proper treatment (Figure 7-1).

The detrimental effects of respiratory or metabolic acidosis are clinically observed when the pH is less than 7.2 and include an increase in serum potassium, depression of the central nervous system, release of catecholamines, cardiac dysrhythmias, and direct myocardial depression. The clinical effects of myocardial depression are often not seen until pH is below 7.1, when the heart is no longer responsive to catecholamines. Respiratory acidosis has a more profound effect when associated with myocardial dysfunction than metabolic acidosis. This is probably because of the high solubility of carbon dioxide in tissue cells, which causes a rapid increase in acid. Patients with ischemic heart disease or with a depressed sympathetic nervous system, such as those on beta-blockers, or under general anesthesia, are especially vulnerable to the negative effects of acidosis.

Clinical Caveat: Myocardial Dysfunction with Acidosis

Clinical effects of myocardial depression are often not seen until pH is below 7.1.
Respiratory acidosis has a more profound association with myocardial dysfunction than metabolic acidosis.

Table 7-1   Characterization of Acid–Base Disturbances

Acid–base Disturbance	pH 7.36–7.44	P_aCO_2 36–44 mmHg	HCO_3^- 24 mEq/L
Respiratory acidosis	Acute ↓ ↓	Acute ↑ ↑ ↑	Acute ↑
	Chronic ± ↓	Chronic ↑ ↑ ↑	Chronic ↑ ↑
Respiratory alkalosis	Acute ↑ ↑	Acute ↓ ↓ ↓	Acute ↓
	Chronic ± ↑	Chronic ↓ ↓ ↓	Chronic ↓ ↓
Metabolic acidosis	Acute ↓ ↓ – ↓ ↓ ↓	Acute ↓	Acute ↓ ↓ ↓
	Chronic ↓	Chronic ↓ ↓	Chronic ↓ ↓ ↓
Metabolic alkalosis	Acute ↑ ↑ ↑	Acute ↑ ↑	Acute ↑ ↑ ↑
	Chronic ↑ ↑ ↑	Chronic ↑ ↑	Chronic ↑ ↑ ↑

±, no change; ↓ slight decrease; ↓ ↓, moderate decrease; ↓ ↓ ↓, severe decrease; ↑, slight increase; ↑ ↑, moderate increase; ↑ ↑ ↑, severe increase.

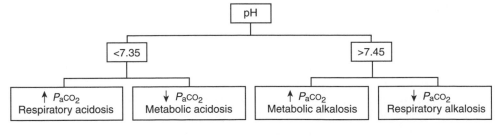

Figure 7-1 Simple acid-base disturbance.

The detrimental effects of respiratory or metabolic alkalosis are decreased serum potassium, decreased ionized calcium availability, excitation of the central nervous system, decreased cerebral blood flow, coronary artery vasoconstriction, increased risk of cardiac dysrhythmias, increased airway resistance, and, in respiratory alkalosis, increased intrapulmonary shunting and a left shift of the oxyhemoglobin dissociation curve, with resulting decreased availability of oxygen to tissues.

ACIDOSIS

Respiratory Acidosis

Respiratory acidosis is defined as an increase in P_aCO_2 above 44 mmHg, with pH less than 7.35. Increases in P_aCO_2 can be due to lack of elimination or increased production of carbon dioxide by a hypermetabolic state. Measuring the pH and HCO_3^- can determine whether this imbalance is acute or chronic. In an acute state, a

CO_2 increase will result in a rapid decrease of pH with little increase in compensation of the HCO_3^-.

Carbon dioxide has high solubility and thus arterial blood and cerebrospinal fluid (CSF) exhibit a similar decrease in pH. The drop in pH will stimulate the carotid bodies and medullary chemoreceptors located in the fourth ventricle to increase ventilation; however, in an anesthetized state, the response of the carotid bodies is depressed.

Acute causes of hypoventilation include central nervous system depression with anesthetics, incomplete muscle relaxant reversal, or rebreathing of exhaled gases. Normally, the compensatory effort of the body will try to maintain the 20:1 ratio of HCO_3^- to CO_2. Carbon dioxide will combine with water to produce plasma $H_2CO_3^-$ immediately and the renal tubules will increase absorption of HCO_3^-; however renal compensation requires many hours. A combination of a normal pH with increased P_aCO_2 is indicative of a chronic condition. Table 7-2 lists the causes of respiratory acidosis.

Table 7-2   Causes of Respiratory Acidosis

Increased CO_2 Production

Malignant hyperthermia		
Intense muscle contraction	Shivering	
	Seizure activity	
Increased carbohydrate load (total parenteral nutrition)		
Thyroid storm		
Burns		

Decreased CO_2 Elimination

Central nervous system depression	Drug-induced	
	Cerebral injury	
	Sleep disorder	
	Obesity hypoventilation syndrome (Pickwickian syndrome)	
Neuromuscular	Inadequate muscle relaxant reversal	
	Myopathies	
	Neuropathies	
Airway obstruction	Upper airway	Laryngospasm
		Sleep disorder
		Foreign body
		Tumor
	Lower airway	Severe asthma
		Chronic obstructive pulmonary disease
		Tumor
Chest wall deformities	Kyphoscoliosis	
	Flail chest	
Pleural	Pneumothorax	
	Pleural effusion	
Parenchymal	Aspiration pneumonia	
	Pulmonary edema	
	Pulmonary emboli	
Iatrogenic	Inadequate mechanical ventilation setting	
	Rebreathing of exhaled gas	

Treatment of marked respiratory acidosis (pH <7.1) include mechanical ventilation and reversing or allowing for elimination of respiratory depressants such as narcotics, benzodiazepines, muscle relaxants, and volatile anesthetics. Capnography can indicate rebreathing by the waveform's failure to return to baseline. Rebreathing of exhaled gases can be due to either exhausted soda lime or an incompetent one-way valve.

Caution should be taken when correcting chronic respiratory acidosis. Renal compensation for this imbalance will increase plasma HCO_3^-; thus rapid decrease of carbon dioxide can result in metabolic alkalosis and central nervous system irritability.

Metabolic Acidosis

Metabolic acidosis is a primary decrease in HCO_3^- to less than 23 mEq/L with build-up of acid other than CO_2 in the body and a resultant pH of less than 7.35. Obtaining a blood gas with measurement of P_aCO_2 will indicate whether this is an acute primary process or a chronic process with compensation (see Table 7-1).

Metabolic acidosis can be classified into two categories by measuring the anion gap. The anion gap is measure by subtracting the major plasma cation from the major plasma anions. The normal range is 9–14 mEq/L.

Anion gap = $[Na^+] - ([Cl^-] + [HCO_3^-])$.

Metabolic acidosis can be due to decreased renal elimination of H^+ with the onset of renal failure, or to liver failure with decreased conversion of acid to renal secreting product. Metabolic acidosis can also be due to increased metabolic production subsequent to decreased delivery of oxygenated blood to the tissues, diabetic ketoacidosis, renal tubular acidosis, iatrogenic – intravenous fluids and total parental nutrition (TPN), and diarrhea. The most common cause of hypercholemic metabolic acidosis is diarrhea. Table 7-3 lists the causes of metabolic acidosis.

The compensatory response to metabolic acidosis initially includes increased alveolar ventilation to maintain the 20:1 ratio of bicarbonate to carbon dioxide. Increased H^+ will also activate the carotid bodies to increase ventilation and renal tubules to increase secretion of H^+. With decreased P_aCO_2, the pH of the CSF will initially increase, which in turn will inhibit the medullary chemoreceptors and blunt the response of the carotid bodies. However, over time the pH of the CSF will normalize, with active recruitment of HCO_3^-, and the effects of the medullary chemoreceptor will increase alveolar ventilation. Patients exposed to volatile anesthetics will have a blunted response of the carotid bodies. The body will also compensate by use of buffers present in bone.

The primary treatment of metabolic acidosis consists of removing and correcting the acid-producing state.

Table 7-3   Causes of Metabolic Acidosis

Elevated Anion Gap		
Ingestion of toxin	Salicylate	
	Sulfur	
	Toluene	
	Ethylene glycol	
	Methanol	
	Paraldehyde	
Increased production of acids	Renal failure	
	Liver failure	
	Lactic acidosis	
	Ketoacidosis	Diabetes insulin dependent
		Starvation
	Mixed	Hyperosmolar coma
		Alcoholic
Normal Anion Gap with Hyperchloremia		
Gastric loss	Diarrhea	
	Ingestion	Calcium chloride
	Bowel obstruction	Magnesium chloride
Renal loss	Renal tubular acidosis	
	Carbonic anhydrase inhibitor	
	Hypoaldosteronism	
	Hydronephrosis	
Total parenteral nutrition		
Intravenous solution	Bicarbonate lacking fluid	

Intravenous bicarbonate can be administered, to increase buffering capacity, in situations with pH less than 7.20. The amount of sodium bicarbonate given is 1 mEq/kg, followed by serial blood gases determinations to measure the impact of therapy. The amount of bicarbonate to be given can also be calculated by: body weight (kg) × base deficit × extracellular fluid volume (30%) and administer half the calculated dose.

Current Controversy: Treatment of Metabolic Acidosis with Bicarbonate

Studies show that treatment of metabolic acidosis with bicarbonate in decreased perfusion states will worsen the acidosis.

Clinical Caveat: Correction of pH

It is not necessary to correct pH to normal range.
Studies have shown that pH corrected above 7.25 is sufficient to overcome myocardial depressant effect of acidemia.

A pH over 7.25 should be sufficient to overcome the detrimental effects of acidemia. The byproducts of sodium bicarbonate will increase production of carbon dioxide; therefore respiratory acidosis should not be treated with bicarbonate – respiratory rate should be increased.

Drug Interaction: Drugs and Acidosis

Opioids have increased sedative and respiratory depressant effects with acidemia that may be due to increased cerebral perfusion with increased carbon dioxide.

The effects of nondepolarizing neuromuscular blockers are prolonged, perhaps because of impairment of the action of anticholinesterase reversal agents such as neostigmine.

Halothane has been noted to increase arrhythmias in the acidotic state.

Succinylcholine will increase the risk of hyperkalemic cardiac dysrhythmias in an acidotic environment.

Anesthetic Impact from Acidosis

Acidemia can increase the sedative and depressant effects of anesthetic agents. In acidic states, opioids, which are weak bases, will decrease the fraction of the non-ionized form; however, the concentration of opioid in the brain is increased. The increase of cerebral perfusion in states of hypercarbia may explain the increased amount of opioids found in the brain. Increased cerebral perfusion may offset the effect of a decreased ratio of the active form of an opioid.

During a state of acidosis, rapid decrease of sympathetic tone should be avoided, as it may leave the myocardium with unopposed circulatory depression from acidosis. Succinylcholine should be used with caution in acidic states, especially when it may be associated with hyperkalemia; and halothane has been known to be arrhythmogenic in acidic states. Nondepolarizing neuromuscular blockers can be potentiated by respiratory acidosis. Although the mechanism is poorly understood, it has been suggested that the potency of reversal agents is impaired in the acidotic state.

Drug Interaction: Drugs and Alkalosis

Opioids are potentiated by increased non-ionic ratio.
Nondepolarizing muscle blocker prolongation, probably due to hypokalemia.

ALKALOSIS

Respiratory Alkalosis

Respiratory alkalosis is present when the P_aCO_2 is less than 36 mmHg. This can be due to hyperventilation or decreased production of carbon dioxide. Measurement of arterial blood gases will give evidence of chronicity and whether this disturbance is a primary or compensatory change (see Table 7-1). An initial decrease in P_aCO_2 and increased pH will depress the stimulus to breathe, which is regulated by the carotid bodies and medullary chemoreceptors. The pH of the CSF is restored to normal by active transport of HCO_3^- out of the CSF. Eventually the stimulation to breathe by the medullary chemoreceptors will return to normal in the presence of a low P_aCO_2.

Increased ventilation or hyperventilation can be caused by central stimulation, peripheral stimulation, and pulmonary disease states, and can be iatrogenic or ventilator-induced. Decreased production of carbon dioxide can be due to hypothermia and skeletal muscle inactivity. Table 7-4 lists the causes of respiratory alkalosis.

The renal tubules will compensate for respiratory alkalosis by decreased reabsorption of HCO_3^-. Increased secretion of bicarbonate in the urine with sodium and potassium ions to maintain electrical neutrality will return the pH to the normal range in chronic states. Therefore, alkalosis is associated with hypokalemia. Think: *al-ka-low-sis* is equivalent to low potassium.

Table 7-4   Causes of Respiratory Alkalosis

Central Stimulation
Pain
Anxiety
Cerebral injury
Fever/ Infection
Pregnancy
Salicylate

Peripheral Stimulation

Hypoxemia	Severe anemia
	High altitude
Pulmonary disease	Asthma
	Congestive heart failure
	Pulmonary edema
	Pulmonary emboli

Iatrogenic
Mechanical ventilator
Self-induced hyperventilation

Other
Sepsis
Liver failure

The primary treatment of respiratory alkalosis is to correct the underlying process. In severe alkalemia, pH above 7.60, intravenous acid can be given, such as ammonium chloride.

Metabolic Alkalosis

Metabolic alkalosis is defined as an increase in HCO_3^- (plasma HCO_3^- >25 mEq/L) and increase in pH above 7.45. Most imbalances can be divided into two categories: chloride-sensitive metabolic alkalosis and chloride-resistant metabolic alkalosis. Chloride-sensitive metabolic alkalosis is associated with sodium chloride deficiency and extracellular volume depletion. The renal tubules will compensate for decreased volume by increasing sodium reabsorption. However, in a chloride deficient state, hydrogen and potassium ions must be secreted in the urine and HCO_3^- absorbed to maintain electrical neutrality. The most common cause of chloride-sensitive metabolic alkalosis is diuretic therapy. Increased loss of gastric secretions through nasogastric drainage is also a common cause of chloride-sensitive metabolic alkalosis.

Chloride-resistant metabolic alkalosis is associated with increased mineralocorticoid activity, which increases sodium reabsorption and the subsequent electrolyte compensation as above; however, it is not associated with extracellular fluid deficiency. Other possible causes of metabolic alkalosis can be related to excessive production of bicarbonate as a byproduct of large volumes of fluids. Citrate in blood products, lactate in lactated Ringer's solution, and acetate in TPN are converted by the liver into HCO_3^-. Table 7-5 lists the causes of metabolic alkalosis.

Compensation by the renal tubules will increase H^+ reabsorption, with consequent excretion of sodium and potassium to maintain electrical neutrality. In depleted states of sodium and potassium, such as are associated with vomiting, the renal compensation is limited and incomplete.

Alveolar hypoventilation is another compensatory mechanism to maintain acid–base balance. In an effort to maintain the 20:1 ratio of HCO_3^- to H^+, the initial compensation mechanism is hypoventilation and an increase in P_aCO_2. However, the medullary chemoreceptor will be activated and hypoventilation suppressed until CSF pH normalizes by active transport of HCO_3^-. Once the CSF pH is normalized, respiratory ventilation will decrease despite an increase in P_aCO_2. Respiratory compensation is typically limited to a P_aCO_2 not greater than 55 mmHg, which will result in a pH slightly above normal.

The primary treatment is to correct the underlying disorder. In chloride-sensitive metabolic alkalosis, intra-

Table 7-5 Causes of Metabolic Alkalosis	
Chloride-sensitive	
Gastrointestinal losses	Vomiting
	Diarrhea
	Gastric drainage
Renal losses	Diuretic
	Chloride-deficient diet
Chloride-resistant	
Primary aldosteronism	
Excessive HCO_3^- Production	
Massive blood product transfusion with citrate preservative	
Lactate, acetate administration	
Renal failure	Sodium bicarbonate therapy
	Antacid
Hypercalcemia	
Bone metastases	

venous saline with potassium is the treatment of choice. H_2-blockers can be administered if there is excessive gastric volume loss. In edematous patients, a carbonic anhydrase inhibitor such as acetazolamide can be given. Patients with increased mineralocorticoid activity can be treated with an aldosterone antagonist such as spironolactone. For severe metabolic alkalosis (pH >7.60), treatment with intravenous hydrochloric acid (0.1 mol/L) or hemodialysis should be considered.

Anesthetic Impact from Alkalosis

The duration of opioid-induced respiratory depression can be prolonged, with associated respiratory alkalosis. This may be due to an increased non-ionic ratio of opioids with an increase in pH, which will facilitate penetration across the blood–brain barrier. Potentiation of nondepolarizing muscle relaxant has been reported; this may be due to the hypokalemia that is associated with alkalosis (Table 7-5). A combination of alkalosis and hypokalemia can lead to cardiac irritability and may precipitate atrial and ventricular dysrhythmias.

SUGGESTED READING

Adrogue HJ, Madias NE. Management of life-threatening acid–base disorders. *N Engl J Med* 1998;338:26–34.

Gabow PA. Sodium bicarbonate: a cure or curse for metabolic acidosis? Acidosis type determines whether administration is appropriate. *J Crit Illness* 1989;4:13028.

Krat JA, Madias NE. Approach to patients with acid–base disorders. *Respir Care* 2001;46:392–403.

CHAPTER 8

Fluid and Electrolyte Therapy

MICHELLE S. KIM

GARY R. STIER

INTRODUCTION

A prerequisite to the optimal administration of therapeutic fluids to patients in the operating room is a fundamental understanding of fluid dynamics. In this section, the following subjects will be discussed:

- The different body fluid compartments
- The distribution characteristic of crystalloids
- The different types of colloids and their characteristics
- Consideration of the hemodynamic benefits of crystalloids and colloids.

BODY FLUID COMPARTMENTS

Total body water (TBW) varies from 45% to 65% of total body weight. For most purposes, 60% of a male's weight is water, and about 55% of a female's weight is water. Therefore, a male weighing 80 kg would have TBW of about 48 L. There are two major body compartments: an intracellular fluid compartment (ICF), roughly two-thirds of TBW, and an extracellular fluid compartment (ECF) comprising about one-third of TBW. The ECF is further subdivided into an interstitial compartment, usually 75% of the ECF, and an intravascular compartment, which is about 25% of the ECF. In the above example, a man with 48 L of TBW would have an ICF of 32 L, an ECF of 16 L, an interstitial compartment volume of 12 L, and an intravascular compartment volume of 4 L.

When water is added into the body, it distributes evenly throughout the entire TBW; therefore, the amount of volume added to any given compartment is proportional to its fractional representation of TBW. If, for example, 3 L of water is added intravascularly, almost instantly the fluid distributes freely throughout the TBW. Therefore, 2 L (two-thirds) goes into the ICF, and 1 L (one-third) goes into the ECF (750 mL into the interstitial space, and 250 mL into the intravascular space). Thus, for 3 L of water, only 250 mL remains intravascular.

How about isotonic fluids? Since there is no difference in osmolarity between the infused fluid and body fluids, there is no driving force to cause water to diffuse into the intracellular compartment. The semipermeable membrane between the interstitial space and the intravascular space is permeable to ions and small particles, whereas the membrane surrounding the ICF space functionally is not. Therefore, the ECF space is the distribution space following the intravascular administration of isotonic fluids. Since isotonic fluid distributes evenly throughout the ECF, only one-quarter of infused fluid remains intravascularly after 20 minutes. Therefore, 20 minutes after the infusion of 3 L of isotonic crystalloid into the intravascular compartment, 2,250 mL of the initial 3,000 mL remains in the interstitial compartment, and 750 mL in the intravascular compartment. Intravascular fluid is the only fluid that has a direct effect on blood pressure, cardiac output, heart rate, and renal blood flow.

DISTRIBUTION OF FLUID

Distribution of fluid is represented by the Starling–Landis equation:

$$J_v = K_h A\{(P_{MV} - P_T) - \delta(COP_{MV} - COP_T)\}$$

where J_v is the net volume of fluid across the capillary wall, K_h is the fluid permeability of the capillary wall, A is the capillary surface area, P_{MV} is the capillary hydrostatic pressure, P_T is the tissue hydrostatic pressure, δ is the reflection coefficient for plasma proteins; COP_{MV} is the colloid oncotic pressure of the capillary wall; and COP_T is the colloid oncotic pressure in tissue.

The difference between the hydrostatic and colloid pressure in the interstitial space is responsible for the movement of water and dissolved solutes. The reflection coefficient greatly varies throughout tissues and represents the ability of semipermeable membrane to prevent movement of solutes. In the case of the lung, as an example of moderately permeable tissue, surgical trauma can increase the capillary permeability or leak, and thus if patient is given colloid (increase oncotic pressure) it is more likely to move into the interstitium and thus increase the likelihood of interstitial edema.

CRYSTALLOIDS

Physiology and Pharmacokinetics

The term "crystalloid" refers to solutions that are isotonic to human plasma. The electrolyte composition of selected crystalloid solutions – dextrose 5% in water, 0.9 saline (normal saline), lactated Ringer's solution, and Plasmalyte B – are shown in Table 8-1.

Indications

Crystalloids are indicated for the following clinical situations:
- Plasma volume expansion
  - Shock (septic, traumatic, hemorrhagic)
- Third space losses
- Diagnosis of oliguria
- Correction of electrolyte deficits
- Daily maintenance fluid requirements.

Plasma Volume Expansion

Crystalloid solutions are used for the treatment of shock of various etiologies in order to restore intravascular volume, interstitial water, and electrolyte deficits. They are inexpensive, easily stored, and readily available. In cases of shock, fluid volume should be restored quickly as "fluid challenge" boluses, in which the fluid (5-7 mL/kg) is given over 1-5 minutes. The volume of crystalloid needed varies but it is about three times the volume of colloid required to reach the same endpoint (because of redistribution of the crystalloid). Acute blood loss of 10-20% can be replaced initially with crystalloid if given in three to four times the volume of blood lost. When hematocrit is less than 30%, and more blood losses are expected, packed blood cells should be considered, as oxygen carrying capacity becomes a consideration.

If the patient is known to have a decreased serum albumin level (i.e., <2.0-2.4 g/dL) before surgery, either pure albumin solutions or synthetic colloid solutions should be added to any crystalloid (3:1 ratio) for fluid replacement in order to maintain colloid oncotic pressure. Remember, with large amounts of crystalloid, peripheral edema is to be expected, and this clinical finding should not be considered to indicate intravascular volume overload. Possible volume overload should always be assessed by serial measurements of urine output, blood pressure, pulmonary artery occlusion pressure (PAOP), central venous pressure, and other clinical indicators.

The first step in managing oliguria (Box 8-1) is to make a quick and accurate assessment of the possible etiologies involved, and then to formulate a diagnostic plan. The initial problem to rule out would be some anatomic/physical malfunction of the urinary drainage system. The next step is to give the patient a "fluid challenge." Fluid challenges are a diagnostic maneuver and crystalloid, not colloid, is recommended. In the postoperative or trauma patient, oliguria (with or without hypotension) almost always (>90%) represents volume depletion. A fluid challenge in

Table 8-1   The Composition of Various Crystalloid Fluids

	Na (mEq/L)	K (mEq/L)	Cl (mEq/L)	Ca (mEq/L)	Glucose (g/dL)	Lactate (mEq/L)	HCO3 (mEq/L)	Osmolarity (mosmol/L)	Mg (mEq/L)	Acetate (mEq/L)
Dextrose 5%					5			253		
0.9% saline	154		154					308		
Ringer's lactate	130	4	109	3		28		273		
Plasmalyte B	140	5	98		23		50	294	3	27

these patients will rapidly expand the intravascular space and result in an increase in urine output to more than 0.5 mL/kg/hr within 20-30 minutes. In the hypotensive patient, this will usually increase blood pressure, although only transiently because of the expected extravascular redistribution of the crystalloid.

Appropriate fluid challenge is safe even in patients with a history of congestive heart failure; the effects of fluid overload will only be transient (the redistribution of crystalloids occurs so rapidly). Colloids, however are poor choices for fluid challenges because their "dwell time" is longer.

Side Effects

Peripheral edema is seen with crystalloid use because three-quarters of the fluid distributes interstitially. However, peripheral edema in a trauma or postoperative patient does not indicate adequacy of intravascular volume.

"Edema safety factors" limit the amount of interstitial pulmonary edema up to a point. If the total crystalloid volume is limited to prevent intravascular volume overload, there is no difference in lung function using either crystalloid or colloid solutions. The development of acute respiratory distress syndrome (ARDS) is related more closely to the presence of sepsis and complement activation than to the particular type of fluid.

Current Controversy: Pulmonary Interstitial Edema

Pulmonary interstitial edema can occur with large amounts of crystalloid. Colloid osmotic pressure is lowered with crystalloid, as a result of dilutional effects. Whether this decreases lung function is controversial.

COLLOIDS

Albumin

Pharmacology and Pharmacokinetics

Albumin is produced in the liver and is the major osmotically active protein, contributing about 80% of the plasma colloid oncotic pressure. A 50% reduction in the serum albumin concentration decreases the colloid oncotic pressure to one-third of normal. Albumin binds cations and anions despite its strong negative charge and is a major transport protein for metals, drugs, fatty acids, hormones, and enzymes.

In the adult, 4-5 g of albumin per kilogram of body weight is present in the extracellular space (30-40% in the intravascular compartment and about 50-60% in the interstitial compartment). Administered albumin distributes freely throughout the ECF; however, the distribution takes much longer to equilibrate than crystalloid. The plasma half-life of albumin is roughly 16 hours (unlike the 20-30 min of crystalloid). One gram of albumin binds 18 mL of water by its oncotic activity. Thus, to determine by how much administered albumin will expand the intravascular space initially, calculate the number of grams of albumin given and multiply by 18.

Recommendations for Use

Albumin therapy can be considered for the treatment of acute intravascular volume depletion, which includes hemorrhage, trauma, acute hemodilution, and acute vasodilation. Colloid should be administered in conjunction with crystalloid to limit edema from large amounts of crystalloid volume resuscitation in the elderly patient with cardiopulmonary disease, or acute blood loss of more than 30% blood volume. Albumin 5% is the most frequent form of albumin administered. Albumin 25% may be given in cases where intravascular volume is low, or in the setting of a hemodynamically stable patient with a large amount of pitting edema. Volume expansion occurs over a period of about 2 hours.

Current Controversy: Colloid for Fluid Resuscitation

There have been recent reports that trauma patients receiving colloid for fluid resuscitation have slightly worse outcomes than patients resuscitated with crystalloid; therefore, limiting the use of colloid in the early resuscitation of trauma patients is probably prudent.

Albumin solutions have been successfully used in patients with extensive "third space" fluid losses, including acute peritonitis, mediastinitis, and postoperative major surgery. Albumin solution is also recommended for patients with burns covering more than 50% of body surface area; however, it is prudent to wait until after the first 24 hours, when the capillary leak has diminished.

Controversial Use of Albumin in Specific Disease States

Patients with chronic protein depletion states such as cirrhosis and nephrotic syndrome should receive albumin solutions only when associated with significant volume depletion (such as after paracentesis, dialysis, or overly aggressive diuresis).

The use of albumin or any colloid other than blood components in patients with established ARDS is very controversial. As a general rule, one should probably avoid administering albumin solutions to patients with documented ARDS. If treating these patients with albumin, measurement of the PAOP and pulmonary artery pressure (PAP) should be used to guide management. Both have an important role in fluid transudation across the pulmonary capillary membrane, with the PAOP slightly more contributory than the PAP in determining interstitial edema. A reasonable endpoint for fluid therapy in patients with ARDS is a PAOP of around 10–14 mmHg.

Side Effects

- Pulmonary edema: The "crystalloid–colloid" debate has produced conflicting animal and human studies. Some studies have shown adverse effects of albumin, while other studies have shown beneficial effects. Most probably, the method of resuscitation, the overall volume used, and the presence or absence of sepsis affects pulmonary function to a much greater degree than does the type of resuscitation fluid used.
- *Depressed ionized calcium levels*: Albumin can lower the serum ionized calcium level, producing a negative inotropic effect and possible coagulopathy.
- *Anaphylaxis*: The incidence is between 0.47% and 1.53% (very low).
- *Hepatitis and AIDS risk*: There is no risk of acquiring either agent secondary to inactivation of the viruses during the preparation of the albumin solution.

Hydroxyethyl Starch

Physiology and Pharmacokinetics

Hydroxyethyl starch (HES) is a synthetic starch that closely resembles glycogen. HES is available as a 6% solution in normal saline (Hespan®). The average molecular weight is 10,000–1,000,000. Some 90% of a single infusion of HES leaves the circulation within 42 days, with a half-life of 17 days. The remaining 10% has a half-life of 48 days. Plasma volume expansion with HES is equal to or greater than that produced by dextran 70 or 5% albumin. Infusion of HES increases intravascular volume by an amount equal to or greater than the volume infused.

Recommendations for Use

Hydroxyethyl starch may be used whenever colloid fluid is indicated to expand the plasma volume. It can also be used in cardiopulmonary bypass as a primer. HES is slightly more effective than 5% albumin expansion on a volume-for-volume basis. One liter of HES will expand the intravascular compartment by about 500–700 mL over 2 hours.

To avoid fluid overload and pulmonary edema, adequate hemodynamic monitoring should be carried out. Following urine output with HES can be misleading, just as with dextran, because of the osmotic diuresis that is produced from the degraded small HES particles. Patients with renal failure are particularly at risk of volume overload when using HES. Serum amylase levels will be about two to three times normal with HES, and are not indicative of pancreatitis.

The advantage of HES over albumin is that it cost about 25–50% as much as 5% albumin solutions; in addition, HES is synthetic and hence the supply is much less limited than albumin.

Current Controversy: Hydroxyethyl Starch in Neurosurgery Patients

Reports have suggested that administration of HES in neurosurgical patients increases the risk of surgical bleeding. Until a prospective study can determine the safety of HES in neurosurgical patients, it should be used with caution.

Side Effects

- *Coagulopathy*: Dilutional effects on cellular and protein elements of the clotting cascade are produced secondary to the blood volume expansion, however, the laboratory effects are not completely explained by dilution alone. Coagulation profile changes include a decrease in platelet count, prolonged prothrombin time and partial thromboplastin time, and a decrease in tensile clot strength. Clinical bleeding is uncommon in doses below 1,500 mL/day.
- *Anaphylaxis*: The incidence of anaphylaxis to HES is less than 0.085%. The incidence of severe reactions resulting in shock and/or cardiopulmonary arrest is 0.008%.
- *Hyperamylasemia*: Serum amylase levels are elevated following HES infusions. This is caused by complexes that form between amylase and hetastarch molecules, creating macroamylase particles, which undergo urinary excretion at a much slower rate than solitary amylase molecules.

A newer formulation of 6% hydroxyethyl starch (Hextend®) has recently been marketed. This colloid solution contains hydroxyethyl starch in a more balanced lactated solution rather than the 0.9 normal saline used in Hespan®. The benefits of this product appear to be that it maintains a more favorable electrolytic profile, primarily avoidance of hyperchloremic acidosis, as well as a reduction in intraoperative blood loss.

Pentastarch

A low-molecular-weight hydroxyethyl starch compound, 10% pentastarch, is currently under clinical investigation as an alternative to avoid blood transfusion and treatment for hypovolemia or as a plasma expander. Preliminary studies show promise as a potential alternative to albumin. Pentastarch should be used with caution in patients with end-stage renal disease.

Dextran

Pharmacology and Pharmacokinetics

Dextran is a large glucose polymer. It is a branched polysaccharide of 200,000 glucose units. There are two forms of dextran and the numbers refer to molecular weights: dextran 40 (mol. wt 40,000 daltons (Da)), and dextran 70 (mol. wt 70,000 Da). Dextran solutions are used clinically not only as volume-expanding agents but also in the prevention of thromboembolism and to increase peripheral blood flow.

Dextran molecules distribute in the extracellular space, mainly in the intravascular compartment. The particle size affects their retention in the intravascular space and the duration of volume expansion accomplished. The major route of elimination of dextran from the intravascular space is via renal excretion. While in the circulation, dextran particles exert osmotic activity. Larger particles remain in the circulation longer but exert less osmotic activity (remember, osmotic activity is related to the number of particles, not to their size). Some 60-70% of dextran 40 and 30-40% of dextran 70 is cleared in 12 hours. Only 20% of dextran 40 and 30% of dextran 70 remains in the circulation after 24 hours. The large particles (dextran 70) are taken up by the reticuloendothelial system and are eventually metabolized to carbon dioxide and water.

Indications for Use

- *Volume expansion*: Dextran solutions are ideal as plasma volume expanders. In shock, numerous studies have shown that dextran increases survival and improves hemodynamic parameters. Dextran infusion is associated with increased renal plasma flow and a fall in serum antidiuretic hormone levels has favorable hemodynamic effects in restoring intravascular volume in shock when compared with other volume expanders. However, the subsequent osmotic diuresis limits the duration of the volume expansion. One gram of dextran will bind 20-30 mL of water to the intravascular space.

A 500 mL bolus of dextran 40 thus produces a 750 mL expansion of intravascular volume at 1 hour and 1,050 mL at 2 hours.

- *Prevention of thromboembolism*: Dextran is effective in reducing the incidence of thromboembolic disease. Compared with controls, dextran is beneficial for the prevention of deep venous thrombosis in general surgery patients and following total hip replacement.
- *Promotion of peripheral blood flow*: Dextran coats the endothelial surfaces of blood vessels, reducing the interaction with the cellular elements in blood, thus potentiating microvascular blood flow. A decrease in viscosity and platelet adherence from dextran therapy limits thrombus formation and activation of the clotting cascade.

Side Effects

- *Renal failure*: Dextran-induced renal failure may occur, especially in the face of undiagnosed hypovolemia. The mechanism for the renal failure is tubular obstruction secondary to concentration and precipitation of dextran in the tubules with cast formation.
- *Anaphylaxis*: The incidence of anaphylactic reactions to dextran is between 1% and 5.3%. Any reactions will occur early, within 30 minutes after beginning the infusion. Symptoms include urticaria, rash, nausea, bronchospasm, shock, and death. Dextran is a potent antigen and has cross-reactivity with bacterial polysaccharide antigens. It is imperative to administer an antibody-binding agent prior to dextran infusion.
- *Osmotic diuresis*: An osmotic diuresis occurs almost immediately upon infusion of any dextran preparation, as the smaller particles are filtered and not reabsorbed. The effect is greater with dextran 40 than with dextran 70. Thus, following dextran therapy, urine volume alone cannot be used to estimate the adequacy of intravascular volume repletion.
- *Type and cross-matching*: Dextran can interfere with the ability to type and cross-match blood. The coating action of dextran on red blood cells causes cells to aggregate, mimicking a cross-match problem.
- *Bleeding diathesis*: Dextran inhibits erythrocyte aggregation *in vivo*. It adheres to vessel walls and cellular elements of the blood, decreases platelet adhesiveness, serum fibrinogen, and other factor levels, and increases bleeding times. At doses less than 1.5 g/kg/day, clinical bleeding is not a problem.

ELECTROLYTE DISORDERS

Sodium

The sodium ion is the principal solute determining osmolarity in the ECF compartment. Changes of extracellular sodium concentration and tonicity are associated

Table 8-2   Categories of Hyponatremia

	Isotonic Hyponatremia	Hypertonic Hyponatremia
Causes	Hyperproteinemic states, hyperlipidemic states	Hyperglycemia, mannitol, glycerol
Diagnosis	Decreased sodium, normal osmolality. Rule of thumb for hyperproteinemia: decrease in Na^+ (mEq/L) = increment of total protein >8 g/dL × 0.25	Decreased sodium, plasma osmolality >290 mosmol/kg
Management	Work up underlying cause	Correct volume deficit: • Insulin to slowly decrease glucose • Hypotonic saline to correct free water deficit • Correct underlying cause
Complications	Related to underlying cause	Hypoglycemia, cerebral edema

with movements of water across cell membranes, the fluid compartment with the higher osmotic gradient determining the direction of fluid movement. The resulting cell volume changes are responsible for the adverse clinical symptoms associated with low (hyponatremia) or high (hypernatremia) extracellular sodium concentrations.

Hyponatremia

Hyponatremia is defined as a serum sodium less than 135 mEq/L; however, clinical significance is not seen until levels reach below 130 mEq/L (Table 8-2). "Tonicity" represents the effective plasma osmolality (that which determines the movement of water between cells):

Tonicity = serum osmolality − blood urea nitrogen (BUN)/2.8.

There are three categories of hyponatremia:
- Isotonic hyponatremia (plasma osmolality 270–290 mosmol/kg)
- Hypertonic hyponatremia (plasma osmolality >290 mosmol/kg)
- Hypotonic "true" hyponatremia (plasma osmolality <280 mosmol/kg).

Clinical Findings

Central nervous system disturbances are the primary manifestations of hyponatremia, relating to the movement of water into the ICF compartment (including brain cells) in order to equalize osmolality differences. With values below 120 mEq/L, weakness, fatigue, somnolence, hyperactive deep tendon reflexes, and muscle twitches are seen. With values below 110 mEq/L, convulsions, coma, areflexia, and death are observed.

Hypotonic Hyponatremia

This category accounts for the vast majority of cases of hyponatremia. It is itself subdivided into three categories differentiated by clinical assessment of volume status (presence or absence of edema, urinary electrolytes, and vital signs): *hypovolemic hypotonic hyponatremia*, *hypervolemic hypotonic hyponatremia*, and *euvolemic hypotonic hyponatremia*. Urinary electrolytes can be helpful in identifying disease processes (Table 8-3).

Table 8-3   Diseases Associated with Hyponatremia and Urinary Sodium Values

Common Cause	Urine Sodium
Syndrome of inappropriate anti-diuretic hormone	>20 mEq/L
Acute H_2O intoxication	<10 mEq/L
Congestive heart failure	<20 mEq/L
Renal failure	>20 mEq/L
Cirrhosis	<20 mEq/L
Diuretics	>20 mEq/L
Adrenal insufficiency	>20 mEq/L
Secretory diarrhea	<10 mEq/L

Treatment

The treatment of hyponatremia is dependent upon which category of hyponatremia is present. For hypovolemic patients, the volume deficit should be corrected with normal saline until euvolemia is established. For hypervolemic (congestive heart failure, liver failure) and euvolemic (syndrome of inappropriate antidiuretic hormone secretion, SIADH) types, free water is usually restricted to less than 1,200 mL/day. In cases of severe or symptomatic hyponatremia (usually values <120 mEq/L), regardless of etiology, the sodium should be corrected with 3% hypertonic saline until the sodium is above 125 mEq/L; thereafter free water should be restricted, allowing the Na^+ to slowly return to normal. A loop diuretic can also be given to increase free water clearance.

The sodium deficit in hyponatremia is calculated by the following formula:

mEq Na^+ needed = (140 − serum Na^+) × (0.6 × weight [kg]).

The serum/blood sodium level should increase by no more than 12 mEq/L in a 24-hour period, with total correction no sooner than 48 hours. Occasionally, life-threatening complications may require a faster correction of serum Na^+ levels; however, too rapid a correction of the serum Na^+ levels may result in central nervous system injury (pontine myelinolysis).

Hypernatremia

Hypernatremia is defined as an elevated serum sodium concentration, which, when clinically significant, is in excess of 150 mEq/L. Life-threatening hypernatremia is seen with a sodium concentration greater than 160 mEq/L. Hypernatremia can be the result of a decrease in body water content secondary to excessive fluid loss or to limited intake of water, or an increased sodium content due to excessive intake or decreased excretion of sodium (Box 8-2).

Clinical Findings

The pathophysiologic consequences of hypernatremia reflect both extracellular dehydration and intracellular volume losses when water is drawn from the intracellular environment in response to extracellular hyperosmolarity. The severity of the clinical presentation is related to the magnitude of the hypernatremia and the rapidity with which it developed. With sodium values greater than 160 mEq/L, symptoms and signs include restlessness, weakness, dry mucous membranes, dry flushed skin, decreased salivation, tachycardia, hypotension, and ultimately delirium, coma, convulsions, and death.

Treatment

The treatment of hypernatremia is correction of the pure water deficit that exists. This deficit can be estimated in a number of ways, but the simplest general rule is the following: For every liter of water deficit, the serum sodium concentration will increase by 3 mEq above normal (140 mEq/L). Another more commonly used rule is:

Box 8-2 Causes of Hypernatremia

DECREASED BODY WATER
EXCESSIVE LOSS OF WATER
Skin
• Sweat
• Increased evaporative loss from altered skin surfaces (e.g., burns)
Lungs – insensible losses
Renal
• Osmotic diuresis
• Diabetes insipidus, hypothalamic or nephrogenic

LIMITED WATER INTAKE
Comatose and disoriented patients
Hypothalamic tumors or disorders with decreased thirst

INCREASED BODY SODIUM CONTENT
Excessive intake of salt
Decreased sodium excretion

$$\text{Water deficit (L)} = 0.6 \times \text{body weight (kg)} \times \left[\frac{\text{Current plasma sodium}}{140} - 1 \right].$$

When the deficit is minimal, simple oral ingestion of water or intravenous administration of 5% dextrose in water to reduce sodium concentrations to normal can be used. With a prolonged and severe hypernatremic state (i.e., serum sodium levels >160 mEq/L), the correction process becomes more difficult. Initial treatment is infusion of normal saline until hemodynamic stability is restored. Treatment should be gradual, over a 36–48-hour period, because of possible intracellular swelling. Brain cells accommodate to extracellular hypertonicity by accumulating additional intracellular solute. A sudden decrease in extracellular osmolarity without time for elimination of this additional intracellular solute will lead to rapid swelling of brain cells, which in turn can cause serious neurologic dysfunction.

An essential part of the treatment of hypernatremia is correction or treatment of the underlying cause whenever possible.

Potassium

Disturbances of potassium balance are common in surgical patients. Their importance relates to the significant role that potassium ion plays in cellular metabolism and the excitation of muscle and nerve. Total body potassium stores equal 50–55 mEq/kg in the average adult. The majority of the potassium, about 140 mEq/L is located intracellularly and roughly 4 mEq/L is present in the ECF.

Hypokalemia

Hypokalemia is defined as a serum potassium concentration below 3.5 mEq/L. Clinically significant hypokalemia is not seen until levels are between 2.5 and 3.0 mEq/L. Major causes of hypokalemia in the surgical patient usually involve increased gastrointestinal and/or renal losses, movement of potassium from the extracellular to the intracellular fluid, and negative potassium balance resulting from inadequate intake or replacement of losses. Box 8-3 lists the causes of hypokalemia.

Clinical Findings

• *Cardiac*: Toxicity may be manifested by serious arrhythmias. Other electrocardiographic changes of hypokalemia include low voltage, prolongation of the P-R interval, T wave depression and prominent U waves.

• *Neuromuscular*: Hyperpolarization of nerve cells slows nerve conduction and muscle contractions, which may contribute to muscle weakness, cramps, and paresthesias. These symptoms are usually not seen until the plasma potassium concentration is less than 2.5 mEq/L. Marked, profound hypokalemia can impair

---

Box 8-3 Causes of Hypokalemia

GASTROINTESTINAL LOSSES

Gastric – nasogastric suction, vomiting
Diarrhea – infectious, *Clostridium difficile*
Fistulas
Obstruction

RENAL LOSSES

Alkalosis
Diuresis and other medications
Nephropathy
Mineralocorticoid excess

INTRACELLULAR SHIFTS

Alkalosis
Total parenteral nutrition
Insulin

INADEQUATE INTAKE

Dietary
Inadequate perioperative K^+-containing fluids

---

respiratory function, leading to hypoventilation. Severe hypokalemia also may cause rhabdomyolysis.

- *Renal*: Manifestations of hypokalemia are polyuria and resistance to antidiuretic hormone action. Chronic hypokalemia can result in chronic interstitial nephritis and a decline in the glomerular filtration rate.

Diagnosis

Excretion of more than 30 mEq/L of potassium per day usually indicates a form of renal potassium wasting. The most common differential diagnosis in normotensive patients with hypokalemia and metabolic alkalosis includes vomiting or diuretic use. Hypertension in the presence of hypokalemia generally indicates that aldosterone or another mineralocorticoid is present in high levels. Measuring plasma renin may be useful.

Treatment

As a general rule of thumb, for each 1 mEq/L decrease in plasma potassium concentration, total body potassium stores decrease by 200–400 mEq, until the potassium is below 2.0 mEq/L. At this point, the total deficit may exceed 1,000 mEq. Oral replacement is preferred whenever possible, usually in doses of 40 mEq every 4-6 hours. If intravenous replacement is needed, then peripheral infusions (containing no more than 40–60 mEq K^+/L of fluid) can be infused at a rate of 10 mEq K^+/hr. In severe hypokalemia, concentrated infusions of potassium may be given via a central line (1 mEq/mL of infusion fluid) not to exceed 0.5 mEq/kg/hr or 25 mEq/hr). Rapid replacement of chronic hypokalemia is dangerous (because of precipitation of dysrhythmias) and replacement should be carried out slowly over a 48–72-hour period.

Hyperkalemia

Hyperkalemia is defined as a serum potassium concentration above 5.5 mEq/L. Clinical significance is reached when values exceed 6 mEq/L. The etiology of increased potassium can be divided into three basic categories: increased potassium load, decreased excretion, and intracellular shifts. Box 8-4 lists the causes of hyperkalemia.

Clinical Findings

Most individuals with hyperkalemia are asymptomatic until the plasma level is above 6.5–7.0 mEq/L. As the plasma potassium increases, the resting membrane potential becomes less negative and moves closer to the threshold for excitation. This change is associated with delayed depolarization caused by a decrease in membrane permeability. Hyperkalemia affects the electrocardiogram as outlined in Table 8-4.

Neuromuscular findings are nonspecific and include paresthesias and weakness, which can progress to paralysis of the respiratory muscles. These symptoms are similar to those seen with hypokalemia.

Diagnosis

The cause of hyperkalemia is usually pinpointed by knowing the etiologic factors most likely at fault (e.g., renal failure, acidemia, renal tubular acidosis, or iatrogenic potassium administration).

Box 8-4 Causes of Hyperkalemia

INCREASED POTASSIUM LOAD

Exogenous
- Excessive dietary intake
- Transfusions of blood
- High-dose potassium penicillin therapy
- Extensive tissue trauma and rhabdomyolysis (crush injuries)
- Hemolysis
- Catabolic breakdown of tissue with trauma, starvation, etc.
- Cellular breakdown with rapid rewarming in severely hypothermic patients

DECREASED POTASSIUM EXCRETION

Renal failure
Adrenal insufficiency and impaired aldosterone activity

EXTRACELLULAR SHIFTS

Acute acidosis, metabolic or respiratory
Insulin deficiency
Digitalis and related cardiotonic drugs

PSEUDOHYPERKALEMIA

Blood sample hemolysis
Blood sample contaminated by infused potassium solution

Table 8-4   Electrocardiographic (ECG) Changes with Hyperkalemia

Serum Level (mEq/L)	ECG Abnormality
6.0–7.0	Peaked T waves (best in precordial leads)
7.0–8.0	Diminished P waves, ↑ P-R interval and heart block, ↓ Q-T interval, widening QRS, depressed ST segments
>8.0	Loss of T waves, asystole

Treatment

The primary goal for treatment of hyperkalemia is to reduce serum potassium concentrations to levels that are not life-threatening. A number of measures can be initiated: restriction of potassium intake; discontinuing of drugs capable of altering potassium homeostasis, such as beta-blockers, angiotensin-converting enzyme inhibitors, and nonsteroidal anti-inflammatory drugs; and administration of potassium-depleting loop diuretic agents, and Kayexalate (sodium polystyrene sulfonate), a cation-exchange resin. Each gram of the resin can bind approximately 1 mEq of potassium.

In most cases these measures will be all that is needed for elevations of potassium up to 6.5 mEq/L. In acute elevations, or with levels greater than 7.5 mEq/L:

- *Insulin*: 10 units given subcutaneously (works within 30–60 min), in conjunction with an intravenous infusion of 25 g of glucose over a 5-minute period. This may reduce serum levels by as much as 1 mEq/L by driving potassium into the cell
- *Sodium bicarbonate*: 50 mEq over 5 minutes induces a metabolic alkalosis with shifting of potassium back into the cells that will decrease serum potassium concentrations lasting up to 2 hours. If the patient is receiving mechanical ventilation, hyperventilation therapy may also be employed
- *Calcium gluconate solution*: 10 mL of a 10% solution should be given. This drug does not lower serum potassium but instead stabilizes the heart's membranes against the effects of hyperkalemia. It should only be given if there is electrocardiographic evidence of hyperkalemia (T-wave peaking, etc.)
- *Dialysis* should be tried if all else fails.

Calcium

Calcium is important in humans for both structural and biochemical integrity. The normal adult body contains approximately 1,000–1,400 g of calcium, of which 99% is located in the skeleton and 1% in the soft tissues and extracellular spaces. Calcium is the most abundant electrolyte in the human body and is essential in humans for proper neuronal and cardiac function, cell division, neurotransmission, hormonal secretion, muscle contraction, and enzyme action. The ionized fraction is the physiologically active form and is homeostatically regulated. A variety of factors are known to alter the total and ionized serum calcium levels:

- *Blood pH*: pH affects calcium binding to serum proteins – acute acidosis decreases protein binding (increasing the ionized calcium level) and alkalosis increases protein binding (lowering the ionized calcium level)
- *Free fatty acids* increase calcium binding to albumin, thus lowering ionized calcium
- *Calcium chelators* (e.g., phosphate, albumin, bicarbonate, radiocontrast agents, and citrate) lower circulating ionized calcium. Citrate may also chelate magnesium, causing hypomagnesemia, which in turn may accentuate hypocalcemia.

Calcium Homeostasis

Calcium is closely regulated by parathyroid hormone (PTH) and vitamin D through their effects on bone, kidney, and the gut. A fall in circulating calcium stimulates an increase in PTH, which stimulates mobilization of calcium from bone as well as renal reabsorption of calcium. PTH also stimulates the 1-alpha-hydroxylation of 25-hydroxycalciferol by the kidney to 1,25-dihydroxycalciferol (vitamin D_3). Vitamin D_3 stimulates reabsorption of calcium from the gut and facilitates mobilization of calcium from bone in response to PTH.

Hypocalcemia

Hypocalcemia is frequently encountered in hospitalized patients, especially patients who are critically ill (Box 8-5). Clinical manifestations are the result of *ionized* hypocalcemia.

Clinical Features

Significant hypocalcemia exists when either the patient demonstrates clinical features or the ionized calcium level is below 0.80 mEq/L. Life-threatening hypocalcemia occurs with levels of less than 0.65 mEq/L.

Neuromuscular manifestations include neuronal membrane irritability and tetany. Latent tetany may be demonstrated by eliciting Chvostek's sign or Trousseau's sign.

Cardiovascular manifestations of hypocalcemia include congestive heart failure, hypotension, dysrhythmias, and insensitivity to digitalis. The electrophysiologic effects of hypocalcemia result in prolongation of the Q-T interval by prolonging the ST interval.

Drug Interaction: Effects of Hypocalcemia

Hypocalcemia diminishes the effects of beta-adrenergic agonists and digoxin, while enhancing the effects of beta-blockers and calcium channel blockers.

Box 8-5 Causes of Hypocalcemia

PRIMARY HYPOPARATHYROIDISM
SECONDARY HYPOPARATHYROIDISM

Neck surgery
Sepsis
Hypo- or hypermagnesemia
Burns
Pancreatitis
Aminoglycosides

CALCIUM CHELATION/PRECIPITATION

Hyperphosphatemia
Citrate
Albumin
Fat embolism
Pancreatitis
Sepsis
Rhabdomyolysis

IMPAIRED VITAMIN D SYNTHESIS OR ACTION

Poor intake
Malabsorption
Hypomagnesemia
Liver disease
Renal failure
Pseudohypoparathyroidism
Sepsis

Box 8-6 Causes of Hypercalcemia

MALIGNANCY

Parathyroid-hormone-like material
Lung, renal cell carcinoma, lymphoma, multiple
    myeloma
Osteoclast-activating factors
Lymphoma, multiple myeloma, prostaglandins, solid
    tumors (lung, breast, kidney)

ENDOCRINOLOGIC

Primary hyperparathyroidism, hyperthyroidism,
    pheochromocytoma, acromegaly

DRUG USE OR INTOXICATION

Thiazide diuretics, low-dose furosemide, hyper-
    vitaminosis A and D, milk–alkali syndrome

GRANULOMATOUS DISEASES

Tuberculosis, sarcoid, histoplasmosis

IMMOBILIZATION

Volume depletion, recovery from acute renal failure,
    phosphate depletion syndrome

Treatment

Therapy of hypocalcemia begins with identifying the cause and then treating appropriately as outlined below:

- Determine magnesium and phosphate levels – effective therapy of hypocalcemia is futile in the presence of severe deficiencies of these ions
- Drugs that may be contributory to hypocalcemia must be identified and withdrawn if possible
- Potassium abnormalities should also be identified and corrected along with the low serum calcium – hyperkalemia and hypomagnesemia potentiate the cardiac and neuromuscular irritability seen in the presence of hypocalcemia
- For severe clinical and symptomatic hypocalcemia (usually levels less than 0.80 mmol/L), intravenous replacement should consist of 100–200 mg of elemental calcium over 10 minutes with electrocardiographic monitoring (1 g of $CaCl_2$ contains 272 mg of elemental calcium, while 1 gram of calcium gluconate consists of 98 mg of elemental calcium). If the cause is hypoparathyroidism, then a maintenance infusion of 1–2 mg/kg/hr of elemental calcium should be started.

Hypercalcemia

Hypercalcemia is defined as an ionized calcium greater than 1.3 mmol/L or a total calcium level greater than 10.5 mg/dL. The majority of hypercalcemia is due to malignancy or hyperparathyroidism (Box 8-6).

Clinical Findings

Common findings in patients with hypercalcemia include loss of appetite, nausea, vomiting, constipation and bone pain. It can cause mental status changes such as lethargy, confusion, and coma. It has also been associated with peptic ulcer disease, pancreatitis, and renal failure. Electrocardiographic changes include prolongation of the P-R interval, widening of the QRS interval, shortening of the ST segment, and a slight flattening of T waves. "Hypercalcemic crisis" involves the triad of intravascular volume depletion, renal failure, and coma.

Drug Interaction: Effects of Hypercalcemia

Hypercalcemia can potentiate the cardiac effects of digoxin.

Treatment

Emergency treatment is indicated for severe hypercalcemia or related mental status changes. Initial intervention should consist of rehydration, followed by diuresis to increase calcium excretion. Magnesium, potassium, sodium, and volume status must be followed closely. This may necessitate placement of a central venous catheter, or pulmonary artery pressure monitoring to manage fluid status, especially in a patient with cardiopulmonary disease. Additional administration of bisphosphonates or calcitonin may be required, as well as dialysis for renal compromised patients.

Clinical Caveat: Severe Hypercalcemia

Severe hypercalcemia is a medical emergency and should be corrected prior to an anesthetic.

Phosphate

Almost all blood phosphorus exists as phosphate anions (PO_4, HPO_4, and H_2PO_4). Phosphate is the major intracellular anion. It is required in protein, fat, and carbohydrate metabolism, and is the source of high-energy bonds in adenosine triphosphate (ATP) and phosphocreatine. Phosphate is also a component of 2,3 diphosphoglycerate (DPG), cyclic nucleotides, nicotinamide diphosphate, phospholipids, and nucleic acids, and participates in buffering of urinary acids.

Phosphate Homeostasis

Phosphate is primarily regulated by the kidney and the adult body contains about 700–800 g of PO_4. The normal serum phosphate level is 0.87–1.45 mmol/L in adults, and 1.29–2.29 mmol/L in children. The average dietary intake of phosphate ranges from 800 to 1,200 mg per day, with most being absorbed in the small intestine. Phosphate is excreted by the kidneys, with parathyroid hormone increasing phosphate excretion by inhibiting the proximal tubular reabsorption. Insulin causes glucose and phosphate to move into the cells and is responsible for the hypophosphatemia seen during insulin administration or high carbohydrate feeding. In addition, ECF volume expansion is associated with decreases in the proximal reabsorption of both phosphate and sodium.

Hypophosphatemia

Hypophosphatemia is a very common problem in perioperative patients. The major causes of hypophosphatemia are categorized into intracellular shifting, gastrointestinal losses, renal phosphate wasting, and drug-induced (Box 8-7).

Clinical Findings

Severe hypophosphatemia is associated with decreased levels of PO_4-containing metabolites (ATP, 2,3 DPG) and membrane phospholipids, and results from a variety of clinical disorders. Patients may develop cardiac insufficiency (resulting in depleted intracellular stores of

Box 8-7   Causes of Hypophosphatemia

INTRACELLULAR SHIFT

Carbohydrate loading
Metabolic alkalosis
Sepsis
Severe burns

GASTROINTESTINAL LOSSES

Malabsorptive states
Diarrhea
Phosphate-binding antacids
Nasogastric suction

RENAL PHOSPHATE WASTING

Excess parathyroid hormone
Diabetic ketoacidosis
Diuretic therapy
Renal tubular defects (myeloma)
Hypokalemia and hypomagnesemia
Vitamin D deficiency
Acidemia
Post renal transplantation
Hypothermia
Drug-induced
Epinephrine
Insulin or glucagon
Saline diuresis
Corticosteroid use
Bicarbonate

PO_4, impaired action of the sodium–potassium ATPase pump, decreased calcium flux, or impaired catecholamine action). With levels of phosphate less than 0.65 mmol/L, muscle pains, anorexia, or tremors can be seen. If the level is less than 0.32 mmol/L, respiratory weakness or failure may supervene. A large number of neurologic syndromes have been observed with low phosphate levels, including ataxia, tremors, paresthesias, myopathy, coma, and even death. Muscle integrity depends upon phosphate, and severe hypophosphatemia (<0.32 mmol/L) may injure muscle cells, resulting in rhabdomyolysis. Severe hypophosphatemia can cause red blood cell hemolysis and platelet and leukocyte dysfunction. Decreased levels of 2,3 DPG causes a left shift of the oxyhemoglobin dissociation curve, which can lead to decreased oxygen delivery to the tissues. In addition, insulin resistance, impaired gluconeogenesis, impaired bone mineralization, and liver dysfunction result from hypophosphatemia.

Treatment

The potential consequences of severe hypophosphatemia necessitate prompt recognition and treatment. If the serum PO_4 is less than 0.32 mmol/L or symptomatic, then intravenous replacement is indicated, with an infusion

---

Box 8-8   Causes of Hyperphosphatemia

REDUCED RENAL PHOSPHATE EXCRETION

Renal failure
Hypoparathyroidism
Hyperthyroidism
Acromegaly

INCREASED PHOSPHATE ENTRANCE INTO THE ECF FROM THE ICF

Chemotherapy for leukemia, lymphoma, multiple myeloma
Rhabdomyolysis
Sepsis
Severe hypothermia
Fulminant hepatitis

INCREASED PHOSPHATE OR VITAMIN D INTAKE

Ingestion of phosphate salts (milk–alkali syndrome)
Intravenous use of phosphate salts
Pharmacologic administration of vitamin D

ECF, extracellular fluid; ICF, intracellular fluid.

of 0.5 mmol/kg for serum phosphate levels less than 0.5 mmol/L, and 0.2 mmol/kg of elemental phosphorus via a 4–6-hour infusion for levels between 0.5 and 1.0 mmol/L. The danger of infusing phosphorus rapidly is primarily that of precipitating hypocalcemia. Parenteral phosphate may be stopped and enteral replacement begun when serum phosphorus levels exceed 0.65 mmol/L. Because coexisting hypomagnesemia is common, magnesium levels should be monitored and magnesium replaced as needed.

Hyperphosphatemia

Hyperphosphatemia is defined by a fasting serum phosphate of more than 1.45 mmol/L. The causes of hyperphosphatemia are listed in Box 8-8.

Clinical Findings

Symptoms of hyperphosphatemia are related primarily to those of hypocalcemia.

Treatment

Treatment consists of eliminating the cause of phosphate elevation and correcting associated hypocalcemia and hyperphosphatemia. Phosphate is lowered by restricting intake, increasing urinary excretion with saline and Diamox (500 mg every 6 hr), and increasing gut phosphate losses with aluminum hydroxide (30–45 mL four times a day).

Magnesium

Magnesium is the second most common intracellular cation, next to potassium. It is required for the activity of phosphatases, which are involved in the function of the sodium–potassium pump, the calcium–ATPase pump, muscle contraction, glucose–fat–protein metabolism, oxidative phosphorylation, and DNA synthesis. Magnesium is also required for the activity of the adenylate cyclase system.

The total body content of magnesium is estimated to be around 2,000 mEq, roughly 50–60% of which is in the skeleton and 20% in muscle. Only around 1% is found in the serum. The total serum magnesium concentration normally varies from 0.7 to 1.0 mmol/L (1.4–2.0 mEq/L) and is composed of three fractions: a protein-bound fraction (30%), a chelated fraction (15%), and an ionized fraction (55%). The ionized fraction is the one that is physiologically active.

The normal dietary intake of magnesium is about 12–15 mmol/day. Magnesium is absorbed in the small intestine and excreted in the urine and stool. Gut absorption occurs by both a vitamin-D-dependent and an independent mechanism. Magnesium reabsorption is linked to the reabsorption of calcium and sodium, and the renal loss of either of these ions results in concomitant loss of magnesium.

Hypomagnesemia

Clinical Findings

It is similar to hypocalcemia with neuronal irritability and tetany. Most patients are symptomatic with levels below 0.4 mmol/L of magnesium. Hypomagnesemia is often associated with hypocalcemia and hypokalemia. The low potassium probably results from renal potassium wasting secondary to decreased function of the sodium–potassium ATPase pump. The cardiovascular manifestations include heart failure, dysrhythmias, hypotension, and coronary artery spasm. Box 8-9 lists the causes of hypomagnesemia.

Drug Interaction: Effects of Hypomagnesemia

Hypomagnesemia increases the sensitivity to digitalis and pressor agents. Standard antiarrhythmic therapy may be ineffective in controlling ventricular dysrhythmias in the presence of magnesium deficiency.

Treatment

Severe magnesium depletion (Mg^{2+} <0.4 mmol/L) requires intravenous replacement of magnesium. An initial dose of 600 mg of elemental magnesium may be required, followed by a maintenance dose of 600–900 mg of elemental magnesium per day. A loading dose of magnesium should not be given faster than 15 mg/min, and the patient should have electrocardiographic monitoring. (1 g of $MgSO_4$ contains 98 mg of elemental magnesium, or 8 mEq). Replacement therapy should be carried out over 5–7 days in order to adequately replenish intracellular stores.

Box 8-9   Causes of Hypomagnesemia

DRUG-INDUCED LOSSES

Diuretics
Aminoglycosides, amphotericin B
Digoxin
Insulin
Saline excess, calcium

RENAL LOSSES

Diuretic phase of ATN – acute tubular necrosis
Hyperthyroidism
Phosphate deficiency
DKA – diabetic ketoacidosis
Hypercalcemia
Syndrome of inappropriate antidiuretic hormone
   secretion

GASTROINTESTINAL DISEASE

Reduced intake
- Malnutrition
- Hyperalimentation
- Prolonged intravenous therapy
Reduced absorption (malabsorption, fistulas)

MISCELLANEOUS LOSSES

Severe burns
Sepsis
Hypothermia
Cardiopulmonary bypass
Administration of glucose or amino acids

Hypermagnesemia

Hypermagnesemia is rare in clinical practice and usually results from iatrogenic causes. The most common etiologies include the administration of magnesium-containing antacids, enemas, or parenteral nutrition solutions to patients with renal failure, and the treatment of pregnancy-induced hypertension (pre-eclampsia) with magnesium sulfate. Excess magnesium inhibits the prejunctional release of acetylcholine and decreases motor end-plate sensitivity to acetylcholine. It may also cause hypotension and vasodilation.

Hypocalcemia may result from the inhibitory effects of hypermagnesemia on parathyroid gland function. The neuromuscular and cardiac side effects of hypermagnesemia can be transiently antagonized by administering intravenous calcium.

Drug Interaction: Effects of Hypermagnesemia

Hypermagnesemia potentiates the effects of neuromuscular relaxants.

SUGGESTED READING

Adrogue H, Madias N. Hyponatremia. *N Engl J Med* 2000;342: 1581–1589.

Choi P, Gordon Y, Quinonez L, *et al*. Crystalloids vs. colloids in fluid resuscitation: a systematic review. *Crit Care Med* 1999;27:200–210.

Doyle J, Davis D, Hoyt D. The use of hypertonic saline in the treatment of traumatic brain injury. *J Trauma* 2001;50:367–383.

Gan T, Bennett-Guerrero E, Phillips-Bute B, *et al*. Hextend, a physiologically balanced expander for large volume use in major surgery: a randomized phase III clinical trial. *Anesth Analg* 1999;88:992–998.

Hankeln K. Comparison of hydroxyethyl starch and lactated Ringer's solution on hemodynamics and oxygen transport of critically ill patients in prospective crossover studies. *Crit Care Med* 1989;17:133–135.

Hauser CJ. Oxygen transport responses to colloid and crystalloid in critically ill surgical patients. *Surg Gynecol Obstet* 1980;150:811.

Khanna S, Davis D, Peterson B, *et al*. Use of hypertonic saline in the treatment of severe refractory posttraumatic intracranial hypertension in pediatric traumatic brain injury. *Crit Care Med* 2000 28:1144–1151.

Porzio P, Halberthal M, Bohn D, Halperin M. Treatment of acute hyponatremia: ensuring the excretion of a predictable amount of electrolyte-free water. *Crit Care Med* 2000;28:1905–1910.

Qureshi A, Suarez J. Use of hypertonic saline solutions in treatment of cerebral edema and intracranial hypertension. *Crit Care Med* 2000;28:3301–3313.

CHAPTER 9

Hemostasis and Transfusion Therapy

JOHN PENNER

INTRODUCTION

This chapter will review the processes of hemostasis and transfusion therapy. It is divided into sections discussing the basic biochemistry of normal coagulation, the laboratory evaluation of coagulation, the blood products available for transfusion therapy, the indications for each of these products, the risks of performing transfusion of these products, and, lastly, the use of autologous transfusion techniques.

Clinical Caveats

Normal saline should be used as the carrier for red cell transfusion as lactated Ringer's solution may cause in-line clotting of the blood as lactate can bind the calcium in the red cell preparations.

Clerical error is the most common reason for all transfusion reactions – if possible, have blood cross-checked by operating room personnel prior to bringing it into the operating room and rechecked again before transfusion.

For cases in which rapid or massive blood loss is anticipated, be sure to warm all blood (and intravenous) products, with the exception of platelets.

In those with pre-existing hyperkalemia or an impaired ability to clear excess serum potassium, request "fresher" packed red cells or washed red cells for transfusion. Transfusion with dialysis is a way to avoid these metabolic complications in patients at risk.

Platelets that are ordered but not immediately transfused should either be returned to the blood bank or gently agitated in the Operating Room to prevent aggregation.

Continued

NORMAL HEMOSTASIS

Injury to a vessel initiates a carefully coordinated
response that first results in a platelet plug being formed,
followed later by formation of a fibrin-linked clot. This
response is coordinated by interactions between blood
vessels, platelets, and circulating clotting proteins. The
role of each of these factors is described briefly below.

The normal vascular endothelium and subendothelium
are active participants in hemostasis. The endothelium
possesses both anti- and prothrombotic proteins. The
antithrombotic components include protein S, thrombomodulin, and heparin-like molecules. These proteins are
involved with the removal of activated clotting proteins,
thus preventing unwanted clot formation in the intact circulation. The pro-thrombotic proteins include tissue factor, von Willebrand factor, and platelet-activating factor, all
of which enhance clotting in the face of injury. Tissue factor is required for the activation of the extrinsic clotting
cascade. It is not normally expressed by the vascular
endothelium but its expression can be stimulated by endo-
toxins, cytokines, and acidosis. Von Willebrand factor is a
protein required for platelet binding to the injured site. In
addition to the endothelium's role, the subendothelium
contains collagen, elastin, and fibronectin, all of which are
thrombogenic. The fibrillar collagen of the subendothelium serves as one of the most potent activators of platelet
aggregation and the intrinsic clotting cascade.

When a vessel is injured, the collagen of the subendothelium becomes exposed, allowing contact with circulating platelets. Platelets that come in contact with the
subendothelial collagen become activated, undergoing
what is known as the "release reaction." In this process, the
contents of the platelet's alpha granules (fibrinogen,
fibronectin, platelet-derived growth factor, and platelet factor 4) and dense granules (adenosine diphosphate [ADP],
ionized calcium, histamine, serotonin, and epinephrine)
are released. The products thus released promote further
vasoconstriction, activate more platelets, and/or serve as

substrate or co-factors for both the clotting cascade and
fibrin cross links. At the same time, both platelet factor
3 and the glycoprotein IIb–IIIa complex become exposed
on the platelet membrane. Platelet factor 3 becomes the
site for binding of calcium and activated factors IX and
VIII, while the glycoprotein IIb–IIIa complex facilitates the
further aggregation of platelets.

The final step in the process of normal coagulation is
activation of the clotting cascade. This cascade describes
the sequential activation of a series of circulating inactive
proenzymes (clotting "factors") into their active enzymatic form at the site of vessel injury. The end result of this
reaction chain is the formation of thrombin, which in turn
acts upon fibrinogen to form fibrin, the protein responsible
for stabilizing the platelet plug.

Each of the inactive proteins of the clotting cascade is
designated by a roman numeral (i.e., factor XI). Once the
factor is activated, a postscript letter a is added after
the numeral (i.e., factor XIa). Most of the factors (I, II, V, VII,
VIII, IX, X, and XIII) are produced in the liver. Of these,
four require a vitamin-K-dependent decarboxylation
reaction. The vitamin-K-dependent factors are factors II,
VII, IX, and X. All the proteins in the cascade are proteolytic proenzymes with the exception of factors V and VIII,
both of which serve as accelerator proteins.

Classically, the clotting cascade is thought to have two
distinct starting points. The first of these is the intrinsic or
"contact activation" pathway. This path begins with the
activation of factor XII when it comes in contact with a
negatively-charged surface. The second path is the extrinsic pathway, which begins with the activation of factor VII
by tissue factor expressed by the damaged endothelium.
These two paths meet at the point of factor X activation.
The common pathway describes the final steps of the
cascade, with the formation of thrombin, which in turn
cleaves circulating fibrinogen to fibrin, which cross-links
and stabilizes the initial platelet plug. This classic view of
the clotting cascade is depicted in Figure 9-1.

The classic breakdown of clotting into the intrinsic
and extrinsic pathways is useful to explain the basic tests
of the clotting process (see below). However, *in vivo*,
these paths do not function as two separate entities but
rather are intertwined and co-dependent. *In vivo*, injury
to a vessel will expose tissue factor. The exposed tissue
factor will activate factor VII, forming factor VIIa. The
activated factor VIIa in turn activates factor X, with the
resultant formation of thrombin. The activation of X by
the factor VIIa–tissue factor complex is short-lived, as the
complex is rapidly inhibited by tissue factor pathway
inhibitor. The sustained activation of factor X depends
upon the continued actions of the factor IXa–VIIIa complex. This is accomplished by the activation of factor XI
by thrombin. In addition, thrombin will also activate
more of factor VII to VIIa. This model of clotting explains
why those with factor VIII and factor IX deficiencies have

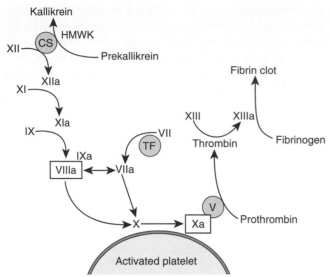

Figure 9-1   The clotting cascade. CS, surface contact; HMWK, high-molecular-weight kininogen; TF, tissue factor. (Redrawn from Hillman RS, Ault KA, eds. *Hematology in clinical practice*, 3rd ed. New York: McGraw-Hill, 2002:304.)

defective clot formation despite an intact factor VII pathway. This integrated approach to the clotting cascade is depicted in Figure 9-2.

There are several regulatory steps in the clotting cascade. These include the removal of activated clotting factors by the liver and the destruction of activated factors and fibrin clot that is no longer needed. Destruction of the circulating factors is accomplished by the circulating anticoagulant system, consisting of antithrombin III, the heparin-like molecules of the endothelium, and the protein C and S system.

Antithrombin III is a protease inhibitor that functions by binding to and inactivating all of the activated proteolytic clotting factors with the exception of factor VIIa. The activity of antithrombin III is potentiated by the heparin-like molecules of the endothelium. In addition,

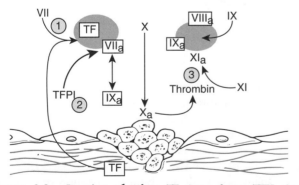

Figure 9-2   *In vivo* clotting. TF, tissue factor; TFPI, tissue factor pathway inhibitor. (Redrawn from Hillman RS, Ault KA, eds. *Hematology in clinical practice*, 3rd ed. New York: McGraw-Hill, 2002:305.)

these heparin-like molecules also inactivate factors IXa, Xa, XIa, and XIIa. Protein C is a vitamin-K-dependent protein that, like other clotting proteins, circulates in its inactive form. Protein C activation occurs when circulating thrombin is bound by the thrombomodulin of the endothelium. The thrombin thus bound loses its procoagulant activity, instead acting on the circulating inactive protein C, cleaving it into its active form. The activated protein C complexes with calcium, phospholipid, and another vitamin-K dependent protein called protein S to destroy the activity of both factors V and VIII.

Fibrinolysis is the process by which fibrin clot is either remodeled or removed. Plasmin, derived from circulating plasminogen, is the protein responsible for fibrinolysis; it also destroys both factors V and VIII. Proteolysis of plasminogen to plasmin is accomplished by two enzymatic systems: tissue plasminogen activator (tPA) and urokinase. tPA is primarily synthesized by the endothelial cell, and is active when attached to fibrin. It thus activates the plasminogen in the clot itself, with little effect on circulating plasminogen. Urokinase is present in the circulation and various tissues, and activates plasminogen in the fluid phase. It helps to keep hollow organs free from clot. These two proteins are secreted in their active forms by appropriately stimulated endothelial cells and mononuclear phagocytes. Urokinase is also secreted by epithelial cells.

The byproducts of the proteolysis of fibrin by plasmin are known as fibrin split or fibrin degradation products. The fibrin degradation products are also potent inhibitors of clotting. They accomplish this by interfering with both the action of thrombin at its fibrinogen-binding site and with fibrin polymerization. The presence of increased fibrin split products can result in clinical bleeding in a variety of common clinical situations.

LABORATORY EVALUATION OF CLOTTING

There are several clinical laboratory tests used to evaluate the integrity of the coagulation system. Each of the more commonly used tests is described in more detail below and summarized in Table 9-1.

Prothrombin Time

The measurement of a prothrombin time (PT) is made by mixing the patient's plasma with a commercially prepared solution of thromboplastin. Thromboplastin contains phospholipid, calcium and tissue factor, which activates the extrinsic pathway. The PT thus tests the integrity of the extrinsic and common pathways. Normal values also vary between institutions, but are in the range of 10–13 seconds. The PT is commonly used to monitor

Table 9-1	Normal Tests of Coagulation		
Laboratory Test	**Evaluates**	**Normal Value**	**Notes**
PT	Extrinsic and common pathways	10–13 sec	Prolonged by deficiencies or functional abnormalities in factor VII (extrinsic path), and factors II, V, VIII, X, and fibrinogen (common path)
INR	Extrinsic and common pathways	1	Compares PT obtained with local reagents to that obtained when standard reagents are used
PTT	Intrinsic and common pathways	28–38 sec	Prolonged by deficiencies or functional abnormalities in factors XII, XI, IX (intrinsic path), and factors II, V, VIII, X, and fibrinogen (common path)
ACT	Intrinsic pathway	110–130 sec	Most commonly used to measure the degree of heparin anticoagulation during cardiac and vascular surgery
Thrombin time	Conversion of fibrinogen to fibrin by thrombin	9–35 sec	Used in conjunction with reptilase test to document the presence of heparin in the patient's plasma or the presence of dysfibrinogenemia (see text)
Fibrinogen	Level of serum fibrinogen	140–410 mg/dL	Also an acute phase reactant. May be decreased in chronic liver disease, congenital deficiencies and consumptive coagulopathy. May be elevated in inflammatory conditions
Fibrin degradation products	Fibrinolysis		Measures the degree of fibrinolysis. Elevated in DIC, pulmonary embolism, deep venous thrombosis, and liver disease and patients 24–48 hr postoperatively
D-dimer	Fibrinolysis	<500 ng/mL	Specific for the product of plasmin's action on fibrin linked by factor XIII. Elevated in DIC, pulmonary embolism, deep venous thrombosis, and liver disease, and in patients 24–48 hr postoperatively
Bleeding time	Platelet function	2–9 min	Poor specificity as affected by technique, factor deficiencies, and systemic diseases

Normal values vary depending upon the laboratory performing the test. The numbers above serve only as a general guide. ACT, activated clotting time; DIC, disseminated intravascular coagulation; INR, international normalized ratio; PT, prothrombin time; PTT, partial thromboplastin time.

the degree of warfarin anticoagulation. Warfarin is an oral anticoagulant that inhibits hepatic vitamin-K-dependent carboxylation reactions. Patients on warfarin therapy therefore have a decreased level of factor VII with a resultant prolongation of the PT.

International Normalized Ratio

Because the reagents used in the PT assay vary between labs, an international normalized ratio (INR), was created in an attempt to standardize anticoagulation values across labs. The INR compares the lab's value to the value one would obtain if using international reference reagents rather than local reagents. The INR is a more consistent way of following anticoagulation therapy.

Partial Thromboplastin Time

The partial thromboplastin time (PTT) is used to screen for the integrity of the intrinsic and common pathways of coagulation. The PTT is measured by exposing the patient's blood to a negatively charged surface in the presence of calcium. This activates the intrinsic (contact) pathway. The time for clot to form is measured and recorded as the PTT. Normal values vary from institution to institution, but are in the range of 28–38 seconds. As heparin acts on antithrombin III to make it 1,000 times more potent, and as antithrombin III inactivates all the factors except factor VIIa (thus has little effect on the PT), the PTT is used to test the degree of anticoagulation of a patient on heparin therapy.

Activated Clotting Time

The activated clotting time (ACT) test measures the integrity of the intrinsic coagulation system. In this test 2 mL of the patient's blood is mixed in a tube containing either celite or kaolin (when aprotinin is used). Both celite and kaolin are negatively charged surfaces that serve to activate factor XII and the intrinsic pathway. The time in seconds for blood to clot in the presence of these negatively charged surfaces is recorded as the ACT. The ACT is commonly employed to measure the degree of anticoagulation by heparin in patients who are anti-coagulated for cardiac and vascular surgery. A normal ACT is 110–130 seconds.

Thrombin Time and Reptilase Time

The thrombin time (TT) and reptilase time (RT) tests measure the time required for fibrinogen to be converted to fibrin. Either thrombin (TT) or reptilase (RT) is added to the patient's plasma and the time for clot formation is measured. A normal thrombin time ranges from 9 to 35 seconds and is dependent upon the concentration of thrombin used by each laboratory. Reptilase is a proteolytic enzyme from snake venom that has a similar action to thrombin but with a different chemical affinity. In the presence of heparin, the thrombin time may be prolonged but the reptilase test will be normal. If the reptilase time is prolonged and the thrombin time normal, then there is probably a dysfibrinogenemia. If both tests are elevated, the patient may have afibrinogenemia.

Fibrinogen

The level of serum fibrinogen can be measured by mixing the patient's plasma with a dilute concentration of thrombin and measuring either the time to clot formation (Clauss assay) or the change in turbidity (Ellis assay). The time to clot formation or change in turbidity is then compared to a standard curve obtained by mixing equal amounts of thrombin with control plasmas of known fibrinogen content. A normal fibrinogen level is 140–410 mg/dL. Fibrinogen, however, is an acute-phase reactant and can be elevated by inflammatory states and post-operatively. It may be decreased in disease states such as disseminated intravascular coagulation (DIC) or liver disease, or with congenital deficiencies.

Fibrin Degradation Products and D-Dimer

The fibrin degradation products (FDP) assay not only measures products of plasmin's action on fibrin, but also reacts with fibrinogen degradation products and fibrinogen itself. Therefore the FDP assay is performed on a sample that has been stored in a tube containing both thrombin (to clot plasma fibrinogen) and soybean tryptase inhibitor (to inhibit *in vitro* fibrinolysis.) The D-dimer is a specific product that results from plasmin degradation of factor-XIII-linked fibrin. Both of these measurements are made using antibody-coated latex beads, mixing serial dilutions of the plasma and comparing the presence of agglutination with samples of known amounts of FDP or D-dimer. A normal serum D-dimer level is less than 500 ng/mL. Elevated levels of FDP and D-dimer suggest increased fibrinolysis.

Bleeding Time

The bleeding time is used to assess platelet function. It is measured by recording the time for a cut of a defined depth and length on the volar aspect of the forearm to stop bleeding, after first inflating a tourniquet on the upper arm to 40 mmHg. A normal bleeding time is 2–9 minutes. While originally thought to be a measure solely of platelet function, the bleeding time has also been shown to be dependent upon many other factors, including deficiencies of factors V, VI, X, XI, and XII. It can also be affected by anemia, hypothyroidism, and Ehlers–Danlos syndrome, as well as anemia and recent drug ingestion (i.e., aspirin). Bleeding times of up to twice normal are not typically associated with an increased risk of bleeding.

In addition to these tests of the integrity or the cascade, there are also assays available for specific clotting factors, which can be useful in sorting out abnormalities not explained by the PT, PTT, or TT.

AVAILABLE BLOOD PRODUCTS

Packed Red Blood Cells

Packed red blood cells (PRBCs) are produced by centrifuging whole blood and removing the plasma. The red cells are suspended in a preservative solution that dilutes the final concentration of red cells to a hematocrit of about 60%. In addition to red cells and preservative solution, PRBC preparations contain most of the leukocyte and platelet debris present in whole blood. There are two primary methods of storage used to extend the useful life of the collected red cells. The first involves suspending them in a preservative solution, while the second is to freeze the cells, thawing them when needed.

Two of the more commonly used preservatives used in the United States are CDPA-1 and Adsol. CDPA-1 consists of citrate, dextrose, phosphate, and adenine. The citrate functions as an anticoagulant by binding free calcium. Dextrose serves as the energy source for the cells. Adenine is used to maintain the stored cells' adenine nucleotide pool which is essential for the generation of adenosine triphosphate (ATP). Finally, phosphate acts both as a buffer and a source of phosphate for ATP. CDPA-1-stored PRBCs may be stored for 35 days without significant decline in their function. Adsol-prepared red cells are collected into a bag containing citrate, dextrose, and phosphate. After separation into plasma and red cells, a nutrient mixture containing dextrose, mannitol adenine, and saline is added. This solution extends the life of the collected red cells to 42 days.

Frozen PRBCs are prepared by mixing packed cells with 40% glycerol and then freezing slowly to a temperature of −65 to −80° C. The glycerol prevents ice crystal formation and the osmotic effects that occur during the freezing process. When the cells are ready to be transfused, they are thawed at 37° C and then washed with progressively less concentrated solutions of saline to remove the glycerol. The washed cells are then resuspended in isotonic saline. Cells can be stored in this manner for up to 10 years; however, once thawed, they must be used within 24 hours. When transfused these cells have the same viability as traditionally stored red cells and have no functioning platelets, leukocytes, or plasma proteins.

Leukocyte-depleted PRBCs are red cells that have had the vast majority of their white cells removed. The presence of leukocytes in red-cell preparations is associated with febrile transfusion reactions, human leukocyte antigen (HLA) alloimmunization, and cytomegalovirus (CMV) transmission. The most common technique to leukodeplete PRBCs is to pass them through a leukocyte adsorption or third-generation filter. These filters decrease the leukocyte levels of the PRBCs to less than 5×10^6. The filters may be used at the bedside or by the blood bank prior to releasing the cells. Another method used to remove leukocytes from red cell preparations is to wash the cells in saline and then resuspend them in an electrolyte solution. Disadvantages of washed red cells include the fact that the method is not as effective at removing leukocytes as the leukodepletion filters and that the PRBCs must be used within 24 hours.

Fresh Frozen Plasma

The supernatant removed after the initial centrifugation of a unit of whole blood is a mixture of platelets and plasma. This supernatant is centrifuged again at a higher speed, resulting in precipitation of the platelets, with the plasma fraction remaining in solution. The plasma fraction thus formed is frozen at −18° C, forming one unit of fresh frozen plasma (FFP). One unit of whole blood will yield about 200-280 mL of FFP, which can be stored in frozen form for up to 1 year. When ready for use, it is thawed over 20-30 minutes. Once thawed, it must be used within 24 hours or it will lose the activity of the labile clotting factors V and VIII. Each unit of FFP contains 0.7-1 unit/mL activity of each of the clotting factors normally present in the circulation, 1-2 mg/mL of fibrinogen, and other plasma proteins.

A new formulation of FFP is solvent–detergent-treated (s/d) plasma. This is prepared from approximately 2,500 units of pooled plasma. The pooled plasma is first sterilely ultrafiltered to remove leukocytes, bacteria, and parasites. Once filtered, it is treated with a detergent that kills all enveloped viruses by dissolving their lipid envelopes. Viruses killed include human immunodeficiency virus (HIV), hepatitis C virus (HCV), hepatitis B virus (HBV), and CMV. The final product is then screened for the presence of unencapsulated viruses such as hepatitis A and parvovirus B19. This product has shown to be effective in treating coagulation abnormalities from DIC, cardiac surgery, and congenital deficiencies of factors VII, X, and XI. It offers the distinct advantage of posing less risk of infection from encapsulated viruses. The concern is that, since it is derived from a large pool, there may be a greater threat from as yet undetectable viruses or prions.

Platelets

Platelets are obtained either by the centrifugation of plasma or via plasmapheresis. Random donor platelets are generated by removing the platelet-rich supernatant from the centrifuged plasma (as described above for FFP). This centrifugation process yields approximately 5.5×10^5 platelets in 30-50 mL of plasma, or a single unit of random donor platelets. These single donor units are then pooled with up to 10 units of other random donor platelets to provide platelets for transfusion (i.e., platelets from 5 donor units are combined to form a "5-pack" of random donor platelets for transfusion).

Single-donor platelets are obtained by plasmapheresis of a single donor's blood. During this procedure the donor's blood is removed and passed through an apheresis machine, in which the blood is separated into red cells, plasma, and platelets. The red cells and the majority of the plasma are then returned to the patient, while the platelets are concentrated and stored in 200-250 mL of plasma. Platelet preparations collected in this manner yield about 3×10^{11} platelets, roughly equal to 6-8 units of random donor platelets.

In order to prevent platelet aggregation after collection, platelets must be continually gently agitated. If the unit is not transfused within 30 minutes, it should be returned to the blood bank so that this agitation can be continued. Platelets are stored at room temperature and can be kept for up to 5 days.

Cryoprecipitate

A white precipitate forms when FFP is thawed to about 5–6° C. Cryoprecipitate is formed by removing this precipitate by centrifugation and then immediately refreezing it at −18° C. The plasma that remains after cryoprecipitate has been removed (cryo-poor plasma) is either discarded or used for factor concentrates. Ordinarily, six to 12 bags of cryoprecipitate are pooled to form a dose of cryoprecipitate. Once unfrozen, the cryoprecipitate must be used within 6 hours. Cryoprecipitate is high in factor VIII (at least 80 IU/mL) and contains 30% of the fibrinogen found in FFP. It also contains von Willebrand factor and factor XIII.

TYPE, SCREEN, AND CROSSMATCH

There are three steps used to decrease the risk of transfusion reaction between the donor and recipient. First, the patient's and donor's blood grouping are determined (both the ABO and Rh status) in a process called the "type." Next, the patient's serum is screened for the presence of commonly encountered anti-erythrocyte antibodies, in a process called the "screen." Finally, the patient's serum is mixed with the intended donor cells *in vitro*, a process called the "crossmatch."

Blood Type

A patient's blood type is determined by both forward (tests the cells for antigen) and reverse (tests the serum for antibody) reactions. In the forward reaction a patient's red cells are combined with sera containing anti-A, and then anti-B, antibodies. Agglutination after mixing with either of the antisera identifies the patient's blood as being of the type of the antisera. For example, if a patient's blood agglutinates with type A antibodies, then the patient's blood is type A, and it is type B if it reacts with anti-B antisera. Blood that reacts with both antisera is type AB, while blood that does not agglutinate with either antiserum is type O.

The reverse reaction involves mixing the serum of the patient with red cells of known type A and B. Agglutination of the cells by the patient's serum indicates the presence of antibodies against the cell type of that particular reaction. For example, if the patient's serum causes agglutination of cells known as type B, but not those of known type A, then the patient's serum contains anti-B antibodies.

Finally, the patient's Rh (or D) status is determined by mixing the patient's red cells with commercially prepared anti-D serum. If this mixture agglutinates, the patient is said to possess the Rh antigen or be Rh-positive. A nonreactive mix indicates Rh-negative status.

The transfusion of blood that is only matched for ABO type and Rh status has a 1 in 1,000 chance of causing an incompatibility reaction. The rare reaction is due to the presence of preformed antibody in the patient's serum. The incidence of this type of reaction is reduced by performing an antibody screen.

The Antibody Screen

The antibody screen tests the patient's serum for the presence of antibodies against common red cell antigens. These antibodies may be naturally occurring or present secondary to prior transfusions or pregnancies. The naturally occurring circulating antibodies are IgM and are able to fix complement. The fixing of complement by these antibodies results in the immediate hemolysis of the transfused cells. Antibodies that are present secondary to prior transfusions or pregnancy are typically IgG and rarely result in immediate hemolysis, but they can cause a significant decrease in survival of the transfused blood. The most commonly used tests to detect these antibodies are the direct and indirect agglutination (Coombs) test.

The direct Coombs test tests the patient's *red cells* for the presence of bound IgG or complement. To perform a direct Coombs test, the patient's red cells are separated from the plasma and then washed and suspended in saline. Antihuman IgG and/or anti-C3 are added to this solution. If the red cells have IgG or complement bound to them, the addition of these anti IgG and anti C3 antibodies will cause the cells to agglutinate. With a positive direct Coombs test, monoclonal IgG is then used to determine which of the antibodies is responsible for the positive test. A direct Coombs test is often used in cases of hemolytic anemia to discover the offending antibody–antigen system.

The indirect Coombs tests the patient's *serum* for the presence of antibodies. The patient's serum is first mixed with normal erythrocytes. The cells are then washed and incubated with the anti-IgG and/or anti-C3 antibodies. If agglutination of these cells occurs, it indicates that the patient's serum contains free anti-erythrocyte antibodies.

Currently, the antibody screen used in a type and screen is an indirect Coombs test using the recipient's serum with a set of standard type O cells with 18 clinically relevant antigens on their surface: D, C, E, c, e, M, N, S, s, P_1, Le^a, Le^b, K, k, Fy^a, Fy^b, Jk^a, and Jk^b. A positive screen indicates the presence of an antibody directed against one of these antigens in the recipient's serum. To identify which antibody is responsible for a positive indirect Coombs test, the patient's serum is reacted with a series of red cells with known antigenic composition to determine which antibody is present. A negative type and screen increases the chance of a compatible transfusion to 99.94%.

The Crossmatch

Once a patient's blood has a negative antibody screen, the blood bank prepares and puts aside blood of that patient's group for the patient should (s)he require transfusion later. If the patient later requires a transfusion, a crossmatch is performed. In the crossmatch, the patient's serum is mixed with potential donor red cells suspended in saline. The mixture is then evaluated for the presence of agglutination. This final test rechecks for incompatibility due to isohemagglutinins in the patient's serum. If the patient's serum was found on the screen to contain atypical antibodies, then donor cells lacking that antigen must be selected and an indirect Coombs test performed on each unit to be transfused. The chance of a compatible transfusion is increased to 99.95% when a full type and crossmatch is performed.

Emergency Transfusion

In emergency situations blood may be needed before the type, type and screen, or type and crossmatch have been completed. In true emergencies type O Rh-negative packed red cells are the blood product of choice. Serum of some O negative donors may contain high titers of hemolytic IgG and IgM anti-A and anti-B antibodies which can be transfused into the recipient when whole blood (as opposed to PRBC) is used. Thus, when type O negative whole blood is used, one should avoid switching to the patient's blood type after two units are transfused, as the transfused titers of anti-A and anti-B antibodies now present in the patient's serum may cause hemolysis of the subsequently transfused cells. Modern units of O negative PRBC contain so little plasma that their use does not typically preclude subsequently switching to typed and crossmatched blood when it becomes available.

If time permits ABO type and Rh status to be established, the transfusion of ABO- and Rh-compatible blood is preferred to the use of O negative blood. For those who have never had a prior transfusion the chance for a serious transfusion reaction using ABO/Rh compatible blood is very small, approximately 1 in 1,000. However, in those with a history of prior transfusion the risks may be an order of magnitude higher, as 1 in 100 of these patients may have an antibody that is detected on the crossmatch.

TRANSFUSION INDICATIONS

Red Blood Cells

The indications for the transfusion of red cells have undergone significant changes over the past 20 years. In the early 1980s the commonly held belief was that patients did better with hemoglobin concentration of at least 10 mg/dL or a hematocrit of greater than 30%. This was called the "10/30 rule." However, with the outbreak of the HIV epidemic in the mid-1980s, and the observation that many patients did well with hemoglobin below this level, this practice was called into question. The debate as to when to transfuse has generated the term "transfusion trigger," referring to the lowest acceptable hemoglobin one accepts before transfusing. Studies trying to identify this elusive trigger have involved both studies evaluating the lowest safe hemoglobin as well as studies evaluating outcomes based upon hemoglobin levels.

Studies have employed acute isovolemic hemodilution techniques both to evaluate the physiologic responses of anemia and to attempt to define the lowest safe hemoglobin. Studies in dogs have looked at the effects of induced anemia on both healthy animals and those with artificially induced coronary stenosis. These studies suggest that, as the hematocrit is decreased, animals are able to compensate for anemia by increasing both cardiac output and the oxygen extraction ratio (ER). However, as the ER increases to more than 50%, the animals show a progressive rise in serum lactic acid, metabolic acidosis, and the concomitant onset of hemodynamic instability and heart failure. In dogs without stenosis, this change occurred at a hematocrit of 8.6%, while in those with a critical stenosis it occurred at a hematocrit of 17%, suggesting that the ability to tolerate anemia is related to underlying cardiac health.

A recent study by Weiskopf et al. studied the effects of induced isovolemic anemia on 32 awake healthy human volunteers and surgical patients. Participants in this study showed no signs of cardiac decompensation and/or organ ischemia as their hemoglobin was reduced from baseline levels to 5 g/dL. Participants were able to compensate for the anemia with a variety of cardiovascular adaptations. There was a fall in systemic vascular resistance, with an increased cardiac output, mediated both via increases in heart rate and stroke volume. Oxygen consumption actually increased slightly with no change in serum lactate levels. This was probably mediated by increased tissue oxygen extraction as mixed venous oxygen fell from baseline levels. Two patients did show electrocardiographic changes. One of these changes was felt to be secondary to change in patient position (the patient needed to urinate), while the other patient's changes were felt to be secondary to a transient tachycardia, which responded to esmolol. Neither of these patients demonstrated any long-term electrocardiographic (ECG) changes or cardiac dysfunction.

These studies suggest that both humans and animals are able to tolerate quite low hemoglobin levels without significant hemodynamic derangements. However, in those with fixed coronary lesions this tolerance appears to be reduced. These studies were not performed in patients who had the added stress of a surgical trespass and/or the cardiac depressant effects of anesthetic agents, imposed upon them. So the question then becomes how low may we safely let the hemoglobin fall before transfusion becomes necessary during surgery and in the perioperative period, with the added physiologic stresses that this period brings.

Perhaps the most interesting data on low hemoglobin levels and morbidity in the perioperative period come from a study by Carson et al. In this study, the investigators retrospectively evaluated the postoperative mortality and morbidity of surgical patients who refused transfusion because of their religious beliefs. This study looked at 300 patients with postoperative hemoglobin levels of less than 8 g/dL. They found that, in the group of patients whose hemoglobin fell to between 7.1 and 8.0 g/dL there were no deaths but there was a morbidity rate of about 9%. In contrast, those whose hemoglobin fell to between 4.1 and 5.0 g/dL had a mortality rate of 34.4%, while 57.7% had either a morbid event or died. Controlling for age, APACHE II score and the presence of cardiac disease, a regression analysis performed suggested a 2.5-fold increased risk of death for each 1 g/dL of decrease in hemoglobin level below 8 g/dL.

Two other interesting studies have investigated the relationship between hematocrit and ischemia in surgical patients at risk for coronary disease. Nelson et al. evaluated 27 high-risk patients undergoing peripheral vascular procedures. The patients were divided into two groups based upon mean postoperative hematocrit (recorded as the mean of hematocrit values recorded for the first postoperative day) – those whose hematocrit was greater than 28% and those with hematocrits below 28%. The results showed a significantly higher risk for both ischemia (77% versus 14%), and cardiac events (46% versus 0%) in those whose hematocrit fell below 28%. Hogue et al. studied a group of men undergoing retropubic radical prostatectomy and found that intraoperative tachycardia, the presence of cardiac risk factors, and an immediate postoperative hematocrit less than 28% were predictive of ischemic cardiac events. Additionally, it was found that postoperative tachycardic episodes and a hematocrit level less than 28% were independently associated with an increased risk of ischemia.

In addition to data in the perioperative patient, there are also studies evaluating the transfusion thresholds in critically ill intensive care unit (ICU) patients, who arguably share some common physiology with the perioperative patient. Perhaps the best data from the ICU populations come from a series of three studies from Canada. The first of these trials was a combined retrospective/prospective cohort study of 4,470 patients admitted to the ICU. This study compared the transfusion practice of those who survived and those who died in the ICU. The results of this study suggested that those who died had lower hemoglobins and were transfused more often. When they compared those with a diagnosis of cardiac disease to those with no cardiac disease, they found a trend towards increased mortality for those with hemoglobin of less than 9.5 g/dL (55% versus 42%; $p = 0.09$). They also found that, in the subgroup of patients with cardiac disease and anemia, increasing the hemoglobin levels was associated with an increase in survival (odds ratio = 0.80 for each 1 g/dL increase in hemoglobin).

The second study from this group was a randomized controlled clinical trial called the Transfusion in Critical Care (TRICC) trial. This study consisted of 838 euvolemic patients admitted to the ICU with hemoglobin levels below 9 mg/dL who were randomly assigned to one of two transfusion strategies. The first group was a restrictive transfusion group in which transfusions were performed only when a patient's hemoglobin fell below 7 g/dL; it was then maintained at between 7 and 9 g/dL. The second group was a liberal transfusion group in which transfusions were performed when a patient's hemoglobin fell below 10 g/dL; it was then maintained at between 10 and 12 g/dL. The study compared overall 30-day mortality between these two groups and divided the results further by age, APACHE score, and the presence of cardiac disease. The major finding was that the overall mortality rate was similar between the two transfusion strategies (18.7% versus 23.3%, $p = 0.11$). Further analysis revealed that the restrictive group actually had an improved outcome in those who were younger (<55 years old; 5.7% versus 13.0%, $p = 0.02$) and less ill (APACHE score less than 20; 9.7% versus 16.1%, $p = 0.03$). In patients with significant cardiac disease, the trend was for mortality to be worse with the restrictive practice, although it did not reach clinical significance (20.5% versus 22.2%, $p = 0.69$).

To further evaluate the issue of a restrictive transfusion policy in those with cardiac disease, the same group reanalyzed the above data using only the subgroup of patients with cardiac or vascular disease as one of their top two admitting diagnoses, as well as those with a known history of acute or chronic coronary artery disease. When the mortality rates of this subgroup of patients were compared based upon transfusion practice, no significant differences were found. The study group was then further divided to evaluate only those patients with ischemic heart disease as a diagnosis. When this group was looked at separately, a decrease in survival in those in the restrictive group was found, although it did not reach statistical significance.

Several criticisms have been directed towards the latter two studies. Chief among them is that only a small number of patients selected actually enrolled in the study (43%), perhaps because of physicians refusing to admit those with significant coronary disease based upon the results of the first study. In fact, there was a higher incidence of patients with coronary disease who did not enroll than of those who did. Even in the study that looked at patients with cardiovascular disease, only 23% of each group had ischemic heart disease as one of their primary diagnoses. Even so, these are the first large-scale, prospective trials to investigate the effect of transfusion practice on outcome. Additionally, the results do suggest that a conservative transfusion threshold is likely to be safe for those without significant coronary disease, especially in young and less sick patients.

What then is the final consensus? Unfortunately there is no clear-cut number one can use to guide transfusion practice in all patients. In 1996, the American Society of Anesthesiologists (ASA) established practice guidelines for transfusion based upon a review of the then current data. These guidelines are summarized in Box 9-1. When one looks at these recommendations, one must keep in mind that, in the operating room in the face of continuing or anticipated further blood losses, and/or in the face of already compromised tissue perfusion, waiting for a patient's hemoglobin to fall to any set level may later result in significant anemia, ischemia, and/or acidosis. It seems prudent to rely not only on hemoglobin level and vital signs, but upon all available data, with particular attention to pH, lactate, and mixed venous oxygenation, as well as anticipated further losses, to determine when the patient is likely to benefit from transfusion.

The transfusion of 1 unit of packed red cells should raise the hemoglobin concentration by 1 g/dL and the hematocrit by 3%.

Fresh Frozen Plasma

Indications for FFP transfusion are situations in which normal levels of coagulation proteins in the serum either have been diluted or depleted or are inherently low. Dilution of clotting factors may occur in the setting of

---

Box 9-1   American Society of Anesthesiologists Task Force Recommendations For Red Cell Transfusion

1. Transfusion is rarely indicated when the hemoglobin concentration is greater than 10 mg/dL and is almost always indicated when it is less than 6 mg/dL, especially when the anemia is acute.
2. The determination of whether intermediate hemoglobin concentration (6–10 mg/dL) justify or require transfusion should be based upon the patient's risk for complications of inadequate oxygenation.
3. The use of a single transfusion trigger for all patients and other approaches that fail to consider all physiologic and surgical factors affecting oxygenation is not recommended.
4. When appropriate, preoperative autologous blood donation, intraoperative and operative blood recovery, acute normovolemic hemodilution and measures to decrease blood loss may be beneficial.
5. The indications for transfusion of autologous red blood cells may be more liberal than for allogenic units because of the lower (but still significant) risks associated with the former.

---

massive blood loss, where plasma-poor fluids (crystalloids, colloids, and/or PRBCs) are used to replace lost blood. Depletion of clotting factors occurs when there is an abnormally high consumption of coagulation factors, as occurs in extensive clinical bleeding and DIC. Inherently low levels of clotting proteins can be found in patients with liver disease or inherited factor deficiencies.

The question becomes: at what point do the clotting factors become so diluted or depleted as to cause a clinically significant coagulopathy that is treatable by the transfusion of FFP? Common tests of the integrity of the coagulation cascade, including the PT, PTT, fibrinogen and platelet count, are useful in determining when such a deficiency is present and can be used as guides to transfusion. If DIC is suspected it is also helpful to obtain D-dimer and factor VIII levels. A summary of laboratory abnormalities suggestive of coagulopathy proposed by Drummond and Petrovich is presented in Table 9-2. Unfortunately, however, these laboratory tests typically are not always available in a timely manner to the anesthesiologist in the operating room.

As these lab results are not always readily available, anesthesiologists have investigated the usefulness of prophylactic FFP transfusions in preventing coagulopathy. There have been several studies that have shown routine

Table 9-2   Laboratory Values Suggestive of Coagulopathy

Laboratory Test (Normal Range)	Value Predictive of Coagulopathy
PT (10–13 sec)	>18 sec
PTT (28–38 sec)	>55 sec
Fibrinogen (140–410 mg/dL)	<100 mg/dL
Platelet count (140,000–440,000/mm³)	<50,000/mm³

Adapted from Drummond JC, Petrovich CT. The massively bleeding patient. *Anesthesiol Clin North Am* 2001.

Box 9-2   American Society of Anesthesiologists Task Force Recommendations for Fresh Frozen Plasma Transfusion

1. Fresh frozen plasma (FFP) is indicated for the urgent reversal of warfarin therapy.
2. FFP is indicated for correction of known coagulation factor deficiencies for which specific factor concentrates are not available.
3. FFP is indicated for correction of microvascular bleeding in the presence of elevated (>1.5 times normal) prothrombin time (PT) or partial thromboplastin time (PTT).
4. FFP is indicated for correction of microvascular bleeding secondary to coagulation factor deficiency in patients transfused with more than one blood volume and when the PT and PTT cannot be obtained in a timely fashion.
5. FFP should be given in doses calculated to achieve a minimum of 30% of plasma factor concentration (usually achieved with administration of 10–15 mL/kg of FFP), except for urgent reversal of warfarin therapy, for which 5–8 mL/kg of FFP will suffice.
6. FFP is contraindicated for the expansion of plasma volume or albumin concentration.

administration of FFP to be ineffective in preventing coagulation abnormalities in patients receiving more than 10 units of PRBCs over 24 hours. Studies investigating the relationship of factor VIII levels to the degree of blood loss have shown weak, if any, correlations. Reed *et al.* investigated the effectiveness of prophylactic transfusion of FFP (2 units/12 units of PRBC), or platelets (12 pack/12 units PRBC), in the prevention of coagulopathy and found no difference in the development of coagulopathy between those transfused prophylactically and those who were not.

Hiippala *et al.* studied the rate of depletion of clotting factors and platelets that occurred in bleeding patients who were kept euvolemic in their resuscitation by the use of PRBCs and colloid. Defining the critical levels as a prothrombin (factor II) or factor VIII level of less than 20% of normal, a factor V level of less than 25% normal, and a fibrinogen of less than 100 mg/dL, the investigators used mathematical modeling to determine at what percentage of blood volume lost these values would be reached. They found that the levels of prothrombin, factor V, and factor VIII would reach critically low levels after 201%, 229%, and 236% of blood volume was lost, respectively; while fibrinogen would reach critically low levels after 129% of blood was lost. This model assumes that the depletion of coagulation factors results only from simple dilution.

In addition to simple dilution of factors, PRBC transfusions, hypothermia, acidosis, excess coagulation protein consumption, and dilutional thrombocytopenia may complicate the assessment of the bleeding patient. Hypothermia decreases the rate of all enzymatic reactions in the body such as coagulation, while end-organ ischemia and acidosis can cause the release of tissue factor and tPA. These in turn can stimulate the coagulation cascade by activating factor VII (via tissue factor) and fibrinolysis (by tPA), increasing the consumption of both clotting factors and platelets. If these events occur, the theoretical calculations of Hiippala are invalid, and trans-

fusion of FFP and platelets may be required when less overall blood loss has occurred.

Thus, determining when the transfusion of FFP is required or indicated is not a simple matter. The ASA position statement guidelines are presented in Box 9-2. In general, it is most effective to transfuse FFP when abnormal laboratory studies indicate insufficient quantities of clotting factors or an inadequacy in clotting. Petrovich and Drummond suggest that coagulation studies be obtained and repeated as each one-half of blood volume is lost so that further treatment may be anticipated. If these laboratory values are not readily available, and there is clinical bleeding after transfusion of large volumes of packed cells, FFP transfusion is likely warranted under the assumption that clotting factor deficits exist.

Each unit of FFP contains 0.7–1 unit/mL activity of each of the clotting factors normally present in the circulation, 1–2 mg/mL of fibrinogen, as well as complement and other plasma proteins. Since each unit of FFP represents about 9% of normal plasma volume, each unit of FFP should raise the serum clotting factors by approximately 9–10%. Normal coagulation requires that approximately 20–30% of normal clotting factor levels are present in the plasma. Hence the transfusion of two units of FFP should be adequate to return coagulation to normal in cases of simple factor deficiency such as occurs with warfarin therapy.

Large quantities of FFP may be required in more complex clinical scenarios. In addition to the restoration of depleted clotting factors, FFP is indicated to acutely correct clotting abnormalities due to warfarin therapy, treat angioedema in those with inherited C1-esterase deficiency, and induce remissions in those with thrombotic thrombocytopenic purpura (TTP), hemolytic uremic syndrome (HUS), and the syndrome of hemolysis, elevated liver enzymes, and low platelets (HELLP).

Compatibility with plasma (FFP) is inverse to that for red cells. The universal donor is type AB, Rh-positive. These donors have no anti-A, anti-B, or anti-Rh antibodies in their plasma to react with recipient red cell antigens. The universal recipient is type O, Rh-negative. These patients have no antigen on their red cells against which the plasma antibodies can react. A variety of reactions to FFP transfusion have been described in the literature, of which transfusion-associated lung injury (TRALI) is the most important. Finally, the likelihood of citrate toxicity is greater with FFP than with other products.

Cryoprecipitate

Cryoprecipitate contains high concentrations of factors VIII and XIII, von Willebrand factor, fibrinogen, and fibronectin. The ASA position statement guidelines for the use of cryoprecipitate are presented in Box 9-3. Its principle use is in the treatment of those with fibrinogen or factor XIII deficiencies, though it can also be used to treat patients with von Willebrand's disease and hemophilia A. Fibrinogen deficiency may be due to consumption, congenital (rare) deficiencies, or disease states such as severe liver disease. Regardless of the cause, as fibrinogen levels fall below 100 mg/dL there is a prolonga-

tion of both the PT and PTT, with the potential for coagulopathy.

Patients with von Willebrand's disease have low levels of active von Willebrand factor, which is required for platelet binding to the vascular endothelium. The treatment of choice for von Willebrand's disease is 1-desamino-8-d-arginine vasopressin (DDAVP or desmopressin), which increases expression of von Willebrand factor; however, cryoprecipitate is sometimes used because it contains both factor VIII:C (the procoagulant activity) and factor VIII:von Willebrand factor (the von Willebrand factor). Recombinant factor VIII is the treatment of choice for hemophilia A; the use of cryoprecipitate is reserved for settings in which factor VIII is unavailable.

Plasma fibrinogen levels of greater than 100 mg/dL are adequate for hemostasis in almost all situations. The dose of cryoprecipitate required to achieve this level is difficult to determine accurately because the concentration of fibrinogen in a unit varies depending on the pooling methods used as well as on the storage volume.

Even though the concentration of ABO antibodies in cryoprecipitate is extremely low, ABO-compatible units should be used. Since cryoprecipitate may contain red cell fragments, it has the potential to sensitize Rh-negative patients. Thus Rh-compatible cryoprecipitate should be used in young women. The reactions to transfusion of cryoprecipitate are similar to those seen for FFP.

Platelets

As with clotting factors, platelets in a bleeding patient become diluted and consumed as volume losses are replaced with platelet-poor products and bleeding continues. So, as with FFP, the question becomes: at what point does the dilution and consumption of platelets manifest as clinically significant bleeding treatable by transfusing platelets?

The simulation performed by Hiippala et al. estimates that platelets will not fall below 50,000/mL until a patient experiences a 230% blood loss. Again, this is based upon the assumption that blood loss is adequately replaced and that acidosis, shock, and hypothermia are minimal or not present. If these criteria are not met, platelet counts may fall at a much faster rate because of increased consumption. Additionally, a variety of conditions may impair platelet functioning, allowing for the evolution of a coagulopathy at seemingly normal platelet counts. These conditions include uremia, sepsis, and treatment with a variety of medications, most notably the nonsteroidal anti-inflammatories.

The ASA guidelines for platelet transfusion are summarized in Box 9-4. Ultimately it is the constellation of the patient's underlying disease process, the surgical procedure, the extent of blood loss, the presence/absence of

---

Box 9-3 American Society of Anesthesiologists Task Force Recommendations for Cryoprecipitate Transfusion

1. Cryoprecipitate is indicated for prophylaxis in non-bleeding perioperative or peripartum patients with congenital fibrinogen deficiencies or von Willebrand's disease not responsive to DDAVP.
2. Cryoprecipitate is indicated for bleeding patients with von Willebrand's disease.
3. Cryoprecipitate is indicated for correction of microvascular bleeding in massively bleeding patients with fibrinogen concentrations of less than 80–100 mg/dL (or when fibrinogen levels cannot be measured in a timely fashion).

Box 9-4   American Society of Anesthesiologists Task Force Recommendations for Platelet Transfusion

1. Prophylactic platelet transfusion is ineffective and rarely indicated when thrombocytopenia is due to increased platelet destruction.
2. Prophylactic platelet transfusion is rarely indicated with thrombocytopenia due to decreased platelet production when the platelet count is greater than $100 \times 10^9/L$ and is usually indicated when the count is less than $50 \times 10^9/L$. The determination of whether patients with intermediate platelet counts ($50-100 \times 10^9/L$) require therapy should be based upon the risk of bleeding.
3. Surgical and obstetric patients with microvascular bleeding usually require platelet transfusion if the platelet count is below $50 \times 10^9/L$ and rarely require therapy if is greater than $100 \times 10^9/L$. With intermediate platelet counts ($50-100 \times 10^9/L$), the determination should be based upon the patient's risk for more significant bleeding.
4. Vaginal deliveries or operative procedures ordinarily associated with insignificant blood loss may be undertaken in patients with platelet counts of less $50 \times 10^9/L$.
5. Platelet transfusion may be indicated despite an apparently adequate platelet count if there is known platelet dysfunction and microvascular bleeding.

---

acidosis, hypothermia, and the potential for DIC and/or platelet dysfunction that must ultimately guide the decision to transfuse platelets.

The dose of platelets required to increase platelet count is dependent upon a host of factors including the presence of active bleeding and the degree of splenic sequestration, fever, and sepsis. In general, a rough estimate of the increase expected can be made by assuming that one unit of platelets transfused into a 70 kg male will increase the platelet count by approximately 5,000–10,000/mL 1 hour after the transfusion and by more than 4,500 /mL 18–24 hours later (see Box 9-4).

While efforts should be made to use ABO-compatible platelets whenever possible, it is not absolutely necessary. Random donor platelets are typically prepared in "packs" of 5–10 units and thus may contain a fair number of anti-A or anti-B isoagglutinins. This can be a cause for acute hemolysis, particularly in those who receive a large number of platelet transfusions.

There is a higher incidence of transfusion reactions seen with platelets than with red cells. Acute symptoms develop in about 2% of all transfused. These reactions include rash, urticaria, fever, chills, wheezing, and hypotension. These reactions were initially thought to result from either antileukocyte antibody or IgE-mediated reactions to plasma proteins. However, recent work has suggested that transfused cytokines may be the cause of some of these reactions. It is felt that these cytokines are either released by leukocytes in the stored platelets as they become damaged over time or result from the activation of stored monocytes.

COMPLICATIONS OF TRANSFUSION

The risks of transfusion are summarized in Table 9-3. Complications of transfusion can be grossly divided into immunologic and nonimmunologic reactions. Immunologic reactions consist of both the recipient's response to the transfused cells (transfusion reactions) and the

---

Table 9-3   Risks of Transfusion

	Estimated Per Million Units	Frequency Per Actual Unit	No. of Deaths per Million Units
Viral Infections			
Hepatitis A	1	1/1,000,000	0
Hepatitis B	7–32	1/30,000–1/250,000	0–0.14
Hepatitis C	4–36	1/30,000–1/150,000	0.5–17
HIV	0.4–5	1/200,000–1/2,000,000	0.5–5
HTLV types I and II	0.5–4	1/250,000–1/2,000,000	0
Parvovirus B19	100	1/10,000	0
Bacterial Contamination			
Red cells	2	1/500,000	0.1–0.25
Platelets	83	1/12,000	21
Immune Reactions			
Acute hemolytic reactions	1–4	1/250,000–1/1,000,000	0.67
Delayed hemolytic reactions	1,000	1/1,000	0.4
Transfusion-related acute lung injury	200	1/5,000	0.2

HIV, human immunodeficiency virus; HTLV, human T-cell lymphotrophic virus.
Adapted from Goodnough LT, Brecher ME, Kanter MH, AuBuchon JP. Transfusion medicine – blood transfusions. *N Engl J Med* 1999;340:438-447.

immunomodulation of the recipient that occurs as a result of the transfusion. The nonimmunologic reactions are further divided into infectious and metabolic complications.

Immune Reactions

Immune transfusion reactions are grossly divided by their time course (immediate versus delayed) and whether or not they cause hemolysis in the recipient. Immediate reactions occur either concomitantly with the transfusion or shortly thereafter (within several hours after the transfusion has completed). Delayed reactions occur within several hours and may not occur for several days to months. There are also febrile and allergic reactions.

Acute Intravascular Transfusion Reactions

Acute intravascular hemolytic transfusion reactions occur when incompatible red cells are transfused into someone with a pre-existing antibody to the incompatible cell. The symptoms of this type of reaction include fever, chills, chest pain, hypotension, dyspnea, and hemoglobinuria, most of which are masked in a patient with a general anesthetic. The mechanism of this reaction is the binding of preformed recipient antibodies to the foreign red cells, resulting in the activation of complement. The most likely cause of this type of reaction is the transfusion of ABO-incompatible blood, although transfusion of blood with any of the complement-fixing antibody–antigen systems can induce the reaction (i.e., Jk^a [Kidd] or Fy^a [Duffy] blood group system). Once complement is activated, C3a and C5a are released into the circulation, causing mast cell degranulation, bronchospasm, hemodynamic instability, $\dot{V}/\dot{Q}$ mismatch and subsequent pulmonary dysfunction, and in some cases DIC. The C5b-9 membrane attack complex of complement causes lysis of the transfused cells, with subsequent hemoglobinuria, hemoglobinemia, and a fall in hematocrit. The antigen–antibody complexes and free hemoglobin in the blood can precipitate renal failure. Finally, the hemolysis of red cells can release potentially large amounts of potassium into the patient's blood, with the potential for complications related to hyperkalemia, especially if renal function is compromised.

The therapy for an acute transfusion reaction is to immediately stop the transfusion, provide cardiopulmonary supportive care, and insure diuresis (goal is 100 mL urine/hour for 24 hours). This therapy is detailed in Box 9-5. At the same time, a repeat blood sample should

---

Box 9-5   Treatment of Acute Hemolytic Transfusion Reaction

1. **Stop the transfusion** – replace all tubing used for the offending transfusion up the hub of the intravenous catheter with a normal saline line.
2. Address the ABCs:
   a. Nonintubated patients may require intubation and mechanical ventilation.
   b. Already intubated patients may require increased ventilatory support (increased F_iO_2, positive end-expiratory pressure).
   c. Support blood pressure.
      i. Primary treatment is increasing plasma volume
      ii. If unresponsive to volume, dopamine is the pressor of choice, as it helps to preserve renal blood flow.
3. Maintain urine output at 75-100 mL/hr.
   a. Insure adequate intravascular volume with generous administration of normal saline (central venous pressure of 10-15 mmHg).
   b. Administer mannitol (12.5-50 g intravenously).
   c. If the above measures are not adequate, furosemide (20-40 mg intravenously) may be used.
4. Alkalinize urine to goal of a pH of 8.
   a. Start with 40-70 mEq/kg sodium bicarbonate intravenously.
   b. Repeat measures of urine pH and treat with additional bicarbonate as needed.
5. Send appropriate laboratory studies. (Ideally these should be sent as soon as transfusion reaction is suspected.)
   a. Send sample of patient's blood with remainder of unit precipitating reaction.
   b. Send baseline coagulation studies including prothrombin time, partial thromboplastin time, platelet count and fibrinogen level.
   c. Send blood and urine for free hemoglobin levels as well as serum haptoglobin.
   d. Send serum potassium.
6. If blood products are needed urgently to treat the symptoms of the reaction (anemia, disseminated intravascular coagulation), type O Rh-negative packed red cells and type AB Rh-positive plasma should be used until the type and screen can be repeated.

be drawn from the patient. The patient's sample, along with the remainder of the unit precipitating the reaction, should be sent back to the lab for a re-crossmatch and identification of the culpable antigen–antibody system. Laboratory findings that support the diagnosis of acute hemolytic transfusion reaction include hemoglobinuria, hemoglobinemia with a low haptoglobin, and a positive direct Coombs test.

Acute Extravascular Hemolytic Reactions

Acute extravascular hemolytic reactions differ from intravascular reactions in that complement is not fixed, or is only fixed to C3b. The presence of the IgG antibody on the red cell results not in intravascular lysis by complement but rather in the clearance of the cells by the reticuloendothelial system. These reactions are the result of either pre-existing alloantibody in the patient's serum that was missed on the antibody screen or clerical error. Patients who have this type of reaction are often clinically stable, demonstrating none of the hemodynamic, pulmonary, and renal manifestations of the acute intravascular reaction. Symptoms can include a low-grade fever, which develops in response to the cytokines generated by the activation of the immune system, and a less than expected rise in hematocrit after transfusion due to the clearance of the antibody-coated cells by the reticuloendothelial system.

The diagnosis is confirmed by a decrease in hematocrit as well as an increase in the byproducts of hemoglobin metabolism; these include an increase in indirect bilirubin, an increase in lactate dehydrogenase (LDH), and an increase in urinary excretion of urobilinogen.

Delayed Intravascular Hemolytic Reactions

Delayed intravascular hemolytic reactions share a common mechanism with the acute intravascular reactions but in this case the antibody–antigen reaction develops slowly over the course of 5–10 days. In this case, the patient has preformed antibodies from prior transfusion or pregnancy that are too low in concentration to be picked up by the type and screen process. As the recipient's immune system generates a higher titer against the transfused cells, the patient slowly develops the symptoms of intravascular hemolysis. This ramping up of the immune system may take up to 30 days. As the reaction occurs gradually, the symptoms are less dramatic than those seen with an acute intravascular hemolytic reaction. Hemoglobinemia and hemoglobinuria are often present, but they are less profound and less abrupt than with the acute reaction. Often all that is required to treat these reactions is a mild diuresis and careful monitoring of the patient and vital signs for any sign of deterioration.

Delayed Extravascular Hemolytic Transfusion Reactions

Delayed extravascular hemolytic transfusion reactions present in a manner similar to an acute extravascular hemolytic reaction. Patients present with a falling hematocrit, mild fever, an increase in indirect bilirubin, and an increase in serum LDH. In this case the antigen complex that is often involved is that of the Rh system. The diagnosis is confirmed by the presence of a new direct Coombs test.

Febrile Nonhemolytic Transfusion

Febrile nonhemolytic transfusion reactions are suspected when patients undergoing transfusion demonstrate an increase in body temperature of at least 1° C without signs of intra- or extravascular hemolysis. In addition to fever, patients often have accompanying shaking chills, headache, myalgia, chest pain, nausea, and a nonproductive cough that begins during or shortly after transfusion. These symptoms result from the actions of cytokines released by the recipient's immune system response to the foreign antigens on the donor's lymphocytes, platelets, and plasma proteins. The symptoms of fever and chills can also be seen with a hemolytic reaction and infection (or transfusion with infected blood products). These two types of reaction are easily distinguished in the lab, as a febrile reaction will not have a positive direct Coombs test since antibodies towards red cells are not involved. Patients at risk for developing this type of reaction are those who have received multiple transfusions in the past and multigravida women, 55% of whom have antileukocyte antibodies.

Treatment of a febrile nonhemolytic transfusion reaction consists of antipyretics, most commonly acetaminophen. If there is a component of shaking chills with the reaction, meperidine in small doses (25 mg intravenously) will often stop these chills immediately. Patients who have a history of febrile reactions with transfusions have a one in eight chance of having a similar reaction when additional blood products are transfused and are thus commonly premedicated with meperidine and acetaminophen prior to further transfusion. If the reactions are severe and/or not responsive to conservative pretreatment therapy, patients may benefit from a dose of corticosteroid (hydrocortisone 100 mg intravenously) prior to therapy. The increasing use of leukocyte-depleted red cells is likely to reduce the incidence of febrile transfusion reactions to red cells.

Allergic Reactions

Allergic transfusion reactions usually begin with skin erythema, pruritus, and the appearance of hives. This can progress to a confluent rash, extensive urticaria, and finally to anaphylaxis with vasomotor instability and bronchospasm. These reactions are most commonly due to the infusion of foreign plasma proteins that induce an antibody response by the host. In mild reactions, the response is primarily mediated by IgE antibody, although IgG can be involved as well.

The treatment of mild allergic reactions is to stop the transfusion and give diphenhydramine, 25–50 mg intravenously. The patient should then be watched carefully to assess whether further symptoms develop. Should the patient's symptoms begin to dissipate, and the rash or urticaria begin to resolve, the transfusion may be reinstituted. It is felt that discontinuing the transfusion and exposing the patient to a different donor unit poses a greater risk to the patient than does worsening of the allergic reaction.

Anaphylactic reactions are rare, occurring most commonly in IgA-deficient patients transfused with blood containing donor IgA. In this case, the reaction is mediated by anti-IgA IgE antibody present in the recipient's serum, which binds to mast cells causing degranulation and the release of cytokines, which in turn are responsible for the symptoms of anaphylaxis. If signs of anaphylaxis such as vasomotor instability, hypotension, bronchospasm, or dyspnea develop, the transfusion should be stopped immediately. If anaphylaxis is suspected, early treatment with epinephrine is essential. Epinephrine not only helps to support blood pressure and relieve bronchospasm, but also, more importantly, stabilizes the mast cells, preventing propagation and/or worsening of the reaction.

Another less common cause of anaphylactic reaction is seen when platelets are transfused through certain leukocyte depletion filters. It is felt that the negatively charged filters may cause contact activation of the intrinsic pathway, ultimately resulting in the formation of bradykinin. The bradykinin is then transfused into the patient with the platelets, resulting in a syndrome characterized by wheezing, hypotension, pain, and flushing. The syndrome is more severe in patients taking angiotensin-converting enzyme inhibitors, as these drugs block the breakdown of bradykinin. The only way to avoid anaphylactic transfusion reactions is to use washed cells; leukocyte-depleted PRBCs are not effective, as plasma proteins are small enough to pass through these filters.

Transfusion-related Acute Lung Injury and Graft-Versus-Host Disease

Transfusion-related acute lung injury and graft-versus-host disease (GVHD) are also immune-mediated responses to transfusion. TRALI presents as a low-pressure pulmonary edema that develops within 4 hours of transfusion of plasma-containing blood products, most commonly FFP. In addition to a low-pressure pulmonary edema, patients with TRALI may have symptoms of fever, chills, cyanosis, hypoxia, dyspnea, hypertension, and/or hypotension. TRALI is felt to result from a reaction between donor white cell or HLA antibodies and recipient leukocytes (as compared to the febrile reaction, in which *recipient* antibodies act against *donor* leukocytes). The activated leukocytes generate an adhesive molecule on their surface, which promotes attachment to the pulmonary epithelium and entry into the pulmonary interstitium. Here, the activated leukocytes degranulate, releasing cytokines, which in turn cause capillary leak and the resultant low-pressure pulmonary edema. When TRALI is suspected, transfusion should be stopped and supportive care initiated. These reactions often do not recur, and transfusion with another unit may be attempted with careful monitoring of the patient's hemodynamic and pulmonary status.

Graft-versus-host disease is seen when immunologically competent white cells are transfused into a patient who is immunocompromised and is therefore unable to destroy the transfused white cells. As a result, the transfused white cells, which recognize the host cells as foreign, initiate an attack on the patient's tissue. This is a rare condition but is associated with a fatality rate of more than 90%. Only irradiated blood products should be used in patients who are considered to be immunocompromised.

Immune System Modulation

A final immune-related complication of transfusion is the modulation of the recipient's immune system after transfusion. This effect of transfusion on the immune system was appreciated as early as the 1970s, when it was noticed that patients who received transfusions prior to renal transplant had a decreased incidence of rejection compared to those who did not. These early observations have been recently confirmed by a large randomized prospective trial in which 5-year renal graft survival was found to be 9% greater in those who had received transfusion compared to those who had not.

The immunomodulatory role of transfusion has also been implicated in tumor recurrence rates, where at least half of retrospective reports have suggested a poorer prognosis in transfused patients when compared with nontransfused patients. This negative effect of transfusion has been seen with soft-tissue sarcomas, colon, renal, lung, head and neck, and prostate cancers. Conversely, few studies have shown any survival benefit from transfusion, other than in a supportive role. The retrospective studies in humans are supported by animal data, most of which suggest that allogenic blood has tumor growth-promoting activity and that this activity may be the result of immune system modulation.

The type of product transfused appears to affect the rate of tumor recurrence. Studies have suggested that transfusion of plasma and leukocyte-containing products (whole blood, FFP) are associated with a higher rate of tumor recurrence and death than transfusion of PRBC.

An additional consequence of immune modulation from transfusion is the apparent increased risk of infection in surgical patients who receive transfusion. While not all studies implicate transfusion as a cause for increased infection, the majority of results suggest an increased risk of infection and/or sepsis in those patients who are transfused. Many of these studies have used regression analysis to control for potentially confounding variables, including length of surgery, shock, and admission hematocrit, and, even when these variables are controlled for, there appears to be a statistically significant contribution to postoperative infection by transfusion.

How transfusion mediates the host immune system is not yet fully understood. However, several changes in the recipient's immune system have been observed after transfusion. These include decreased numbers of lymphocytes, natural killer T cells, and T helper cells as well as a decrease in cytokine production. In addition, T suppresser cells are increased. Changes in B-cell function, with downregulation of antigen-presenting cells, has also been observed. A role for transfused white cells as contributory to these changes is supported by recent studies that suggest postoperative infections, and rates of morbidity and mortality may be reduced when leukocyte depletion filters are employed during transfusion, although there are also data to suggest that there is no difference when leukodepleted products are used.

Infectious Complications

The infectious complications of transfusions include the risk of acquiring HIV, hepatitis A, B, C, and Delta, human T-cell lymphotrophic virus (HTLV)-1 and -2, and parvovirus B19; in addition, several bacterial and parasitic infections can be transmitted, most commonly *Yersinia enterocolitica*, syphilis and malaria. The risks of transfusion-related infection have greatly decreased over the past 20 years. Initially this decrease was due to a more careful screening of the donor pool. More recently, the development of more sensitive tests, which allow for the detection of virus while still in the latent phase (or "window period") of infection, has reduced this incidence even further. Unfortunately these window periods have not been completely eliminated and there are still significant window periods between infectivity and the ability to detect infection for HIV, hepatitis B and C, and HTLV-1. Currently, all blood collected in the United States is tested for the presence of hepatitis C antibody, hepatitis B core antigen, HIV-1, HIV-2, HIV p24 antigen, HTLV-I, and HTLV-II, as well as serum markers of *Treponema pallidum* infection (syphilis). The most recent estimates of these risks are summarized in Table 9-3.

Human Immunodeficiency Virus

The presence of HIV in the donor blood pool has decreased dramatically as the donor pool was first screened, then tested sequentially for the HIV antibody, elevations in serum transaminases, and finally the presence of p24 antigen. Current testing has reduced the window of HIV infection to seropositivity to a mean of 16 days. The risk of transfusion-related infection has been estimated to be approximately 1 in 670,000. The newest concern is for HIV 1 strain O, which is found primarily in western and central Africa and France. This virus

is not reliably detected by the current enzyme-linked immunosorbent assay (ELISA) test.

Hepatitis B

Hepatitis B is responsible for about 10% of all transfusion-related hepatitis. The risk of acquiring hepatitis B from transfusion is estimated at 1 in 63,000. This number is expected to fall as a greater portion of the population is immunized. Of those who receive a unit of blood infected with hepatitis B, 35% will develop an acute infection while an even smaller portion, 1–10%, develop chronic infection.

Hepatitis C

The risk of receiving a unit containing hepatitis C varies depending upon whether one includes the remote possibility of transfusing blood in a chronic, silent immunologic state. If one disregards this possibility, the risk is about 1 in 103,000 using the second-generation ELISA; if the immunologically silent state is considered, the risk increases to 1 in 30,000. The use of ribonucleic acid polymerase chain reaction (RNA PCR) analysis should reduce this risk even further, to about 1 in 121,000. The current window period is about 70–80 days. Unlike hepatitis B, more than 90% of those transfused with a hepatitis-C-infected unit will develop clinical infection. Of those infected, 85% develop chronic infection, with a 20% incidence of cirrhosis and 1–5% incidence of hepatocellular carcinoma. The combined mortality for these states is 14.5% over 21–28 years.

Human T-cell Lymphotrophic Viruses 1 and 2

Human T-cell lymphotrophic viruses 1 and 2 are retroviruses that infect a patient's leukocytes. HTLV-1 infection is associated with both adult T-cell leukemia/lymphoma and myelopathy/tropical spastic paraparesis. HTLV-2 infected patients may have an increased risk for bacterial, mycobacterial and fungal infections. Since both these viruses reside in white cells, they can only be transmitted via cellular blood component therapy; transfusion-related infection should not occur with the use of FFP or cryoprecipitate. The current window of infection is 51 days using enzyme immunoassay (EIA). The rate of transmission of HTLV by transfusion of an infected unit is estimated to be between 20% and 60%. The actual risk is related to the number of white cells transfused and the length of storage. Red cells stored over 14 days have very little risk of causing a transfusion-related infection. The current risk of receiving either of these viruses from transfusion is estimated to be 1 in 640,000.

Parvovirus B19

Parvovirus B19 infection normally occurs via the respiratory route but may be transmitted via transfusion. In healthy patients, parvovirus B19 infection results in erythema infectiosum, an infection characterized by fever, arthralgia, headache, malaise, and itching as well as a confluent ("slapped cheek") rash on the face that later spreads to the exposed surfaces of the arms and legs. Serious complications of this infection are extremely rare. In addition, parvovirus B19 infection can suppress normal erythropoiesis. In otherwise healthy patients this effect is trivial. However, in those patient populations who are at risk for hemolysis (those with sickle cell anemia, thalassemias, autoimmune diseases), or in those who are immunosuppressed (HIV infection, solid organ transplant recipients, and children with malignancies), this can cause acute aplastic or hypoplastic anemia. Additionally, infection of pregnant women can result in hydrops fetalis. The risk of transmission of parvovirus B19 varies depending upon the prevalence in the blood donor pool, which varies from year to year, and is greater when pooled products (random donor platelets, factor concentrates, and cryoprecipitate) are used. The virus is not readily inactivated by normal methods of viral inactivation.

Cytomegalovirus

Cytomegalovirus is a herpesvirus that rarely causes symptomatic illness in immunocompetent patients, although it has been associated with a mononucleosis like syndrome in young adults. However, in the immunocompromised patient, CMV infection may cause devastating sequelae, including interstitial pneumonia, chorioretinitis, encephalitis, hepatitis, esophagitis, and cholecystitis. Congenital infection of a fetus also can result in significant long-term consequences. Patients at high risk from complications of CMV infection thus include immunocompromised patients, pregnant women, and babies under 1,200 g. It is recommended that CMV-negative blood be used for these patient populations. The risk of seroconversion even after using seronegative donor blood is 0–6% because of the insensitivity of serologic testing. Since the virus is carried by the leukocytes, leukocyte-depleted products should be also used in the high risk patient.

Bacterial Infection

Bacterial infection is generally felt to be the result of contamination rather than collection of already infected blood. Contamination may occur during the donation, storage, or transfusion processes. The primary risk factor for bacterial contamination is the length of storage. The bacterial contaminant varies depending upon the product infected.

The most common bacterial agents contaminating red cells are *Yersinia enterocolitica* and *Pseudomonas fluorescens*. Together these account for over 75% of all contaminated red cell transfusions. Infection from *Y. enterocolitica* contamination is directly related to storage time, with most cases presenting after blood stored for more than 21 days is used. There have,

however, been reports of patients developing *Yersinia* sepsis after receiving blood that was stored for only 7–14 days. These organisms have enhanced growth at the 4° C temperature in which red cells are stored. It is estimated that the risk of receiving a contaminated unit of red cells is less than 1 per 1,000,000 units in the United States.

The symptoms of *Yersinia* sepsis often begin at the time of transfusion and the disease progresses rapidly. Of the 20 reported cases of transfusion-related *Yersinia* sepsis, 12 have resulted in death, with a median time to death of 25 hours.

It is conceivable that asymptomatic donors may donate *Yersinia*-infected blood. These donors will report having a diarrheal illness 1 month prior to their donation. The use of this as a screening question has not been implemented, as it would exclude up to 10% of donors from the donor pool.

The bacteria commonly associated with platelet contamination are different from those associated with contamination of red cells, probably a reflection of the fact that platelets are stored at room temperature. The most commonly reported bacteria associated with platelet contamination are *Staphylococcus aureus*, *Klebsiella pneumoniae*, *Serratia marcescens*, and *Staphylococcus epidermidis*. The risk of receiving a contaminated platelet transfusion is estimated at 1 in 12,000. The risk, as with red cells, is greater with increased storage time. In addition, risk is higher for those who receive pooled platelets. Apheresis platelets are typically stored for briefer periods and are collected from single donors, and are therefore safer.

The course of platelet-related sepsis is more variable than that of red-cell sepsis. It ranges from mild fever to septic shock with hypotension, capillary leak, and death. The overall mortality rate for sepsis secondary to platelet transfusion is estimated at 26%. Platelet-transfusion-related sepsis is probably under-reported as the organisms involved are similar to those associated with line sepsis.

Metabolic Complications

Metabolic complications of transfusion are secondary to the effects of storage and the storage medium on the composition of the stored blood. These changes can result in coagulopathy, potassium abnormalities, pH disturbances, and altered oxygen-carrying capacity in the patient being transfused.

Citrate Toxicity

The anticoagulant used to prevent clotting in stored blood is citrate. Citrate functions as an anticoagulant by binding the free calcium, a factor necessary for normal clotting. When a patient is transfused with citrate-preserved blood, the transfused citrate is rapidly metabolized to bicarbonate, with each millimole of citrate metabolized to 3 mEq of bicarbonate. However, if the patient has significant liver dysfunction, is transfused rapidly, or receives a large number of units, the transfused citrate can accumulate, binding the patient's ionized calcium, thus decreasing the patient's ionized calcium level. The decrease in serum ionized calcium can predispose the patient to hypotension and interfere with normal coagulation. In an awake patient, hypocalcemia may manifest as mild circumoral numbness or tetany. In an anesthetized patient, the only signs may be a prolongation of the QT interval, hypotension, and clotting abnormalities. The treatment is to give either calcium gluconate or calcium carbonate.

Hyperkalemia

The Na–K ATP-ase is essentially nonfunctional at the temperature in which red cells are stored. This, coupled with the normal hemolysis of cells as they age, results in a progressive increase in the plasma potassium concentrations of red cell preparations. At expiration, the plasma concentration of potassium in stored units can reach 40–70 mEq/L. As stored cells only contain between 40 and 60 mL of plasma, the total potassium load per unit transfused is between 2 and 7 mEq at expiration. Most patients can tolerate this potassium load; however, in patients who receive massive transfusion, who have pre-existing elevated serum potassium, or who have renal failure, this excess potassium load may cause hyperkalemia. In these patients it may be advisable to use "fresher" blood or washed cells. Washed cells are resuspended in saline and centrifuged repeatedly, removing the high levels of potassium from the unit.

Treatment for hyperkalemia is aimed at stabilizing the cardiac membranes to prevent arrhythmia (calcium chloride), driving the serum potassium intracellularly via increasing serum pH (bicarbonate and hyperventilation), and, finally, by clearing the excess potassium using loop diuretics.

Hypokalemia

Transfusion may also result in hypokalemia. Hypokalemia results from both the reuptake of the recipient's plasma potassium by the transfused cells and from the change in serum pH that can occur as citrate is converted to bicarbonate. The increased level of bicarbonate may increase serum pH, which in turn drives serum potassium intracellularly.

Acidosis

Red cells are obligate anaerobes and produce lactic acid as a byproduct of anaerobic metabolism. In addition, the PCO_2 of the stored blood rises over time as the bags used to store cells are not permeable to CO_2. Despite the presence of buffers in the storage solution, this accumulation of lactic acid and carbon dioxide causes a decrease in the pH of stored blood; a fresh unit of blood stored in CDPA-1 has a pH of less than 7.5 units, whereas at 35 days this pH has dropped to less than 6.7. Normal patients have no trouble eliminating the excess acid load via increasing alveolar ventilation to remove excess CO_2 and via hepatic and renal clearance of the lactic acid. However, patients with limited pulmonary reserve or hepatic insufficiency may develop a substantial acidosis as a consequence of red cell transfusion.

Decreased 2,3-diphosphoglycerate Levels

The final metabolic consequence of the storage of blood is the fall in 2,3-diphosphoglycerate (2,3-DPG) that occurs over time in stored blood. After 35 days of storage, CDPA-1-stored blood contains less than 10% of the original level of 2,3-DPG. This shifts the oxygen dissociation curve to the left, with the potential for a fall in the oxygen delivery of the transfused red cells. However, after transfusion, *in vivo* the 2,3 DPG level rapidly rises again towards normal and is greater than 50% of normal at 6 hours and at 100% by 24 hours. Practically, this means that most patients with adequate cardiac reserves can compensate in the short term for the decreased oxygen delivery of these cells by increasing cardiac output. However, patients with cardiac compromise may suffer adverse consequences from this phenomenon and may receive benefit by being transfused with fresher blood.

Hypothermia

Refrigerated blood has a temperature of 1–6° C. As such there is the potential for hypothermia when large volumes of blood are transfused. There are data showing that the rapid transfusion of cold blood can drop the temperature of the sinoatrial node to less than 30° C, which may cause ventricular irritability and even fibrillation. The drop in whole-body temperature also causes a decline in the rate of normal enzymatic reactions, with the result that basic functions such as metabolism and coagulation are slowed. As patients waken from anesthesia, this hypothermia can also result in shivering and an increase in oxygen consumption of up to 400%. These consequences of hypothermia can place a significant strain on the cardiovascular system. Transfusion-associated hypothermia may be prevented by the use of fluid warmers for the transfusion of blood products (with the notable exception of platelets). In addition to the benefits of improving enzymatic efficiency, warming the blood has a beneficial effect on viscosity, allowing a greater flow rate than cold blood.

Microaggregates

There is some concern that the transfusion of stored blood may lead to the transfusion of microaggregate debris that accumulates in the bag of the stored cells. Microaggregates are composed of dead platelets, granulocytes, and fibrin strands that accumulate in the storage medium over time. It was felt that the passage of these particles with transfusion might lead to the development of acute respiratory distress syndrome by occluding the small pulmonary capillaries. It has been shown, however, that this is an unlikely event, and that the occurrence of acute respiratory distress syndrome after transfusion is more probably due to the pre-existing sepsis and hypotension than to the transfusion itself.

AUTOLOGOUS TRANSFUSIONS

Perhaps the biggest change in transfusion practice since the acquired immunodeficiency syndrome (AIDS) epidemic raised concerns about the safety of the blood supply is the use of autologous transfusion. The theoretical advantage of using autologous blood is that it virtually eliminates the risks of viral transmission and immunologically mediated transfusion reactions, including the risk of immunomodulation. There are three strategies used for autologous blood transfusion. These are autologous predonation, acute isovolemic hemodilution, and cell salvage techniques.

Autologous Predonation

Autologous predonation involves collecting units of the patient's blood preoperatively for infusion intra- or postoperatively. The donor criteria for autologous predonation are less stringent than those for allogenic donation. Patients must have a hemoglobin of at least 11 g/dL before each donation and must not have, or be in the process of treatment for, an active bacterial infection. Patients who have unstable angina, congestive heart failure, left main coronary disease, or myocardial infarction within 3 months are generally not considered suitable candidates for predonation. The precollection process is commonly combined with iron and/or erythropoietin therapy, which helps to augment the rate of replacement of the predonated cells. Most centers do not allow the collection and storage of blood from patients who have tested positive for hepatitis B and C, and HIV, as these units pose potential threats to the safety of lab and operating room personnel. Some centers, however, will perform predonation on patients with these diseases, arguing that to not do so may violate the American with Disabilities Act.

Collection of the predonated blood begins 3–5 weeks prior to the scheduled surgery date. During these phlebotomy sessions, about 250–500 mL of blood are removed and stored in a bag containing citrate, phosphate, adenine, and dextrose. The shelf life of this blood is 35 days. Unlike most allogenic blood, autologous blood is stored as whole blood, rather than its constituents (PRBC, FFP, platelets, and cryoprecipitate).

Disadvantages of autologous predonation include complications that can occur during donation, the potential for ischemia in patients with silent or known coronary disease, the accidental transfusion of an allogenic unit, and a higher likelihood of requiring a transfusion intraoperatively, as well as cost and logistical issues.

During donation the most common adverse event is a vasovagal response. The incidence of these reactions appears to be similar in autologous and first-time allogenic donors. Studies evaluating the risk of ischemic events during autologous donations in those with a history of coronary disease via Holter monitoring, have shown that a nontrivial number (up to 37% in one study) of those with coronary disease are at risk for developing ECG-detectable ischemia either during and/or after the donation process. These results suggest that caution should be used when recommending this technique for this patient population.

Clerical error can result in the patient receiving allogenic rather than his autologous blood, thus subjecting that patient not only to the risks of autologous donation but also to those of allogenic transfusion. The cost of using autologous blood has been estimated to be considerably higher than when using allogenic blood, primarily because of the added administrative costs. In addition, many patients who do predonate do not receive all of their autologous blood before discharge, resulting in wastage of the non-used unit(s). Lastly, this strategy involves several additional clinic visits for the patient, as well as the issue of transfer of the units from the site of donation to the site of surgery.

Added to these risks is the fact that patients who predonate will have a lower starting hematocrit and will therefore require transfusion earlier in a procedure than had they not predonated. The actual degree of preoperative anemia induced by predonation varies depending upon the time from donation to surgery, the degree of erythropoiesis, and the degree of iron supplementation. Mathematical modeling suggests that a 70 kg male who predonates 2 units of blood and has a replacement by erythropoiesis of 60% of that loss will be able to tolerate approximately 200 mL less blood loss before requiring a transfusion than if he had not predonated.

The question becomes: do the risks of autologous predonation (reactions during donations, ischemia, higher likelihood of requiring transfusion, clerical error, and cost) outweigh its benefits (potential to avoid the transfusion of an allogenic unit)? Algorithms have been developed to try and stratify patients at higher risk of requiring transfusion and those who would benefit from autologous predonation based upon patient history and type of procedure but these are not yet widely applied. What does seem clear is that those who have a less than 50% chance of requiring transfusion should not be encouraged to donate units preoperatively. There is some discrepancy as to whether the transfusion threshold should be raised in those who have donated preoperatively. According to the ASA guidelines, the raising of the threshold is acceptable when using autologous blood. However, the Canadian Medical Association recommends that the same transfusion threshold be used in both populations.

Intraoperative Acute Normovolemic Hemodilution

The second autologous technique is that of intraoperative acute normovolemic hemodilution. In this technique, the patient is brought to the operating room, where 1-4 units of blood are withdrawn and the lost volume is replaced with an equal volume of colloid or three times the volume in crystalloid (or a combination thereof). This technique has certain advantages over autologous predonation. First, during the donation process, the patient is in a closely monitored situation, under anesthesia, which should allow for early detection of any hemodynamic or ischemic change, while also decreasing the stress of donation. Since the patient's blood does not leave the operating room, the chance for clerical error is virtually eliminated. Lastly, as the blood is stored at room temperature and only for only a minimal period of time before being reinfused, platelet function and 2,3-DPG levels are maintained, while the pH, P_{CO_2}, and potassium are virtually unchanged.

This technique is recommended for those patients expected to lose more than 20% of their blood volume who have a preoperative hemoglobin of more than 10 mg/dL. It is estimated that hemodilution to a hematocrit of 28% saves about 100-200 mL of red cells when compared to normal techniques. This manifests as a saving of 0.5-1 unit of packed cell transfusion. There have been more dramatic results when hemodilution to hematocrits of 20-24% have been performed. However, the potential for ischemic complications increases substantially when hematocrits this low are induced and there is sudden, unexpected surgical blood loss. Recent data using this technique in patients undergoing hepatic resections has demonstrated a decreased need for allogenic transfusion.

Intraoperative Cell Salvage

The last of the autologous techniques is cell salvage. The automated devices used for this process consist of a double-lumen suction port that infuses an anticoagulant (heparin or citrate) at a constant rate while blood lost from the patient (now mixed with the anticoagulant) is suctioned via the other port into a reservoir. Once in the reservoir, the blood passes through a filter that functions to remove the cellular debris. After passing through the filter the blood is centrifuged to concentrate the red cells. The concentrated cells are then washed with saline and re-suspended in saline. The concentrated and washed cells are then placed in storage bags for reinfusion into the patient. The process of filtering and washing removes most of the white cells, platelets, activated clotting factors, plasma hemoglobin, and cell fragments.

The contraindications to this technique are situations in which tumor cells, bacteria, and/or other debris (amniotic fluid, ascitic fluid) might be aspirated into the salvage reservoir. The reinfused blood has oxygen transport properties similar to that of allogenic units. The advantage of this technique is that it can provide a large volume of autologous blood for transfusion. In a severely hemorrhagic patient, it can provide the equivalent of up to 10 units of allogenic blood per hour. The disadvantage of this technique when compared to other autologous techniques is that the reinfused cells contain none of the coagulation proteins or platelets lost, and thus cell-saver use may potentiate the development of dilutional coagulopathy (unlike the whole blood that is collected for both autologous predonation and isovolemic hemodilution). For cell salvage to be cost effective, at least 2 units of washed cells need to be recovered, meaning that its use should be considered when blood losses in excess of 1-2 L are anticipated.

SUMMARY

The first portion of this chapter served as a review of the basic science of transfusion medicine, including the processes of normal coagulation and the basic immunology of the hematopoietic system. The standard laboratory tests of the hemostasis were discussed, as were the preparation and composition of each of the commonly used blood products.

We then discussed the major changes that have occurred in the field of transfusion therapy. Many of these changes began in the mid-1980s when the realization that HIV was transmissible by the transfusion of blood products occurred. This realization led first to changes in the screening of the blood donor pool and then later prompted increasingly complex tests designed to immunologically detect the transmissible infectious agents while still in their latent period. As a result of these advances, the risks of receiving an infected blood product are now lower than ever. The latest estimates for risks of the major viral and bacterial infections as well as the metabolic consequences of transfusion were reviewed. Lastly the immunomodulatory effects of transfusion were discussed.

Current Controversies

What is the appropriate transfusion trigger (minimal acceptable hemoglobin) for transfusion of red blood cells.

In settings of massive blood loss and unavailable lab data, when is transfusion indicated/helpful in the treatment or prevention of coagulopathy.

- Fresh frozen plasma
- Platelets
- Cryoprecipitate

Should new screening tests be employed for emerging infectious diseases (i.e. West Nile Virus, Creutzfeldt-Jakob disease)? If so, for which diseases should we screen, and how can it be done in a cost effective manner?

Should all units to be transfused be screened for bacterial contamination? If so, what are cost effective ways to do this?

What are the clinically significant affects of immune modulation by transfusion?

- Increased risk of infection?
- Increased risk of tumor recurrence?
- Is there a potential to reduce these risks by using leukodepleted products?

What and who are the appropriate procedures and surgical patients for autologous techniques:

- Autologous predonation
- Acute isovolemic hemodilution
- Intraoperative cell salvage techniques

Is the use of leukodepleted blood products cost effective?

The fear of transfusing infected allogenic blood products also prompted changes in the practice of transfusion therapy. These changes include both a greater use of autologous techniques and a re-evaluation of the transfusion triggers for available blood products. The current strategies for autologous transfusion and the advantages and disadvantages of each have been discussed. The use of autologous techniques has decreased recently as it has become increasingly evident that they are not appropriate for all situations and, while the risks of transfusion-related infection from allogenic units may be decreased, the risks of donation and clerical error, cost, and logistics make their universal use inappropriate. However, in the properly selected patient undergoing select procedures, the use of these techniques may decrease the patient's exposure to allogenic blood products and the risks thereof.

A greater understanding of the risks of transfusion has also prompted more study of the appropriate transfusion indications. The current ASA guidelines and data regarding transfusion indications were reviewed in some detail for each of the commonly used blood products. The general theme of the data, with the noticeable exception of the patient with known or suspected coronary disease, is that patients seem to do at least as well, if not better, when lower transfusion thresholds are employed than were previously accepted.

In general, what does this all mean to the practicing clinician? The bottom line is that transfusion of allogenic blood is as safe as it has ever been but is still not without risk. These risks are not only from the classic infective agents clinicians worry about (HIV, HCV, HBV) but also from emerging and, as of now, untested for infectious agents including prions and viruses such as the West Nile virus as well as bacterial contaminants. There are also noninfectious risks, which include metabolic derangements, transfusion reactions, and immunomodulation.

The question of when to transfuse remains a difficult one to answer precisely, and all the data available should be reviewed as carefully as possible before a decision is made. Data to be reviewed include not only the patient's hematocrit but also the patient's past medical history, the surgical procedure, and the likelihood of additional intra- or postoperative bleeding, as well as measures of tissue oxygenation including pH, serum lactate, serum bicarbonate, and mixed venous oxygen content, and finally laboratory evaluation of coagulation (PT, PTT, fibrinogen, platelets, and FDP).

Case Study

Mr Jones is a 65-year-old male who presents for radical retropubic prostatectomy. This patient has a history of hypertension, non-insulin-dependent diabetes mellitus, non-Q-wave myocardial infarction, osteoarthritis, and peripheral vascular disease. His past surgical history includes an open inguinal hernia repair at the age of 21 under general anesthesia and a cataract repair performed under monitored anesthesia care at age 51; he reports no anesthesia complications with either surgery. His current medications include Lisinopril, Metformin, Glucophage, Atenolol, and aspirin.

His review of systems is remarkable for being only able to walk a block before needing to stop secondary to pain in his knees and mild shortness of breath; he denies chest pain, orthopnea, and symptoms of gastroesophageal reflux. On examination the patient is 6 feet tall, 245 pounds (111 kg). Vital signs include a heart rate of 68, a blood pressure of 158/90, and a respiratory rate of 16. His cardiorespiratory and airway examination is unremarkable. Preoperative workup revealed the

Continued

Case Study—cont'd

following: hematocrit 41%, normal electrolytes with a creatinine of 1.2, PT of 13 seconds with an INR of 0.98, a PTT of 28.7 seconds. ECG shows a sinus rhythm, normal axis, Q waves in the anterior leads, and nonspecific ST segment changes; this is unchanged from an ECG done 1 year ago.

Given Mr Jones's cardiac history, a preoperative cardiology consult was obtained and a stress echocardiogram was ordered. The stress echocardiogram shows preserved systolic function with an ejection fraction of 55%, decreased diastolic relaxation, and a reversible defect in the distribution of the left anterior descending coronary artery. The cardiologist says that the results of this test were consistent with the patient's prior stress echo, done 1 year previously. At that time, cardiac catheterization was performed that revealed diffuse coronary disease with no lesions that were amenable to angioplasty and/or stenting. The cardiologist feels that no further cardiac workup is in order, and recommends that the patient have a postoperative ECG and be monitored via Holter monitoring for the first 24 hours postoperatively.

What are the recommendations for stopping a patient's aspirin therapy prior to an elective surgery? What about the other common anticoagulant therapies ticlopidine, clopidogrel, and warfarin?

Are there specific anesthetic techniques that are associated with decreased blood loss intraoperatively. Is there a specific technique that may be useful in this patient?

Which, if any, of the autologous techniques would be appropriate in this patient to decrease the use of allogenic blood products?

Given this patient's history, what do you think the lowest safe post/intraoperative hematocrit is? Is there a way to estimate the volume of blood that can be lost before the patient reaches that hematocrit?

During the dissection the patient is bleeding more than the surgeons expect. Are there any pharmacologic techniques that you might employ to try and decrease the degree of blood loss?

SUGGESTED READING

ASA Task Force of Blood Component Therapy. Practice guidelines for blood component therapy. *Anesthesiology* 1995;84:732-747.

Carson JL, Noveck H, Berlin JA, Gould SJ. Mortality and morbidity in patients with very low postoperative hemoglobins who decline blood transfusion. *Transfusion* 2002;42:812-818.

Drummond JC, Petrovich CT. The massively bleeding patient. *Anesthesiol Clin North Am* 2001;19:633-649.

Goodnough LT, Brecher ME, Kanter MH, AuBuchon JP. Transfusion medicine. First of two parts - blood transfusions. *N Engl J Med* 1999;340:438-447.

Goodnough LT, Brecher ME, Kanter MH, AuBuchon JP. Transfusion medicine. Second of two parts - blood conservation. *N Engl J Med* 1999;340:525-533.

Hebert JC, Wells G, Blajchman MA *et al*. A multicenter, randomized, controlled clinical trial of transfusion requirements in critical care. *N Engl J Med* 1999;340:409-417.

Hebert PC, Wells G, Tweeddale M, *et al*. Does transfusion affect mortality in critically ill patients? *Am J Respir Crit Care Med* 1997;155:1618-1623.

Hebert PC, Yestiser E, Martin C *et al*. Is a low transfusion threshold safe in critically ill patients with cardiovascular disease? *Crit Care Med* 2001;29:227-234.

Hiippala T, Gunnar GJ, Vahtera EM. Hemostatic factors and replacement of major blood loss with plasma-poor red cell concentrates. *Anesth Analg* 1995;81:360-365.

Hogue CW, Goodnough LT, Monk TG. Perioperative myocardial ischemic episodes are related to hematocrit level in patients undergoing radical prostatectomy. *Transfusion* 1998;38:924-931.

Landers DF, Hill GE, Wong KC, Fox IJ. Blood transfusion-induced immunomodulation. *Anesth Analg* 1996;82:187-204.

McFarland JG. Perioperative blood transfusions, indications and options. *Chest* 1999;115:113S-121S.

Nelson AH, Fleisher LA, Rosenbaum SH. Relationship between postoperative anemia and cardiac morbidity in high risk vascular patients in the intensive care unit. *Crit Care Med* 1993:21:860-866.

O'Connor MF, Apfelbaum JL. Update on transfusion therapy. *Semin Cardiothorac Vasc Anesth* 2000;4:236-243.

Spahn DR, Cusutt M. Eliminating blood transfusions: new aspects and perspectives. *Anesthesiology* 2000;93:242-255.

Weiskopf RB, Viele MK, Feiner J, *et al*. Human cardiovascular and metabolic response to acute severe isovolemic anemia. *JAMA* 1998;279:217-221.

ANESTHETIC MANAGEMENT

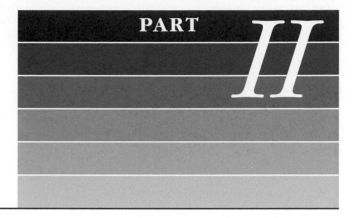

PART

II

CHAPTER 10

Anesthesia for Thoracic Surgery

ANNIE V. CÔTÉ

JOANNE D. FORTIER

MICHEL-ANTOINE PERREAULT

ANNIE PHARAND

With increasing experience and the development of better techniques for administering anesthesia, a greater number of patients are now coming to the operating room for surgical treatment of previously considered incurable diseases. The most common indication for thoracic surgery today is the resection of lung cancer. Other indications include mediastinal mass biopsy or resection, pulmonary lavage for alveolar proteinosis and esophagectomy for carcinoma.

Patients presenting for thoracic surgery must undergo proper preoperative evaluation. A thorough investigation of their thoracic disease and associated manifestations, as well as other comorbidities, is essential to providing safe anesthetic care.

History

In patients with a history of thoracic disease, special attention should be given to bronchopulmonary symptoms. Dyspnea occurs when pulmonary reserve is inadequate for ventilation requirements. The severity of the dyspneic symptoms can be assessed by evaluating exercise tolerance. Ischemic cardiac disease can also manifest with dyspnea, underlying the importance of taking a good history. Increasing cough, secretions and hemoptysis are frequently found in this patient population. Concomitant infection, use of antibiotics and associated anemia must be determined. Wheezing and stridor may be strong indicators of intra/extrathoracic obstruction, possibly requiring additional investigation (see below).

Patients presenting with thoracic disease often have a long history of cigarette smoking with associated lung parenchymal disease. All patients should be encouraged to stop smoking, although it may have significant effects, good or bad, on respiratory physiology. Within 12–48 hours of stopping smoking, the level of carboxyhemoglobin returns to normal and the oxyhemoglobin dissociation curve is shifted back to the right, allowing better oxygen availability to the tissues. The incidence of nicotine-induced tachycardia is also lessened.

Ischemic cardiovascular disease is frequently found in this patient population. Symptoms such as chest pain and shortness of breath with or without exertion should be sought. An understanding of the patient's functional exercise capacity is necessary to determine the need for further investigation with more invasive cardiac testing.

Nonspecific symptoms and signs such as fever, weight loss and anorexia are encountered, especially in patients with neoplasms, and may have significant impact on anesthetic management. Pre-existing comorbidities, including severity, associated complications and treatments, deserve attention and thorough questioning.

Physical Examination

Inspection, palpation, percussion and auscultation help in determining the overall severity of the thoracic disease causing the patient to require surgical treatment. Respiratory distress, bronchospasm, areas of consolidation and atelectasis are examples of problems that may be identified by physical examination. A patient's physical examination should be as complete as possible and, in the context of preoperative thoracic evaluation, should include detailed heart and lung examination, as well as evaluation of musculoskeletal limitations that may influence positioning of the patient.

Investigations

Laboratory studies should include a complete blood count to rule out the presence of anemia (hemoptysis, chronic disease), polycythemia (low hemoglobin oxygen saturation) and leukocytosis (active pulmonary infection). Basic electrolytes, creatinine levels, liver enzymes and urinalysis may help with diagnosis of paraneoplastic syndromes and renal/hepatic dysfunction.

Chest radiograph and computed tomography (CT) scans can provide information on tumor location, extent of disease and spread, bronchial compression, atelectasis, tracheal deviation, bullas, pulmonary edema and cardiac enlargement.

Associated with obstructive pulmonary disease, electrocardiographic signs of right axis deviation, right ventricular enlargement and right bundle branch block can be seen. Low voltage QRS complexes may be present in cases of lung hyperinflation, as well as diffuse ST changes in cases of pericarditis.

Arterial blood gases are indicated in patients with on-going respiratory distress or chronic obstructive pulmonary disease causing carbon dioxide retention. Baseline blood gas values may also serve as predictors of postoperative pulmonary function.

Pulmonary function tests are useful for the evaluation of pulmonary resectability.

- *Spirometry*: The volume of air passing through an airway opening can be measured by a spirometer. Measurements obtained are all effort-dependent and include: vital capacity, inspiratory reserve volume and expiratory reserve volume (Table 10-1 and Figure 10-1).
- *Functional Residual Capacity* (FRC) can be measured by several methods, including an equilibration method using helium, the washout method calculated from lung washout of a tracer gas, or plethysmography using a technique based on Boyle's law. When combined with measurements obtained by spirometry, the FRC measurement allows calculation of total lung capacity and residual volume.
- *Forced Expiratory Spirography*: This forceful expiration is obtained after maximal inspiration. Expiratory flow and volumes are measured: forced vital capacity (FVC) and forced expiratory volume in 1 second (FEV_1). A low FEV_1 is the hallmark of chronic obstructive pulmonary disease.

$FEV_1 = 60–70\% \rightarrow$ mild obstruction
$FEV_1 = 40–60\% \rightarrow$ moderate obstruction
$FEV_1 < 40\% \rightarrow$ severe obstruction

Forced expiratory flow from 75–25% of vital capacity (FEF_{25-75}) is less effort-dependent and is a sensitive indicator of obstruction of small airways (Figure 10-2).

Table 10-1 Lung Volumes and Capacities

Measurement	Definition	Average Adult Values (mL)
Tidal volume (V_t)	Each normal breath	500
Inspiratory reserve volume (IRV)	Maximum additional volume that can be inspired above V_t	3000
Expiratory reserve volume (ERV)	Maximum volume that can be expired below V_t	1100
Residual volume (RV)	Volume remaining after maximal exhalation	1200
Total lung capacity (TLC)	RV + ERV + V_t + IRV	5800
Functional residual capacity (FRC)	RV + ERV	2300

From Morgan GE, Mikhail MS, Murray MJ. *Lange's clinical anesthesiology*, 3rd ed. New York: Lange/McGraw Hill, 2002:787.

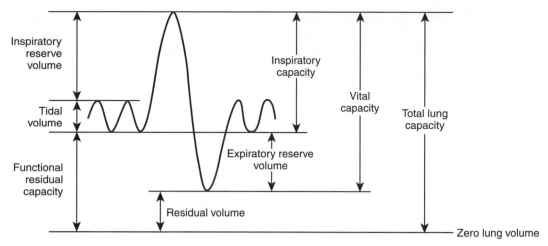

Figure 10-1   Spirogram showing static lung volumes. (Redrawn from Lumb A, ed. *Nunn's applied respiratory physiology*, 5th ed. Oxford: Butterworth-Heinemann, 2000.)

If maximal inspiratory flows are also measured, flow–volume loops can be obtained and are useful in identifying sources of airway obstruction. In patients with obstructive disease, forced expiratory spirography may be done after bronchodilator inhalation to assess reversibility of airway obstruction (>10% change in FEV_1).

• *Diffusion Lung Capacity* (D_LCO) measures diffusion of carbon monoxide across the alveolar-capillary membrane. Reduced D_LCO is an indicator of parenchymal loss as in emphysema or thickening of the alveolo-capillary membrane, as in pulmonary fibrosis. In cases

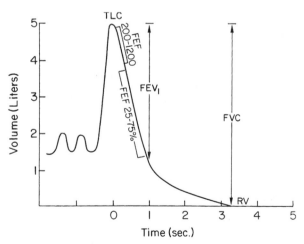

Figure 10-2   Forced vital capacity (FVC) maneuver in a subject with a normal lung. Exhaled volume is plotted against time as the subject expires forcefully, rapidly, and completely to residual volume (RV) after a maximal deep inspiration to total lung capacity (TLC). FEV_1, forced expired volume in 1 second; $FEF_{200-1200}$, forced expiratory flow between 200 and 1200 mL of expired volume; $FEF_{25-75\%}$, forced expiratory flow over the midportion of vital capacity, i.e., from 25% to 75% of expired volume. (From Gal TJ. Pulmonary function testing. In: Miller RD, ed. *Anesthesia*, 5th ed. New York: Churchill Livingstone, 2000:886.)

of pulmonary resection, predicted postoperative D_LCO (ppo D_LCO) may be an important predictor of mortality.

Split lung function tests are regional lung function studies done to help predict the function of the remaining lung tissue after parenchymal resection. Hence, they should always be performed in patients in whom pulmonary function is impaired and thought to be at greater risk of having higher postoperative morbidity and mortality.

Regional ventilation/perfusion scans allow assessment, using radioactive gas, of proportional degrees of ventilation and perfusion in each lung.

The regional bronchial balloon occlusion test simulates the situation following lung tissue resection. Spirometric and arterial blood gas measurements are thus obtained and values are compared with original ones.

A pulmonary artery balloon occlusion test simulates postoperative stress on the right ventricle and the remaining vasculature by occluding the pulmonary artery of the lung to be resected. This test can be performed at rest or on exertion.

Exercise tolerance is an easy measure and gives great indication of early cardiac and respiratory complications. The simplest exercise test is to determine the number of flights of stairs that can be climbed by the surgical patient preoperatively. The ability to climb fewer than three flights of stairs is associated with increasing risk of complications. An indicator of oxygen consumption ($\dot{V}O_{2\,max}$) can also be used to predict outcome. A preoperative $\dot{V}O_{2\,max}$ of more than 20 ml/kg/min is associated with a good outcome, while a $\dot{V}O_{2\,max}$ of less than 10 ml/kg/min is an absolute contraindication to pulmonary resection.

Several measures and factors have been associated with increasing risk of morbidity and mortality after pulmonary tissue resection and are summarized in Box 10-1.

> ### Box 10-1   Factors Associated with Poor Prognosis After Pulmonary Resection
>
> P_aCO_2 >45 mmHg, P_aO_2 <50 mmHg on arterial blood gas
> FEV_1 <2 L
> ppo FEV_1 <0.8 L or <40% predicted
> FEV_1/FVC <50% predicted
> RV/TLC >50%
> MBC <50% predicted
> $\dot{V}O_{2\,max}$ <10 mL/kg/min
> ppo D_LCO <40%

MBC, maximal breathing capacity.

Preoperative data may also be used to anticipate a patient's ventilation management. Conservative ventilatory management is recommended when patients are older than 80 years of age or have a history of cardiac ischemic disease or renal dysfunction. Patients with ppo FEV_1 of more than 40% may be extubated immediately after the procedure. When ppo FEV_1 is 30–40%, the results of exercise tolerance, ppo D_LCO, ventilation/perfusion ($\dot{V}/\dot{Q}$) scan and the presence of other existing comorbidities need to be considered in deciding when to extubate the patient. Staged weaning is considered a safer route when ppo FEV_1 is less than 30%.

Specific Anesthetic Risks

To complete the preoperative evaluation and formulate an anesthetic plan, the anesthesiologist must consider the anesthetic risks associated with a patient's specific diagnosis and existing comorbidities. The following section deals with the diagnoses most frequently encountered in thoracic surgical patients, along with their anesthetic implications.

Lung Carcinoma

1. *Compression of surrounding structures* by a growing mass:
   - Distortion of the tracheobronchial tree
   - Obstructive pneumonia
   - Esophageal compression (dysphagia, dehydration, malnutrition)
   - Recurrent laryngeal nerve compression (hoarseness)
   - Phrenic nerve compression (hemidiaphragm palsy)
   - Pancoast tumor (shoulder/arm pain C7–T2)
   - Superior vena cava syndrome (to consider in choosing invasive monitoring placement sites)
   - Bernard–Horner syndrome
2. *Paraneoplastic syndromes* with their metabolic effects:
   - Lambert–Eaton myasthenic syndrome (proximal myopathy, weakness unresponsive to anticholinergics or steroids, and improving with activity, sensitivity to both depolarizing and nondepolarizing neuromuscular blockers)
   - Cushing's syndrome
   - Hypercalcemia
   - Syndrome of inappropriate secretion of antidiuretic hormone (SIADH)
3. *Other considerations*:
   - Metastatic disease (brain, bone, liver and adrenal)
   - Side effects of radiation therapy or chemotherapeutic agents:
     - Pulmonary toxicity (bleomycin)
     - Cardiac toxicity (adriamycin, doxorubicin)
     - Renal toxicity (cisplatin)
4. *Pain control*.

Lung Bullae

1. *Etiology or underlying pathology*:
   - Emphysema
   - Alpha-1 antitrypsin deficiency (associated liver disease)
2. Potential association with *right ventricular hypertrophy and pulmonary hypertension*
3. *Risk of bulla rupture*, causing a tension pneumothorax:
   - Careful use of positive-pressure ventilation
   - Awake intubation or general anesthesia, keeping the patient spontaneously breathing, may be required.

Bronchiectasis

Bronchiectasis is an irreversible dilation of a localized area of bronchus caused by destructive inflammatory processes involving the bronchial walls.

1. Presence of a large amount of purulent secretions at risk of spilling into areas of normal lung (double-lumen tube indicated)
2. Frequent hemoptysis (anemia, risk of massive bleeds)
3. Possible association with cystic fibrosis (autosomal recessive disease due to a mutation on chromosome 7, causing impaired clearance of secretions):
   - Sinusitis
   - Bronchiectasis
   - Pancreatic insufficiency
   - Hepatic cirrhosis with portal hypertension

Empyema

An empyema is an infectious, consolidated process.

1. Need to protect the nonaffected lung from soiling (double-lumen tube indicated)
2. Tuberculosis must be ruled out.

Anterior Mediastinal Masses

1. *Potential airway compression*, indicating possible need for awake intubation or general anesthesia, keeping the patient breathing spontaneously (Table 10-2)

Table 10-2 Evaluation of Patients with Anterior Mediastinal Masses

General anesthesia	Criteria	Anesthetic plan
Safe	Asymptomatic patient Tracheal/bronchial diameter >50% on CT	Proceed
Unsafe	Symptomatic patient (dyspnea, orthopnea, paroxysmal nocturnal dyspnea)	Consider: Biopsy of the mass under local anesthesia
	Child with tracheal/ bronchial diameter <50% on CT or with abnormal flow–volume loops	Preoperative radiation therapy or chemotherapy
Uncertain	Mildly symptomatic patient	
	Asymptomatic adult patient with abnormal flow–volume loops or tracheal/bronchial diameter < 50% on CT	Proceed* with: Awake fiberoptic intubation Inhalation induction with spontaneous breathing

* With a surgeon available in the operating room, equipped with a rigid bronchoscope.
CT, computed tomography.

2. Considerations associated with *the etiology of the mass*:
   - *Thymoma* is frequently associated with myasthenia gravis, an autoimmune disease affecting the postsynaptic receptors of the neuromuscular junction. Considerations associated with this disease include the weakness of proximal muscles (worsening with exertion), the risk of pulmonary aspiration, especially when respiratory or bulbar muscular involvement is present, the risk of respiratory depression with sedation, sensitivity to nondepolarizing muscular blockers and the risk of postoperative respiratory failure. The side effects of anticholinesterase therapy include vagal reflexes, increased bowel peristaltism, and a longer duration of action with succinylcholine and ester local anesthetics (Box 10-2).
   - *Goiter* associated with thyroid disease
   - *Hyperplasia of Parathyroid Glands*
   - *Lymphoma*
   - *Teratoma*

Pulmonary Alveolar Proteinosis

This is a disease of unknown etiology characterized by deposition of lipid-rich proteinaceous material in the alveoli. Patients often present with significant dyspnea and arterial hypoxemia. A $\dot{V}/\dot{Q}$ scan is indicated to identify the more affected lung, which will be lavaged first. There is a strict need for lung isolation during lavage.

Box 10-2 Risk Factors Associated with Postoperative Respiratory Failure in Myasthenia Gravis

Diagnosis >6 years
Concomitant pulmonary disease
Peak inspiratory pressure ≥25 cmH2O
Vital capacity <4 mL/kg
Pyridostigmine dose >750 mg/day

A subsequent return to the operating room for lavage of the opposite side usually occurs 3–10 days later.

Esophageal Disease

Patients with esophageal disease have a higher incidence of acid reflux disease and aspiration pneumonia with subsequently reduced pulmonary reserve. Premedication with antacids is recommended followed by rapid sequence induction.

In the patient population with esophageal carcinoma, there is a frequent association with cardiovascular disease and an increased incidence of alcohol abuse with its associated problems: alcohol-induced liver disease, upper gastrointestinal bleeding, coagulopathy and challenging pain control issues.

PHYSIOLOGY

This section will review the indications and methods of lung isolation, particularly the ones that apply to thoracic surgery. We will closely examine the cardiorespiratory effects of one-lung ventilation (OLV) on the awake versus the anesthetized patient, with a closed or an opened chest. Finally, we will briefly elaborate on the ventilation management of a patient on OLV.

Thoracic surgery raises unique anesthetic considerations, one being lung isolation. Absolute and relative indications for lung isolation are listed in Box 10-3.

Many tools have been developed over the past few decades to facilitate lung separation. There are only a few situations in which we cannot isolate one lung from the other, even in patients with a potentially difficult airway. Double-lumen endotracheal tubes (DLTs) are the most commonly used means for lung isolation. Their safety, easiness of insertion and efficacy for rapid lung inflation and deflation and for lung suctioning make them the standard of care when lung isolation is required (Figures 10-3 and 10-4).

As suggested in Figure 10-4, right-sided DLTs are less convenient to use than left-sided ones. The location of the right upper lobe bronchial orifice 2–3 cm from the carina requires precision and confirmation of proper positioning. Great care must be taken not to occlude the orifice with

Box 10-3   Indications for Lung Isolation

Absolute

Isolation of one lung from the other to avoid spillage or contamination
- Infection
- Massive hemorrhage

Control of the distribution of ventilation
- Bronchopleural fistula
- Bronchopleural cutaneous fistula
- Surgical opening of a major conducting airway
- Giant unilateral lung cyst or bulla
- Tracheobronchial tree disruption

Unilateral bronchopulmonary lavage for alveolar proteinosis

Relative

Surgical exposure – high priority
- Thoracic aortic aneurysm
- Pneumonectomy
- Upper lobectomy

Surgical exposure – low priority
- Middle and lower lobectomies and subsegmental resections
- Esophageal resection
- Thoracoscopy
- Procedures on the thoracic spine

Post-cardiopulmonary-bypass status after removal of totally occluding chronic unilateral pulmonary emboli

From Benumof JL. *Anesthesia for thoracic surgery*, 2nd ed. Philadelphia: WB Saunders, 1995.

the endobronchial cuff. This problem is easily avoided with the insertion, if appropriate, of a left-sided tube, as the opening of the left-upper lobe is about 5 cm from the carina.

Some situations make the use of a DLT difficult or impossible. In those cases, lung isolation can be achieved by fiberoptically placing a bronchial blocker (BB) alongside a single-lumen tube. A Fogarty occlusion catheter with a 3 ml balloon can be used as a BB (Figure 10-5). The Arndt blocker, a new wire-guided endobronchial blocker, has recently been designed. Campos *et al.* tested it and compared its use to that of a DLT. They found that, although surgical exposure was as good, it took longer to position and longer to deflate the isolated lung.

Using the BB principle, the Univent tube has emerged as the alternative of choice when a DLT cannot be placed. Instead of placing the BB alongside the endotracheal tube, the BB is built into the Univent tube. Once the tube is placed endotracheally, the BB can be pushed either into the right or left bronchus (Figures 10-5 and 10-6).

Although indicated to prevent spillage of blood or pus from one lung to the other, the BB and the Univent tube are not as effective as the DLT for quickly deflating and reinflating the lung. The small lumen diameter of the BB makes for a high resistance to airflow (Figure 10-7).

Thoracic anesthesia raises two particular physiologic considerations: lateral positioning and OLV with an open chest. In the following, we will explain, step by step, the circulatory, ventilatory and oxygenation changes caused by operating on an open deflated lung with a patient in the lateral decubitus position.

An awake patient in the lateral position creates changes in blood flow and ventilation distribution in a beneficial way: gravity makes for better perfusion in the dependent lung and decreases the portion of lung in the physiologic West zone 1, the vertical hydrostatic gradient being less in the lateral decubitus position than in the standing position. Moreover, ventilation is also increased in the dependent lung because of a vertical gradient in pleural pressure and

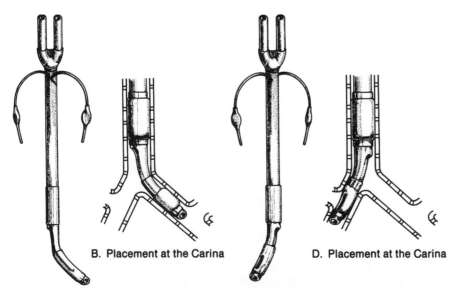

Figure 10-3   Sketch of the red rubber Robertshaw double-lumen tube. (From Benumof JL. *Anesthesia for thoracic surgery*. Philadelphia: WB Saunders, 1997.)

A. Left Robertshaw Tube

B. Placement at the Carina

C. Right Robertshaw Tube

D. Placement at the Carina

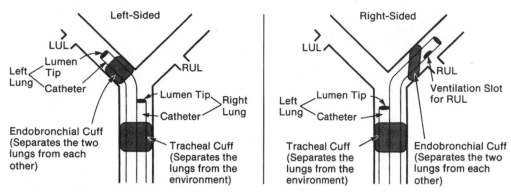

Figure 10-4   Essential features and parts of right-sided and left-sided double-lumen tubes. (From Benumof JL. *Anesthesia for thoracic surgery*. Philadelphia: WB Saunders, 1997.)

diaphragmatic muscle efficacy. The dome of the lower diaphragm is being pushed higher in the thoracic cavity, and its contraction is more efficient. Ventilation ($\dot{V}$) and perfusion ($\dot{Q}$) are thus properly matched in the awake patient in the lateral decubitus position (Figures 10-8 and 10-9).

On anesthetizing the patient, the distribution of blood flow doesn't change, with gravity being the major determinant. However, with the loss of FRC secondary to anesthesia, the nondependent lung moves to the steeper portion of the pressure–volume curve and the dependent lung is now on the lower, flatter portion. The compliance of the nondependent lung is therefore greatly enhanced, and it will receive more ventilation than the lower lung (Figure 10-10). Another important factor is the weight of the mediastinum and the abdominal contents now pushing more on the lower lung than on the upper lung, impeding ventilation of the lower lung. Ventilation is now directed towards the more compliant nondependent lung, resulting in an increased degree of $\dot{V}/\dot{Q}$ mismatching, as blood flow distribution is still greater to the dependent lung.

Opening the chest in an awake patient results in the same clinical picture as an open pneumothorax. Stable, spontaneous ventilation cannot be contemplated. The loss of pleural pressure on the nondependent, opened chest cavity causes atmospheric pressure to collapse the upper lung and push on the mediastinum, exerting pressure on the dependent lung. On inspiration, negative pressure in the dependent cavity causes more mediastinal

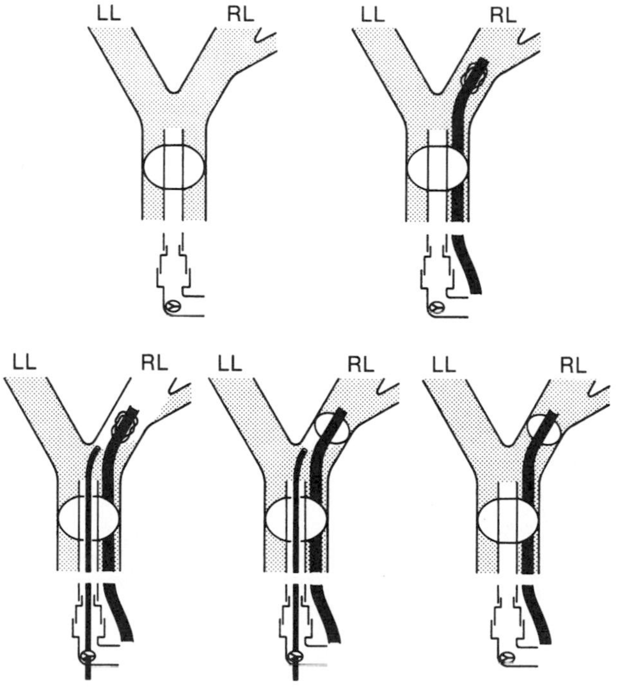

Figure 10-5   Lung separation with a single lumen tube, fiberoptic bronchoscope, and right lung bronchial blocker tube (From Benumof JL. *Anesthesia for thoracic surgery*. Philadelphia: WB Saunders, 1997.)

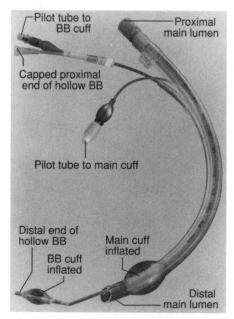

Figure 10-6   The Univent tube. (From Benumof JL, Alfery DD. Anesthesia for thoracic surgery. In: Miller RD, *Anesthesia*, 5th ed. New York: Churchill Livingstone, 2000.)

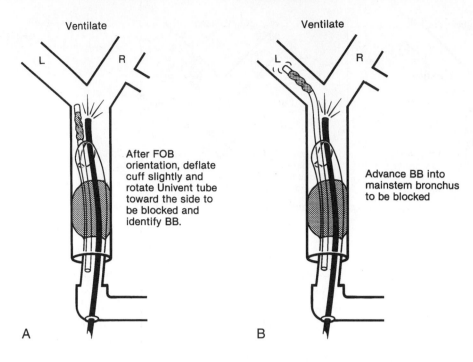

Ventilate

L   R

After FOB orientation, deflate cuff slightly and rotate Univent tube toward the side to be blocked and identify BB.

A

Ventilate

L   R

Advance BB into mainstem bronchus to be blocked

B

Figure 10-7   Isolating a lung with a Univent tube and a bronchoscope. FOB, fiberoptic bronchoscope; BB, bronchial blocker. (From Benumof JL. *Anesthesia for thoracic surgery*. Philadelphia: WB Saunders, 1997.)

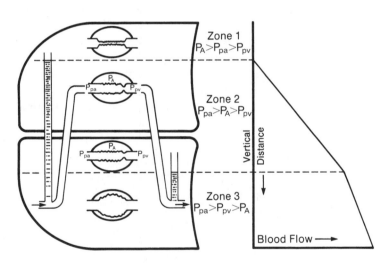

Zone 1
$P_A > P_{pa} > P_{pv}$

Zone 2
$P_{pa} > P_A > P_{pv}$

Zone 3
$P_{pa} > P_{pv} > P_A$

Vertical Distance

Blood Flow →

Figure 10-8   Effects of gravity on the distribution of pulmonary blood flow in the lateral decubitus position. (From Benumof JL. *Anesthesia for thoracic surgery*. Philadelphia: WB Saunders, 1997.)

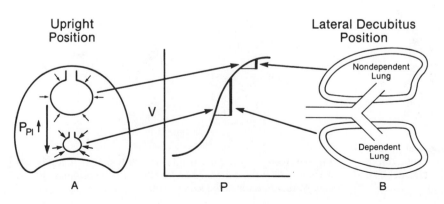

Upright Position

P_{Pl}

A

Lateral Decubitus Position

Nondependent Lung

Dependent Lung

V

P

B

Figure 10-9   Awake, closed-chest distribution of ventilation related to the pressure–volume curve. (From Benumof JL. *Anesthesia for thoracic surgery*. Philadelphia: WB Saunders, 1997.)

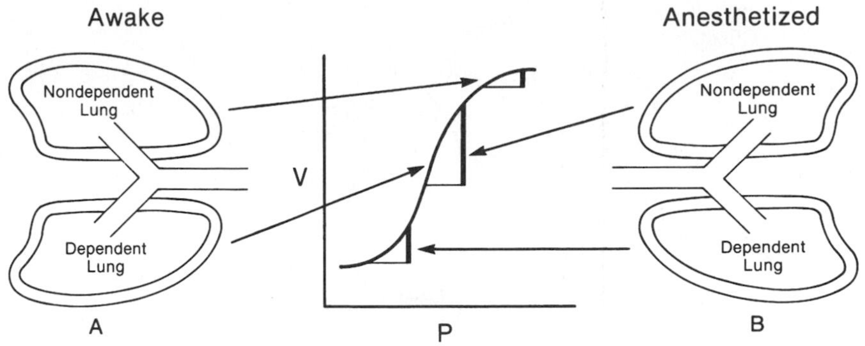

Figure 10-10   Distribution of ventilation in the awake and the anesthetized patient, in lateral decubitus, closed chest. (From Benumof JL. *Anesthesia for thoracic surgery*. Philadelphia: WB Saunders, 1997.)

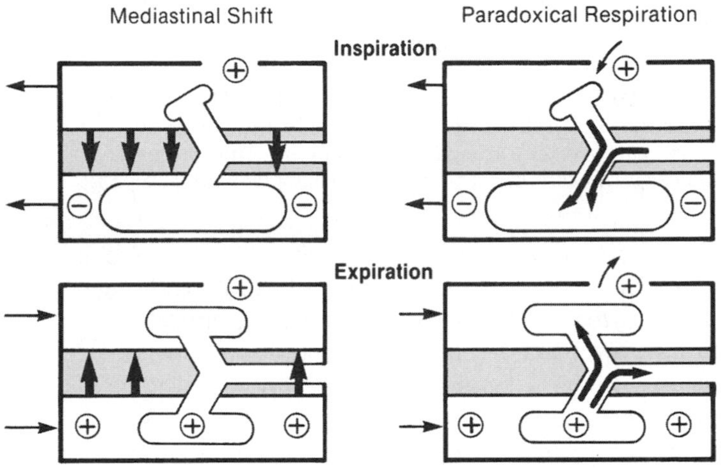

Figure 10-11   Schematic representation of mediastinal shift and paradoxical respiration. (From Benumof JL. *Anesthesia for thoracic surgery*. Philadelphia: WB Saunders, 1997.)

shift and more upper lung collapse. Moreover, on expiration, part of the expired tidal volume expands the nondependent lung. This phenomenon is called paradoxical respiration (Figure 10-11).

Positive-pressure ventilation thus appears as the only way to conduct open-chest surgery safely. As we have seen, anesthetizing the patient shifts the nondependent lung to a steeper portion of the pressure–volume curve. Mechanical ventilation will therefore go preferentially to the upper lung. However, gravity still favors blood flow to the lower lung. The mismatch persists, unless surgical retraction or compression redirects some respiratory volume to the non-operated dependent lung. Muscle paralysis may further

aggravate the mismatch. Flaccid paralysis of the diaphragm creates more resistance to lung expansion in the dependent thoracic cavity because of the pressure exerted by the abdominal contents. The less ventilated lung continues to receive more perfusion. Suboptimal positioning may also aggravate the mismatch, putting more pressure on the lower lung (Figures 10-12 and 10-13).

One-lung Ventilation

When ventilation to the nondependent lung is stopped, an obligatory shunt is created, resulting in an increased alveolar-to-arterial oxygen tension gradient

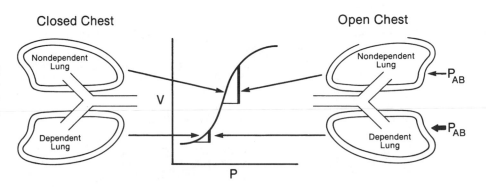

Figure 10-12   Anesthetized, lateral decubitus position distribution of ventilation. (From Benumof JL. *Anesthesia for thoracic surgery*. Philadelphia: WB Saunders, 1997.)

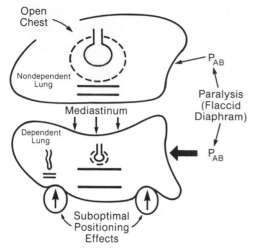

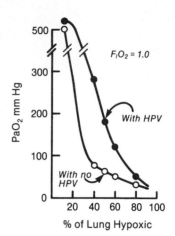

Figure 10-13   Summary of ventilation–perfusion relationships in the anesthetized patient in the lateral decubitus position with an open chest, paralyzed, and suboptimally positioned. (From Benumof JL. *Anesthesia for thoracic surgery*. Philadelphia:WB Saunders, 1997.)

Figure 10-14   Effect of hypoxic pulmonary vasoconstriction (HPV) on P_aO_2 as a function of the percentage of hypoxic lung. (From Benumof JL. *Anesthesia for thoracic surgery*. Philadelphia: WB Saunders, 1997.)

($P_{A-a}O_2$). One would expect to have a $\dot{Q}_s/\dot{Q}_t$ ratio of at least 50% because only half of the total lung parenchyma is ventilated while being entirely perfused. Nevertheless, this is not exactly the case since passive (gravity, surgical compression and degree of pre-existing disease in the nondependent lung) and active compensation mechanisms, the most important of which being hypoxic pulmonary vasoconstriction (HPV), come into play to redirect blood flow to the dependent, ventilated lung (see Figure 10-14). HPV re-directs blood flow from the atelectatic, hypoxic, non-ventilated lung towards the remaining normoxic lung. This mechanism is only capable of diminishing blood flow to the hypoxic lung by half. The upper/lower lung perfusion ratio is already 40/60% because of gravity, when both lungs are ventilated. Considering that an obligatory shunt of 10% is distributed equally between both lungs, the fractional blood flow to the nondependent lung on one lung ventilation is now 5 + 35/2 = 22.5% and the total shunt fraction is: 10 + 35/2 = 27.5% (Figure 10-15).

These are only theoretical values. One must not assume that the dependent lung is entirely perfused. General anesthesia, circumferential compression, absorption atelectasis from high fractional inspired oxygen (F_iO_2) and secretion accumulation all contribute to decreasing the dependent lung volume and creating shunt areas. HPV in these atelectatic zones will therefore increase blood flow to the nondependent lung.

Many intrinsic or extrinsic factors affect HPV. Hypocapnia is thought to directly inhibit HPV. Conversely, hypercapnia enhances regional HPV. However, hypocapnia and hypercapnia are often associated with hyper- and hypoventilation respectively, both of which have a direct effect on airway pressures in the ventilated lung and can act positively or negatively on vascular resistance.

Extrinsic factors include systemic vasodilator drugs such as nitroglycerin, nitroprusside, and dobutamine. Vasoconstricting medications indirectly inhibit HPV by constricting preferentially normoxic lung vessels. As a result, blood is shunted towards atelectatic lung, with a negative effect on HPV.

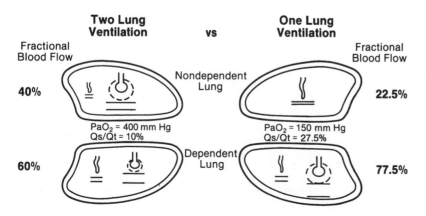

Figure 10-15   Shunt fraction when comparing one-lung ventilation with two-lung ventilation. (From Benumof JL. *Anesthesia for thoracic surgery*. Philadelphia:WB Saunders, 1997.)

Box 10-4   Overall One-lung Ventilation Plan

1. Maintain two-lung ventilation until pleura is opened
2. Dependent lung
   - $F_iO_2 = 1.0$
   - TV = 10 mL/kg
   - RR = so that $P_aCO_2 = 40$ mmHg
   - Positive end-expiratory pressure (PEEP) = 0.5 mmHg
3. If severe hypoxemia occurs
   a. Check position of double-lumen tube with fiberoptic bronchoscopy
   b. Check hemodynamic status
   c. Nondependent lung continuous positive airway pressure
   d. Dependent lung PEEP
   e. Intermittent two-lung ventilation
   f. Clamp pulmonary artery as soon as possible (for pneumonectomy)

From Miller RD, *Anesthesia*, 5th ed. New York: Churchill Livingstone, 2000.

Anesthetic agents and their effect on HPV have been studied over the last few years. Although there is a tendency to believe that volatile anesthetics inhibit HPV and that intravenous anesthesia, especially propofol, preserves HPV, the clinical data are not consistent. Abe *et al*. compared the effects of sevoflurane against propofol, and isoflurane against propofol during OLV, each patient serving as his own control. They found a rise in P_aO_2 and a reduced shunt fraction with propofol compared to both volatile agents. On the other hand, Beck *et al*. studied two groups undergoing OLV, comparing the effects of propofol and sevoflurane. They could not find a significant difference in P_aO_2 or shunt fraction between the two groups.

The suggestion to change from a volatile-based anesthetic to a total intravenous anesthetic may be made if oxygenation problems arise during OLV, although no clear clinical evidence exists that it will significantly reduce the shunt fraction. There are more efficient ventilation strategies that may be used when desaturation occurs on OLV. These are listed in Box 10-4.

If desaturation remains after an initial check on the position of the DLT, continuous positive airway pressure (CPAP) on the upper lung should be applied, after delivering an initial tidal volume. CPAP is the first approach to desaturation on OLV because it allows some degree of oxygen uptake in the distended alveoli and, because of increased vascular resistance, diverts blood flow to the lower ventilated lung, thus diminishing shunt fraction. The second step is to apply positive end-expiratory pressure (PEEP) to the dependent lung in an attempt to recruit atelectatic alveoli. This maneuver may increase shunt fraction by overdistending some alveoli, thereby increasing vascular resistance and redirecting blood flow to the nondependent lung.

ANALGESIA FOR THORACIC SURGERY

A well known correlation exists between postoperative thoracotomy pain and morbidity (cardiac, pulmonary, and gastrointestinal). The release of stress hormones and a restrictive lung disease pattern are probably involved. Smaller incisions, as used in video-assisted thoracoscopic surgery (VATS) and other muscle-sparing incisions, are associated with less postoperative pain than the standard posterolateral thoracotomy incision. In performing an esophagectomy, an isolated left thoracotomy incision results in fewer complications than the Ivor Lewis approach, which itself leads to lower morbidity than the transhiatal technique.

The goals of analgesia after thoracic surgery are to minimize postoperative pain, to facilitate coughing and mobilization, to diminish pulmonary complications and overall morbidity and mortality, and to prevent chronic post-thoracotomy pain.

A patient's postoperative care involves much more than analgesia itself. For analgesia to have significant impact, it must be part of a multimodal approach, including respiratory physiotherapy, early mobilization and early feeding.

Regional anesthesia offers several alternatives for intra- and postoperative pain control in patients undergoing thoracic surgery. Contraindications to each procedure must be well known by the practitioner and reviewed in each case, to insure each patient's safety. The risks and benefits of such procedures must be properly explained to the patient and informed consent must be obtained before performing a technique.

Thoracic Epidural Analgesia

Thoracic epidural analgesia (TEA) has become the first choice for post-thoracotomy pain management. In addition to providing better analgesia, there is growing evidence that TEA, along with a multimodal approach, may improve clinical outcome. When compared with systemic analgesia, TEA was associated with fewer perioperative myocardial infarctions, postoperative arrhythmias, and pulmonary complications. Ileus has been found to be less frequent and of shorter duration in patients receiving TEA. Epidural analgesia has also been associated with a decreased incidence of thromboembolic events following hip, knee, and prostate surgery, but the data have not been yet confirmed in thoracic anesthesia. Improved outcome with TEA is probably greater in patients with multiple or severe comorbidities, such as patients undergoing esophagectomy for carcinoma.

Techniques

Median and paramedian approaches are commonly used. An anesthesiologist's experience often dictates the choice of approach. Because of the steeper angle of the thoracic spinous processes, the paramedian approach might prove to be easier. Postdural puncture headache caused by inadvertent dural puncture is thought to be less frequent with the paramedian approach, possibly because it creates a flap rather than a hole through the dura mater. Interestingly, it seems that TEA is not associated with a greater incidence of neurologic injuries when compared to the lumbar approach. This may be due to more experienced anesthesiologists performing thoracic epidural placement and by the tangential trajectory of the needle toward the spinal cord.

Pharmacology

A combination mixture of local anesthetic and opioids is current practice in TEA. While the effect of opioids is primarily analgesic, sympathetic blockade by local anesthetics is the mechanism proposed to explain the beneficial effects of TEA on clinical outcomes mentioned earlier. The use of both medications allows potentiation of their individual analgesic effects through different mechanisms of action. Smaller drug doses are therefore needed to provide pain relief. Side effects are not as frequent and tachyphylaxis to local anesthetic is diminished. Adding patient-controlled epidural analgesia is an option that improves the individual patient's pain control and satisfaction and lowers the total dose of medication administered.

In TEA, lipophilic opioids are preferred since cephalad migration is not needed and drug duration is shorter, allowing for easier titration. Opioids alone provide analgesia that is comparable to mixtures of opioids and local anesthetic, with the exception of the first few hours following surgery, when adjunct local anesthetic may improve analgesia. The use of opioids alone in TEA is an option in cases of known allergy to local anesthetic or if hypotension is a major concern. Neuraxial opioids side effects include pruritus, nausea, vomiting, urinary retention, sedation, and respiratory depression.

Low-dose preservative-free epinephrine (2 μg/ml) may be added to local anesthetic to enhance analgesia. The presumed mechanism of action is the activation of spinal cord alpha-2 receptors.

Lumbar epidural analgesia (LEA) is an alternative option to TEA. When compared to LEA using hydrophilic opioids, TEA with lipophilic opioids is thought to be easier to titrate and to be associated with a lower risk of delayed respiratory depression. While TEA often contains local anesthetic, these are not often used in LEA, thus withholding their potential benefits on outcome. In thoracic anesthesia, placement of a lumbar epidural catheter is considered a good alternative measure in cases of unsuccessful thoracic epidural catheter placement, and an alternative way to provide analgesia in cases where a

thoracotomy incision was unplanned. Contraindications to epidural techniques include patient's refusal, coagulopathy or anticoagulants, infection at the puncture site, systemic infection, uncorrected hypovolemia, and intracranial hypertension. In these cases, other means to provide analgesia must be evaluated.

Systemic Opioids

Systemic opioids are an alternative in providing analgesia for patients undergoing thoracic surgery, especially when anatomical variations or contraindications preclude placement of a thoracic epidural catheter. When compared to systemic analgesia, TEA is thought to offer better analgesia with fewer narcotic-related side effects.

Patient-controlled analgesia seems to provide better pain control, along with lower opioid overall doses and reduced incidence of side effects when compared to intermittent bolus administration by a health care provider. Other advantages of patient-controlled analgesia include simplicity of installation and a patient's sense of control over pain.

Nerve Blocks

Paravertebral, intercostal, and interpleural blocks with local anesthetic are other alternative methods of post-thoracotomy pain management. These blocks act at the intercostal nerve level but the thoracic sympathetic chain may also be involved in interpleural blocks. Placement of a catheter is favored since it allows for continuous infusions and administration of subsequent boluses. Their use can be combined with patient-controlled analgesia or intermittent narcotic injections, helping to limit narcotic doses. Advantages linked to the use of these blocks in thoracic analgesia include improvement in respiratory function and lower incidence of hypotension due to sympathetic blockade. These blocks may be performed while the patient is under general anesthesia, although there is a potential risk for epidural or spinal injection with paravertebral and intercostal approaches. These same techniques may be performed by the surgeon, under direct vision, reducing the risk of misplacement.

Pneumothorax is an uncommon complication and is of minimal concern since a chest tube is often already in place. Toxicity to local anesthetic is of greater concern, especially with intercostal blocks, where systemic absorption is greatest. The addition of epinephrine limits vascular reabsorption of local anesthetic, thus reducing systemic toxicity and prolonging the duration of the block. Another concern with this method of analgesia is the variability of block level obtained with interpleural analgesia, caused by the loss of local anesthetic in chest tube drainage. Clamping of the chest tube for 10–15 minutes to retain local anesthetic is not always possible, as a tension pneumothorax may develop. Alternatively, two interpleural catheters may be inserted at distant sites, providing a more extended block. Patients with pleural fibrosis or pleural effusions have greater systemic absorption of local anesthetic from inflammatory or infected pleura and therefore a higher incidence of local anesthetic toxicity.

Contraindications are the same as those for epidural analgesia – patient's refusal, anticoagulation, and infection at puncture site.

Cryoanalgesia consists of intercostal nerve blocks with the use of a cryoprobe, under direct vision, by the surgeon. Multiple rib fractures from chest trauma are the most often cited indication for this particular technique.

Transcutaneous Electrical Nerve Stimulation

Transcutaneous electrical nerve stimulation (TENS) analgesia involves endorphin release. Successful use is limited to light or moderate types of pain, as after VATS. However, it is a noninvasive means of providing analgesia, with minimal side effects. It is therefore considered to be a useful adjunctive therapy.

Pain at Other Sites

Patients with thoracotomy incisions often complain about pain related to chest tube sites or pain located in the ipsilateral shoulder. This shoulder pain is thought to originate from phrenic afferents. There is a paucity of data on how to treat these entities. Brachial plexus blockade is thought to be ineffective, while phrenic nerve infiltration with local anesthetic alleviates the pain. Although beneficial, phrenic nerve infiltration is likely to cause diaphragmatic dysfunction. Nonsteroidal anti-inflammatory agents such as ketorolac may help both shoulder and chest tube pain. Eutectic mixture of local anesthetic (EMLA) cream has been reported to lessen pain during chest tube removal when compared to systemic opioids. Local anesthetic infiltration directly at the chest tube site is another option. Paravertebral, intercostal or interpleural blocks at the chest tube level could also be considered.

INTRA-OPERATIVE CONSIDERATIONS FOR THORACIC ANESTHESIA

With all the methods available to isolate lungs, we can now look at the specific considerations of various thoracic procedures.

Thoracotomy

Pulmonary resection, including lymph node dissection, is the mainstay of curative treatment for carcinoma of the lung. Depending on the extent of the disease, a single lobectomy or bilobectomy is carried out, or even a pneumonectomy. Positioning is in the lateral decubitus position, usually with flexion of the table. Care must be taken to insure proper alignment of the spine. An axillary roll is placed under the dependent arm and there should be no hyperextension of the upper arm. The incision will be a posterolateral thoracotomy in the fifth or sixth intercostal space with possible rib resection (Figure 10-16). A DLT or BB is used to deflate the operative lung. Standard chest tube placement involves one placed anteriorly and the other posteriorly. Most patients have either an infectious process or a lung neoplasm, with a high incidence of associated cigarette smoking and chronic bronchitis and/or emphysema.

Premedication with sedatives must be titrated according to the pulmonary reserve. Baseline monitors include electrocardiography, noninvasive blood pressure, pulse oximetry, end-tidal CO_2 and temperature. An arterial catheter is usually placed. A central venous pressure (CVP) line may be considered in higher-risk patients.

Complications of this type of surgery include malpositioning of the tube, hypoxemia due to shunt, hypotension due to manipulation of heart or great vessels, and airway rupture. Postoperative injuries related to the lateral decubitus position may occur, such as pressure damage to the ear, eyes, nose, deltoid muscle, iliac crest, or brachial plexus as well as to the radial, ulnar, common peroneal, and sciatic nerves. Deep venous thrombosis prophylaxis with subcutaneous heparin and/or anti-embolic stockings is common.

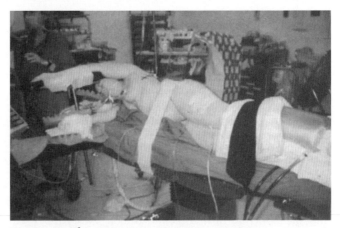

Figure 10-16   The lateral decubitus position, most commonly used for thoracic surgery. In this position, the most common thoracic incision, the posterior lateral incision, is performed. (From Cohen E. *The practice of thoracic anesthesia.* Philadelphia: Lippincott Williams & Wilkins, 1995:262.)

Lobectomy and Wedge Resection

A surgical lobectomy is performed under general anesthesia, often with a thoracic epidural catheter placed preoperatively and used intraoperatively. Monitoring is standard with the addition of an arterial line and a urinary catheter. Intubation is either directly with a DLT or first with a single-lumen tube if a bronchoscopy is initially required to evaluate the tumor.

Wedge resection of the lung is defined as removal of a mass with 1 cm negative margins, in a manner that does not remove an entire anatomical segment. It can be appropriate in patients with limited pulmonary reserve who would not tolerate a lobectomy. Wedge resection can also be performed in cases of single or multiple metastatic lesions. A single metastasis can be removed through a limited thoracotomy incision but bilateral lesions may require a sternotomy. Incisions may thus be either a standard thoracotomy, limited, or median sternotomy, and the positioning lateral decubitus or supine. Lung isolation with a DLT is usually required. The anesthetic considerations are those of a surgical thoracotomy, bearing in mind that candidates for wedge resection are often the ones with the least pulmonary reserve.

Pneumonectomy

Surgical pneumonectomy is indicated for complete removal of lesions involving a main bronchus, those with spread or fixation to the hilum, and those that cross the lobar fissure. It is associated with a 30-day mortality of 5–15%, cardiac morbidity being significant. One should be concerned about the pulmonary reserve after resection, potential pulmonary hypertension, concomitant cardiovascular disease, pulmonary edema, and frequent postoperative cardiac arrhythmias, as well as thromboembolic events.

Pneumonectomy is carried out under general anesthesia with or without associated epidural anesthesia. Monitoring should include an arterial line. A CVP line may be more useful postoperatively than intraoperatively. A pulmonary artery catheter has to be placed under fluoroscopy to insure positioning into the nonoperative side. Transesophageal echocardiography is a good option. A left-sided DLT is usually the first choice, unless the tumor involves the left main bronchus, when a right-sided DLT can be used. For either side, a BB can be used and removed when the surgeon sutures the main bronchus. Another option is to use a single-lumen tube advanced into the opposite bronchus and pulled back after resection. Attention must be paid to ventilation pressures to avoid damage to or rupture of the bronchial stump.

Intravenous fluid administration should be limited intraoperatively because of the high risk of pulmonary edema, atrial fibrillation, and left atrial dilation. Blood loss is usually slight (<500 mL). The stump seal is usually tested with positive pressure breaths. Chest tubes are not placed. Air may be aspirated to a pleural pressure of –4 to –10 cmH$_2$O to prevent mediastinal shift.

Thoracoscopy

Video-assisted thoracoscopic surgery is most often used for assessment of pleural processes of unknown etiology. It is also used for the treatment of spontaneous pneumothorax due to bullae, biopsy of peripheral infiltrates or nodules, and for drainage of pleural effusions. Small, accessible tumors may also be removed. VATS has also been used for lung volume reduction surgery, Heller myotomy, and upper dorsal sympathectomy.

Anesthetic considerations are those of the underlying disease. Positioning is in the lateral decubitus position. Three or four small portal incisions are made. A DLT is highly recommended as a well collapsed lung is essential for good visualization. A chest tube will be left in place at the end of the surgery.

General anesthesia with use of a DLT or BB to isolate the diseased lung is the preferred technique. Monitoring includes American Society of Anesthesiologists (ASA) standard monitors and an arterial line may be considered. As the chest is opened, air enters the pleural cavity, causing a partial pneumothorax, with potential for dyspnea and visceral discomfort. Regional anesthesia is an option – the incision site is infiltrated with local anesthetics and intercostal nerve blocks are placed at the level of the incision and also at several levels above and below. Thoracic epidural anesthesia may also be used.

Complications include air leak from the operative lung, hemorrhage, injury to thoracic structures, and air embolism. There is approximately a 4% risk of conversion to open thoracotomy. Pain is less than with an open thoracotomy.

Tracheal Resection

Indications for tracheal resection are primary tumors (malignant and benign), secondary tumors by direct extension or metastasis, inflammatory lesions including postintubation and post-traumatic lesions, connective tissue disease, and compressive lesions. Rigid bronchoscopy is the key to determining the nature, length, location, and degree of obstruction. Therapeutic options for obstruction of the airway include radiation, dilation, laser, stents, tracheostomy (in the most damaged area), and surgery.

The chosen surgical approach will depend on the location of the lesion. High and mid-tracheal lesions are done with the patient supine, with an inflatable bag between the scapulas to provide full neck extension

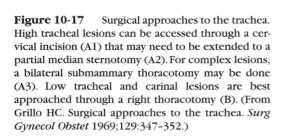
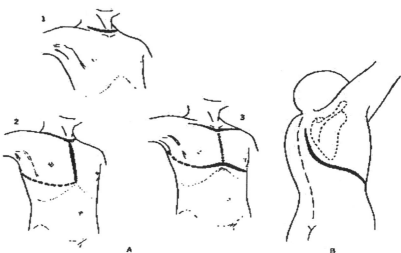

Figure 10-17 Surgical approaches to the trachea. High tracheal lesions can be accessed through a cervical incision (A1) that may need to be extended to a partial median sternotomy (A2). For complex lesions, a bilateral submammary thoracotomy may be done (A3). Low tracheal and carinal lesions are best approached through a right thoracotomy (B). (From Grillo HC. Surgical approaches to the trachea. *Surg Gynecol Obstet* 1969;129:347-352.)

which can be reversed at the end. An alternative approach is through a collar incision with or without an upper sternotomy. Low tracheal lesions may be done supine or in the left lateral decubitus position, with the neck flexed. The proposed surgical approach is then through a right posterolateral thoracotomy in the fourth intercostal space. For carinal lesions, a right posterolateral approach or a median sternotomy may be chosen. A bilateral submammary trans-sternal approach may be required for extensive resections (Figure 10-17)

One of the main challenges of tracheal resection lies in sharing the airway with the surgeon. The decision to premedicate with sedative agents must be carefully weighed. Monitoring will include standard ASA monitors with an arterial line on the left side, as compression of the innominate artery during surgery is possible and should be monitored. A CVP or pulmonary flow catheter should be used if indicated by the general status of the patient. Induction must not be rushed. A rigid bronchoscope should be available in case of critical obstruction.

Many techniques have been used, dictated by each patient's condition and their preoperative evaluation (see above). In most cases reported, an inhalation induction was chosen as the safest method. An adequate preoxygenation period is followed by introduction of the inhalation agent. Spontaneous ventilation is maintained. As the depth of anesthesia increases, the airway is topicalized with local anesthetic and ventilation is resumed until intubation. A full range of endotracheal tube sizes (cuffed and uncuffed) must be available. The tip of the tube can be above or below the lesion. Maintenance agents must be chosen, taking into consideration that the patient will ideally be extubated at the end of the procedure.

When the trachea is opened, ventilation can be accomplished by various methods (Table 10-3).

Cardiopulmonary bypass was popular for carinal resection in the 1960s but the bleeding risks are high. It can also be used to secure the airway, especially in pediatric patients.

After the trachea is resected, the patient's head is flexed at 35° and a guardian stitch is placed between the chin and anterior chest, which will remain in place for 7-10 days. Extubation should take place as early as possible. If reintubation is required, it is best done with a fiberoptic bronchoscope. Complications include dehiscence of the anastomosis and, rarely, infection. Tetraplegia has also been reported, due to hyperflexion of the neck.

Table 10-3	**Methods of Ventilation for Tracheal Resection**
Ventilation Method	**Comment**
Manual oxygen jet ventilation (low-frequency jet ventilation)	High tidal volumes
	Gas trapping can cause barotraumas
High frequency ventilation:	Can ventilate both lungs independently
High-frequency positive-pressure ventilation (HFPPV)	V_t size of anatomic dead space at 1-2 Hz (60-120 bpm)
High-frequency jet ventilation (HFJV)	Pulses of small jet of gas derived from a high pressure source (50 psi) at 1.7-6.7 Hz
High-frequency oscillation ventilation (HFOV)	Air entrainment
	V_t 50-80 ml at 6.7-40 Hz
Distal tracheal intubation and intermittent positive pressure ventilation	Most frequent – sterile endotracheal tube inserted by surgeon into distal trachea and pulled back for suturing during short apneic periods

Bronchopulmonary Lavage

This procedure is performed in patients with pulmonary alveolar proteinosis. Indication for lavage is a P_aO_2 less than 60 mmHg at rest, or hypoxemic limitation of normal activity. Rarely, lavage has been performed for asthma, cystic fibrosis, and radioactive dust inhalation.

Unilateral lavage is done under general anesthesia with a DLT, as isolation of the two lungs is imperative. The most affected side will be done first. Patient monitoring will include standard ASA monitors plus an arterial line and often a CVP or pulmonary flow catheter, depending on the general condition of the patient. The procedure can take several hours and care must be taken to monitor and maintain body temperature. After adequate preoxygenation, general anesthesia is induced and the largest possible DLT is placed. Precise placement is confirmed by fiberoptic bronchoscopy. A leak test must be performed to insure a tight seal.

Patient positioning is also important. The lateral decubitus position with the lavaged lung in the dependent position minimizes the risk of spillage but worsens $\dot{V}/\dot{Q}$ mismatch. The supine position can be used to balance the risks of aspiration and hypoxemia.

The operating room ventilator should be able to deliver high ventilatory pressures. Airway pressures, compliance, and volumes should be measured and recorded. Blood gases should be obtained. The fluid used to lavage the lung is warm isotonic saline and is infused by gravity, from 30 cm above midaxillary line. Drainage is accomplished by clamping the inflow line and unclamping the drainage line in a collection bottle placed 20 cm below the patient (Figure 10-18). Each filling is accompanied by chest percussion. When the fluid is infused, a decrease in perfusion of the diseased lung decreases the shunt fraction, thus improving oxygenation temporarily. The opposite occurs when the lung is drained. Total volume infused is usually between 10 and 20 liters. Complications include hypoxemia, variations in cardiac output, and massive spillage. Adequate muscle relaxation is recommended.

Mediastinoscopy

Mediastinoscopy is carried out to evaluate extrapulmonary spread of tumors, to diagnose and resect anterior mediastinal masses, and to place electrodes for atrial pacing of the heart. It is contraindicated in cases of thoracic aneurysm or obstructed superior vena cava, as the

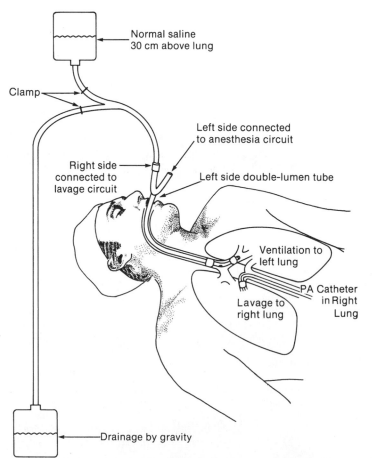

Normal saline
30 cm above lung

Clamp

Left side connected
to anesthesia circuit

Right side
connected to
lavage circuit

Left side double-lumen tube

Ventilation to
left lung

Lavage to
right lung

PA Catheter
in Right
Lung

Drainage by gravity

Figure 10-18 Technique for providing unilateral pulmonary lavage. A left clear plastic double-lumen endotracheal tube allows ventilation to the left lung during lavage of the right lung (and vice versa). Normal saline is infused and drained by gravity; clamps on the connection tubes determine direction of fluid flow. PA, pulmonary flow. (From Benumof JL. *Anesthesia for thoracic surgery*, 2nd ed. Philadelphia: WB Saunders, 1995:549.)

endoscope may puncture the distorted vessels. The endoscope is inserted into the upper mediastinum through a small transverse incision just above the sternal notch. This allows access to the lymph nodes anterior and to the right of the trachea. Proximity to major vessels raises the risk of massive hemorrhage. For nodes on the left side, an anterior mediastinotomy is performed through the second interspace with the patient supine.

Anesthetic considerations for patients with mediastinal masses include the potential for complete airway obstruction or cardiovascular collapse on induction of general anesthesia. The anesthetic plan should be established according to the preoperative airway evaluation and the expected risk of obstruction on induction. Even when the patient is considered at low risk of airway obstruction, a careful approach is still indicated. Options for induction include initial awake fiberoptic intubation or a mask induction with sevoflurane with the patient spontaneously breathing. If muscle relaxants are chosen, it is best to start with a short-acting agent like succinylcholine.

The presence of an experienced surgeon equipped with a rigid bronchoscope in the operating room during induction is prudent. Monitoring is standard. In cases of superior vena cava syndrome, a large-bore intravenous or CVP line should be placed in the femoral vein. The blood pressure cuff should be placed on the left arm and the pulse oximeter or arterial line on the right arm, as the mediastinoscope or mass may compress the innominate artery. Arterial compression can lead to compromised cerebral perfusion and subsequent cerebrovascular ischemia.

Complications associated with mediastinoscopy are rare but can be life-threatening. Bleeding may be due to a major vessel rupture, requiring emergency thoracotomy or sternotomy. Air embolism is possible when the patient's head is elevated. Airway rupture or obstruction may require immediate thoracotomy and tracheal collapse may require rigid bronchoscopy to open the airway. Phrenic or recurrent laryngeal nerve damage is also possible. Postoperatively all patients should have a chest radiograph to rule out a pneumothorax.

Esophagogastric Fundoplasty

Esophagogastric fundoplasty represents a variety of surgical procedures designed to prevent acid reflux by wrapping the fundus of the stomach around a 3–4 cm segment of the lower esophagus, which reinforces the lower esophageal sphincter. The approach may be transabdominal, transthoracic, or laparoscopic. The most frequent approach is the open or laparoscopic Nissen fundoplication.

Positioning for this procedure is supine. The incision is midline or through multiple laparoscopic ports. A nasogastric tube is required, as are Hurst dilators. Anesthetic considerations include the need for premedication with H_2 antagonists, metoclopramide, and sodium citrate. Rapid sequence induction is indicated.

Mortality is low (<0.5%) and morbidity includes recurrent hernia (20%), gas bloat syndrome (10–20%), temporary dysphagia (5–10%), and gastric fistula (<2%).

Esophagectomy

Esophagectomy is commonly performed for malignancies of the middle and lower thirds of the esophagus. Barrett's esophagus is another common cause. The mortality rate is less than 5% but the complication rate is 10–27% and includes anastomotic disruption with sepsis, pulmonary insufficiency, diaphragmatic herniation, and massive aspiration.

The surgical approach varies according to lesion site. Lesions in the lower third of the esophagus are usually approached via a left thoracoabdominal incision. Lesions of the middle third are usually approached via the abdomen and right chest (Ivor Lewis approach). Another variation is to go through the abdomen and the neck by blunt dissection. A total esophagectomy can also be performed via an abdominal incision and right thoracotomy with a colonic interposition and anastomosis in the neck. Endoscopic resection is being developed.

Premedication should include acid reflux prophylaxis. Preoperative dehydration and malnutrition are frequent concerns. General anesthesia is used, often in combination with thoracic epidural anesthesia. When a cervical incision is made, this will need to be supplemented with systemic opioids. Induction must be planned considering the aspiration risk of the patient. A rapid-sequence induction or awake technique should be used when appropriate.

Monitoring should include an arterial line, a urinary catheter, and a CVP or pulmonary flow catheter when indicated. Large-bore intravenous access is needed, as blood loss can be significant. Measures to prevent hypothermia should be undertaken, as the surgery will take several hours. Positioning (Table 10-4) can change during surgery and care must be taken to protect all pressure points. Intraoperative complications include those related to OLV, possible important blood loss, hypothermia, hypotension due to compression of vena cava, and dysrhythmias.

Postoperatively, these patients generally go to the intensive care unit (ICU) and many require postoperative ventilation, depending on the extent of the surgical procedure and their preoperative condition. When ventilation is to be continued in ICU, the DLT must to be changed to a single-lumen tube. A tube exchanger should be considered, as edema is frequent after prolonged surgery and reintubation may be challenging. The most feared complication in such cases is an anastomotic leak.

Table 10-4   Anesthetic Considerations for Thoracic Procedures

	Esophagectomy	Blind esophagectomy	Esophago-gastrectomy	Total esophagectomy + colonic interposition
Position	Supine + left/right lateral decubitus	Supine	Left lateral decubitus	Supine and right? lateral decubitus
Incision	Midline abdominal + right or left chest and/or cervical	Cervical and midline abdominal	Thoracoabdominal	Midline + right thoracic and cervical
Intubation	Double-lumen	Standard single lumen	Double-lumen	Double-lumen
EBL	200–300 mL	500–600 mL	200–300 mL	500–600 mL

EBL, estimated blood loss.
From Jaffe RA, Samuels SI. Thoracic surgery. In: *Anesthesiologist's manual of surgical procedures*, 2nd ed. Philadelphia: Lippincott Williams & Wilkins, 1999:171–212.

COMPLICATIONS FOLLOWING THORACIC SURGERY

Anesthesiologists are involved in the postoperative care of patients and a thorough knowledge of the potential complications that may occur during this period is essential. Those more specifically related to the post-thoracic-surgery period will be discussed.

Cardiac Herniation

Cardiac herniation occurs after pneumonectomy and is due to a residual pericardial defect. Precipitating factors include turning the patient from the lateral to the dorsal position, placing the operative lung in a dependent position, active suctioning of the chest tube, using high positive ventilation pressures, and coughing.

Cardiac herniation manifests with sudden cardiorespiratory instability and displacement of the cardiac apex, which is seen pointing towards the lateral chest wall at a right angle on chest radiograph. Twisting of the great vessels and airways results in inferior vena cava syndrome, cardiovascular collapse (inferior vena cava), wheezing (trachea), pulmonary edema (pulmonary veins), or arrhythmia and myocardial ischemia (pericardium).

In this situation, rapid surgical re-exploration is mandatory (mortality rate 50%). The patient must be placed in the lateral decubitus position, with the non-operative side in the dependent position. Suction on the chest tube is stopped. High tidal volumes and PEEP are avoided. A total of 1–2 L of air may be injected into the operative hemithorax and the circulation is supported with vasoactive and antiarrhythmic medications.

Pulmonary Torsion

Pulmonary torsion is caused by increased mobility of the remaining lobes after a lobectomy. Atelectasis or an expanding mass on chest radiograph and severe thoracic pain are suggestive of this complication. Reintervention is necessary to avoid pulmonary infarction. Isolation of the lungs with a DLT is mandatory as massive bleeding from injured lung vessels and airways may occur. The use of PEEP helps in re-expanding the atelectatic lung. Saline lavage removes residual blood and clots. Intravenous steroids may reduce the amount of pulmonary inflammation.

Major Hemorrhage

The incidence of this complication is as high as 3% and the mortality rate is about 23%. Pulmonary, bronchial, or intercostal vessels all are potential sources. Raw surfaces may also bleed. Blood loss will be obvious if the chest tube is patent (the hematocrit value of the chest tube drainage will be higher than 20%). Red blood cell transfusions, correction of coagulation abnormalities, pharmacologic hemodynamic support, and rapid reintervention are the mainstays of treatment.

Acute Respiratory Insufficiency

This is the most common major complication after lung surgery. The incidence is about 4% and the mortality rate is high (50%). Causes specific to lung surgery include diminished residual pulmonary function, lung soiling with blood during surgery, and edema of the remaining parenchyma. Atelectasis from pain, causing splinting, and pulmonary infections are also involved. Adult respiratory distress syndrome (ARDS) is another cause of respiratory insufficiency after thoracic surgery.

Ipsilateral pulmonary edema may occur after re-expansion of the atelectatic lung. Increased vascular permeability is thought to result from hypoxic injury or from mechanical trauma due to rapid re-expansion. Gradual re-expansion of the lung is a preventive measure. Established re-expansion edema is treated with positive pressure ventilation, PEEP, fluid restriction, and diuretics.

Bronchopleural Fistula

Acute rupture of the bronchial stump may be secondary to inadequate surgical closure or to high airway pressures during mechanical ventilation. Risk factors for chronic bronchopleural fistula after lung surgery include radiation therapy, presence of residual cancer tissue at the surgical site, infection, and a long or avascular stump. Symptoms are a large or persistent air leak via the chest tube, hypoxemia, and hypercarbia. When a chest tube is not in place (postoperative pneumonectomy) or not properly functioning, a pneumothorax will build up. In chronic bronchopleural fistula, infected sputum or infected chest tube drainage is often present.

Supportive treatment includes placing a chest tube, discontinuing suction on the chest tube, 100% oxygen therapy, maintaining spontaneous ventilation, placing the affected lung in a more dependent position, and placing a DLT. A DLT is used to prevent lung soiling, to selectively ventilate the healthy lung, or to ventilate both lungs independently. If positive-pressure ventilation is necessary, tidal volumes, inspiratory pressure, and inspiratory period must be reduced. PEEP on the patient's chest tube or occlusion of the chest tube during inspiration may be tried, but a pneumothorax may result. High-frequency jet ventilation has been tried with variable results and requires the use of muscle relaxants. Definitive closure of a bronchopleural fistula necessitates either bronchoscopy, pleurodesis, or surgery.

Contralateral Pneumothorax

The most frequent causes include high airway pressures during re-expansion of the operated lung, damage to the contralateral pleura during surgery, and pleural puncture during CVP line placement.

Chylothorax

Chylothorax occurs from thoracic duct lesion during surgery. Therapeutic intervention includes repeated thoracocentesis, chest tube drainage, parenteral nutrition, pleuroperitoneal shunting, and surgical repair.

Right Heart Failure

There are multiple causes of right heart failure, including:
- increased pulmonary vascular resistance secondary to loss of pulmonary vascular bed
- increased pulmonary blood flow from fluid overload or from sympathetic nervous system activation (stress, pain)

- pulmonary vasoconstriction secondary to hypoxemia (e.g. atelectasis, pneumonia, ARDS), hypercarbia, acidosis, and vasoactive amines
- increased pulmonary vascular resistance secondary to mechanical ventilation (PEEP) or bronchospasm (auto PEEP)
- left heart failure with right septal shift
 Diagnosis and treatment will not be discussed here.

Supraventricular Arrhythmia

Atrial fibrillation is the most common supraventricular arrhythmia, with an incidence of about 20%. Supraventricular tachycardia and atrial flutter are also frequent. Pneumonectomy and bilobectomy are associated with higher rates of supraventricular arrhythmia. Dissection near the mediastinum and distention of right heart cavities with high pulmonary artery pressure are probably involved. Supraventricular arrhythmias are associated with increased morbidity and, perhaps, increased mortality.

Treatment of atrial fibrillation begins with pain control and correction of hypoxemia and hypercarbia. Epidural analgesia has been associated with a reduced incidence of supraventricular arrhythmias. The efficacy of amiodarone and beta-blockers for both prevention and treatment of atrial fibrillation is well documented.

Myocardial Ischemia

Electrocardiographic ischemic changes have been associated with the diminished oxygen saturation observed during the first days after lung surgery. Moreover, stress- or pain-related tachycardia augment myocardial oxygen consumption, increasing the risk of perioperative myocardial ischemia.

Systemic Tumor Embolism

This may arise from surgical manipulation of a pulmonary vein invaded by the lung neoplasm. The most frequent site of embolization is the femoral artery.

Patent Foramen Ovale (PFO) with Right-to-Left Shunt

At least 20% of the adult population have a patent foramen ovale. Right-to-left shunt through a PFO may occur whenever right heart pressures exceed left heart pressures. Causes of right heart failure (discussed earlier) that increase right heart afterload also lead to a rise in right heart pressures. If shunting occurs, hypoxemia is the primary manifestation. Transesophageal echocardiography confirms the diagnosis. Treatment is aimed at treating the cause of the elevated right heart pressure. Of note: air bubbles in intravenous lines should be avoided as systemic embolization is an issue.

Neurologic Complications

Nerve injuries occur during hilar dissection or resection of mediastinal masses. Paralysis is usually not permanent but may take months to resolve.

Phrenic nerve palsy may lead to flail chest and the inability to wean a patient from mechanical ventilation. Gas exchange may be normal, while chest radiographs show one-sided elevation of the diaphragm. Diagnosis is made with fluoroscopy, which shows paradoxical diaphragm movement. Phrenic nerve stimulation and diaphragm plication may be used when normal function does not resume. Vagus nerve palsy leads to gastric atony.

Of interest is the bilateral partial lesion of recurrent laryngeal nerves. This leads to vocal cord adduction with airway occlusion and the need to maintain mechanical ventilation until recovery of normal function occurs. The use of steroid or Teflon injections to improve vocal cord function has been described.

The dreaded complication of paraplegia is related to clamping of the thoracic aorta and/or surgical damage to the spinal branches of the intercostal arteries. Intraoperatively, compressive blood clots or gauzes compressing the epidural space due to inadvertent surgical dissection or aggressive hemostatic packing near the spinal structures may also be contributing factors.

SUMMARY

Anesthesia for thoracic surgery is challenging. Proper care of the patient requires thorough knowledge of several considerations, physiologic principles and potential complications. Keeping ourselves informed about new devices and research findings may help to improve our anesthetic strategies.

SUGGESTED READING

Benumof JL. *Anesthesia for thoracic surgery*, 2nd ed. Philadelphia: WB Saunders, 1995.

Benumof JL, Alfery DD. Anesthesia for thoracic surgery. In: Miller RD, *Anesthesia*, 5th ed. New York: Churchill Livingstone, 2000:1665-1752.

Cohen E. *The practice of thoracic anesthesia*. Philadelphia: Lippincott Williams & Wilkins, 1995.

Jaffe RA, Samuels SI. Thoracic surgery. In: *Anesthesiologist's manual of surgical procedures*, 2nd ed. Philadelphia: Lippincott Williams & Wilkins, 1999:171-212.

Morgan GE, Mikhail MS, Murray MJ. *Clinical anesthesiology*, 3rd ed. New York: Lange/McGraw Hill, 2002:525-551.

Neuroanesthesia

PIYUSH M. PATEL

INTRODUCTION

In the clinical practice of anesthesia, anesthetic agents are targeted at the brain and the spinal cord. Anesthetic agents have a profound influence on the function of both the normal and abnormal central nervous system. Suppression of synaptic function results in a spectrum of effects that range from mild sedation to deep anesthesia and unconsciousness. Simultaneously, anesthetics can modulate cerebral blood flow, either indirectly by suppression of metabolism or directly by the alteration of vascular tone. Anesthetic effects on the brain are also influenced by central nervous system (CNS) pathology. Although the CNS effects are common to all forms of general anesthesia, they are of particular relevance to neuroanesthesia and neurological surgery. An understanding of the physiology and pathophysiology of the CNS, and of CNS anesthetic pharmacology, is therefore essential to the sound and scientific practice of neuroanesthesia.

In this chapter, the discussion of the basic anatomy and physiology of the CNS is followed by the presentation of anesthetic pharmacology. Aspects of neuroanesthesia care, which are common to most neurosurgical conditions, are then presented. Finally, the anesthetic considerations of the major categories of neurosurgical procedures are discussed. It should be noted that the sound neuroanesthesia care can be provided by a number of different approaches and that these approaches depend upon the experience and personal preference of the anesthesia care provider. Therefore, emphasis is placed on a consideration of the pathophysiology of the disease processes and the anesthetic interactions with these processes rather than on the mechanics of anesthetic management. The practical anesthetic approach can then be easily developed.

ANATOMY OF THE CEREBRAL CIRCULATION

Blood flow to the brain is supplied by the carotid and vertebral arteries. The vertebral arteries unite to form a single basilar artery. The paired carotid arteries and the basilar artery provide inflow into the Circle of Willis. The vertebrobasilar circulation provides perfusion primarily to the posterior fossa. The carotid-internal arterial system supplies the remainder of the brain. Although the Circle of Willis can form a conduit through which blood from the carotid and basilar arteries can mix, very little admixture occurs because the blood pressure in these vessels is similar. Furthermore, there is little side-to-side mixing of blood. If a focal occlusion in one of the feeding arteries occurs, the Circle of Willis can serve as a channel through which blood can be shunted between the internal carotid and the vertebrobasilar systems and between the left and right sides.

The superficial and deep cerebral veins are valve-less structures that drain blood from the cerebral cortex and the deeper brain regions respectively. These veins eventually empty into the non-elastic and thick walled dural sinuses. Confluence of the dural sinuses leads to the internal jugular veins. Approximately 60% of the blood in the jugular bulb is derived from the ipsilateral hemisphere and the remainder is derived from the contralateral hemisphere. Admixture of blood from the extracranial venous drainage can occur but is usually less than 5%.

REGULATION OF CEREBRAL BLOOD FLOW (CBF)

Under normal circumstances, the brain, which represents 2% of total body weight, receives about 15% of the cardiac output. The brain's oxygen consumption, about 3.5 ml/100 gm/min, is significantly greater than most other tissues and the high blood flow rate is necessary to support the high metabolic rate (Table 11-1). Electrical activity accounts for approximately 60% of the brain's

Table 11-1   Normal Cerebral Physiologic Parameters

$CBF \ ml^{-1} \cdot 100 \ gm^{-1} \cdot min^{-1}$	50
Grey matter	40
White matter	10
$CMRO_2 \ ml^{-1} \cdot 100 \ gm^{-1} \cdot min^{-1}$	3.5
CBF to CMR ratio	15
ICP mmHg	5-12
PvO_2 mmHg	>35
Energy consumption	
Electrical activity	60%
Basal metabolism	40%

energy consumption. Maintenance of the cellular homeostasis and integrity accounts for the remaining 40% of the energy expenditure. The brain's high metabolic rate and its dependence upon a steady blood flow mandate strict regulation of cerebral blood flow. CBF is normally under chemical and metabolic, myogenic and neural control.

CHEMICAL REGULATION OF CBF

Metabolic Control

Local CBF is tightly coupled with local neuronal metabolic activity. Increases in neural activity result in a coupled increase in blood flow. Conversely, a reduction in metabolic activity is accompanied by a corresponding reduction in local blood flow. The underlying physiologic mechanisms that mediate flow and metabolism coupling have not been clearly defined. By-products of increased metabolism, which include K^+, H^+, adenosine and phosphate, probably play an important role in producing vasodilation. Glutamate, an excitatory neurotransmitter that activates neurons, can result in the production of nitric oxide (NO); NO is a potent vasodilator and its role in flow-metabolism coupling is supported by a considerable amount of experimental evidence. More recent data also implicate glial cells. During increased neuronal activity, uptake of glucose by glia has been demonstrated. Metabolism of glucose to lactate and the subsequent release of lactate from glia can lead to local vasodilation. Finally, both sympathetic and parasympathetic nerves have been implicated in flow-metabolism coupling; however, their precise role remains to be determined.

$PaCO_2$

Carbon dioxide (CO_2) is a potent cerebral vasodilator and is one of the most important modulators of CBF. Within a $PaCO_2$ range of 25 to 80 mmHg, there is a linear relationship between $PaCO_2$ and CBF (Figure 11-1). A change in $PaCO_2$ of 1 mmHg results in a change in CBF of about 1–2 ml/100 gm/min (2–4%). Increases in CO_2 tension above 80 mmHg result in only modest increases in CBF whereas reductions in $PaCO_2$ below 25 mmHg do not result in further decreases in CBF. The effect of CO_2 on CBF is mediated primarily by changes in cerebrospinal fluid (CSF) pH. An increase in CSF pH produced by hypocapnia results in cerebral vasoconstriction. Conversely, a hypercapnia induced decrease in CSF pH is accompanied by cerebral vasodilation. Nitric oxide has been implicated as important mediator of hypercapnia induced vasodilation. The effects of $PaCO_2$ on CBF are not sustained beyond 8 hours because of corresponding changes in CSF pH. With sustained hypocapnia, the initial increases in CSF pH will be moderated by the gradual

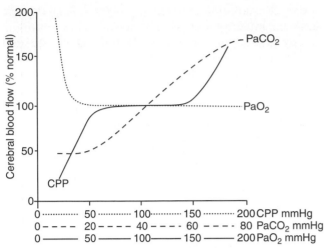

Figure 11-1 The effect of cerebral perfusion pressure, $PaCO_2$ and PaO_2 on cerebral blood flow. (Redrawn from Michenfelder. *Anesthesia and the brain.* Churchill Livingstone, New York, 1988.)

reduction in CSF bicarbonate and CBF will return to normal levels. Acute normalization of $PaCO_2$ levels in patients who have been subjected to sustained hyperventilation therefore has the potential to cause CSF acidosis, thereby leading to dramatic increases in CBF.

PaO_2

The arterial oxygen (O_2) tension has little effect on CBF under normal circumstances. However, reductions in PaO_2 below a level of about 50 mmHg effect dramatic increases in CBF. Further reductions in PaO_2 can lead to CBF increases of more than 400% of baseline flows. Hypoxemia induced increases in CBF are mediated by a direct vasodilator effect of hypoxia on vascular smooth muscle. Increases in NO and adenosine also contribute to vasodilation. Neurons of the rostral ventral medulla are oxygen sensors and their stimulation by hypoxemia can increase CBF significantly. The vasodilatory response to hypoxemia is augmented by simultaneous hypercarbia.

MYOGENIC CONTROL OF CBF

Autoregulation is a physiologic mechanism by which CBF is maintained in a relatively narrow range (~50 ml/100 gm/min) over a wide range of mean arterial pressures. CBF is held constant by an alteration of cerebrovascular resistance; an increase in blood pressure is accompanied by an increase in resistance while resistance will decrease with reduction in blood pressure. Like most physiologic processes, autoregulation is effective only within a certain range of mean arterial pressure (MAP). The upper limit of autoregulation is a MAP of

about 150 mmHg. Increases in MAP beyond 150 mmHg result in a progressive increase in CBF. Conversely, a reduction in MAP below 70 mmHg, the lower limit of autoregulation, will lead to a gradual reduction in CBF. Below the lower limit, cerebral blood flow is essentially pressure passive. Current thinking about autoregulation posits that vascular smooth muscle responds by contraction to an increase in MAP and by dilation to a reduction in MAP.

NEUROGENIC CONTROL OF CBF

Cerebral vessels, both arteries and veins, receive dense sympathetic innervation from the superior cervical ganglion. Stimulation of sympathetic nerves results in relatively modest constriction of cerebral arterioles with little, if any, effect on smaller penetrating vessels. By contrast, sympathetic stimulation can lead to venous constriction and a reduction in cerebral blood volume (CBV). Although the role of sympathetic innervation has not yet been clarified, the available data indicate that this innervation may serve to limit increases in blood flow when arterial pressure exceeds the upper limit of autoregulation. Norepinephrine and neuropeptide Y are the major neurotransmitters in the synaptic vesicles of sympathetic nerve endings. Parasympathetic innervation is derived primarily from the pterygopalatine ganglion. While acetylcholine is the principal neurotransmitter of this system, vasoactive intestinal peptide and nitric oxide also play significant roles. Stimulation of the pterygopalatine ganglion can lead to cerebral vasodilation.

EFFECT OF TEMPERATURE

Brain temperature has a profound effect on brain metabolism. Induction of mild to moderate hypothermia can result in a reduction of cerebral metabolic rate (CMR) by about 5–7%/° C. Electroencephalogram (EEG) silence is observed at a core temperature of about 18–20° C. With mild to moderate hypothermia, flow-metabolism coupling and cerebral vessel responses to $PaCO_2$ and PaO_2 are preserved. By decreasing CMR, hypothermia produces coupled reduction in CBF and CBV. Hyperthermia increases CMR and therefore increases CBF.

EFFECT OF VISCOSITY

Viscosity is a major determinant of laminar flow rate of fluids. One of the major contributors of viscosity to blood is the red cell mass and changes in hematocrit can alter CBF. Within a hematocrit range of 35–45%, little alteration of CBF occurs. With a reduction in hematocrit, blood viscosity is reduced, CBF increases. Conversely, increases in hematocrit beyond 50% can lead to significant reductions in CBF. The ideal hematocrit, one that results in a CBF that optimizes oxygen delivery, is in the range of 30–35%.

EFFECT OF VASOACTIVE AGENTS

α1 Agonists

These agents are potent constrictors of the systemic circulation. However, their effect on the cerebral circulation is limited. Administration of phenylephrine and norepinephrine do not produce vasoconstriction and do not reduce cerebral blood flow. In the presence of hypotension at a level below the lower limit of autoregulation, α1 agonists can increase CBF by increasing MAP.

β Agonists

When administered in low doses, β agonists have little effect on CBF. However, these agents have the propensity to cause anxiety. Increases in CMR that accompany this anxiety can increase CBF indirectly. Their effect on CBF is more pronounced in the setting of a blood–brain barrier that permits entry of parenterally administered β agonists into the brain parenchyma. β receptor mediated increases in neuronal activity can, via flow-metabolism coupling, increase CBF.

Dopamine

Within the dose range of 2.5–10 μg/kg/min, dopamine has little effect on CMR and CBF.

Vasodilators

Both nitroglycerin and nitroprusside are cerebral vasodilators. In low doses, both can increase CBF. With increasing doses, these agents produce systemic hypotension. The corresponding reduction in cerebral perfusion pressure can lead to decreases in CBF.

The effects of vasoactive agents on the cerebral circulation are summarized in Table 11-2

ANESTHETICS AND CNS PHYSIOLOGY

Anesthetic agents have profound effects on cerebrovascular and neuronal physiology. An understanding of these effects is important to the proper use of anesthetic agents for neuroanesthesia and neurosurgery. CNS pharmacology of anesthetic agents is summarized in Table 11-3.

Table 11-2   Effect of Vasoactive Agents on Cerebral Blood Flow

Agent	CPP	CMR	CBF
α1 agonists	↑ ↑ ↑	0	0
α2 agonists	↑ ↑ ↑	↓	↓ ↓
β1 agonists	↑ to 0	0	↑ to 0
β2 agonists	↑ to 0	0	↑ to 0
Dopamine	↑ ↑	0	↑ to 0
Nitroprusside *	↓ ↓ ↓	0	↑ ↑ to ↓ ↓
Nitroglycerin *	↓ ↓ ↓	0	↑ ↑ to ↓ ↓

The values listed in the table pertain to situations in which the blood–brain barrier is intact. * The effect of the vasodilators nitroprusside and nitroglycerin are dependent upon their effects on systemic blood pressure. In doses in which the systemic blood pressure is maintained, cerebral vasodilation will result in increased CBF. In larger doses, a reduction in systemic pressure will decrease CPP, thereby reducing CBF.

Volatile Agents

The volatile agents isoflurane, enflurane, sevoflurane and desflurane produce dose related suppression of CMR. In doses of 1.5 MAC, these agents can produce burst suppression of the EEG. Halothane also reduces CMR but in clinically used doses, it does not produce EEG burst suppression. The effect of volatile agents on CBF is a combination of two opposing influences on the cerebral vasculature. Volatile agents suppress CMR and can reduce CBF. However, this effect is offset by their ability to produce direct cerebral vasodilation. The net effect on CBF is relatively small when administered in doses of 1 MAC or less. Beyond 1 MAC, the direct vasodilation of both the arterial and venous cerebral circulation predominates. Vasodilation mediated increases in CBV can lead to increases in intracranial pressure (ICP). The elevation in ICP is relatively small and its clinical significance in patients with normal intracranial compliance* is questionable. Moreover, volatile agents do preserve the CBF response to $PaCO_2$ and the increase in ICP can be blunted by simultaneous hyperventilation. Nonetheless, in patients with significant intracranial hypertension, anesthetic induced increases in ICP can potentially reduce cerebral perfusion pressure. In these patients, volatile agents should be used with due consideration of their potentially adverse effects on ICP.

Volatile agents cause dose related suppression of somatosensory evoked potentials (SSEP). In sub MAC doses, a gradual increase in the latency and a reduction in the amplitude of SSEP can be observed. In doses of 1 MAC and beyond, complete suppression of SSEP can occur. Limitation of the dose of volatile agents to 1 MAC or less (0.5 MAC is preferable) permits reliable SSEP recording and interpretation. By contrast, transcranial motor evoked potentials (tc-MEP), elicited by transcranial

Table 11-3 Effect of Anesthetic Agents on Cerebral Physiology

	EEG	CMR	Coupling Ratio	CBF	CBV	ICP	CO$_2$ React	SEP Amp	Lat	MEP
Halothane	↓↓	↓↓	↑↑	↑↑↑	↑↑↑	↑↑	0 – ↑	↓	↑	↓↓↓
Isoflurane	↓↓↓ BS	↓↓↓		0 – ↑	0 – ↑	0 – ↑	0 – ↑	↓	↑	↓↓↓
Desflurane	↓↓↓ BS	↓↓↓	↑	0 – ↑↑	0 – ↑↑	0 – ↑↑	0 – ↑	↓	↑	↓↓↓
Sevoflurane	↓↓↓ BS	↓↓↓	↑	0 – ↑	0 – ↑	0 – ↑	0 – ↑	↓	↑	↓↓↓
Nitrous Oxide	0	↑↑	↑	↑↑	↑↑	↑	0	↓	0	↓↓
Barbiturates	↓↓↓ BS	↓↓↓	0	↓↓↓	↓↓↓	↓↓	0	0	↑	↓↓
Propofol	↓↓↓ BS	↓↓↓	0	↓↓↓	↓↓↓	↓↓	0	0	↑	↓↓
Etomidate	↓↓↓ BS	↓↓↓	0	↓↓↓	↓↓↓	↓↓	0	0	↑	0 – ↓
Ketamine	↑	↑ – 0 – ↓	↑	↑	↑	↑	0	0	↑	0 – ↓
Narcotics	↓	0 – ↓	0	0	0	0	0	0	0	0 – ↓
Benzodiazepines	↓	0 – ↓	0	0 – ↓	0 – ↓	0 – ↓	0	0	↑	↓↓
Succinyl Choline*	↑	↑	0	↑	↑	↑	0	0	0	0
Atracurium^a	0	0	0	↑	↑	0 – ↑	0	0	0	0
Cisatracurium	0	0	0	0	0	0	0	0	0	0
Mivacurium^a	0	0	0	↑	↑	0 – ↑	0	0	0	0
Vecuronium	0	0	0	0	0	0	0	0	0	0
Rocuronium	0	0	0	0	0	0	0	0	0	0
Pancuronium	0	0	0	0	0	0	0	0	0	0

* Succinylcholine increases EEG activation primarily due to activation of afferent input from muscle spindles; this increase in metabolism coupled blood flow can be attenuated by the prior administration of a pre-curarizing dose of a non-depolarizing muscle relaxant. ^{a} Effects on cerebral physiology are manifest upon drug induced histamine release.

electrical or magnetic stimulation of the cortex, are completely suppressed by volatile agents in doses as low as 0.2–0.3 MAC. In most cases, reliable MEP monitoring is incompatible with the administration of volatile agents.

Nitrous Oxide (N$_2$O)

When administered alone, N$_2$O is a potent cerebral vasodilator and can increase CBF substantially. The increase in CBF is accompanied by a modest increase in CMR. These cerebrovascular effects of N$_2$O are attenuated by the simultaneous administration of barbiturates, propofol and opiates. In the presence of volatile agents, N$_2$O can lead to further increases in CBF, CBV and ICP. While it is generally agreed that N$_2$O can increase CBF and potentially ICP, the clinical relevance of these effects of N$_2$O is questionable in most neurosurgical patients. In certain patients with intracranial hypertension and in those situations in which surgical brain relaxation is inadequate, the vasodilatory effects of N$_2$O should be taken into consideration.

Barbiturates

Barbiturates produce dose dependent suppression of the EEG, and when administered in relatively large doses, can produce EEG burst suppression. At this level of EEG activity, CMR is suppressed by about 60%. Flow-metabolism coupling is preserved and a reduction in CMR is accompanied by corresponding reductions in CBF, CBV and ICP. Autoregulation and the CBF response to CO$_2$ are preserved. Barbiturates have little effect on SSEP. However, tc-MEP can be attenuated or even abolished by barbiturates.

Propofol

The effects of propofol on the CNS are remarkably similar to those produced by barbiturates. Dose dependent suppression of the EEG, including burst suppression, can be observed. CMR suppression then leads to decreases in CBF, CBV and ICP. Like the barbiturates, autoregulation is maintained and the CBF-CO$_2$ relationship is not altered. Propofol is an ideal agent for purposes of SSEP monitoring. However, tc-MEP can be abolished by propofol.

Narcotics

The synthetic narcotics fentanyl, sufentanil, alfentanil and remifentanil have minimal effects on the cerebral vasculature. Although reductions in CBF and CMR have been demonstrated, these are modest at best. In the absence of a reduction in blood pressure, these narcotics do not increase ICP. The use of high dose narcotics is attended by a shift in the frequencies of the EEG to the delta range. SSEP and tc-MEP monitoring is compatible with the administration of narcotics. Autoregulation and the CBF-CO$_2$ relationship are preserved.

Benzodiazepines

Diazepam and midazolam produce moderate reductions in CMR and CBF. SSEP monitoring, but not tc-MEP monitoring, is compatible with their use. Benzodiazepines do not alter autoregulation or the CBF-CO_2 relationship.

Ketamine

Dose related increases in CMR and CBF have been demonstrated after the administration of ketamine. These effects are effectively blunted by the simultaneous administration of barbiturates, propofol and benzodiazepines. Ketamine administration is compatible with both SSEP and tc-MEP monitoring. Autoregulation and the CBF-CO_2 relationship are preserved.

Muscle Relaxants

The non-depolarizing muscle relaxants do not have significant effects on the cerebral circulation or on ICP. The only concern with the use of these agents is the potential release of histamine and a histamine induced reduction in cerebral perfusion pressure (CPP). With modern relaxants, this is much less of a concern. The administration of the depolarizing muscle relaxant succinylcholine has been shown to produce modest increases in ICP. This increase in ICP, which is most likely due to a fasciculation induced arousal and an increase in CMR, can be effectively blunted by the prior administration of a "pre-curarization" dose of a non-depolarizing muscle relaxant. In the absence of the usual contraindications to its use, succinylcholine can be safely administered in patients with intracranial hypertension.

INTRACRANIAL PRESSURE AND INTRACRANIAL HYPERTENSION

The contents of the cranial vault, brain tissue, CSF and blood, are encased by the dura mater and by the rigid bones of the skull and the skull base. The ICP is therefore determined by the relationship between the volume of the intracranial contents and the volume of the cranial vault. The ICP under normal circumstances, which by definition implies a volume homeostasis between the components of the cranial vault, is approximately 8–12 mmHg. An idealized intracranial pressure volume curve is presented in Figure 11-2.

In pathologic conditions, the volume of the intracranial components, alone or in combination, can rise significantly. Owing to the rigidity of the encasing bone, an increase in the volume of any one component must be offset by a corresponding reduction in the volume of the other compo-

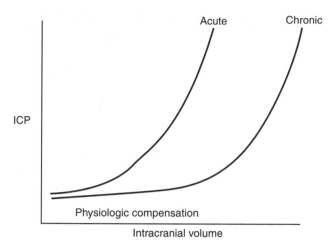

Figure 11-2   The intracranial compartment has a limited ability to compensate for increases in intracranial volume (ICV). When the physiologic compensation capacity is exhausted, an increase in ICV will be accompanied by significant increases in ICP. Compensatory capacity is limited with acute increases in ICV. However, with a slowly progressive increase in ICV, such as might occur with a slowly growing tumor, physiologic compensation can be more effective in limiting increases in ICP.

nents for ICP to remain constant (Monroe Kellie doctrine). With a relatively slow increase in intracranial volume (ICV), as might occur with a slowly growing tumor, translocation of CSF and venous blood from the cranial vault serve as effective volume compensation measures and the rise in ICP is minimized. However, when the volume compensation ability of the brain is exhausted, further increases in ICV can produce dramatic increases in ICP. Since CPP is determined by the difference in the MAP and ICP, increases in ICP can reduce CPP and can lead to the development of ischemia. The reflex response to intracranial hypertension is an increase in MAP that is accompanied by a reduction in heart rate (Cushing response). Further, increases in ICP may result in herniation of brain tissue from one compartment to another. Brain tissue distortion and ischemia, in addition to the primary cause of intracranial hypertension, cause severe neurologic injury. Effective surgical and medical management, to reduce ICP and to improve cerebral perfusion, can mitigate neuronal damage.

Treatment of intracranial hypertension is directed at a reduction in brain bulk, a reduction in cerebral blood volume, modulation of CSF formation and CSF drainage, and surgical evacuation of intracranial mass lesions.

Cerebral Blood Volume

Although CBV comprises about 5% of the intracranial contents, even slight reductions in CBV can effect dramatic changes in ICP. CBV can be manipulated by the following interventions:

1. Maintenance of normal arterial oxygenation. Hypoxemia, with a PaO_2 of less than 60 mmHg, is

a potent cerebro-vasodilator. The importance of maintaining adequate oxygenation is quite self-evident.

2. Hypocapnia. Acute reductions in arterial PCO_2 produce cerebral vasoconstriction and the corresponding reduction in CBV can reduce ICP quite effectively. There are two caveats about hyperventilation that one must be cognizant of. First, sustained hypocapnia leads to compensatory changes in CSF bicarbonate concentrations and its effectiveness in producing cerebral vasoconstriction is significantly reduced by 24 hours. Second, hypocapnia can reduce local blood flow in regions of the brain in which perfusion is already compromised. As such, hypocapnia can potentially aggravate cerebral ischemia. Accordingly, it is recommended that hypocapnia be used as any pharmacologic intervention. Its indications should be defined and the minimum amount of hyperventilation that is necessary to achieve the desired effect should be used. Further, when these indications are no longer present, hypocapnia should be withdrawn. Restoration of normal arterial CO_2 concentrations must be accomplished slowly and with caution given the potential of a rebound increase in CBF (see above).

3. Facilitate venous drainage. Moderate head elevation can facilitate venous drainage and can reduce ICP. Head elevation of about 30° is ideal. Further elevation can reduce MAP and can compromise CPP. Obstruction of venous drainage can occur by kinking of the neck veins (malposition of the head) and by significant increases in intrathoracic pressure. The latter can easily occur with the presence of a pneumothorax or by patient coughing. Attention to proper head position and the judicious use of muscle relaxation can facilitate management.

4. Blood pressure management. In pathologic conditions, cerebral autoregulation may be defective. In these situations, both arterial hypertension and hypotension can produce deleterious effects. Systemic hypotension can further reduce CPP and lead to an exacerbation of cerebral ischemia. Hypertension, particularly in the setting of defective autoregulation, can produce cerebral hyperemia. Clearly, appropriate blood pressure control is an important aspect of the management of intracranial hypertension. A CPP of about 60-70 mmHg is a reasonable target in most patients.

5. Anesthetic management. Volatile agents and nitrous oxide can produce vasodilation. However, under most circumstances, their use is safe and can be easily justified. In situations in which the increase in ICP is severe, consideration should be given to the implementation of an intravenous anesthetic technique. Such situations, which usually arise with traumatic brain injury or in patients in whom the level of consciousness is significantly reduced, are fortunately uncommon. Intravenous anesthetics such as propofol

can reduce CMR substantially and indirectly effect a reduction in CBF, CBV and ICP. Barbiturates have also been used for the treatment of intracranial hypertension. Their use, however, is usually restricted to situations in which the intracranial hypertension is unresponsive to other treatment modalities.

Brain volume

Osmotic and loop diuretics are the primary means by which intracellular and interstitial fluid can be removed.

1. Mannitol. Mannitol, administered in doses that range from 0.25 gm/kg to 1 gm/kg, is an osmotic diuretic that effectively reduces ICP. The onset of its effect can be observed in about 15 minutes and lasts about 2-3 hours. Intravascular volume is initially increased by the osmotic translocation of fluid from the intracellular and interstitial pools. Osmotic diuresis subsequently can reduce intravascular volume. Repeated use of mannitol can lead to a rebound increase in intracranial hypertension. Part of this rebound effect is due to the extravasation of mannitol into the brain tissue in regions where the blood-brain barrier (BBB) is damaged. In addition, the generation of idiogenic osmoles within neurons leads to neuronal swelling once serum osmolarity decreases upon mannitol excretion.

2. Loop diuretics. Loop diuretics reduce ICP primarily by reducing intravascular volume and the formation of CSF. The administration of a loop diuretic simultaneously with mannitol may help in the prevention or attenuation of the rebound increase in ICP. The combination of the two diuretics, however, can produce severe dehydration and attention to appropriate hydration is mandatory.

3. Steroids. Corticosteroids are quite effective in reducing cerebral edema surrounding brain tumors. Steroids are most effective when they are administered at least 48 hours prior to surgery. The available evidence does not favor the use of steroids for the treatment of intracranial hypertension in head injured patients.

CSF drainage

Drainage of CSF from catheters placed in the ventricular system can rapidly reduce ICP. These catheters can also be used to improve visibility in the surgical field, thereby reducing the need for brain retraction.

The approach to the management of intracranial hypertension and inadequate intraoperative brain relaxation is summarized in Table 11-4.

CEREBRAL ISCHEMIA AND BRAIN PROTECTION

One of the most feared complications of anesthesia and surgery is the occurrence of cerebral ischemia and neuronal injury. This has fostered a considerable amount of interest

Table 11-4   Approach to the Swollen Brain

Action	Rationale
Correct hypotension	Hypotension can cause cerebral vasodilation
Correct hypertension	Uncontrolled hypertension can ↑ CBV, ICP
Check PaO₂	Hypoxemia ↑ CBF, CBV, ICP
Check PaCO₂	Hypercarbia ↑ CBF, CBV, ICP Check ABG, don't rely simply on Et-CO₂ Hyperventilation to PaCO₂ ~ 25–30 mmHg
Elevate head	Head elevation facilitates venous drainage, ↓ ICP
Check neck position	Impedance of venous drainage can ↑ CBV, ICP
Muscle relaxation	Coughing, straining ↑ ICP
Check inspiratory pressure	Rule out pneumothorax (CVP placement)
Mannitol	Osmotic diuretic, ↓ brain volume
Furosemide	Loop diuretic, ↓ CSF production, ↓ brain volume
CSF drainage	
Discontinue N₂O	N₂O is a cerebral vasodilator
Discontinue volatile anesthetic	Volatile anesthetics can ↑ CBF, CBV, ICP
Switch to TIVA technique	Propofol ↓ CBF, CBV, ICP
Barbiturate coma	Barbiturates ↓ CBF, CBV, ICP
Brain amputation	Maneuver of last resort

Routine maneuvers are listed in the upper part of the table. In the event that brain relaxation is not achieved with those maneuvers, suggestions in the bottom half of the table can then be followed.

in not only evaluating measures designed to prevent cerebral ischemia but also in identifying anesthetic agents that might decrease the brain's vulnerability to ischemia.

PATHOPHYSIOLOGY

The brain is metabolically very active and its oxygen consumption is about 3.5–4.0 ml/100 gm/min. Electrical activity of neurons (transient depolarization and repolarization with their attendant ionic shifts) consumes about 60% of the total energy production of neurons. Thus, energy consumption can be reduced significantly by agents that can render the EEG isoelectric (e.g., barbiturates). The remaining 40% is used to maintain basal cellular homeostasis. Although this portion of the total energy consumption is not amenable to reduction by anesthetic agents, hypothermia can reduce it substantially.

The normal CBF in humans is about 50 ml/100 gm/min. The response of the brain to ischemia has been well characterized. With a moderate reduction of CBF, slowing of the EEG is observed (Figure 11-3). When CBF reaches

about 20 ml/100 gm/min, EEG isoelectricity occurs. At a flow of about 15 ml/100 gm/min, evoked responses can no longer be obtained. Although neurons do not immediately die at this flow rate, death will eventually occur if flow is not restored. Below a flow of 10 ml/100 gm/min, ATP levels decline rapidly (within 5 minutes) and the neuron is unable to maintain ionic homeostasis. At this point, the neuron undergoes depolarization (anoxic depolarization) and neuronal terminals release massive quantities of neurotransmitters. These neurotransmitters (such as glutamate) activate post-synaptic receptors which results in the neuron being flooded with calcium. By activating several biochemical cascades in a haphazard manner, calcium ultimately leads to neuronal death.

Cerebral ischemia is broadly classified into two categories: global ischemia and focal ischemia. Global ischemia is characterized by a complete cessation of CBF (e.g., cardiac arrest). In this situation, neuronal depolarization occurs within 5 minutes. Selectively vulnerable neurons within the hippocampus and cerebral cortex are the first to die. The window of opportunity for the restoration of flow is very small because death of neurons is rapid. Focal ischemia is characterized by a region of dense ischemia (the so called "core") that is surrounded by a larger variable zone that is less ischemic (the penumbra). Within the core, flow reduction is severe enough to result in relatively rapid neuronal death. Flow reduction in the penumbra is sufficient to render the EEG isoelectric but not severe enough to kill neurons rapidly. If, however, the flow is not restored, death and infarction will also occur in the penumbra albeit at a much slower rate. Because of this slow rate of neuronal death, the window of opportunity for therapeutic intervention that is designed to salvage neurons is considerably longer in the setting of focal ischemia. Most episodes of ischemia in the operating room are focal in nature.

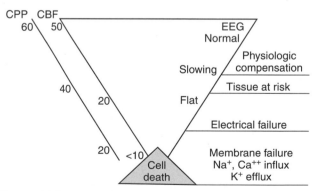

Figure 11-3 The effect of a reduction of cerebral perfusion pressure on cerebral blood flow and EEG. Rapid membrane failure and ionic flux, with attendent cell swelling and death occur when CBF is less than 10 ml/100 gm⁻¹/min⁻¹. CPP: cerebral perfusion pressure in mmHg; CBF: cerebral blood flow in ml/100 gm⁻¹/min⁻¹. (Adapted from Shapiro HM.)

INFLUENCE OF ANESTHETICS ON THE ISCHEMIC BRAIN

The approach to the problem of cerebral ischemia was initially focused on reducing the brain's requirement for energy. The rationale was that by reducing ATP requirements, the brain would be able to tolerate ischemia for a longer time. Such a supply and demand concept had already been proven to be relevant in the case of cardiac ischemia. Therefore, the agents investigated first were those that could render the EEG isoelectric (such agents would be capable of reducing ATP requirements by 60%).

Barbiturates

Barbiturates can produce isoelectricity of the EEG and they have been studied extensively. In the setting of global ischemia, barbiturates in EEG burst suppression doses do not reduce ischemic injury. Barbiturates have been found to be efficacious in the treatment of focal ischemia. In humans, thiopental loading has been demonstrated to reduce post-cardiopulmonary bypass neurologic deficits. As a result, barbiturates have been considered to be the "gold standard" cerebral protectants among anesthetics. More recent studies, while having confirmed the protective efficacy of barbiturates, have shown that EEG burst suppression may not be necessary to achieve maximal protection with barbiturates.

Volatile Anesthetics

There is little doubt that volatile agents can reduce ischemic cerebral injury. In doses of 1–1.5 MAC, isoflurane, halothane and sevoflurane have demonstrated neuroprotective efficacy. More recent studies indicate that volatile agents produce only transient protection and that neuronal survival is not sustained. It should be noted that, by delaying neuronal death, volatile agents might increase the duration of the therapeutic window for the administration of other agents that have neuroprotective efficacy.

Propofol

Propofol shares a number of properties with barbiturates. In particular, propofol can also produce burst suppression of the EEG, thereby reducing $CMRO_2$ by 50–60%. Experimental studies have shown that propofol has neuroprotective efficacy that is similar to that of barbiturates and volatile agents. Nonetheless, given the long history of their use, barbiturates are still considered to be the standard for anesthetic mediated brain protection.

Etomidate

On paper, etomidate appears to be the ideal neuroprotective agent. It can reduce $CMRO_2$ by up to 60% by producing EEG burst suppression. Furthermore, unlike the barbiturates, etomidate is cleared rapidly and it does not cause myocardial depression or hypotension. Experimental studies in models of focal ischemia revealed, surprisingly, that etomidate actually increased the volume of brain infarction. Furthermore, etomidate administration in the setting of cerebral ischemia in humans can actually reduce cerebral blood flow. This injury enhancing effect of etomidate has been attributed to its ability to reduce nitric oxide levels in ischemic brain tissue (either by inhibiting nitric oxide synthase or by directly scavenging nitric oxide). Since nitric oxide is thought to be important in the maintenance of blood flow during ischemia, it is conceivable that etomidate might increase the severity of ischemia. The available data indicate that etomidate should be avoided in situations in which the risk of cerebral ischemia exists.

CEREBRAL ISCHEMIA – INFLUENCE OF PHYSIOLOGIC PARAMETERS

Physiologic parameters, such as MAP, $PaCO_2$, blood glucose and body temperature, have a significant influence on the outcome after cerebral ischemia. In fact, greater emphasis should be placed on the maintenance of physiologic homeostasis than on the administration of anesthetic agents for their putative neuroprotective effects.

Body Temperature

The effect of deep and moderate hypothermia on the brain's tolerance is well known. For example, while the normothermic brain undergoes injury after 5 min of ischemia, the brain made hypothermic to a temperature of 16° C can tolerate ischemia for up to 30 minutes (and longer in certain situations). Similarly, cardiopulmonary bypass (CPB) is usually conducted at a temperature of 28° C in part to reduce the potential of ischemic brain injury. What has only recently been appreciated is that temperature reduction of only a few degrees (~33–34° C) can substantially reduce the brain's vulnerability to ischemic injury. Experimental work has consistently demonstrated the neuroprotective efficacy of mild hypothermia in a wide variety of animal models. In light of this dramatic protective effect of mild hypothermia, its use in the operating room setting has been advocated. Proponents of its use argue that hypothermia is readily achieved and it is not accompanied by significant myocardial depression or arrhythmias. In addition, the patient can be readily rewarmed in the operating room after the risk of ischemia has subsided. However, the efficacy of mild hypothermia in humans who have incurred ischemic cerebral injury has not been extensively evaluated. A randomized prospective trial in which the neuroprotective efficacy of mild hypothermia will be evaluated is currently being performed. Results of a pilot study clearly demonstrated a trend toward improved neurologic outcome in hypothermic patients undergoing intracranial aneurysm surgery. These data provide strong support for more frequent use of intraoperative mild temperature reduction in the management of neurosurgical cases in which there is a significant risk of cerebral ischemia (intracranial neurovascular surgery).

By contrast, increases in brain temperature during and after ischemia aggravate injury. An increase of as little as 1° C can dramatically increase injury. It therefore seems prudent to avoid hyperthermia in patients who have suffered an ischemic insult or those who are risk of cerebral ischemia.

Cerebral Perfusion Pressure

Cerebral blood flow is normally autoregulated over a CPP range of 60 to 150 mmHg. In hypertensive patients, the lower limit of autoregulation is shifted to the right. In most patients, maintenance of CBF can be assured with a CPP in excess of 50 mmHg. The question is whether this CPP is adequate to maintain perfusion in a brain that has undergone ischemic injury. The ideal CPP in such patients has not been adequately studied. In head injured patients however, a higher than normal CPP is required to maintain normal CBF. In the absence of firm data, a target CPP of 65–70 mmHg is reasonable. By contrast, hypotension has been shown to be quite deleterious to the injured (ischemic or traumatic) brain. Hypotension can increase cerebral infarct volumes significantly and should be avoided in patients who have suffered a stroke. Similarly, hypotension has been demonstrated to be one of the most important contributors to a poor outcome in patients who have sustained head injury. Maintenance of an adequate MAP and CPP is therefore critical. Elevation of MAP by alpha agonists such as phenylephrine is appropriate (with the assumption that the patient's intravascular volume is normal).

Blood Glucose

In the normal brain that is adequately perfused, glucose is metabolized aerobically. When the brain is rendered ischemic, oxygen is no longer available and glucose then undergoes glycolysis. The resultant production of lactic acid contributes to the acidosis that occurs in many ischemic tissues.

With hyperglycemia, the amount of lactic acid produced is considerable and the cerebral pH decreases. This acidosis contributes significantly to neuronal necrosis. In many laboratory and human studies, pre-existing hyperglycemia has been shown to be associated with increased neurologic injury. As a corollary, treatment of hyperglycemia with insulin has been shown to reduce neurologic injury. Consequently, it has been suggested that hyperglycemia be treated in patients at risk of cerebral ischemia and in those who have suffered an ischemic insult. Although the threshold at which insulin treatment should be initiated has not been defined, treatment with a blood glucose in excess of 250 mg/dl is reasonable. Hypoglycemia, however, should be avoided when insulin treatment is initiated.

Seizure Prophylaxis

Seizures commonly occur in patients with intracranial pathology. Seizure activity is associated with increased neuronal activity, increased cerebral blood flow and cerebral blood volumes (consequently increased ICP) and cerebral acidosis. Untreated seizures can actually produce neuronal necrosis even with normal cerebral perfusion. Prevention of and rapid treatment of seizures is therefore an important goal. Seizures can be rapidly treated with benzodiazepines, barbiturates, etomidate and propofol. For more long lasting anti-epileptic activity, phenytoin and pentobarbital are often used.

CURRENT INSIGHTS INTO THE PATHOPHYSIOLOGY OF CEREBRAL ISCHEMIA

As described above, our concepts of brain protection have been derived primarily from the viewpoint of the supply and demand balance of oxygen. From this perspective, agents most likely to protect the brain against ischemic injury are those that reduce $CMRO_2$ to the greatest extent. However, more recent data suggest that CMR reduction per se is not the major determinant of cerebral protection. In fact, drugs that normally *increase* $CMRO_2$ have been shown to *reduce* ischemic brain injury. These data have forced a re-evaluation of our understanding of the pathophysiology of cerebral ischemia.

Current thinking about ischemic brain injury is based upon the concept of excitotoxicity (Figure 11-4). There are a number of neurotransmitters in the brain that serve a multitude of functions. These can be classified broadly as inhibitory (e.g., GABA, glycine) and excitatory (glutamate, dopamine). Inhibitory neurotransmitters reduce the excitability of the post-synaptic neuron by producing hyperpolarization. The excitatory neurotransmitters, on the other hand, enhance the excitability of the post-synaptic

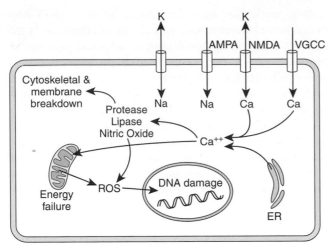

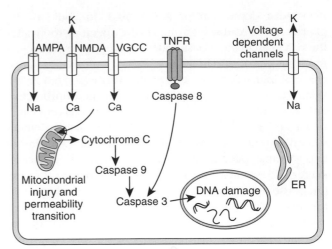

Figure 11-4   Exitoxicity. Ischemia induces the release of the excitatory neurotransmitter glutamate. Glutamate activates its receptors (NMDA, AMPA) and results in Ca^{++} influx into the cell. Ca^{++} also enters the cell from voltage gated calcium channels (VGCC). Release of Ca^{++} from intracellular stores also contributes to the rise in intracellular Ca^{++} concentration. High intracellular Ca^{++} concentrations lead to the activation of a number of enzymes within the neuron and mitochondrial injury. The latter releases reactive oxygen species (ROS) which further serve to exacerbate injury. The net result is neuronal death.

Figure 11-5   Apoptosis. Ischemia-induced mitochondrial injury results in the release of cytochrome C from the mitochondria. Cytochrome C release leads to the activation of caspases 9 and 3. Caspase 3 proteolytically cleaves a number of protein substrates within the neuron. This results in neuronal apoptosis. Caspase 3 activation can also occur by tumor necrosis factor receptor (TNFR) signaling via caspase 8 activation.

neuron and often lead to its depolarization. These neurotransmitters are stored in synaptic vesicles that are located in nerve terminals. Under normal circumstances, the release of these neurotransmitters is followed rapidly by their uptake. Consequently, their duration of action is very brief.

During cerebral ischemia, depletion of ATP results in massive depolarization of neurons. This leads to the release of neurotransmitters, particularly glutamate. Glutamate stimulates glutamatergic receptors (NMDA-, AMPA and metabotropic receptors). Excessive stimulation of these receptors causes neuronal depolarization, K^+ efflux and Na^+ and Ca^{++} influx into the neuron. Calcium is an activator of a number of enzyme systems in neurons. Unregulated increases in cytoplasmic calcium lead to the simultaneous and uncoordinated activation of enzymes such as lipases, proteases and endonucleases. Under normal circumstances, these enzymes are tightly regulated. Their uncontrolled activation causes "molecular havoc" and ultimately causes neuronal death. More recent data also indicate that a number of neurons that survive the initial ischemic insult will undergo a delayed death. One of the mechanisms by which this delayed death occurs is apoptosis (Figure 11-5). A number of pathways that lead to apoptosis have been defined. Of particular importance is mitochondrial injury and the subsequent release of cytochrome c. The released cytochrome c from mitochondria leads to the activation of caspases. Caspases, which cleave proteins that are essential for cell survival and repair, lead to apoptotic neuronal death.

A fundamental difference between excitotoxic and apoptotic death is that the former triggers an inflammatory response, which in turn can cause a significant amount of collateral injury. By contrast, apoptotic neurons form apoptotic bodies; these are gradually removed from the brain without injury to neighboring neurons.

From the above discussion, it is apparent that agents that reduce excitotoxicity might also reduce post ischemic injury. Pharmacologic approaches that are being actively investigated include measures to inhibit glutamate release, pharmacologic antagonism of postsynaptic glutamate receptors and calcium channel blockade. With the exception of calcium channel blockers, used in the setting of subarachnoid hemorrhage, these agents have not shown any neuroprotective efficacy in the clinical setting. It is quite apparent that our ability to "protect" the brain is rather limited. However, the extent to which the brain can be injured during anesthetic mismanagement is almost unlimited. Approaches to brain "protection" should focus more on the prevention of injury (by appropriate physiologic homeostasis management) rather than on the reliance of pharmacologic magic bullets that might minimize neuronal injury.

THE NEUROLOGIC EXAM

A thorough neurologic evaluation forms the foundation upon which appropriate anesthetic management of the neurosurgical patient is based. Pre-operative evaluation of patients is covered elsewhere in this volume and only aspects of this evaluation that are pertinent to the neurosurgical patient are reviewed. Neurosurgical patients undergo extensive clinical and laboratory investigation prior to their presentation to the operating room and the results of this investigation should be reviewed.

Clinical Evaluation

The patient's presenting symptoms are caused either by the primary pathologic condition or the effect of this pathology on intracranial pressure. The region of the brain in which the surgical lesion is present should be identified. The position in which the patient will be placed in the operating room can be inferred from this information. Lesions that involve eloquent regions (e.g., the motor cortex) of the brain will produce characteristic symptoms and focal deficits. Symptoms of headache, nausea, vomiting and visual disturbance may indicate the presence of intracranial hypertension. Severe intracranial hypertension can result in somnolence, oculomotor palsy, pupillary dilation and contralateral paresis. These symptoms are characteristic of uncal herniation and are often accompanied by hypertension and bradycardia. Brain stem compression, loss of brain stem reflexes and apnea indicate brain stem ischemia and impending brain death.

Patients with degenerative disease of the spine often manifest symptoms of reduced neck and spine mobility. The presence of paresthesia, weakness and muscle wasting indicate nerve root compression. When possible, the freedom of movement of the neck and spine, as well as the ability of these patients to tolerate the planned intraoperative surgical position, should be evaluated. Manifestations of spinal cord compression (upper motor neuron compromise), which include weakness, spasticity, ataxia and clonus, imply limited spinal cord perfusion and therefore the need to maintain adequate spinal cord perfusion pressure. Lower motor neuron compromise produces flaccidity and areflexia. Succinylcholine is best avoided both in patients with upper and lower motor neuron compromise. In hemiplegic patients, if one chooses to monitor neuromuscular function on the side affected by previous interruption of upper motor neurons, one may grossly overestimate the amount of relaxant needed. Following general anesthesia normal patients may exhibit all of the typical upper motor neuron lesion signs. When these signs occur in response to anesthesia, they tend to be bilateral and they regress upon patient recovery from anesthesia. The presence of post-traumatic neck pain should immediately raise the suspicion of a spine fracture and an unstable C-spine.

The examination of the eyes is an important part of the physical examination. In addition to the primary neurologic condition, anesthetic agents can also alter papillary size. It is therefore essential to establish a baseline against which future examinations of the eyes can be compared. The most important thing to observe is pupil size and reaction to light. Unequal pupil size (anisocoria) is a frequent finding in normal individuals. Anisocoria that occurs with an intracranial mass indicates the compression of the ipsilateral 3rd cranial nerve by herniation of the uncus. The function of the parasympathetic papillary constrictor fibers, which are located in the mantle of the 3rd cranial nerve, is attenuated. Unopposed sympathetic activity therefore produces mydriasis. Typically, the pupillary response to light is diminished on that side. In this case the pupil is an early warning sign. Most anesthetic techniques will impair the pupillary response to light, but the effects are nearly always bilateral and tend to disappear as the patient awakens. Narcotics probably directly stimulate the 3rd nerve nucleus to cause miosis and it may be difficult to determine the response to light. However, if ischemia of the 3rd nerve is produced by an expanding mass lesion, the ipsilateral pupil will dilate regardless of the presence of narcotics. Dilation of both pupils and with loss of light reactivity is a grave sign that is indicative of significant ischemia of the brain and possible brain death.

In patients who are comatose both the oculocephalic (doll's eyes) and oculovestibular (caloric) maneuvers may be used to assess brainstem integrity (***never perform if cervical injury is suspected***). In awake, noncomatose patients, the eyes follow passive turning of the head, and irrigation of the tympanic membrane with cold water causes nausea and vomiting and is therefore not done. However, in the comatose patient, the presence of the oculocephalic and oculovestibular responses usually indicates that the brainstem is intact. It should be noted that some anesthetic agents such as barbiturates can completely suppress these responses in a dose dependent manner. Obviously, neuromuscular blockade will also abolish these signs.

Patients with limited cardiovascular reserve may not be able to tolerate both intravascular volume expansion attendant with mannitol administration and the potential intravascular volume depletion that follows diuresis. Appropriate cardiovascular monitoring of these patients should be considered.

The medication list of neurosurgical patients often includes anticonvulsants and corticosteroids. Neurosurgical procedures are often of long duration and these medications may have to be administered in the operating room. Anticonvulsants accelerate the metabolism of several commonly used anesthetic agents and a shorter duration of action of these agents should be expected. Of particular concern is the rapid metabolism of steroidal muscle relaxants in patients who take carbamazepine chronically. Steroids are often administered to patients with intracranial and spinal tumors and these agents can produce hyperglycemia.

Laboratory Evaluation

Fluid and electrolyte abnormalities are often present in neurosurgical patients. Reduced fluid intake due to debilitating neurologic conditions, use of diuretics with the attendant volume and electrolyte loss and neuroendocrine abnormalities contribute to this imbalance. Renal function may be adversely impacted by radiologic studies that entail the use of contrast agents. Resuscitation of the patient and the correction of these abnormalities are essential prior to anesthesia and surgery.

Radiologic Evaluation

Computed tomography and magnetic resonance imaging are standard imaging techniques that are widely employed. The results of these investigations should be reviewed. Particular attention should be paid to the location of the primary lesion and the potential existence of intracranial hypertension. Indications of the latter include primary mass lesions, edema, ipsilateral ventricular effacement, brain distortion, midline shift and possible enlargement of the contralateral ventricle (due to obstruction of CSF outflow). The basal cisterns should be identified; obliteration of these cisterns signifies significant intracranial hypertension. Recent pneumoencephalography may contraindicate the use of nitrous oxide; fortunately, this study is seldom conducted. CT and MRI scans of the spine should also be reviewed in appropriate patients. The presence of spinal cord compression, particularly of the cervical spinal cord, has implications for neck manipulation during laryngoscopy and tracheal intubation.

Electrocardiography

The presence of intracranial pathology, such as subarachnoid hemorrhage, intracerebral hemorrhage, ischemia, head trauma and tumors, often results in abnormalities of the EKG that mimic those seen with cardiac disease. The most dramatic changes are often seen in the setting of subarachnoid hemorrhage: deep, symmetrical, inverted "canyon" T waves. Other EKG changes include flat or inverted T waves, u waves, tall peaked or notched T waves, elevated or depressed ST segments, Q waves, etc. Rhythm disturbance may also be evident. The EKG abnormalities do not indicate the presence of cardiac disease per se. Nonetheless, a thorough cardiovascular evaluation is necessary to rule out cardiac disease.

POSITIONING OF THE PATIENT

The general principles that are applicable to patient positioning for all anesthetized patients also apply to neurosurgical patients. Pre-operative evaluation of the patient should include an assessment of the range of mobility of the cervical and lumbar spines and the ability of the patient to assume the anticipated position in the operating room. This maneuver will provide information about the position limitations that are imposed by the patient's anatomy and physiology. Although non-anesthetized patients may be able to assume the intraoperative position without difficulty, position related injury cannot be assured. The use of anesthetic agents and muscle relaxants permit a range of motion that may not be possible when the patient is awake. This is of specific concern in patients who manifest evidence of neural compression (e.g., radiculopathy with cervical and lumbar spine degenerative disorders).

The patient should be placed on a well padded, preferably with gel pads, operating table. Pressure points should be cushioned with appropriate pads. A foam "donut" is used to support the patient's head. Venous compression stockings provide mechanical support for venous return and assist in the prevention of circulatory instability. Automated inflatable leg wraps, which inflate intermittently, minimize venous blood stasis in the lower extremities and they reduce the incidence of venous thrombosis. Attention to proper support and padding is of particular importance in patients, such as those with spinal cord injury, who are prone to skin breakdown.

The four basic positions that are employed in neurosurgery include the supine, lateral, prone and sitting positions.

Supine Position

The supine position is used for frontal, parietal and/or temporal craniotomy, transsphenoidal approaches, cerebrovascular surgery, and anterior approaches to the cervical spinal cord. The patient is placed in a "lounging" chair position in which the back is elevated and the legs are dropped. The table is then placed in a slight Trendelenburg position. Such a position will relieve back strain and sciatic nerve stretch. The back of the bed is elevated to facilitate venous drainage. The patient's head is positioned to permit optimal surgical access. Extreme flexion-extension or rotation of the head can impede cerebral venous egress and lead to brain swelling and increased surgical bleeding. Seemingly minor changes in head position accomplished by the surgeon intraoperatively may be responsible for acute brain swelling and should always be considered in this situation. Carotid and vertebrobasilar arteries can also be occluded by extreme neck and thorax positions. The degree of head rotation and flexion-extension should be guided by the preoperative evaluation of the patient. In general, the ability to place two fingers between the chin and chest for head flexion and between the chin and the shoulder tip should be ensured.

Lateral and Semi-Lateral Positions

The indications for lateral and semi-lateral positions include laminectomy, lateral posterior fossa craniectomy, posterior parietal and occipital procedures, and cranial nerve decompression. The lateral position can provide an alternative to the sitting position especially with surgery not requiring mid-line posterior fossa exposure. The semi-lateral position is easily achieved by elevating the shoulder with padding, minimal head rotation, and rotation of the table to achieve the proper viewing angle for the operating microscope. Side rotation of the table requires that the patient be secured to the table. Extreme head-up positioning can potentiate venous air embolism in the lateral positions. Improved mechanical stability in the lateral position can be attained by using the moldable "bean bag" which is evacuated after conforming to the patient and the position. An axillary pad is required in the lateral position. Pillows placed between the knees provide padding and stability, and the patient is securely fastened to the table.

Prone Position

The prone position may be used for spinal column/cord procedures and provides an alternative to the sitting position for posterior fossa surgical approaches. The prone position and its variants can be achieved in many ways and requires advance preparation of the operating table. The head can be supported with foam pillows, the newer Prone-View head support, the horse shoe shaped Mayfield head rest or the head may be secured in pins. Compression of the eyes must be prevented and the ability to observe the eyes during surgery should be maintained. The neck is usually flexed slightly and the bed is placed in a reverse Trendelenburg position to facilitate venous drainage. To prevent caudad patient movement, the legs are flexed upward. An umbilical tape sling for support of the endotracheal tube and other airway related devices can be fashioned using the head rest as its base. Depending on surgical needs the arms can be at the patient's side or placed on arm boards or slings. In order to reduce the possibility of brachial plexus compression, a degree of ventral displacement of the arms relative to the chest, should be attained. This is usually accomplished by the use of chest bolsters or a support frame. Extreme abduction of the shoulder joint should also be avoided. Management of the prone position requires minimizing intrathoracic pressure increases due to restriction of chest wall motion and compression of the abdomen with resultant upward diaphragmatic displacement. This may be accomplished with the use of parallel chest bolsters and elevation of the hips. Alternatively, an adjustable padded frame may be used with the added benefits of improved mechanical stability and the ability to adjust the frame to reverse lumbar lordosis with resultant opening of the interspinous spaces. Prone position checkpoints for neurovascular-cutaneous compression include forehead, eyes, arms, axilla, breasts, male genitalia, iliac crests, knees and feet.

The major advantage of the prone position over the sitting position is circulatory stability and a reduced risk of venous air embolism. Disadvantages include pooling of blood and CSF in the wound, compression of chest and abdominal contents, possible extreme rotation or extension of the head, and lack of access to the face for observation and/or adjustments. When head support devices are not used extreme head rotation and/or extension may occur with the possible consequence of cervical muscle strain or even spinal cord compression. The latter is most likely to occur in individuals with a narrowed spinal canal due to congenital or degenerative conditions. Unexpected extubation, endotracheal balloon rupture or cardiovascular collapse can create an emergent need to reposition the patient. For this reason, solid surface transport should readily available. Vision loss is one of the most dreaded complications of the prone position. Pressure on the globe must be avoided. The greatest stress to circulatory integrity during attainment of the prone position occurs as the patient is rolled from the supine to face down position, often accompanied by a transfer from the transport cart to the operating table. The motion necessitated by prone positioning renders cardiovascular monitoring difficult at precisely the moment when it is most needed. In healthy individuals continuous monitoring can be provided by an esophageal stethoscope which remains in the axis of the rotation. The EKG and blood pressure cuff can be checked immediately before and after positioning, as well as peripheral pulses. This monitoring approach minimizes the confusion of a twisted array of intravenous and monitoring lines, which can be a hazard. In sicker patients arterial pressure can be continuously recorded as an additional guide to cardiovascular stability during prone positioning.

The complications associated with the prone position are listed in Table 11-5.

Sitting Position

The sitting position is employed for posterior fossa explorations and posterior cervical laminectomies. Its application remains controversial among neurosurgeons. However, those that have trained with it are likely to continue using this position and anesthesiologists should understand how it is accomplished and its risks. Advantages of the sitting position include improved access to midline posterior fossa lesions, facilitation of blood and CSF drainage, unobstructed facial visualization, lack of abdominal-thoracic compression, access to

Table 11-5   Potential Problems Associated with the Prone Position

Problem	Management
Airway Security – ET tube may dislodge due to weight of tubing, may advance or kink because of neck flexion, tape may be loosened by saliva.	- tape carefully - support weight of tubing - consider armored tube - constant awareness
Ventilation – abdominal or chest compression decrease lung compliance.	- careful positioning, keep abdomen clear
Circulation – hypotension if abdomen compressed or if legs pendulant.	- check BP immediately after turning
Urgent Access to Patient – may need to turn urgently e.g. to reintubate or perform CPR.	- make sure gurney or bed readily available
Difficult Access to Patient – difficult to start iv or arterial lines after turning. Hard to check pulse oximeter on hand.	- place all lines and secure well before turning - consider foot for pulse oximeter
Pressure Injuries:	
Eyes – unilateral blindness can occur due to retinal ischemia from ocular compression. Especially likely with hypotension and anemia and where there may be elevated venous pressure.	- avoid direct pressure on the globe - support head on headrest with eyes completely clear - check and document that position is OK
Forehead, Nose, Ears, Face – pressure necrosis/blistering	- soft headrest, ears not folded over, no cables etc. in contact with face
Neck – excessive flexion or extension, especially in the elderly or those with narrowed spinal canal. Brachial plexus injury from excessive and prolonged rotation.	- keep in neutral position - avoid over extension or prolonged rotation to one side
Chest – breast compression, implant rupture, coronary graft occlusion	- support should be as lateral as possible - breasts should lie within support device
Genitalia – compression injury in male	- check carefully
Knees and Feet – pressure necrosis	- use ample padding, check pulses in feet
Bony Prominences – compression at iliac crest, olecranon process	- use ample padding
Peripheral Nerves – stretch or compression of brachial plexus, femoral and lateral femoral cutaneous nerves	- maintain neutral position - avoid pressure or stretch on nerves

the chest for cardiovascular resuscitation, and rare occurrence of sudden extubation. Complications of the sitting position include circulatory instability, air embolism, pneumocephalus, kinking/migration of endotracheal tubes, and neurologic damage (cervical cord, sciatic and peroneal nerves).

The standard sitting position is attained by several maneuvers and requires constant monitoring of circulatory stability during positioning. With the patient in the supine position and the head-holder frame attached to the table, full-flexion of the table is achieved, followed by elevation of the back. When the clamp device equipped with pins is used it should be attached to the patient after induction of anesthesia and prior to head elevation. This maneuver usually results in sufficient noxious stimuli to increase arterial pressure and facilitate cardiovascular stability during positioning. Care should be taken to prevent injuries due to inadvertent punctures by the pins especially in ocular areas. When the Gardner clamp is not

used various modifications of the horseshoe headrest can be used to stabilize the head. Despite apparently adequate fixation with adhesive tape to the headrest, patients usually slip from its fixation to some degree. This can result in ocular compression or loss of suitable surgical positioning. Various degrees of reverse Trendelenburg are then achieved to position the knees and slightly flexed legs at the heart level. This is done to elevate venous pressure and reduce the potential for air embolism. The foot portion of the table is lowered to ease back strain and keep the patient from sliding downward. At this juncture the headclamp is attached to the holder and final adjustments made. When this is accomplished the holder-clamp frame can be used to support airway and other equipment via umbilical tape slings. The bed is placed in the Trendelenburg position in a manner that the vertical distance between the head and the heart is reduced.

After attaining the sitting position several checks must be performed. The forehead must not rest directly on the bar of the head clamp and there should be sufficient space between the chin and the chest to permit easy insertion of a finger. The endotracheal tube and airway monitoring devices can be suspended from the head clamp frame with a loop of umbilical tape. The position of the endotracheal tube must be carefully ascertained as head movement can alter its relationship to the carina and larynx. Endotracheal tube kinking may occur in this position, and the use of an armored tube for the sitting position is recommended by some authorities. Neurovascular compression points particular to the sitting position should be checked and include elbows, buttocks, thighs, legs and heals. Sciatic nerve stretching can occur when thigh flexion is extreme. Clearance of the head clamp frame from the area of the lateral peroneal nerve must be assured. The most comfortable position for the arms can be accomplished by crossing the hands in the lap and securing them with adhesive tape.

The sequence of head clamp removal is important as removal with the patient's head elevated has resulted in air embolism. Therefore, the head clamp should be disconnected from the support frame, the patient's back lowered to the horizontal plane, and the clamp removed from the head when the patient is supine. Care should be taken not to inflict ocular injury with the tips of the pins as the clamp is removed from the skull. Bone wax applied to the skin around the pins after their insertion may help to prevent air entrainment in the head elevated position.

The sitting position conveys a risk of impaired cardiovascular function. Changing from the supine to sitting position results in a reduction of pulmonary capillary wedge pressure (PCWP), stroke volume (SV) and cardiac index (CI), and increase in systemic vascular resistance (SVR). In the majority of healthy subjects these changes are not of significant consequence. Consequently, routine insertion of a pulmonary artery catheter (PAC) is not necessary. The decision to insert a PAC should be based upon the evaluation of the patient's cardiovascular status rather than on the decision to utilize the sitting position per se.

VENOUS AIR EMBOLISM (VAE)

Entrainment of air into the venous system can occur in situations in which the surgical site (and therefore the open vein) is about 5 cm or higher than the heart. During surgery in the sitting position, VAE has been reported to occur in 35–100% of patients. VAE can also occur with spinal instrumentation procedures.

Pathophysiology

The consequences of VAE, which can range from the inconsequential to sudden cardiovascular collapse and cardiac arrest, depend upon the volume and rate of air entrainment. With small volume air entrainment (less than 0.2 ml/kg in small bubbles), air bubbles are readily transported to the pulmonary circulation. Over a period of time, these air bubbles are eliminated. This type of VAE can lead to transient increases in pulmonary vascular resistance and pulmonary arterial pressures. In instances in which a patent foramen ovale is present (~15% of the population), air can gain access to the arterial circulation and lead to the development of stroke.

Entrainment of large volumes of air (greater than 1 ml/kg), as can occur during the inadvertent opening of a dural sinus, produce an air lock within the caval veins and in the right heart chambers. The consequences of this type of VAE can be devastating. A sudden reduction in cardiac output, with hypotension and tachycardia, occurs. Pulmonary dead space increases, ET-CO$_2$ decreases and pulmonary vascular pressures may rise. The mixture of air and blood can lead to the activation of a variety of mediators which can produce further bronchoconstriction and hypotension. Arterial hypoxemia and hypercarbia are common. If uncorrected, this type of VAE rapidly leads to cardiopulmonary collapse, dysrhythmias and cardiac arrest.

Detection of VAE

Doppler ultrasonography is one of the most sensitive detectors of VAE. The presence of air, even very small bubbles, within the venous system produces turbulence. This turbulence is converted into a characteristic sound of VAE. The characteristic sound of venous air embolism is readily identifiable, even when the anesthesiologist is attending to other tasks in the operating room. The Doppler ultrasound monitor is useful because it detects air before it enters the pulmonary circulation. The Doppler detector is placed on the chest in the 3rd–5th interspace along the right parasternal border. The position of the detector should be adjusted to provide the most optimum audible signal. It should be noted that the precordial Doppler is not quantitative and that it may be difficult to place on some patients, especially those who are obese or those who have a chest wall deformity. The Doppler is overly sensitive and does not differentiate between a massive air embolism and a physiologically insignificant embolism. Further, the Doppler does not function during electrocautery because of radio frequency interference, and is unable to detect air embolism during that time. Nonetheless, it is a highly cost effective and non-invasive monitor and it represents the first line monitor for VAE detection.

Transesophageal echocardiography (TEE) is more sensitive than Doppler ultrasound. However, it is a little more invasive, and is technically more difficult to place (especially with head flexion). It does, however, allow determination of the volume of air aspirated. Transesophageal echocardiography will also show air passing through a patent foramen ovale into the left atrium and into the systemic circulation. At the present time, placement of TEE for the detection of VAE is not routine.

Air entering the pulmonary circulation causes mechanical obstruction and reflex vasoconstriction. The resultant increases in pulmonary vascular pressures and pulmonary vascular resistance can be readily detected by a PAC. The pulmonary artery catheter is easy to place in experienced hands, but is invasive. Its disadvantages are that its small lumen makes air aspiration difficult and increases in pulmonary artery (PA) pressure are not specific for air.

Mass spectrometry for end-tidal nitrogen is as sensitive as the pulmonary artery catheter. It is highly specific for air. However, end-tidal N_2 detection requires an anesthesia circuit that does not contain any leaks, even ones that are considered to be insignificant. This is difficult to achieve in the clinical situation. In addition, with the wide availability of end-tidal capnometers and agent analyzers, mass spectrometers have fallen into disuse.

End-tidal carbon dioxide ($ETCO_2$) is commonly used, widely available, and sensitive. It is not specific for air embolism, however. Hyperventilation and low cardiac output can also decrease $ETCO_2$. With the monitoring of the trend of $ETCO_2$, the diagnosis of VAE is relatively easy within the appropriate clinical circumstance.

The least sensitive monitor is the precordial or esophageal stethoscope. A "millwheel murmur" indicates a massive air embolism. When a millwheel murmur is heard, significant cardiovascular compromise is imminent. The relative sensitivity of the various detectors of VAE is listed in Table 11-6.

Management of VAE

Treatment is largely supportive. The surgeon should be informed as soon as the diagnosis is made. N_2O diffuses into air bubbles faster than nitrogen can diffuse out, and increases the size of the bubble. If N_2O is used, it should be discontinued when an air embolism occurs. FiO_2 should be increased to 1.0. The surgeon should flood the surgical field with saline. This maneuver

Table 11-6   Sensitivity of Detectors of VAE
Cardiac echocardiography
Pre-cordial Doppler
End-tidal N_2
Pulmonary arterial pressure
End-tidal CO_2
Arterial pressure and heart rate
Esophageal stethoscope

reduces further air entrainment and assists in the detection of open veins, which can then be cauterized. If significant amounts of air have entered the circulation, the jugular veins should be manually occluded. This will prevent additional air from being entrained while the surgeons obtain hemostasis. The blood pressure should be supported by the administration of fluid and appropriate vasopressors. If possible, the operative site should be positioned below the level of the heart. This can be done by tilting the table into the Trendelenburg position. This will increase venous pressure at the operative site and reduce air entrainment. If a large volume of air has been entrained, and surgical conditions permit (i.e., the head is not in pins), positioning the patient in the left lateral decubitus position will help to keep air in the right atrium from entering the ventricle. The application of positive end-expiratory pressure (PEEP) can increase the risk of paradoxical air embolism. In addition, it can reduce venous return further and exacerbate cardiovascular instability. Consequently, PEEP should be avoided when VAE occurs.

In many institutions, the placement of a central venous catheter with its tip located at the junction of the superior vena cava and the right atrium is routine during surgery conducted in the sitting position. Such a catheter will permit rapid aspiration of air from the SVC. Catheters can be inserted into the large central veins (internal jugular, subclavian and femoral veins) or into the antecubital veins. If the latter is chosen, preference should be given to the cannulation of the medially located basilic vein rather than the laterally located cephalic vein. The ideal location of the tip of the catheter is at the junction of the SVC and right atrium. Electrocardiographic guidance can be used to place the catheter tip close to this junction. Currently available multi-orifice catheters utilize a stylet. When the catheter has been inserted to the appropriate depth, the stylet is withdrawn 1 cm and the right arm lead of an electrically isolated EKG monitor is attached to the stylet with an alligator clip. A characteristic bi-phasic P wave is indicative of the placement of the tip of the catheter within the right atrium (Figure 11-6). The catheter can then be withdrawn until the P wave becomes monophasic (deep and negative P wave). This placement can then be verified by pressure wave transduction or the detection of a rapid fluid infusion by a Doppler probe. It is important that the CVP catheter position be rechecked after the patient is in final position for surgery, as ventricular irritability may result from incidental catheter migration. Radiographic confirmation of the catheter tip is not necessary in most cases. The right atrial catheter should be aspirated until no more air can be obtained. The approach to VAE is summarized in Table 11-7.

Prevention measures include elevating the head only as much as necessary to obtain adequate exposure.

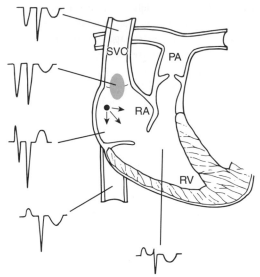

Figure 11-6   Intravascular and intracardiac electrocardiography. The positive electrode of lead II is attached to the central venous catheter and lead II is monitored. The presence of a biphasic P wave indicates the presence of the catheter tip in the right mid-atrium. The catheter is then withdrawn 1–2 cm so that the tip is located at the junction of the right atrium and the superior vena cava (indicated by the grey oval). To prevent microshock, an isolated EKG monitoring system is recommended. (Adapted from Drummond CA, Patel PM. Cerebral physiology and the effects of anesthetics and techniques. In, Miller RD, *Anesthesia,* 5th Edition, Chapter 19, pp 695–734. Churchill Livingstone, New York, 2000.)

Meticulous surgical attention to cauterization of open veins and the application of bone wax to the edges of the craniotomy is essential. The patient should be well hydrated and euvolemia should be assured.

SUPRATENTORIAL TUMORS

Craniotomy for the excision of supratentorial tumors is one of the most common neurosurgical procedures. The majority of intracranial tumors are comprised of gliomas, astrocytomas and meningiomas. These tumors generally tend to grow slowly and produce specific

Table 11-7   Approach to the patient with VAE
1. Inform the surgeon
2. Discontinue N$_2$O
3. Administer 100% oxygen
4. Place patient in "head-down" position
5. Surgical field should be flooded with saline
6. Aspirate the CVP line and remove air if possible
7. Monitor (and support) the cardiopulmonary status
8. Manual jugular vein compression
9. Consider change of patient position for completion of surgery
10. CPR if necessary

symptoms by compression of surrounding brain tissue and general symptoms by producing increases in intracranial pressure. Variable degrees of cerebral edema surrounding the tumor exacerbate the mass effect produced by tumors. In rare situations, hemorrhage into the tumors can acutely increase ICP. The rapid increase in ICP represents a neurosurgical emergency, and if uncorrected, can lead to brain tissue herniation. The latter symptoms include headache, nausea, vomiting and visual disturbances.

Pre-operative evaluation of patients should be focused upon two aspects. First, the degree of intracranial hypertension should be determined. Clinical symptoms of raised ICP include headache, nausea, vomiting, visual disturbances and alterations in the level of consciousness. Specific neurological symptoms, produced by compression of brain tissue by the tumor, may be evident. CT and MRI scans should be reviewed. Radiological evidence of intracranial hypertension includes ventricular effacement, midline shift and obliteration of basal cisterns. Second, the size and location of the tumor and the degree of cerebral edema should be determined. Tumors that are adjacent to dural sinuses deserve special attention. The risk of inadvertent entry into the dural sinuses and subsequent venous air embolism is not insignificant. In these cases, appropriate monitoring for VAE and the placement of a VAE aspiration catheter at the junction of the SVC and right atrium is recommended. Resection of tumors that are located in close proximity to the hypothalamus (e.g., craniopharyngioma) may produce hemodynamic and temperature instability.

Dexamethasone reduces tumor edema and produces an improvement in symptoms; its administration is almost routine in patients with intracranial tumors. Patients with severe intracranial hypertension may benefit from mannitol administration prior to anesthesia induction. The prophylactic administration of anticonvulsants should be discussed with the surgical team. For long duration procedures, repeat administration of these agents may be necessary.

Anesthetic Management

Insertion of an arterial catheter for blood pressure monitoring is quite routine. Additional invasive monitoring is dictated by the nature of the tumor, the anticipated blood loss and the general cardiopulmonary condition of the patient. Head elevation, usually 10–20°, is often employed to facilitate venous drainage and improving exposure in the surgical field. The choice of anesthetic agents is governed by the understanding of their effects on intracranial dynamics. In general, most agents can be used safely and effectively and there are no data to indicate superiority of one anesthetic regimen over another. A possible exception to this generalization is the patient in whom the intracranial hypertension is severe enough to produce a reduction in the level of consciousness. In these patients, the ability of the brain to compensate for increases in ICP is almost exhausted and they will be intolerant of further increases in ICP. In such patients, the use of an intravenous technique with agents that do not produce any cerebral vasodilation may be more judicious. Once the dura has been opened, the condition of the brain can be examined and the anesthetic regimen can be adjusted accordingly. Modest hyperventilation, with a $PaCO_2$ target of about 25–30 mmHg, and mannitol may be of benefit in reducing brain bulk and facilitating surgical exposure.

Management of the Tight Brain

An increase in brain bulk during surgery can reduce surgical exposure and necessitates more aggressive brain retraction. In extreme cases, the brain can actually herniate through the open craniotomy. In these situations, a rapid reduction in brain bulk is necessary. Modest head elevation should be maintained to facilitate venous drainage. Muscle relaxation should be achieved in order to prevent patient bucking and straining. Adequacy of hyperventilation and of oxygenation should be confirmed by measurement of arterial gas tensions. Auscultation of the lungs should alert one to the presence of a pneumothorax. Additional doses of mannitol and furosemide may be administered to reduce brain bulk. Drainage of CSF by the opening of the cisterns or by the insertion of a ventricular catheter can be quite effective. If these measures are not adequate, the anesthetic regimen should be altered. Although nitrous oxide, when administered together with opiates, does not produce vasodilation, it should be discontinued to remove any vasodilatory effect that it may produce. Similarly, volatile agents should be discontinued and anesthesia should be maintained by an intravenous technique. Intravenous infusions of propofol or thiopental reduce cerebral metabolism, blood flow and brain bulk. If the increase in brain bulk has been rapid, the possibility of intra-tumor hemorrhage should be considered. Finally, in rare cases, herniated brain may have to be amputated.

Emergence

Many neurosurgical patients manifest hypertension upon emergence from anesthesia. Anti-hypertensive therapy, when instituted in the operating room, prevents uncontrolled hypertension that often occurs in the PACU. Tracheal extubation should be accomplished as soon as is feasible. This is followed by a brief neurologic exam to insure that the patient does not manifest any evidence of further neurologic injury. In the event that the patient does not regain consciousness after termination of anesthesia (after a reasonable amount of time has elapsed), a CT scan, which may reveal the presence of a pneumocephalus or hemorrhage, should be considered. Patients who undergo incomplete tumor resection, particularly meningiomas, have a higher incidence of postoperative intra-parenchymal hemorrhage at the site of surgical resection. Blood pressure control in these patients is required.

POSTERIOR FOSSA SURGERY

Surgery in the posterior fossa necessitates the consideration of patient position for surgical access to the structures in the posterior fossa and the potential hemodynamic and respiratory aberrations attendant with stimulation/manipulation of the brain stem. By far the majority of the surgery in the posterior fossa is performed with the patient in the prone position. The risks of venous air embolism, as well as those of quadriplegia and macroglossia, are reduced substantially in comparison to the sitting position. Nonetheless, the sitting position is still employed under certain circumstances. The anesthetic considerations and complications of the sitting position have been presented in the section on patient positioning and will not be discussed further.

Manipulation of the cardiovascular and respiratory control centers in the medulla, either by direct surgical manipulation or by electrical stimulation with cautery, can cause intense cardiovascular and respiratory changes in patients. Traction of the cranial nerves that carry a sensory component (trigeminal and glossopharyngeal nerves) can produce similar hemodynamic aberrations. Profound hypertension and bradycardia are most commonly observed. However, combinations of hypotension, bradycardia and tachycardia can also be seen. Alterations in respiratory pattern, which include apnea and irregular breathing, are sensitive indicators of irritation of the respiratory centers in the medulla. These cardiorespiratory changes are brief and they dissipate rapidly once the stimulus has been discontinued. Close monitoring of hemodynamic variables and of the EKG is essential during these procedures and the neurosurgeon should be kept apprised of any changes. Changes in respiratory pattern are observed only during spontaneous ventilation. The monitoring of spontaneous respiration has been advocated for procedures that entail a risk of damage to the respiratory center. However, in most centers, spontaneous ventilation is not employed.

Surgery in the posterior fossa entails a risk of injury to various cranial nerves. Injury to CN V renders the cornea insensate. Precautions to prevent corneal drying and irritation should be taken; an eye patch is usually all that is necessary. Of greatest concern is injury to the cranial nerves that are involved in the motor and sensory control of the airway. These are the CN IX, X and XII. Lack of sensation within the oropharynx and laryngeal inlet and poor motor control of muscles of the oropharynx and larynx render patients prone to aspiration pneumonia. Vocal cord paresis reduces airway caliber and can produce frank obstruction. Inability to protrude the tongue due to CN XII injury precludes maintenance of a patent airway. The decision to extubate the trachea must therefore be made after due consideration of the extent of surgical trauma, the development of edema in the posterior fossa and a subjective evaluation of injury to the cranial nerves. Frequent hemodynamic aberrations, described above, indicate substantial manipulation of the brain stem and argue against tracheal extubation upon emergence from anesthesia.

The posterior fossa is relatively small and is not able to accommodate increases in volume caused by edema or hematoma. Compression of the brain stem can rapidly lead to cardiorespiratory instability and collapse. It is therefore important to prevent hypertension as increases in blood pressure can exacerbate edema development and can lead to hemorrhage. The patients at greatest risk of hematoma development are those in whom resection of tumor is incomplete.

Surgery in the posterior fossa is occasionally associated with complications that are not often observed during other surgical procedures. These include:

Macroglossia

Edema of the tongue, soft palate and oropharynx has been reported as an uncommon complication of the sitting position. The etiology of the problem is most likely due to the combination of flexion of the head onto the chest and the simultaneous placement of anesthesia equipment (oral airways, esophageal stethoscopes, orogastric tubes and TEE probe). With surgical procedures of long duration, either direct trauma or occlusion of the venous drainage from the structures in the mouth can lead to substantial edema. In such cases, extubation of the trachea at the conclusion of surgery may not be possible. For purposes of prevention, head flexion should be minimized (one should be able to place at least two fingers between the chin and the chest) and oral airways should be removed once the patient has been placed in the sitting position.

Quadriparesis

The etiology of this rare complication has been attributed to significant head flexion; such flexion can cause direct trauma to the spinal cord and can also compromise vascular perfusion. The risk is clearly the greatest in patients who have cervical spine stenosis and in these patients, the head should be flexed with caution. In addition, maintenance of perfusion of the cord, with the administration of vasoactive agents if necessary, is essential.

Pneumocephalus

Posterior fossa procedures that are conducted with the patient in the sitting position can lead to excessive drainage of the CSF. As the CSF is drained, air can enter the cranial vault. In circumstances where this air is in direct communication with the atmosphere, air trapping will not occur. However, during cranial closure, air in the cranial vault may no longer be in continuity with the atmosphere and significant air trapping can occur. The pneumocephalus can be further enlarged by the use of N_2O. It is therefore reasonable to discontinue N_2O administration before the commencement of cranial closure. A large pneumocephalus can increase ICP significantly and can delay or even prevent the return of consciousness upon the discontinuation of anesthetic administration. Should this occur, emergent CT scan should be obtained. If a pneumocephalus is detected, a burr hole with a needle puncture of the dura can help remove the air and decompress the cranial vault.

SURGERY FOR INTRACRANIAL ANEURYSMS

The patient with a ruptured cerebral aneurysm poses unique challenges to anesthetic management. Therefore, expert anesthetic management requires an understanding of the pathophysiology of aneurysmal rupture and subarachnoid hemorrhage. This is what the present discussion is focused upon.

PATHOPHYSIOLOGY OF SUBARACHNOID HEMORRHAGE (SAH)

Classification

The severity of SAH is categorized according to the Hunt-Hess neurologic classification Table 11-8). The grade of SAH is an important determinant of the neurosurgical management approach. Patients with grades I, II and III SAH often undergo early clipping of the aneurysm (within 72 hr of the rupture). Early clipping of good grade SAH prevents aneurysmal rebleeding and permits the utilization of induced hypertension as a modality to treat vasospasm (see below). In patients with grades IV and V hemorrhage, surgery is delayed for at least two weeks after the initial rupture.

Table 11-8 Classification of subarachnoid hemorrhage

Hunt-Hess Classification of Post-SAH Neurologic Status

Grade I:	Minimal headache, slight nuchal rigidity
Grade II:	Moderate to severe headache, nuchal rigidity, no neurologic deficits with the exception of cranial nerve palsies
Grade III:	Decreased LOC, confusion, focal neurologic deficits
Grade IV:	Stupor, hemiparesis, early decerebrate posturing
Grave V:	Deep coma, decerebrate rigidity, moribund

World Federation of Neurological Surgeons SAH Scale

Grade	GCS	Motor Deficit
I	15	Absent
II	14-13	Absent
III	14-13	Present
IV	12-7	Present or absent
V	6-3	Present or absent

GCS: Glasgow Coma Score (Table 11-9)

Rebleeding

Rebleeding of the aneurysm is one of the most feared complications of aneurysmal rupture. The incidence of rebleeding is the greatest during the first 24 hrs (incidence 5-6%) and then stabilizes to about 1-2% per day. Blood pressure management is important in the preoperative period. Antihypertensive agents and sedatives are used judiciously to minimize sudden increases in blood pressure. Caution must be exercised in order to avoid hypotension. A reduction in blood pressure is not well tolerated by the injured brain and hypotension can increase ischemic brain injury. As a general rule, the mean arterial pressure is maintained within 20% of the patient's normal blood pressure.

Vasospasm

Vasospasm is thought to occur because of the breakdown products of hemoglobin that are present in the vicinity of the intracranial blood vessels. Although the initial arterial constriction does represent spasm of the vessels, the delayed narrowing of the arteries is caused by an obliterative endarteritis. Vasospasm may become evident 3 days after SAH and peaks at about 7 days. In most instances, vasospasm resolves 2 weeks after SAH. The administration of calcium channel blockers (nimodipine and nicardipine) has become routine. These agents do not reduce the degree of vasospasm. Their beneficial effects have been attributed to their ability to protect neurons against ischemic injury. The time course of vasospasm has dictated the timing of surgery. During the first 3 days, vasospasm is not a significant concern and patients with a good grade SAH (I–III) undergo surgery during this time. Beyond three days, vasospasm increases the risk of surgery. Consequently, in patients with poor grade SAH, surgery is delayed until vasospasm has resolved.

Hydrocephalus

The presence of blood within the subarachnoid space can cause obstruction of CSF absorption by the arachnoid villi. Hydrocephalus is usually present in patients who undergo delayed surgery. This is treated preoperatively by the removal of CSF via a ventriculostomy.

Neurogenic Pulmonary Edema

The sudden increase in ICP that accompanies SAH causes a dramatic increase in sympathetic outflow and in serum catecholamine levels. The resultant increase in blood pressure can increase pressures in the left side of the heart and in the pulmonary veins. Pulmonary edema can be a consequence of this. Neurogenic pulmonary edema, which can produce hypoxemia, is usually self-limited and resolves spontaneously. One must also be cognizant of the risk of pulmonary aspiration. Patients with acute SAH often lose consciousness and are prone to aspiration of gastric contents. These patients often develop ARDS.

Cardiac Complications

Patients with SAH often manifest abnormalities of the EKG. These can range from minor, non-specific ST segment and T wave abnormalities to the classic symmetrical T wave inversion that is characteristic of subendocardial ischemia. These changes however *do not* portend ischemic myocardial injury. Some degree of myocardial injury does occur (focal microscopic necrosis) but it does not correlate well with EKG abnormalities. Wall motion abnormalities have been demonstrated by echocardiography. These tend to occur in patients with high grade SAH. In fact, the presence of these wall motion abnormalities correlates well with the grade of SAH. In patients who have sustained severe SAH, close evaluation of cardiac function is warranted. Echocardiography in these patients is often obtained.

Electrolyte Abnormalities

Hyponatremia is commonly seen in patients with SAH. This reduction in serum sodium (Na^+) levels was initially attributed to the syndrome of inappropriate antidiuretic hormone (SIADH). Increased levels of ADH reduce renal free water clearance. As a result, water is retained and serum Na levels are reduced. The treatment of SIADH is usually *water restriction*. Recent studies have indicated that the cause of hyponatremia in most patients with SAH is probably due to cerebral salt wasting. Naturetic peptides are synthesized and released by the brain. These peptides then cause a loss of sodium within the urine. Cerebral salt wasting is characterized by intravascular volume contraction, hyponatremia and relatively high urine sodium levels (greater than 50 mmol/liter). This syndrome is treated by *volume expansion* with saline. The differentiation of SIADH from cerebral salt wasting is very important because the treatment approach for these conditions is diametrically opposed. Hypovolemia is associated with greater cerebral infarction in patients who have sustained SAH.

INTRAOPERATIVE MANAGEMENT

This part of the discussion is focused primarily upon the physiologic parameters that have to be controlled. Anesthetic agent selection is less relevant because anesthesia can be provided with almost any combination of agents. The most important consideration is the management of arterial blood pressure and the ability to precisely manipulate this pressure should the need arise.

Blood Pressure Management

The injured brain is vulnerable to ischemic injury. This is particularly so in patients with vasospasm. Therefore, the MAP is maintained in the high normal range for the patient. Patients with SAH are monitored in the ICU and baseline pressures are easily obtained. However, it is important to realize that sudden increases in MAP can increase the risk of rebleeding. To facilitate rapid reduction in MAP should the need arise, a nitroprusside infusion should be prepared and the infusion tubing should be connected to a functioning intravenous cannula. After aneurysm clipping, the MAP is increased by about 10-15% above the patient's baseline to augment cerebral perfusion in case the patient has vasospasm.

Management of Intraoperative Aneurysm Rupture

Manipulation of a previously ruptured aneurysm can cause sudden rebleeding. The traditional approach to prevent this occurrence was to reduce MAP to decrease the transmural pressure gradient across the aneurysm. This approach is not favored today. Hypotension can cause brain injury and generally should be avoided. To decompress the aneurysm, temporary clipping is used. A temporary clip is placed on the feeding artery proximal to the aneurysm. This reduces the pressure within the aneurysm and thereby decreases the risk of rupture.

There is, however, a potential risk of causing ischemic injury during the period of temporary clipping. To minimize this risk, the MAP is often increased (by about 5-10% above baseline) judiciously after the temporary clip has been applied. The increased MAP should improve collateral blood flow. In the event that the aneurysm does rupture, the MAP might have to be decreased to reduce bleeding from the aneurysm and to improve visibility in the surgical field. The MAP is usually reduced only when the neurosurgeon requests hypotension. The MAP can be reduced by nitroprusside infusion. The least amount of hypotension that provides adequate visibility in the field should be used. Once the bleeding is controlled, the MAP should be restored.

PaCO$_2$ Management

The PaCO$_2$ is usually maintained in the normal range (35-38 mmHg). Hyperventilation is not induced because cerebral blood flow can be compromised in regions of the brain that are injured (direct effect of hemorrhage) or ischemic (vasospasm). If brain relaxation is a concern, then hyperventilation can be induced judiciously. If hyperventilation is instituted, the PaCO$_2$ should be restored as soon as the aneurysm is clipped.

Mannitol

Mannitol is a staple means by which brain relaxation is achieved. Mannitol has also been shown to improve cerebral perfusion in compromised regions of the brain. Clearly, mannitol can reduce ICP. As a consequence, there is a small theoretic risk that a reduction in ICP can increase the transmural pressure gradient across the aneurysm (pressure gradient = MAP − ICP). To mitigate this risk, mannitol is usually administered after the dura has been opened. At that time, the ICP is essentially atmospheric.

CSF Drainage

Lumbar CSF drainage is occasionally employed to reduce CSF accumulation in the surgical field. This has the effect of improving visibility within the surgical field. The standard epidural catheters are not large enough to allow adequate CSF drainage. Large catheters, specifically designed for CSF drainage, are inserted into the lumbar CSF space via 14 gauge Tuohy needles. The catheter is clamped after placement and CSF is drained only after the dura has been opened.

Brain Protection

In patients who have sustained a SAH, the brain is clearly at risk of ischemic injury. This is particularly true in patients who have vasospasm. To reduce the risk of ischemic neuronal injury, all patients with SAH are given calcium channel blockers (nimodipine or nicardipine). Unfortunately, other agents that can reduce ischemic injury are not currently available. In patients who are at high risk of cerebral ischemia or who develop ischemia because of intraoperative vessel occlusion, barbiturates can be administered in the *hope* of reducing neuronal injury. Pentobarbital or thiopental, administered to the point of EEG burst suppression, can theoretically protect the brain. Administration of these agents can cause myocardial depression and hypotension. Therefore, appropriate intravascular volume expansion and the use of inotropic agents may be warranted. The need for barbiturates is rare.

Temperature Management

Of the many interventions that have been employed for the purposes of brain protection, the most effective has been hypothermia. Mild hypothermia, in the range of 33–34° C, is remarkably effective in preventing ischemic brain injury. A preliminary multicenter trial has indicated that this degree of hypothermia can reduce the incidence of perioperative neurologic abnormalities in patients undergoing aneurysm clipping. At this temperature, the risk of cardiac complications (arrhythmias) is extremely low. Furthermore, rewarming of the patient can be readily accomplished within the operating room. Patient cooling may be accomplished by a water-cooled blanket (10° C) and by reducing the temperature in the operating room. A heated air blanket is placed on the patient. This is used to rewarm the patient. A potential complication of hypothermia is the increased incidence of myocardial ischemia. In extubated patients with core body temperatures of less than 35.5° C, shivering can dramatically increase body metabolism. This increases the demand of oxygen and as a result, both cardiac output and blood pressure rise. In patients who have coronary artery disease, this can precipitate ischemia. To prevent ischemia, susceptible patients should be rewarmed to a core temperature of at least 35.5° C before tracheal extubation is contemplated. If the patient is not sufficiently warm, rewarming is continued in the intubated and sedated patient in the ICU.

SURGERY FOR ARTERIOVENOUS MALFORMATIONS

Arteriovenous malformations (AVM) are characterized by aberrant connections between arteries and veins without the presence of an intervening capillary network. AVMs are usually of congenital origin and have a preva-

lence of about 0.5%. Approximately 50% of patients with AVMs present with hemorrhage and 25% present with seizures. The remaining patients present with non-specific symptoms such as headaches or with specific neurologic deficits that can be attributed to the physical presence of the AVM.

AVMs are composed of the nidus of abnormal vessels, the feeding arteries and the draining veins. The morbidity associated with surgical resection of the AVM is greatest in those patients in whom the AVM is large (greater than 4 cm), the venous drainage is deep within the substance of the brain and the location of the AVM is within eloquent regions of the brain. Low grade AVMs are ideal candidates for microsurgical resection. High grade AVMs, particularly those that are large, require a multimodality approach. Embolization and radiosurgery of the AVM can reduce flow within the AVM. In addition, staged resection of the AVM can reduce the risk of neurologic complications.

The anesthetic considerations for AVM surgery are similar, in large measure, to those outlined for aneurysm surgery. The mean arterial pressure is maintained within the normal limits for the patient; a CPP of about 60-70 mmHg is adequate in most patients. Mild hyperventilation ($PaCO_2$~35 mmHg) may be employed to reduce brain bulk. Aggressive hyperventilation entails the risk of cerebral ischemia and should generally be avoided unless catastrophic brain swelling (see below) occurs. The institution of mild hypothermia may be of benefit, not only in reducing brain bulk and improving surgical exposure, but also by reducing the vulnerability of the brain to ischemic injury. Osmotic diuresis will facilitate brain relaxation.

A phenomenon that is unique to AVM resection is that of perfusion pressure breakthrough. The AVM represents a low resistance circuit and blood will preferentially flow through the AVM. The surrounding brain may therefore be deprived of some perfusion. Autoregulation within this region is maintained. However, the curve is shifted significantly to the left. With surgical resection, the flow within the AVM is reduced while that in the surrounding brain is increased. With small AVMs, the flow redistribution is relatively small and is rapidly accommodated by the brain. In high flow AVMs, flow redistribution may exceed the capacity of the surrounding brain to accept the blood flow. In this situation, brain swelling, caused by increased regional brain blood volume and the development of cerebral edema, can be catastrophic. The increase in brain bulk can result in herniation of the brain though the craniotomy. Should this occur, measures to reduce brain bulk must be initiated rapidly. Gentle pressure on the brain by the neurosurgeon may be of benefit. Osmotic diuresis and hyperventilation may be necessary. An anesthetic technique that minimizes brain bulk should be considered. Volatile agents and nitrous oxide are cerebrovasodilators and their use should be curtailed. An intravenous technique with propofol and opiates is ideal.

Barbiturates have been advocated for control of the brain volume in this circumstance. Pentobarbital or thiopental can be administered under EEG guidance until burst suppression is achieved. The barbiturates reduce cerebral metabolism and via flow-metabolism coupling, will also reduce cerebral blood volume. Given the vasodilatory and negative inotropic effects of barbiturates, their administration in large doses can result in significant hypotension. Euvolemia should be assured and the means to support the blood pressure (phenylephrine, dopamine) should be at hand. Another advantage of barbiturate use is that their effects are dissipated rather slowly. This allows for a more gradual and controlled emergence from anesthesia and is attendant with reduced hemodynamic instability.

Blood pressure control is critical during and after AVM resection. High blood pressure will increase blood flow within the AVM and will make surgical resection more difficult. It will also increase the risk of perfusion pressure breakthrough and intracerebral hemorrhage. In most patients, a CPP of 60 to 70 mmHg should be sufficient. Antihypertensive medications that are often utilized for BP control include beta blockers (labetolol, esmolol, metoprolol), calcium channel antagonists (nifedipine, nicardipine), arterial dilators (hydralazine) and angiotensin converting enzyme inhibitors (enalapril). These agents are available in a parenteral form and can be used to minimize the risk of hypertension. Nitroprusside can be used to rapidly decrease BP should uncontrolled hypertension occur. The antihypertensive therapy should be continued well into the post-operative period to reduce the risk of perfusion pressure breakthrough and of intracerebral hemorrhage.

HEAD INJURY

Traumatic brain injury (TBI) represents a major public health problem. The incidence of head TBI has been estimated to be about 500,000 patients per year. About 10% of these patients perish prior to admission. Of the remaining 450,000, 80% are classified as having mild, 10% moderate and 10% severe TBI. The greatest incidence is in the age group 18–24 yrs. A secondary peak occurs in middle aged and young children. The overall mortality from TBI is significant and is the chief cause of death of young adults. A significant proportion of head injured patients will require surgical intervention sometime during the course of their hospitalization. An understanding of the pathophysiology of head injury is therefore required for the optimal anesthetic management of these

patients. In the present discussion, the classification and pathophysiology will be presented first followed by a discussion of the common types of head injury that are likely to require surgical intervention.

CLASSIFICATION

A number of classifications of brain injury, based upon pathologic findings at autopsy, have been proposed. Of these, categorization of brain injury into primary and secondary damage has gained wide acceptance.

Primary Injury

This type of injury is defined as that occurring at the moment of the head injury and is determined by the biomechanical forces exerted upon the head. Skull fractures, brain contusions and lacerations, diffuse axonal injury and diffuse vascular injury are examples of primary head injury. Diffuse axonal injury is the result of shearing forces upon the brain at the moment of impact and is the cause of 35% of deaths from severe head injury. Diffuse vascular injury is characterized by the presence of multiple petechial hemorrhages in the brain.

Secondary Injury

The importance of secondary injury to the brain has been highlighted by reports of head injured patients who "talk and die." In these patients, the primary injury is not sufficient to result in death. However, insults to the brain that occur after the initial injury result in an exacerbation of the injury and lead eventually to death or severe disability. Causes of secondary deterioration of brain function include intracranial hemorrhage, raised intracranial pressure, hypoxia, hypercarbia, hypotension and infection. Contemporary management of head injured patients has been focused upon the prevention and treatment of secondary brain injury.

The above classification is based upon pathologic findings. A more clinically appropriate and applicable classification is the one based upon the Glasgow Coma Scale (GCS). Originally described by Teasdale and Jennett, the GCS is a practical numeric score that is assigned to patients who have been head injured. The score has three major components: eye opening, motor response and best verbal response (see Table 11-9). The GCS score is used not only to classify head injury clinically (severe, moderate and mild) but also to assess head injury upon initial presentation for purposes of triage and transport to tertiary care facilities, to follow the clinical course of the patient and to predict outcome in individual patients.

Table 11-9 The Glasgow Coma Scale	
Eye Opening	
Spontaneous	4
To speech	3
To pain	2
No response	1
Best Verbal Response	
Oriented	5
Confused	4
Inappropriate words	3
Incomprehensible sounds	2
No response	1
Motor Response	
Obeys commands	6
Localizes	5
Withdraws	4
Flexes	3
Extends	2
No response	1
Classification	
Mild injury	13–15
Moderate injury	8–12
Severe injury	<8

PATHOPHYSIOLOGY

Cerebral Blood Flow

CBF is reduced in the early stages after head injury (HI). This reduction in CBF is accompanied by increases in the $AVDO_2$, indicating that CBF may be insufficient to meet the needs of the brain. In patients who recover, the CBF tends to return to normal. The CBF in HI patients is also influenced by age. In children and young adults, CBF is increased, often to levels that are considered hyperemic. Conversely, CBF in older patients is reduced.

CO_2 Reactivity

The reactivity of the cerebral vasculature to changes in $PaCO_2$ is well preserved in HI patients. Immediately after HI, a reduction in the CO_2 reactivity may be seen. However, the CO_2 reactivity recovers soon after the initial impact. Although global CO_2 reactivity is preserved, there is a regional heterogeneity in the response of CBF to changes in $PaCO_2$. In general, regions in which the flow is increased demonstrate either normal or increased CO_2 reactivity whereas poorly perfused regions do not respond as well. Loss of CO_2 reactivity portends a poor prognosis and reflects the severity of the injury.

Autoregulation

Autoregulation of CBF after HI is maintained in about half of adult patients. In children, in whom hyperemic CBF is more common, autoregulation is maintained in 59% of patients. The status of autoregulation is not related to the resting CBF and does not correlate with outcome. However, the status of autoregulation is important in determining which therapeutic interventions are indicated in specific patients with intracranial hypertension (see below).

Intracranial Hypertension

Intracranial hypertension occurs in more than 75% of severely head injured patients and a considerable amount of evidence suggests that sustained elevation in ICP is associated with poor outcome. Indeed, ischemic brain damage that occurs in HI patients has been partly attributed to ICH. Treatment and control of ICH is therefore a priority in the management of HI patients. A number of factors contribute to the increase in ICV in head injured patients. These include:

1. **Increased blood volume**: An increase in blood volume is one of the most important contributors to ICH early after HI. Hypoxia, hypercarbia and venous outflow obstruction can rapidly increase both ICV and ICP. Cerebral vasodilation in response to a reduction of CPP also increases ICV. Finally, hyperthermia and convulsions can increase $CMRO_2$, CBF and ICV.

2. **Edema formation**: Traumatic brain edema usually occurs 24–48 hrs after HI. There are four basic mechanisms that lead to the formation of traumatic brain edema:

   i. Vasogenic edema: Impairment of the BBB results in the transfer of proteins from the vascular space into the interstitial space of the brain. Accompanied water movement results in the formation of edema. With a disruption of the BBB, transient increases in MAP can lead to enhanced vasogenic edema formation.

   ii. Hydrostatic edema: With an intact BBB, increases in MAP can lead to the transfer of a greater hydrostatic pressure to the capillaries in the brain. This can lead to enhanced transport of water into the brain by Starling forces. This type of edema is thought to occur after surgical evacuation of intracranial hematomas.

   iii. Cytotoxic edema: Ischemic neurons are unable to maintain normal ionic gradients across their cell membranes. This results in the movement of Na^+ into the cells. Osmotically obligated water follows and leads to cellular or cytotoxic swelling.

iv. Osmotic edema: This type of edema usually occurs after a reduction in serum osmolarity (i.e., as occurs in SIADH). Inappropriate administration of hypotonic fluids can lead to the formation of osmotic edema, usually in normal parts of the brain.

3. **Intracranial Hematomas**

TREATMENT OF INTRACRANIAL HYPERTENSION

1. **Oxygenation**: Maintain PaO_2 greater than 60 mmHg. A reduction in PaO_2 below 50-60 torr can lead to cerebral vasodilation and a corresponding increase in ICV.

2. **Hyperventilation**: Hyperventilation results in a reduction of CBF, CBV and ICP. Arterial CO_2 tension can be safely reduced to about 25-28 torr. The effects of hyperventilation on CBV and ICP are rapid. In patients with life threatening intracranial hemorrhage (ICH), hyperventilation can be a life saving measure. However, recent data suggest that hyperventilation is not entirely benign and it can cause cerebral ischemia. Hyperventilation is more likely to provoke ischemia in patients in whom CBF is below normal and in whom cerebral vasospasm exists. Arbitrary hyperventilation in HI patients, in the absence of ICH, leads to worse outcome 3 and 6 months after the HI. Another potential drawback to sustained hyperventilation is that the cerebral vasculature adapts to a reduction in CO_2 tension in about 24 hours. Thereafter, hyperventilation is not effective. This adaptation occurs because the level of bicarbonate (HCO_3^-) in the CSF decreases. There are two consequences of this adaptive process. First, the utility of hyperventilation as a therapeutic measure is exhausted and becomes ineffective. Second, because of the reduction of the HCO_3 buffer, small increases in $PaCO_2$ can lead to dramatic increases in CBF and CBV and consequently, ICP. Therefore, hyperventilation, like all other therapeutic interventions, should be used cautiously and the minimum amount of hyperventilation that is effective should be utilized.

3. **Mannitol**: The osmotic diuretic mannitol reduces ICV (intercranial volume) by osmotically drawing water from brain tissue and CSF. It was initially thought that water was drawn primarily from regions in which the BBB was intact. More recent data, obtained by magnetic resonance imaging, suggest that water is drawn primarily from regions adjacent to the sites of primary injury. A second mechanism by which mannitol might reduce ICP is by improving CBF. Mannitol reduces blood viscosity and secondarily can increase CBF. In patients with intact autoregulation, this increase in CBF can lead to a compensatory vasoconstriction and a reduction in ICV. Mannitol should be administered over 10-15 min in doses of 0.25-1.0 mg/kg. The smallest effective dose should be used. If serum osmolarity is greater than 320 mOsm, mannitol is ineffective and should not be used.

4. **Furosemide**: Loop diuretics reduce ICP by brain dehydration and by reduction in CSF formation. Its use may be particularly effective in patients with marginal cardiopulmonary reserve. An added advantage of the use of loop diuretics is that they reduce the severity of a "rebound" increase in brain edema that occurs after prolonged use of mannitol.

5. **Sedation**: A reduction in $CMRO_2$ might decrease CBF, CBV and ICP.

6. **Paralysis**: Increases in intrathoracic pressure in a struggling mechanically ventilated patient can be transmitted to the cerebral veins. This can lead to increased CBV and ICP. Judicious use of muscle relaxants can obviate this problem.

7. **Patient position**: Head elevation by 30° can reduce cerebral venous pressure, CBV and ICP. In addition, it is important to maintain the head in a neutral position in order to avoid venous outflow obstruction.

8. **Barbiturates**: These agents reduce $CMRO_2$ by about 50% and secondarily reduce CBF and CBV. In HI patients with preserved EEG activity, they are particularly effective in the treatment of ICH. However, they can also produce hypotension and can reduce CPP. If their use is contemplated, aggressive hemodynamic monitoring, including pulmonary artery pressure monitoring, may be indicated. Although barbiturates can reduce ICH, their use has not been shown to improve outcome in HI patients.

SPECIFIC TYPES OF HEAD INJURY

1. **Acute extradural hematoma (EDH)**: Although EDH is an infrequent finding in HI patients (2.7%), it represents a neurosurgical emergency. Direct trauma to the skull results in the tearing of the meningeal vessels and the consequent separation of the dura from the skull. The majority of patients with EDH have an underlying skull fracture. The expanding hematoma can cause a rapid increase in ICP and can result in transtentorial herniation of the brain. This produces the classic syndrome of ipsilateral pupillary dilatation and contralateral hemiparesis. The treatment consists of emergent craniotomy and hematoma evacuation. The mortality from EDH has been reported to be 5-43%. Age, rate of development and associated intracranial injury influence outcome greatly.

2. **Acute subdural hematoma (SDH)**: In patients with severe HI, SDH have been reported to occur in

22%. Acceleration-deceleration injuries of the brain result in a tearing of the bridging veins that drain blood from the surface of the brain into the dural sinuses. This results in bleeding into the subdural space and the accumulation of a hematoma. In a significant number of patients, SDH is complicated by the presence of other intracranial lesions such as cerebral contusion, intracerebral hematoma and extradural hematoma. Owing to the associated parenchymal brain injury, the mortality from SDH is high (between 50 and 85%). Treatment consists of evacuation of the hematoma. This is usually accomplished by wide craniotomy. Emergency decompression can also be performed by the drilling of burr holes. After the evacuation of the SDH, a malignant swelling of the underlying brain can occur. This swelling, which can be severe enough to result in herniation of the brain through the craniotomy site, has been attributed to an increase in CBV due to vasoparalysis of vessels in the underlying brain. The mortality in these cases is exceedingly high.

3. **Cerebral concussion and diffuse axonal injury**: In the absence of intracranial hematoma and depressed skull fractures, patients who have sustained either concussion or diffuse axonal injury seldom require neurosurgical intervention. However, many of these patients have sustained other injuries (e.g., extremity fracture, abdominal trauma) that require surgical intervention. Serial neurological examinations in these patients (under anesthesia) is not possible. Therefore, the occurrence of delayed intracranial hematoma and increased ICP may go undetected for a prolonged period of time. In these patients, the placement of an ICP monitor (ventricular catheter or Camino catheter) will facilitate early detection and management of potentially treatable conditions.

EMERGENCY MANAGEMENT

The emergency management of the head injured patient is not different than the management of traumatized patients. Initial attention must be paid to the establishment and maintenance of an airway, adequate ventilation and circulatory support. Thereafter, a neurologic exam should be performed and a GCS score should be assigned to the patient. If the patient is considered to have a severe head injury (GCS < 8), then the probability that the patient will require either surgical intervention or will have raised ICP is considerable. In these patients, endotracheal intubation should be performed and mechanical ventilation established. The management of the airway in patients who may have sustained a cervical spine injury has been discussed above.

Hypoxia and hypotension have been identified as independent factors that are associated with secondary brain injury. It is therefore imperative that both hypoxia and hypotension be treated aggressively. In HI patients, hypoxia may due to associated airway and pulmonary injuries, aspiration and a reduced ventilatory drive due to the ingestion of alcohol and other illicit drugs. Establishment of an airway and mechanical ventilation with supplemental oxygen is generally sufficient. Endotracheal intubation can be facilitated by the induction of anesthesia and the use of muscle relaxants. Succinylcholine is preferable as all patients with HI are considered to have a full stomach. The choice of the induction agent is determined by the condition of the patient. In patients with normal blood pressure, most induction agents can be used safely; the use of ketamine in these patients may lead to increases in ICP. However, etomidate and ketamine may be preferable in patients who are hemodynamically unstable.

Hypotension, defined as systolic blood pressure less than 95 mmHg, should be treated with intravenous fluids and blood as necessary. There continues to be a controversy as to the optimum choice of fluid in HI patients. Both crystalloids and colloid solution have their proponents. A reduction of serum osmolarity will lead to increased edema formation primarily in the normal brain. Therefore, maintenance of serum osmolarity is considered an important goal of fluid resuscitation. In this regard, resuscitation with normal saline may be ideal. Recent studies indicate that a reduction in serum oncotic pressure can also increase cerebral edema. Accordingly, the administration of albumin has been advocated. Glucose administration can lead to increased brain injury and should generally be avoided in the acute setting of HI. In the event that the patient is anemic, blood transfusion should be considered.

ANESTHETIC MANAGEMENT

The goals of anesthetic management include the maintenance of an adequate CPP, prevention of anesthetic mediated increases in ICP (and in most situation, a reduction of ICP), minimization of increases in CBV and, as required, brain relaxation (to facilitate surgical exposure). A wide variety of anesthetic regiments can be employed to provide adequate anesthesia. There are no data to indicate that one regimen is superior to another. A possible exception to this generalization may be the patient in whom intracranial hypertension is severe enough to produce a reduction in the level of consciousness. The compensatory capability of the brain is exhausted and further increases in ICP can lead to cerebral ischemia and possibly brain herniation. The administration of volatile agents and nitrous oxide may produce vasodilation and by so doing, increase ICP. In such patients, the use of an intravenous technique (such as a combination of propofol and narcotic) should be considered. Once the dura has been opened, the status of the brain can be examined directly. Thereafter, the anesthetic regimen can be adjusted accordingly.

MANAGEMENT OF INTRAOPERATIVE BRAIN SWELLING

Malignant brain swelling can occur in patients in whom an intracranial hematoma (usually SDH) has been evacuated. Occasionally, this swelling can result in herniation of the brain through the craniotomy site, necessitating brain amputation. The management of this distressing complication has been discussed previously (see Table 11-4).

Occasionally, brain swelling may be caused by a second lesion that was not evident prior to surgery. Such lesions include the development of an intracerebral hematoma, and SDH and EDH in the contralateral hemisphere. Intraoperative ultrasonography can aid in the diagnosis of these lesions. Appropriate surgical treatment may then lead to a reduction of brain swelling.

Management of the Head-Injured Patient for Non-Neurological Surgery

The head injured patient may require surgical intervention for other non-neurologic injuries. Patients who have not sustained transient loss of consciousness, whose neurologic exam is entirely normal and whose CT scans do not demonstrate any abnormality may undergo surgery safely. However, surgery in patients with LOC, a GCS score of less than 15 and CT evidence of brain injury should be deferred until the full extent of the head injury is determined. Neurologic deterioration can occur well beyond 2 days post injury. In addition, neurologic lesions that were not apparent upon initial examination may be manifest at later time intervals. The injured brain is exquisitely vulnerable to subsequent secondary insults that might be imposed by hypoxemia and hypotension. In the event that the surgical intervention is emergent and necessary, ICP should be monitored. Measurement of ICP is a poor substitute for clinical examination for the assessment of neurologic function. Nonetheless, under general anesthesia, ICP monitoring may assist in the detection of intracranial problems. In the presence of sustained intracranial hypertension that is unresponsive to the treatment regimen discussed above, a prompt CT scan should be obtained. Definitive intervention can then be based on radiologic findings.

PITUITARY SURGERY

Pituitary tumors account for 8–10% of all intracranial tumors. The pituitary gland is located within the sella turcica. The roof of the sella is formed by the diaphragm sella, a dural fold, which is pierced by the pituitary stalk and a cuff of arachnoid. The optic chiasm lies above the diaphragm and is anterior to the stalk. The cavernous sinuses are located lateral to the sella and contain the intracavernous portion of the carotid artery and cranial nerves III, IV, VI and V. The carotid arteries are usually 2–7 mm lateral to the gland. Anatomically, the pituitary gland is separated into the anterior adenohypophysis and the posterior neurohypophysis. Prolactin, corticotrophin hormone (ACTH), growth hormone (GH), thyrotropin (TSH), follicle stimulating hormone (FSH) and luteinizing hormone (LH) are released from the adenohypophysis in response to releasing factors from the hypothalamus. Oxytocin and antidiuretic hormone (ADH) are stored in and released from the neurohypophysis.

Pathology

Pituitary tumors are termed "microadenomas" if they are less than 10 mm in diameter. Larger tumors, "macroadenomas", may erode into the bone of the sella or laterally into the cavernous sinus. Extension superiorly leads to compression of the optic chiasm and tumors can impinge upon the hypothalamus and the third ventricle. Approximately 10% of pituitary tumors are locally invasive, but it is rare for these tumors to metastasize. Prolactin and GH secreting tumors tend to be located laterally in the gland while ACTH secreting adenomas are usually located centrally.

Clinical Presentation

Clinical manifestations of pituitary tumors arise primarily from compression of surrounding brain structures or from the physiologic derangements produced by alteration of physiologic pituitary hormone secretion (Table 11-10). Compression of the optic chiasm produces visual field deficits. Extension of tumors superiorly from the sella can also produce deficits of cranial nerves that are located within the cavernous sinus. Headache is a common symptom.

Corticotrophin

Hypersecretion of ACTH results in a characteristic clinical presentation that is called Cushing's syndrome. The features of importance to anesthesia that may be present in such patients are obesity, diabetes and glycosuria, hypertension, easy bruisability and osteoporosis.

Table 11-10   Classification of Pituitary Tumors

Hormone Secreted	%	Features
Prolactin	40	Commonest in females and causes amenorrhoea, galactorrhoea and infertility. Often become large in males until hypopituitarism or visual problems develop.
Growth hormone	20	Acromegaly, hypertension, diabetes mellitus, cardiac hypertrophy, headaches. Visual symptoms are present in 15%.
Null cell (no hormone)	20	Mild hyperprolactinemia may occur. Aggressive tumor, often large and presents with visual symptoms.
ACTH	15	Cushingoid body habitus, glucose intolerance, hypokalemia and hypertension.
Others	5	TSH, FSH/LH, acidophil stem cell, or GH/Prolactin combination. All are rare.

Growth Hormone

Acromegalic patients have enlarged facial bones and tissue, a large protruding mandible, thickened tongue and lips, bulbous nose, and hypertrophy of nasal turbinates, soft palate, tonsils, epiglottis and arytenoids. While the larynx and vocal cords might be enlarged there is often glottic stenosis due to soft tissue overgrowth. This predisposes to post extubation edema. Vocal cord paralysis may occur due to recurrent laryngeal nerve stretching, thyroid enlargement or impaired motility of the crico-arytenoid joints. The presence of these abnormalities convey the possibility of difficulty with endotracheal intubation. A thorough evaluation of the airway is therefore mandatory and appropriate plans for airway management should be decided upon preoperatively. Patients with acromegaly often have hypertension, atherosclerosis and coronary artery disease. Appropriate evaluation and treatment of these conditions may be necessary. A high incidence of carpal tunnel syndrome has been reported in acromegalic patients. The possibility of arterial insufficiency after radial arterial cannulation should be considered.

Prolactin

Women with prolactinomas present with amenorrhea and galactorrhea, men with parasellar compression, headache, panhypopituitarism, gynecomastia, galactorrhea, and impotence. Relevant to anesthesia are weight gain, emotional lability and osteoporosis.

Endocrine Inactive Tumors

Patients with these tumors present with headache and panhypopituitarism. Loss of ADH release results in impaired renal concentrating ability and excessive free water loss. Diabetes insipidus (DI) is characterized by plasma hyperosmolarity and intravascular volume depletion. Arginine vasopressin has been used for the treatment of diabetes insipidus. In adults, hormone replacement therapy should include corticosteroids and thyroxine.

Anesthetic Management

The primary anesthetic consideration should be a proper medical evaluation of the patient with pituitary tumors (discussed above). The documentation of basal function of the patient can be of assistance in the evaluation of the patient in the post-operative period. Surgery is usually performed under general anesthesia and a transsphenoidal approach to the sella is employed. A frontal craniotomy may be necessary in patients with large tumors that extend significantly above the sella. The endotracheal tube is secured to the left side of the mouth. The placement of saline soaked gauze in the posterior oropharynx prevents drainage of blood into the esophagus and stomach; this serves to reduce the incidence of post-operative nausea and vomiting. Head elevation in excess of 20° increases the risk of venous air embolism and pre-cordial Doppler should be utilized for its detection. Injection of air into the subarachnoid space may be employed to permit the surgeon to better delineate the pituitary tumor on fluoroscopic images. The injected air may also push the pituitary tumor toward the sella base, helping the surgeon in tumor removal. If this approach, which is quite uncommon now, is used, the administration of nitrous oxide should be discontinued. Injury to the carotid arteries is extremely rare. In the event of dural violation, a small amount of fat tissue, obtained from the patient, is packed into the base of the sella. The nose is packed with lubricated gauze. Coughing and straining during emergence and extubation should be minimized to prevent the dislodgement of fat tissue from the sella. Appropriate adjustments to hormonal replacement therapy have to be made following pituitary surgery.

Table 11-11   Characteristics of Diabetes Insipidus

1. Urine specific gravity 1.005 or less for 2 consecutive hours
2. Urine output >250 ml in any 60-minute period or 1000 ml in any 4-hr period
3. Serum osmolality >300 mOsm/kg
4. Urine osmolality <200 mOsm/kg
5. Serum Na >150 mEq/L

Diabetes Insipidus

DI after pituitary surgery is of variable occurrence. Damage to the neurohypophysis results in transient loss of ADH secretion. In time, ADH is released directly from the stalk and DI abates. DI usually occurs 12–24 hours after surgery and is characterized by polyuria, increased serum osmolarity and hypernatremia (Table 11-11). With the loss of renal concentrating ability, urine osmolality is quite low (usually less than 1.002). Treatment consists of volume replacement with a hypotonic fluid at a rate of about two thirds of urine volume. Saline, 0.45%, is a reasonable choice. Replacement of the entire urine volume prevents normalization of plasma volume and carries with it the risk of fluid overload. The administration of pitressin or DDAVP can significantly reduce urine output.

THERAPEUTIC AND INTERVENTIONAL NEURORADIOLOGY (TINR)

The last decade has seen significant advances in therapeutic neuroradiology. The development of equipment specific to neuroradiology has allowed the interventionalist to treat a variety of neurosurgical problems that previously required neurosurgery. Anesthesia services are often requested for procedures in which either conscious sedation or general anesthesia induced immobility is required. Although the routine considerations for anesthesia are also germane to TINR, considerations specific to TINR should be kept in mind. These include patient immobility, manipulation of blood pressure and carbon dioxide tension, anticoagulation and the management of complications. A wide variety of diseases is amenable to treatment by TINR. This section will focus upon neurologic conditions that are of relevance to neuroanesthesia; these are listed in Table 11-12.

Conscious Sedation

A major advantage of conscious sedation is the ability to perform a neurologic examination of the patient. The sedation regimen employed should therefore permit rapid neurologic evaluation. A variety of sedation techniques are suitable for TINR. A combination of opiate analgesics and droperidol is a popular technique. Benzodiazepines may also be administered to provide not only sedation but also amnesia and anxiolysis. Sedation with propofol is gaining popularity. This is best attained by initiating sedation with relatively small doses of propofol and then increasing the dose as required to maintain patient immobility. It should be noted that, in most patients, a minimum time period of 15–20 mins after the discontinuation of propofol infusion is required to permit a thorough neurologic evaluation of the patient. The maintenance of immobility is essential during certain TINR procedures. In the event that immobility cannot be assured, the induction of general anesthesia is warranted.

Table 11-12   Interventional Neuroradiologic Procedures and Primary Anesthetic Considerations

Procedures	Anesthetic Considerations
Therapeutic embolization of vascular malformation	
Intracranial AVMs	Deliberate hypotension, post-procedure NPPB
Dural AVM	Deliberate hypercapnia
Extracranial AVMs	Deliberate hypercapnia
Cerebral aneurysms	Aneurysmal rupture, blood pressure control*
Balloon angioplasty of occlusive cerebrovascular disease	Cerebral ischemia, deliberate hypertension, concomitant coronary artery disease
Balloon angioplasty of cerebral vasospasm secondary to aneurysmal SAH	Cerebral ischemia, blood pressure control*
Therapeutic carotid occlusion for giant aneurysms and skull base tumors	Cerebral ischemia, blood pressure control*

AVM = arteriovenous malformation; NPPB = normal perfusion pressure breakthrough; SAH = subarachnoid hemorrhage; ICH = intracerebral hemorrage.
* Blood pressure control refers to deliberate hypo- and/or hypertension.
Adapted from Young and Peil-Spellman

General Anesthesia

The basic principles that apply to general anesthesia conducted in the operating room also apply to the situation in the radiology suite. A variety of anesthetic techniques can be employed to provide general anesthesia and the available data do not favor one approach over another. The use of the laryngeal mask for airway maintenance during general anesthesia is one aspect that differs from routine neuroanesthesia in the operating room. It should be noted, however, endotracheal intubation is necessary if manipulation of arterial carbon dioxide tension is required (see below).

Anticoagulation

Thrombosis of a cerebral artery and subsequent clot propagation or distal embolization is a major potential complication of TINR. In many centers, routine anticoagulation with heparin is instituted. In the average adult patient, the administration of 5,000 IU of heparin is usually sufficient. The efficacy of heparinization can be easily monitored by the measurement of the activated clotting time; the target ACT is about 2–3 times the baseline value. Protamine should be immediately available to reverse the effect of heparin should intracranial hemorrhage occur.

Induced Hypotension

Extirpation of AVMs with glue is made difficult by the high flow within the AVM. This blood flow can be reduced substantially by reducing arterial blood pressure. The consequent flow reduction will facilitate the precise placement of the glue such that the AVM is extirpated and that the glue does not interfere with the vascular supply in normal regions of the brain. Hypotension can be achieved with beta blockers (esmolol, labetolol, metoprolol), angiotensin converting enzyme inhibitors (enalapril) and direct arterial dilators such as hydralazine, nitroprusside and nitroglycerin. Careful titration of these agents will minimize the risk of excessive blood pressure reduction.

Induced Hypertension

Blood pressure augmentation can be of major benefit in situations in which a reduction in blood flow results in cerebral ischemia. These situations are most likely to arise when vascular occlusion occurs. Augmentation of mean arterial pressure will increase collateral blood flow to the ischemic brain and can prevent or minimize ischemic brain injury. An infusion of phenylephrine that results in an increase of blood pressure of about 10–20% above the resting blood pressure is usually sufficient in most patients. If the patient is awake, the neurologic status can be monitored and the blood pressure can be adjusted accordingly. In patients with poor left ventricular function, the afterload increase imposed by phenylephrine induced systemic vasoconstriction may not be well tolerated. A dopamine infusion may be the more appropriate choice in these patients.

Induced Hypercapnia

Injection of occlusive glues or sclerosing agents into facial and dural venous malformations entails the risk of the entry of these agents into the intracranial venous sinuses. To minimize this risk, blood flow to the brain can be increased by inducing hypercapnia. The rationale for this approach is that, by augmenting brain blood flow, the venous outflow from the brain can exceed that from the extracranial circulation. As a result, the pressure within the dural sinuses exceeds that in the extracranial veins and the risk of the drainage of potentially deleterious agents into the intracranial sinuses is minimized. Deliberate hypoventilation to an arterial PCO_2 tension of about 50–60 mmHg is usually sufficient. If hypoventilation is not feasible, the admixture of carbon dioxide in the inspiratory limb of the anesthesia circuit can raise $PaCO_2$ to the desired level.

SPECIFIC PROCEDURES

Intracranial AVMs

In the majority of cases, occlusion of the feeding vessels is accomplished to reduce flow through the AVM temporarily in order to facilitate surgery. As such, embolization of feeders by pellets or extirpation of part of the AVM with cyanoacrylate is utilized as an adjunct for surgery. In high flow AVMs, precise placement of the occluding material can be quite difficult. In these situations, intentional hypotension can be induced to reduce flow through the AVM. With reduced flow, the interventional radiologist can precisely place the occluding materials and the risk of passage of the occluding material to normal areas of the brain is minimized. Occlusion of feeding vessels can lead to a redistribution of blood flow to the surrounding areas of normal brain. These regions, which often have adapted to lower perfusion because of AVM induced steal, may not be able to accommodate the increased blood flow. There is a potential for the development of cerebral edema and hemorrhage due to perfusion pressure breakthrough. Management of intracranial hemorrhage is discussed below.

Intracranial Aneurysms

Occlusion of the sac of the aneurysm by balloons or coils is, in many centers, becoming the procedure of choice in patients with intracranial aneurysms. Patients with fusiform aneurysms and aneurysms with wide necks are probably best treated by surgical clipping of the aneurysm. The risks of the balloon or coil occlusion of the aneurysmal sac include the perforation of the parent vessel, rupture of the sac with consequent subarachnoid hemorrhage, and thrombosis and distal embolization. Obliteration of the sac may not be complete immediately after the placement of the coil and strict attention to the blood pressure, with a view to the prevention of hypertension, should be maintained in the post-operative period. In patients with subarachnoid hemorrhage induced vasospasm, therapeutic angioplasty of the affected vessels may be performed to improve perfusion to the ischemic regions of the brain. If the aneurysm sac has been obliterated, the blood pressure may be safely increased to improve cerebral perfusion.

Carotid Angioplasty

In patients with occlusive atherosclerotic carotid disease who are at increased risk of complications from anesthesia and surgery, angioplasty and stenting of the affected vessel is an option. Anticoagulation with heparin is routinely employed. In addition, antiplatelet agents such as abciximab may be administered. Inflation of a balloon within the carotid artery can elicit a baroreceptor reflex mediated bradycardia. Treatment with atropine or glycopyrrolate is sufficient in most patients. In the rare patient, bradycardia may be refractory to anticholinergic agents and external transthoracic pacing may be required. Such a pacing modality should be readily available in the radiology suite. Other potential complications include vessel rupture, dissection, thrombosis and distal embolization and stroke. Several reports have indicated that post-angioplasty cerebral hyperperfusion may be more common with carotid angioplasty than with carotid endarterectomy. In rare instances, intracerebral hemorrhage has been described. It is therefore essential that the blood pressure be controlled in patients who undergo carotid angioplasty and that uncontrolled hypertension be prevented. Measures to rapidly reverse anticoagulation, such as protamine and platelets, should be readily available.

MANAGEMENT OF COMPLICATIONS

The development of a new neurologic deficit should prompt a rapid evaluation of the cause of the deterioration. A central question that must be answered is whether the deficit is due to vessel occlusion or to cerebral hemorrhage. For vessel occlusion, perfusion pressure to the ischemic brain can be improved by augmenting mean arterial pressure (described above). In case of hemorrhage, rapid normalization of coagulation can be accomplished by the administration of protamine. In the event that abciximab is used, the transfusion of platelets may be necessary to restore normal coagulation. In addition, the blood pressure should be rigidly controlled and hypertension prevented. Neurosurgical consultation and immediate operative intervention may be required.

SPINAL CORD INJURY

There are 10,000 new cases/year of spinal cord injury (SCI) in the United States. Early mortality is about 50%; less than 10% of survivors experience a neurologic improvement. Perioperative strategies which prevent an injury, limit the extension of an existing injury, or salvage of even a few dermatomal levels can have a significant influence on morbidity, mortality, long-term disability, quality of life, and health care costs. There is an equal distribution of SCI between incomplete quadriplegia, complete quadriplegia, incomplete paraplegia, and complete paraplegia. Common causes of SCI include motor vehicle accidents, falls, violence, and sports injuries. Most injuries occur at the midcervical or thoracolumbar region, and are often associated with other concomitant injuries.

Surgical treatment for SCI is directed at immobilization, medical stabilization, spinal alignment, operative decompression and spinal stabilization. The scope of this section will focus on the perioperative care of the patient with, or at risk for, acute SCI. Specific issues pertaining to an intermediate or chronic phase of injury are also briefly presented.

Anatomy of the Spine

The vertebral column is composed of seven cervical, twelve thoracic, five lumbar, five sacral (fused), and four coccygeal (fused) bones. Individual vertebra are composed of a ventral vertebral body and a dorsal arch composed of a pedicle on either side of the vertebral body. The laminae combine posteriorly into a spinous process. The vertebral foramen is bounded anteriorly by the posterior surface of the vertebral body, laterally by the pedicles and posteriorly by the lamina. The neural laminar arches bear lateral transverse processes and superior and inferior articular facets. The vertebral column is stabilized by ligaments (from posterior to anterior): supraspinous, interspinal, ligamentum flavum, posterior longitudinal, and anterior longitudinal ligaments. The spinal cord begins at the foramen magnum and terminates as the conus medullaris (L_2 in adults). Below the termination of the spinal cord, the lumbar and sacral roots form the cauda equina.

The anterior spinal artery originates from the vertebral arteries and receives about 6 to 8 radicular arteries along the length of the cord. The largest of these is the artery of Adamkiewicz, which in the majority of people, originates from the aorta between spinal segments T5 and T9. The anterior spinal artery supplies blood flow to the anterior 2/3rd of the spinal cord. The distances between the radicular arteries can be large and variable. Consequently, regions of the spinal cord that are within the watershed area between two radicular arteries are at risk of cerebral ischemia in the event of vascular occlusion of the arterial supply to the cord. The paired posterior spinal arteries arise from the posterior inferior cerebellar arteries and they supply the posterior 1/3rd of the spinal cord. Spinal cord blood flow is autoregulated between perfusion pressures of 65–120 mmHg and its responses to changes in PO_2 and PCO_2 are similar to that of the cerebral circulation. Autoregulation may impaired or abolished after SCI.

Pathology of SCI

Primary SCI results from direct mechanical forces. Histologic changes consist of hemorrhage and protein extravasation into the central gray matter which spread to adjacent white matter. Spinal cord edema peaks at 3 days and may persist for 2 weeks. *Secondary SCI* is the result of the activation of biochemical, enzymatic, and microvascular processes which cause ischemia and cell death in adjacent "normal" areas of the spinal cord.

Flexion injuries cause anterior subluxation or fracture-dislocations of the vertebral bodies (Table 11-13). Hyperextension is associated with transverse fractures of the vertebra, disruption of the anterior longitudinal ligaments, and posterior dislocations. Vertical compression produces burst fractures and ligamentous rupture. Rotational injuries may result in fractures of the vertebral peduncles and facets.

SCI may result in complete (total loss of function distal to the injury) or incomplete (the presence of any non-reflex function distal to the injury, see Table 11-14) loss of neurologic function. The prognosis for complete recovery of cord function is very low (<10%) with complete spinal cord injury. The outcome of incomplete cord injury is more favorable; about 60–75% of patients recover some of the lost function.

A summary of cardiac and respiratory function, dependent on the site of acute SCI, is detailed in Table 11-15.

Acute Care of the Patient with SCI

The immediate management of the spine injured patient should be directed at stabilization of the spine to prevent extension of cord injury and the management of medical problems attendant with SCI. External splinting and immobilization of the spine is performed

Table 11-13   Types of Spinal Injury and their Management

Spinal Injury	Clinical Finding	Treatment
Atlanto-occipital dislocation	Usually unstable; commonly fatal	Reduction, immobilization, fusion
Atlanto-axial injury		
Isolated atlas fracture	Usually stable/no neurologic injury	Philadelphia collar
Isolated odontoid fracture	Usually neurologically intact	Immobilization
Displaced fracture C_{1-2}	Commonly fatal or quadriplegic	Immobilization & reduction
Posterior subluxation C_{1-2}	Usually neurologically intact	Immobilization
Axis pedical fracture	May be neurologically intact	Immobilization
Hyperflexion dislocation C_3–T_1	Any subluxation is unstable	If neurologic deficit decompression
Dislocated facets	Neurologically variable	
Flexion-rotation injuries	Neurologically variable	Traction & surgery if anterior subluxation & jumped facet
Compression fractures C_3–T_1		
Wedge compression/burst fractures	Frequent neurologic damage	Surgical decompression
Teardrop fractures	Usually unstable	Posterior fusion
Hyperextension injuries	Geriatric patients with spondylosis producing central cord syndrome	Immobilization; if significant spinal canal narrowing decompression
Thoracic spine injuries	Incomplete neurologic injury	Realignment & stabilization
Thoracolumbar injuries	Neurologic deficits complex	Decompression & fusion
Lumbar injuries	Incomplete neurologic injury	Realignment & decompression
Penetrating injuries	Neurologic deficit variable	Decompress/foreign body removal

Table 11-14   Spinal Cord Injury Syndromes

Syndrome	Clinical Findings
Anterior Cord Syndrome	Motor and some sensory function, temperature & pain sensation lost; vibration/position intact
Central Cord Syndrome	Motor impairment of upper more than lower extremities
Posterior Cord Syndrome	Loss of fine, vibratory & position sensation; preserved motor function
Brown-Séquard (hemicord) Syndrome	Ipsilateral paralysis, loss of proprioception, touch & vibration; contralateral loss of pain & temperature
Conus Medullaris Syndrome	Areflexic bladder, bowel, & lower extremities; sacral reflexes may be preserved; reduced rectal tone & perirectal sensation
Cauda Equina Syndrome	Sensory loss with flaccid weakness. Sacral reflexes abnormal or absent

in the field by placing the patient on a spine board with sandbags on either side of the head to prevent rotation. Adhesive straps can also be used to stabilize the head. SCI leads to the dysfunction of a number of organ systems, the severity of which depends upon the level of the spine injury.

Airway Management

Tracheal intubation in patients who have sustained a cervical spine injury can be particularly challenging. Movement of the cervical spine, which normally occurs during laryngoscopy, can further injure the spinal cord. The potential for intubation related injury is greatest in patients who have sustained an upper cervical spine injury (C1–3) than those who have a lower injury.

Table 11-15   Physiologic Effects of SCI

Cardiovascular
- reduced preload, cardiac output and blood pressure, vasodilation
- bradycardia
- reduced myocardial contractility
- susceptible to DVT

Respiratory
- reduced mechanical power for respiration
- poor cough, inability to clear secretions
- viscous mucous

Gastrointestinal
- gastric dilation and atony
- prone to aspiration

Genitourinary
- bladder distention

Electrolytes
- hypercalcemia
- hyperphosphatemia
- hyponatremia
- hyperkalemia

Unfortunately, it is often difficult to determine the level of injury in the trauma room. Lateral and antero-posterior x-rays do not reveal injury in a small number of patients who do in fact have injured cervical spines. When possible, flexion-extension x-rays of the spine should be performed. The absence of neck pain and tenderness of the spine on palpation is strongly suggestive of a normal spine in unmedicated patients who do not have another source of pain that may mask neck pain. If the evaluation of the spine indicates the presence of an injury, alternate means to direct laryngoscopy for airway management are advocated provided the time latitudes permit such time consuming approaches. Although a variety of means to secure the airway have been advocated, the available data indicate that laryngoscopy and endotracheal intubation by skilled care providers are appropriate maneuvers if emergent airway control is necessary. Manual in-line stabilization minimizes spine movement. Traction of the spine can distract the spine further and should generally be avoided. The decision to use hypnotics and muscle relaxants must be based upon the nature of associated injuries, hemodynamic status, respiratory compromise and whether patient cooperation can be assured. Succinylcholine can be used safely in the acutely spine injured patient provided that there are no other contraindications to its use. The presence of increased ICP per se is not viewed as a contraindication. The administration of "pre-curarizing" doses of non-depolarizing muscle relaxants can prevent the relatively small increases in ICP that may occur after succinylcholine administration. An approach to the management of the airway in patients with cervical spine injury is presented in Figure 11-7. The best outcome often occurs when care providers employ a technique with which they are most familiar and have the greatest expertise in.

Blind nasal-tracheal intubation has been advocated because of minimal head and neck movement. However, this procedure occasionally can be time consuming. The presence of a basilar skull fracture or extensive facial

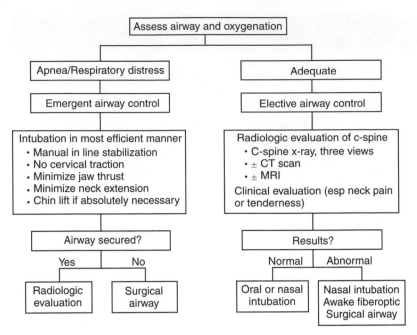

Figure 11-7 Airway management algorithm for the patient with suspected C-spine injury.

trauma is a relative contraindication to the instrumentation of the nares.

The application of cricoid pressure in patients who have the potential for C-spine injury and who are at risk for pulmonary aspiration remains controversial. It has been reported that neck displacement of up to 9 mm can occur with the application of cricoid pressure. The risk of causing or exacerbating C-spine injury should be judged against the risk of pulmonary aspiration.

Cardiovascular Function

Within the first few minutes after a SCI, a brief and intense autonomic discharge due to direct compression of neural tissue and sympathetic fibers can produce hypertension and dysrrhythmias. In susceptible patients, left ventricular failure, myocardial infarction, and pulmonary capillary leak with the development of neurogenic pulmonary edema can occur. This transient phase is usually not apparent by the time the patient arrives in the hospital. At this time, spinal shock is commonly seen. The effects that SCI has on the cardiovascular system depend upon the level of injury (see Table 11-16). For levels of SCI below T_6, hypotension produced by reduced venous return and arterial vasodilation is the major problem. Spinal shock is a condition which occurs with cord transection above C_6 and is manifested by complete loss of sensory and motor function and autonomic dysfunction. Loss of sympathetic function decreases arterial and venous tone. A reduction in venous return, with the consequent decrease in cardiac output, reduces blood pressure. Interruption of the cardiac sympathetic fibers (T1-4) leads to decreases in cardiac contractility and bradycardia. Bradycardia usually resolves over a 3-5 week period. More profound degrees of bradycardia as well as cardiac arrest may occur during stimulation of the patient (e.g., tracheal suctioning). An awareness of the factors precipitating bradycardia can lead to preventive interventions (sedation, anticholinergics, 100% oxygen prior to suctioning, and limiting the time allowed for suctioning).

Early intervention to maintain mean arterial pressures greater than 65-70 mm Hg is necessary to preserve neurologic function as autoregulation is impaired. Hypovolemia in patients with spinal shock should be treated with prompt intravascular volume resuscitation. Caution should be exercised in limiting the overall volume of fluid administered as pulmonary edema and cardiac decompensation can occur, especially with high SCI. If hypotension persists despite adequate fluid administration, vasopressor therapy should be instituted. The decision to use invasive central hemodynamic monitoring should be based upon the nature of injury, preexisting cardiovascular and pulmonary disease and the failure to achieve the targeted blood pressure with simple volume expansion and vasopressor support.

Cardiac rhythm disturbances are commonly observed in SCI, and include bradycardia, primary cardiac arrest, supraventricular dysrrhythmias (atrial fibrillation, re-entry supraventricular tachycardia), and ventricular dysrrhythmias. These dysrrhythmias are probably caused by an acute autonomic imbalance produced by disruption of sympathetic pathways and the maintenance of vagus function.

Table 11-16 Level of SCI and Pulmonary and Cardiac Function. Scale is 0 (no Function) to +++ (Normal)

| Level of SCI | Pulmonary Function | | Cardiovascular Function | |
	Mechanics	Cough	Sympathetic Function	Cardiovascular Reserve
$C_{1,2}$	0	0	minimal	minimal
$C_{3,4}$	0	0	minimal	minimal
$C_{5,6}$	+	+	minimal	minimal
C_7	+-++	+-++	minimal	+
High Thoracic	++	++	+-++	++
Low Thoracic	++-+++	++-+++	++-+++	++-+++
Lumbar	+++	+++	+++	+++
Sacral	+++	+++	+++	+++

Pulmonary Function

The impact of SCI on pulmonary function is dependent upon the spinal level of the injury. Disruption of C3–5 is not compatible with adequate ventilation and mechanical ventilation is required. Some degree of respiratory failure is invariably present with injury at levels above C7. Intact diaphragmatic innervation by the phrenic nerve is sufficient to maintain adequate gas exchange. Loss of innervation to the intercostals and abdominal muscles prevents adequate stabilization of the chest during spontaneous ventilation. In addition, the patient is unable to cough. Consequently, these patients are at risk for pulmonary aspiration. Neurogenic pulmonary edema, if present, further exacerbates gas exchange. It is therefore imperative that patients be frequently evaluated as significant declines in pulmonary reserve may occur before overt clinical signs of respiratory failure are apparent. Serial measurements of vital capacity (VC) and negative inspiratory force can provide an early warning of impending respiratory failure. The decision to institute mechanical ventilation of the lungs should be based upon the level of injury, serial evaluation of the patient's pulmonary status, pre-existing pulmonary disease and concomitant injuries. In patients with acute cervical SCI, weaning from mechanical ventilation should be considered when the respiratory muscles develop spasticity (~3 weeks); this stabilizes the chest wall sufficiently to improve overall ventilatory function. Respiratory dynamics often improve when patients are placed in the supine position due to the more cephalad position of the diaphragm; this position should be used when weaning from mechanical ventilation is attempted.

Pulmonary edema may be observed in patients with acute SCI. Neurogenic pulmonary edema has been attributed to an intense sympathetic discharge at the time of the injury. Cardiogenic pulmonary edema may also occur due to reduced myocardial contractility and overzealous fluid administration. Pneumonia is observed in 70% of cervical and high thoracic spinal cord injuries. Pneumonia may also result from aspiration of gastric contents at the time of the initial injury. Chest trauma resulting in hemothorax, pulmonary contusions, pneumothorax, and rib fractures may be present in patients with SCI. These injuries may result in prolonged mechanical ventilation with difficulty weaning, and delay operative spinal intervention.

Gastrointestinal Function

During the acute stages of SCI, the GI tract loses sympathetic input and becomes atonic. Gastric dilation can adversely affect ventilation by causing a cephalad movement of the diaphragm and also places the patient at risk for aspiration. Insertion of a nasogastric tube will help limit distention and reduce the risk of regurgitation. As hypochloremic metabolic alkalosis may occur with excessive gastric suctioning, appropriate fluid and electrolytes must be administered. Ileus is common after SCI in the thoracic and lumbar areas. Gastritis, stress ulceration and hemorrhage may occur. The administration of histamine H_2 receptor antagonists can ameliorate some of these problems.

Genitourinary Function

During the acute stages of SCI, the bladder is flaccid. Insertion of an indwelling urinary catheter is often necessary. Bladder flaccidity is followed by spasticity. The abnormalities with bladder emptying predispose the patient to recurrent urinary tract infections, bladder stones, nephrocalcinosis, and recurrent urosepsis. Although an indwelling drainage catheter is required in the initial 2–3 weeks to prevent urinary retention and reflex vagal responses, intermittent straight catheterization of the bladder should be instituted as soon as feasible.

Thermoregulation

SCI injury patients are essentially poikilotherms because of their inability to vasoconstrict the cutaneous circulation to conserve heat. Conversely, the inability to vasodilate substantially reduces their ability to dissipate heat. Environmental temperature control is of particular importance for these patients.

Venous Thrombosis and Pulmonary Embolism (PE)

Deep vein thrombosis (DVT) and PE occur in 12–24% and 10–13% of SCI patients, respectively. 75% of PE occur in the first month after SCI but rarely after 3 months and is more common in patients with complete SCI and concomitant thoracic injury. The high incidence of DVT necessitates some form of prophylaxis.

Neuroprotective Strategies

It is rather obvious that movement of the injured segment leads to exacerbation of the initial injury. Thus, an important neuroprotective strategy is to prevent further neurologic compromise by immediate and effective immobilization of the spine. Failure to accomplish this may lead to loss of residual neurologic function or even ascension of the patient's neurologic level of injury.

Pharmacologic protection of the injured spinal cord may be achieved by the administration of relatively high doses of methylprednisolone. The protocol entails high-dose methylprednisolone administration with an intravenous bolus of 30 mg/kg over 15 minutes followed by a 23 hour intravenous infusion at a rate of 5.4 mg/kg/hr. The National Acute Spinal Cord Injury III study, published in 1997, demonstrated that, if methylprednisolone is started within 3 hours of SCI, the steroid infusion need only be continued for 24 hours, whereas if therapy is started between 3–8 hours of injury, 48 hours of the steroid infusion should be administered. Hypertension is advocated as a means to improve blood flow to the injured and hypoperfused spinal cord. Definitive human data to support this practice are not available. Maintenance of normal perfusion pressure is recommended.

MEDICAL PROBLEMS ASSOCIATED WITH CHRONIC SCI (TABLE 11-17)

Autonomic Hyperreflexia

Autonomic hyperreflexia occurs in 85% of patients with spinal cord injury above T_6. Autonomic hyperreflexia is secondary to abnormal autonomic vascular reflexes which usually begin to appear about 2–3 weeks after injury. Afferent impulses originating from bladder or bowel distention, childbirth, manipulations of the

Table 11-17   Summary of Medical Problems in the Patient with Chronic SCI

System	Abnormality	Relevant Comment
Cardiovascular	• autonomic hyperreflexia • ↓ blood volume • orthostatic hypotension	Susceptible to hypertensive crisis if SCI level above T_5. Positional changes and intrathoracic pressure may cause hypotension.
Respiratory	• muscle weakness • ↓ respiratory drive • ↓ cough	SCI patient susceptible to post-op pneumonia and may be difficult to wean from mechanical ventilation.
Muscular	• proliferation of acetylcholine receptors • spasticity	Hyperkalemia from succinylcholine.
Genitourinary	• recurrent urinary tract infections • altered bladder emptying	May lead to renal insufficiency, pyelonephritis, sepsis, or amyloidosis.
Gastrointestinal	• gastroparesis • ileus	Susceptible to aspiration.
Immunologic	• urinary tract infection • pneumonia • decubitus ulcers	Watch for subtle signs of infection and sepsis. Questionable risk of seeding an infection from invasive monitoring.
Skin	• decubitus ulcers	Prevention.
Hematologic	• anemia • risk of DVT	DVT prophylaxis.
Bone	• ↓ bone density	Osteoporosis, hypercalcemia, heterotopic ossification and muscle calcification.
Nervous System	• chronic pain	Perioperative pain can be difficult to manage.

urinary tract, or surgical stimulation are transmitted to the isolated spinal cord and elicit a massive sympathetic response from the adrenal medulla and sympathetic nervous system; the latter are no longer modulated by the normal inhibitory impulses from the brainstem and hypothalamus. Vasoconstriction occurs below the lesion and blood pressure increases. Reflex activity of carotid and aortic baroreceptors produces vasodilation above the lesion and bradycardia. Common symptoms include headache, palpitations, diaphoresis, pallor and nasal congestion. Symptoms less frequently observed include Horner's syndrome, pupillary changes, anxiety, and nausea. Systolic pressures of >260 mmHg and diastolic pressures of 220 mmHg have been reported. Adverse sequelae include myocardial ischemia, intracranial hemorrhage, pulmonary edema, seizures, coma, and death. Removal of the offending stimulus is one of the first steps in the treatment. Pharmacologic treatment includes direct-acting vasodilators, combination of α and β-blockers, calcium channel blocking agents, or ganglionic blocking agents. β-blockers can reduce the vasodilation produced by β2 receptor activity and they also leave unopposed the α-receptor activity of catecholamines. The administration of β-blockers only should be avoided.

ANESTHETIC MANAGEMENT OF THE SCI PATIENT

Preoperative Assessment

1. Suggested laboratory tests include a complete blood count, serum electrolytes, BUN, creatinine, glucose, liver function tests and a urinalysis. A preoperative ECG, ABG, chest x-ray, and pulmonary function tests may also be indicated.

2. Examination of the airway must include the oropharynx with a Mallampati classification, range of motion of the neck with particular attention to any limitation of motion, stimulation of pain, or neurologic symptoms. If movement elicits any abnormality, the offending position should be avoided. Airway problems are most frequently encountered in patients with atlantoaxial subluxations, traumatic C-spine injuries in combination with facial trauma, severe kyphoscoliosis or spinal deformities, and spinal stabilization devices. If the patient is in a halo brace or other cervical fixation device, plans for either an awake tracheal intubation or another technique of securing the airway safely should be made well in advance of anesthetic induction.

3. Neurologic evaluation should be performed preoperatively and any preexisting neurologic deficits documented. Regional anesthesia should be chosen only after careful evaluation and review of any preexisting deficits.

4. Pulmonary evaluation must take into consideration the level of SCI. For instance, patients with C-spine injury have restrictive pulmonary defects with marked reductions in lung volumes which predispose the patient to hypoxemia. Patients with spinal injuries involving the cervical and high thoracic spine also have difficulties with secretion clearance which may predispose patients to hypoxemia and hypercarbia.

5. Cardiac evaluation is essential to elicit evidence of cardiovascular dysfunction due to acute SCI, or preexisting abnormalities. In addition, an assessment of orthostatic hypotension and autonomic hyperreflexia should be made.

Monitoring

Decisions regarding the utilization of advanced monitoring are based on the level of injury and neurologic deficit, the complexity and length of the surgical procedure, and any preexisting underlying medical diseases. Neurophysiologic monitoring is often indicated for patients who either have no neurologic injuries but are at high risk due to the instability of their spinal abnormalities, or those patients with incomplete neurologic injuries who are undergoing spinal stabilization surgery. Neurophysiologic monitoring usually consists of either an intraoperative "wake-up" test, somatosensory evoked potential (SSEP) monitoring, or motor evoked potentials (MEP) monitoring. SSEP monitors the posterior columns of the spinal cord, while MEP monitor the anterior portion of the spinal cord.

Anesthetic Induction

The principal concern is securing the airway without causing or exacerbating SCI. Options include:

1. An awake intubation. The advantage is that the patient acts as a monitor to avoid worsening of the spinal cord condition. In addition, a neurologic evaluation can document the absence of any new changes.

2. A *blind* nasal endotracheal intubation is often recommended as one of the best means to avoid spinal manipulation during intubation. This approach is contraindicated if there is facial trauma or a basilar skull fracture. When used, topical application of 0.2% phenylephrine hydrochloride in 4% lidocaine is essential to shrink nasal tissues and limit bleeding. Anesthesia of the tongue can be achieved using 2% lidocaine ointment or local anesthetic sprays. Vocal cord and laryngeal anesthesia is provided with the combination of transtracheal injection of 4% lidocaine via a percutaneous puncture of the cricothyroid membrane, and superior laryngeal nerve blocks

applied by bilateral injection of 2 ml of 1% lidocaine into the thyrohyoid membrane off the lateral wings of the thyroid cartilage.

3. Fiberoptic endotracheal intubation may be used in a controlled fashion using local anesthesia of the airway as mentioned above. If using the oral route, a bite block or large oral airway with a central passageway for the fiberoptic scope is essential.

4. In skilled hands, direct laryngoscopy may be chosen if the previous methods do not seem feasible; however, further SCI may occur if extension of the neck is not avoided. Many maneuvers employed for intubation can result in displacement and worsening of the original SCI. Inline manual cervical immobilization appears to be the safest method to minimize spinal column motion. It should be noted that cricoid pressure has been reported to cause neck displacement of up to 9 mm.

5. In situations where severe facial trauma or neck instability exist, or if the airway is lost, a surgical airway via cricothyrotomy or tracheostomy may be indicated. The method chosen for intubation depends on perceived airway difficulties, coexisting disease and trauma, or other factors including facial trauma or soft tissue swelling. During induction of general anesthesia, particular attention should be given to agents and doses which allow maintenance of a perfusion pressure of at least blood 50 mmHg (ideally 70–90 mmHg). If the patient is in the early phase of spinal shock with a high cord injury, the patient is at risk of developing bradycardia or asystole. Some have advocated the use of an anticholinergic agent to avoid this complication.

Succinylcholine

After 24 hours, the possibility of excessive K^+ release after succinylcholine administration must be considered. With muscle denervation, the number of postsynaptic acetylcholine receptors increases, especially in the extrajunctional muscle cell membrane. Binding of succinylcholine to these extrajunctional receptors leads to significant egress of K^+. Lethal levels of K^+ have been reported (>14 mEq/L) after neurologic injury. The administration of succinylcholine should be avoided in patients with SCI.

Positioning

Spinal surgery is most often performed in the prone position. Patients can be anesthetized on the gurney bed or stretcher and then log-rolled onto the operating table. Important goals include maintaining the head and neck in a neutral position, providing adequate padding to the chest, abdomen, head, extremities, and avoiding excessive flexion or extension. Special attention should be

given to the endotracheal tube as significant movement or obstruction can occur with positional changes.

Anesthetic Maintenance

The anesthetic regimen should be based upon the considerations for evoked potential monitoring and for hemodynamic stability. In general, for adequate SSEP monitoring, the dose of volatile agents should be limited to 0.5 MAC or less. If MEP monitoring is planned, a technique that consists of an opiate, nitrous oxide and etomidate or ketamine is suggested.

Fluid Management

Administration of fluids should be based on estimated preoperative fluid deficits, intraoperative blood and fluid losses, and a knowledge of the effect that the level of spinal injury will have on cardiac and pulmonary function. Meticulous fluid management is essential as it is well known that patients with high thoracic and C-spine injuries have an increased propensity for developing pulmonary edema. In addition, patients with C-spine injury may have cardiac dysfunction manifesting by decreased inotropy and chronotropy (due to reduced sympathetic input to the heart). These factors will dictate decisions regarding the placement of arterial pressure catheters, central venous or pulmonary artery catheters, and indwelling urinary catheters. Decisions about whether to use crystalloid or colloidal solutions for volume resuscitation are of less importance than the decision to avoid glucose containing solutions which are known to worsen spinal cord injury.

Temperature Regulation

SCI patients have impaired thermoregulation below the level of injury. Aggressive prevention of intraoperative hypothermia should be prophylactically instituted. These measures include a warm environment, warm intravenous fluids, standard warming mattresses, humidification of the respiratory circuit, and forced hot air blankets.

Postoperative Care

Vigilance for adequacy of the airway should be maintained in the postoperative period.

SPINAL CORD PROCEDURES

Kyphoscoliosis

Important considerations relate to the stability of the spinal column and pulmonary function. An appreciable degree of spinal column instability is justification for awake intubation and positioning. The pulmonary status of scoliosis patients should be reviewed. Severe scoliosis is associated with limitation of pulmonary function and pulmonary hypertension. Correction of the spinal curvature may not necessarily lead to an improvement in pulmonary function immediately after surgery. There should be rigorous attention to the preoperative treatment of bronchospasm, infection and right heart failure prior to undertaking these procedures. Curvatures of less than 50° are usually associated with normal pulmonary function tests. Patients with curvatures of 50–100° will in general have a mild to moderate limitation in exercise tolerance and comparably modest abnormalities in PFTs. Patients in whom the curvature is greater than 100° are at risk for cardiorespiratory failure.

Monitoring for these procedures usually includes arterial and CVP catheters. Posterior tibial SSEPs are usually also recorded. The choice of anesthetic agents is not critical with exceptions related to the interaction of muscle relaxants with neuromuscular diseases. The selection of agents is usually made with reference to 1) the need to perform a prompt and controlled "wake-up test" and 2) to the constraints imposed by the effects of anesthetic agents on somatosensory evoked responses which are recorded intraoperatively. The anesthetic is designed to provide a stable SSEP. Induction is accomplished with fentanyl (or its equivalent) and thiopental. Muscle relaxation is achieved with nondepolarizing agents.

Substantial blood loss may occur at the time of decortication, which is performed prior to placing the bone graft. Blood loss can continue to occur into the wound in the post operative period. The use of induced hypotension has been advocated to reduce the extent of blood loss. The application of induced hypotension should be tempered by a certain knowledge of what benefits accrue as a result of its use. Surgery may be facilitated by a dryer field and the importance of this consideration will certainly vary with the procedure and the surgeon performing it. The available literature, however, suggests that the use of induced hypotension for scoliosis in adult patients, results in a surprisingly small reduction in the total perioperative transfusion requirement. By contrast the efficacy of induced hypotension in younger patients is apparently much greater. The potential for hypotension, especially when combined with anemia, to contribute to retinal ischemia and postoperative vision loss should be considered. Given the limited benefits of hypotension and the potential serious complications of spinal cord and retinal ischemia, the available data do not support the routine use of induced hypotension during scoliosis surgery.

Anterior Cervical Discectomy

The important preoperative consideration is a thorough assessment of the patient's range of neck motion. The presence of long tract signs (lower extremity hyper-

reflexia, clonus spasticity) indicate significant spinal cord compression. If radiologic evidence is consistent with cord compression, then the control of the airway should be obtained by means other than direct laryngoscopy. In patients who present with radicular symptoms only, direct laryngoscopy may be feasible. Attention should be paid to the placement of retractors in the surgical field. Aggressive retraction of the carotid sheath can compress the carotid artery, thereby reducing ipsilateral carotid flow. In patients with spinal cord compression, maintenance of normal perfusion pressure (measured at the level of the cord) is essential. Hypotension induced reduction in blood flow in a spinal cord in which perfusion is already compromised increases the risk of ischemic injury. Consideration should be given to the placement of an arterial catheter and careful monitoring of the blood pressure.

The important postoperative considerations relate to the airway. There is a 5% incidence of recurrent laryngeal nerve injury. The incidence is somewhat higher when the procedure is performed from the right side. The recurrent laryngeal nerve is more tightly opposed to the esophagus as it travels cephalad on the left side and, hence, is less likely to traverse the operative field when the procedure is performed from the left. A unilateral recurrent laryngeal nerve palsy in isolation should not cause airway obstruction. It will manifest itself as hoarseness and a weak voice. The most important airway hazards are the result of bleeding. Careful observation of the dressings and repeated neck circumference measurements are appropriate. Progressive neck swelling requires early intervention. If a patient with progressive neck swelling develops stridor of any degree, compression and distortion of the airway is far advanced; this mandates immediate airway control and tracheal intubation. In a few situations, opening the wound in the recovery room has been necessary and lifesaving. An additional infrequent complication is esophageal perforation. This complication usually declares itself some hours later as substernal pain with mediastinal air on chest x-ray.

Anterior Vertebrectomy

This procedure is performed to relieve compression of the spinal cord from the anterior aspect. Trauma is the most common etiology. Commonly, a flexion injury will result in a burst fracture of a lower thoracic or upper lumbar vertebra with retropulsion of fragments into the spinal cord. Occasionally the compression is the result of metastatic tumor. The approach to the spinal column is similar to that used for anterior discectomy. Multiple anterior discectomies may be performed in a severely scoliotic patient to facilitate some straightening of the vertebral column by traction prior to a posterior instrumentation procedure. These procedures are performed in the lateral position. The approach is almost invariably

Case Study

A 56 year old female with a prior history of moderate hypertension and type II diabetes mellitus, presented with a frontal occipital headache that was gradually increasing in severity. She had noticed slight weakness of her left arm and leg and she had experienced difficulty with walking over the past three weeks. The headache was accompanied by occasional nausea and vomiting. Her vision, especially in the right eye, had deteriorated considerably. The patient's husband had noticed that she was somnolent. Physical examination revealed a well nourished female. Her blood pressure was 190/100 and heart rate was 75 beats/min. Weakness and a slight reduction in the briskness of reflexes in the left lower and upper extremities was noted. Fundoscopy revealed moderate papilledema in the right eye.

1. *Describe the clinical symptomology of increased intracranial pressure. What is the etiology of papilledema?*
2. *What does the clinical findings of left sided weakness and hypo-reflexia indicate about the location of the lesion?*
3. *A CT scan was performed. What aspects of the CT scan should the anesthesia care provider pay particular attention to?*

The CT scan revealed a 5 × 5 cm right fronto-parietal mass that was close to the falx cerebri. The lesion was surrounded by a significant amount of edema. Effacement of the right lateral ventricle was evident and a mid-line shift of about 14 mm was noted.

4. *What do the CT scan findings indicate about the intracranial compliance?*
5. *Describe the therapeutic maneuvers that might reduce ICP.*

Dexamethasone was prescribed. Three days after initial presentation, the severity of the headache had decreased and the patient was more awake. A tentative diagnosis of a right fronto-parietal glioma was made and craniotomy for excision of the tumor was scheduled. The remainder of her work-up, which included serum chemistry, hematology, chest x-ray and EKG, were unremarkable.

6. *Describe the monitors that may have utility in the anesthetic management of the patient. Should a central venous catheter be placed?*
7. *Should the patient receive mannitol prior to anesthetic induction?*
8. *What should the target mean arterial pressure be during and after surgery?*
9. *What is the ideal anesthetic technique? How can the selection of the anesthetic technique be justified?*

In view of the fact that the patient's level of consciousness had improved considerably, mannitol was not administered prior to anesthetic induction. In addition to standard monitors, an arterial line catheter was inserted. There were no specific cardio-pulmonary indications for the placement of a CVP catheter. However, the lesion was close to the superior sagittal sinus and the risk of venous air embolism was present. A "long arm" CVP catheter was inserted into the right antecubital vein and the tip was advanced to the junction of the superior vena cava and right atrium; location of the catheter tip was confirmed by intracardiac electrocardiography. A pre-cordial Doppler was placed along the right parasternal border in the 3rd interspace. The patient's blood pressure had stabilized in the range of 170-190/70-95. A target mean arterial pressure of about 90-100 mmHg was selected. Even though the patient did not have coronary artery disease, peri-operative beta blockade with metoprolol was initiated to facilitate peri-operative blood pressure control.

Anesthesia was induced with fentanyl, propofol and vecuronium. Maintenance anesthesia consisted of nitrous oxide (65%), isoflurane 0.5 MAC and a fentanyl infusion. The head was secured in a Mayfield pin device. Upon removal of the craniotomy bone flap, mannitol 1 gm/kg was administered to facilitate brain relaxation. Moderate hyperventilation was initiated.

10. *A risk of venous air embolism was present. Is the use of nitrous oxide appropriate?*
11. *What should the target $PaCO_2$ be? Can the use of sustained hyperventilation produce detrimental effects?*
12. *Shortly after the removal of the tumor, the surgeon noticed that the surrounding brain was swollen. Closure of the dura was difficult. More aggressive "brain relaxation" was requested.*
13. *What is the etiology of brain swelling during neurosurgery?*
14. *What should a practical differential diagnosis of brain swelling include?*

The blood pressure was 130/70 and the heart rate was 70 beats/min. Arterial oxygen saturation was 99% and the end-tidal CO_2 was 30 mmHg. An arterial blood gas was performed; the PaO_2 was within normal limits and the $PaCO_2$ was 34 mmHg. Auscultation of the chest was normal. Adequate neuromuscular relaxation was confirmed. In spite of further hyperventilation to a $PaCO_2$ of 28 mmHg and the additional administration of 0.25 mg/kg of mannitol, the brain swelling was not controlled. The administration of nitrous oxide and isoflurane was discontinued and a propofol infusion was initiated. Although an improvement in brain swelling was evident, dural closure was still not possible.

15. *What is the rationale behind the discontinuation of nitrous oxide and isoflurane?*
16. *What advantages might a propofol based anesthetic have in this particular situation?*

The patient's head was raised by about 30° to facilitate venous drainage. At that time, the anesthesia care provider noticed that the head was flexed and rotated to the left. The head was re-positioned in a more neutral position and shortly thereafter, the brain swelling abated. The remainder of the surgery was uneventful.

17. *What is the impact of head position on venous outflow from the brain?*
18. *What should the disposition of the patient be? Should be patient be monitored in an intensive care unit during the post-operative period?*

through the patient's right side. For access to L1 and the thoracic vertebrae, the exposure is made via the chest and retroperitoneum. Procedures at L2 and below are performed without entering the chest.

The relevant anesthetic considerations outlined above for anterior cervical discectomy are also relevant to cervical vertebrectomies. A double lumen tube may be necessary in patients who undergo thoracic disectomy and vertebrectomy. The magnitude of blood loss is likely to be greater with vertebrectomy than a simple disectomy. Accordingly, preparations for rapid fluid and blood volume resuscitation should be made prior to the commencement of surgery. Patients in need of an anterior vertebrectomy will often also require posterior stabilization. It is common practice to perform both procedures during the same anesthetic. In such patients, a need for airway control and post operative mechanical ventilation may arise. The decision to institute postoperative mechanical ventilation of the lungs should be based on the extent and site of surgery, blood loss and fluid management and on the pre-operative airway examination. A double lumen tube, when used, should be replaced with a single lumen tube in the operating room prior to transport to the intensive care unit.

Note that, as is the case with the posterior instrumentation procedures, the postoperative blood loss into the wounds (both the vertebrectomy and graft-donor sites) may be substantial. The intraoperative fluid administration may be substantial in these procedures. The patients are not uncommonly "puffy" at the end of the procedure. This in general resolves very rapidly and is of little clinical significance except that airway structures may be similarly edematous and the second laryngoscopy on occasion is somewhat more difficult than the first.

Posterior Cervical Fusion

Cervical instability may be justification for awake intubation with or without awake positioning. When there is instability related to fracture/dislocation, when the neck is too immobile to achieve a reasonable intubating position, or when attempts to achieve the sniffing position result in neurologic symptoms, awake intubation is appropriate. If the procedure involves the high cervical region, the suboccipital muscles must be taken down. There are substantial veins from the occipital bone to the suboccipital musculature. Entrainment of air through these veins has been described. A Doppler on the precordium, for the detection of air embolism, should be considered when the procedure involves C_3 or above.

SUMMARY

The brain and the spinal cord are the primary targets of anesthetic agents, and anesthetics have a profound impact on the physiology and pathophysiology of the CNS. As a result, the choice of anesthetic agents and the conduct of anesthesia has a significant impact upon the conditions under which the neurosurgeon has to operate. The goals of neuroanesthesia include the provision of excellent surgical conditions, facilitation of brain relaxation, prevention of brain and spinal cord injury, minimization of interference with neurophysiologic monitoring and the recovery from anesthesia that is prompt enough to permit early postoperative neurologic examination. It is therefore quite apparent that an understanding of the underlying pathophysiology of the CNS and of the physiologic impact of anesthetic agents is essential to the proper and safe conduct of neuroanesthesia. It should be recalled that there are no clinical or experimental data that provide support for the use of one anesthetic technique over another. The focus therefore should be upon the selection of anesthetic agents that best match the patient's underlying disease condition and the surgeon's requirements, rather than a strict adherence to one technique. Finally, one should note that our capacity to protect the brain against injury is extremely limited. By contrast, our capacity to produce irreparable harm to the brain and spinal cord is almost limitless. Maintenance of CNS homeostasis, therefore, is of paramount importance.

REFERENCES

Albin MS: *Textbook of neuroanesthesia with neurological and neuroscience perspectives.* McGraw-Hill, New York, 1997.

Cottrell JE, Smith DS: *Anesthesia in neurosurgery*, 4th edition. C.V. Mosby, St Louis, 2001.

Cucchiara RF, Michenfelder JD: *Clinical neuroanesthesia.* Churchill Livingstone, New York, 1990

Drummond JC, Patel PM: Cerebral physiology and the effects of anesthetics and techniques. In, Miller RD, *Anesthesia*, 5th Edition, Chapter 19, pp 695-734. Churchill Livingstone, New York, 2000.

Drummond JC, Patel PM: Neurosurgical anesthesia. In, Miller RD, *Anesthesia*, 5th Edition, Chapter 52, pp 1895-1933. Churchill Livingstone, New York, 2000.

Young WL, Pile-Spellman J: Anesthetic considerations for interventional neuroradiology. *Anesthesiology* 80(2):427-456, 1994.

CHAPTER 12

Anesthesia for Urologic Surgery

CHARLES LEE

INTRODUCTION

The majority of adult patients undergoing renal and genitourinary procedures are elderly. Because of advanced age and the association of cigarette smoking with urologic malignancies, many of these patients have concomitant cardiovascular and pulmonary disease in addition to the physiologic changes of aging. A thorough medical history, physical examination, and appropriate diagnostic and laboratory tests are necessary to evaluate coexisting disease.

To add to the challenges of anesthetizing elderly patients, advances in minimally invasive surgical techniques have made it possible to treat a population of patients who were once considered to be poor candidates for open surgical procedures. In fact, open surgical procedures in urology have largely been replaced by endoscopic procedures, laparoscopy, and lithotripsy. Many urologic diseases are now diagnosed, evaluated, and treated endoscopically through the urethra using specialized instruments such as cystoscopes and resectoscopes. Continuing improvements in instrumentation, along with economic considerations and patient convenience, have furthered this trend. Today, nearly 70% of urologic procedures are performed endoscopically (Boxes 12-1 and 12-2).

INNERVATION OF THE GENITOURINARY SYSTEM

Genitourologic procedures are well suited to regional anesthesia, as the genitourinary system receives segmental sensory nerve supply from the thoracolumbar and sacral outflow. The abdominal components of the genitourinary system, the kidneys and ureters, receive their nerve supply from the autonomic nervous system via both sympathetic and parasympathetic pathways. The pelvic components and the genitalia are innervated by somatic as well as autonomic nerves (Figures 12-1 and 12-2).

The kidneys and ureters are retroperitoneal structures that receive sympathetic innervation from T8–L1. Preganglionic fibers from these segments converge to the celiac plexus and aorticorenal ganglia, from which postganglionic fibers proceed to the kidney. Sympathetic nerves originating from T10–L1 conduct sensations of renal pain. Some sympathetic fibers may also reach the kidney via the splanchnic nerves. Parasympathetic innervation of the kidneys is provided by the vagus nerve, while the parasympathetic fibers from S2–S4 supply the abdominal ureters. Because these spinal segments also provide somatic innervation to the flank, lumbar area, ilioinguinal area, and scrotum or labia, pain from the kidney and ureter is referred to these areas.

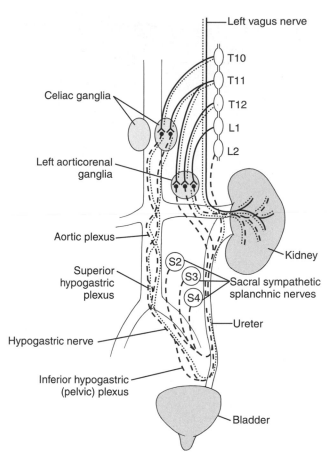

Box 12-1 Common Endourologic Procedures

Cystourethroscopy
Ureteroscopy
Ureteral stent placement
Ureteral stone manipulation
Laser lithotripsy
Transurethral resection of the prostate (TURP)
Transurethral resection of bladder tumors

Box 12-2 Common Urologic Disorders Evaluated Endoscopically

Hematuria
Benign prostatic hypertrophy
Urinary tract stones
Hydronephrosis
Cancer of the prostate
Cancer of the bladder
Cancer of the urethra
Cancer of the ureter
Cancer of the renal pelvis
Strictures of the ureter and urethra
Ureteropelvic junction obstruction
Hemorrhagic or interstitial cystitis

Figure 12-1   Autonomic and sensory innervation of the kidney and ureters. Solid line, preganglionic fibers; dashed line, postganglionic fibers; dotted line, sensory fibers. (Redrawn from Gee WF, Ansell JF. Pelvic and perineal pain of urologic origin. In: Bonica JJ, ed. *The management of pain*, 2nd ed. Philadelphia: Lea & Febiger, 1990:1368-1378.)

The bladder receives sympathetic innervation from the T11–L2 segmental levels. These fibers, which conduct pain sensation, travel through the superior hypogastric plexus and supply the bladder via the right and the left hypogastric nerves. Bladder stretch and fullness sensation, on the other hand, is transmitted via parasympathetic fibers from spinal cord segments S2-S4. These nerve fibers form the pelvic parasympathetic plexus, which is joined by the hypogastric plexus. Vesical branches then innervate the bladder and the proximal urethra. The majority of the bladder's motor innervation, with the exception of the trigone, is provided by the parasympathetic pathways.

The prostate, penile urethra, and penis receive both sympathetic and parasympathetic fibers from the T11–L2 and S2-S4 segments, respectively. Fibers from the pelvic parasympathetic plexus and hypogastric plexus converge at the prostatic plexus, which then supplies the prostate, the penile urethra, and the cavernous tissue of the penis. The primary sensory supply to the penis is via the dorsal nerve of the penis, the first branch of the pudendal nerve (S2–S4).

The scrotum is innervated anteriorly by the ilioinguinal and genitofemoral nerves (L1–L2) and posteriorly by the perineal branches of the pudendal nerve. During

fetal development, the testes descend into the scrotum from their intra-abdominal location. The nerve supply to the testes is similar to that of the kidney and upper ureter because of a shared embryologic origin. Therefore, regional anesthesia should extend up to the T10 sensory level for testicular surgery (Table 12-1).

ENDOUROLOGIC PROCEDURES

Cystoscopy

Cystoscopy is one of the most commonly performed urologic procedures (Figures 12-3 and 12-4). It allows examination and treatment of lower urinary tract disease through direct visualization of the urethra, bladder neck, and bladder. It is commonly performed for the evaluation of hematuria, recurrent urinary tract infections, and urinary obstruction. Either a rigid or flexible endoscope is used. Flexible endoscopes are associated with less discomfort than rigid endoscopes and are useful for diagnostic procedures. A rigid cystoscope is used to perform

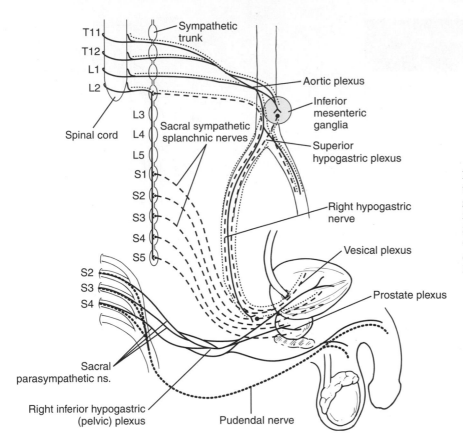

Figure 12-2 Segmental nerve supply to the bladder, penis, and scrotum. Solid line, preganglionic fibers; dashed line, postganglionic fibers; dotted line, sensory fibers. (Redrawn from Gee WF, Ansell JF. Pelvic and perineal pain of urologic origin. In: Bonica JJ, ed. *The management of pain*, 2nd ed. Philadelphia: Lea & Febiger, 1990:1368–1378.)

therapeutic procedures such as bladder biopsy, removal of bladder and prostatic tumors, extraction or laser lithotripsy of renal stones, retrograde pyelography, and placement or manipulation of ureteral stents.

Brief flexible or rigid cystoscopy can often be performed with topical anesthesia in the form of viscous lidocaine instilled into the urethra prior to the procedure, especially in women because of their short urethra. Intravenous sedation is beneficial when a rigid cystoscope is used. Cystoscopies involving therapeutic procedures require regional or general anesthesia. General anesthesia with muscle paralysis should be considered if extensive use of electrocautery is anticipated. Stimulation of the obturator nerve by electrocautery current through the lateral bladder wall may elicit the obturator reflex, which causes external rotation and adduction of the thigh. This sudden musculoskeletal response may cause the surgeon to perforate the bladder with the cystoscope. Central neuraxial anesthesia does not abolish the obturator reflex. General anesthesia with muscle paralysis is the

Table 12-1   Pain Conduction Pathways and Spinal Segment Projection of Pain of the Genitourinary System

Organ	Sympathetics, Spinal Segments	Parasympathetics	Spinal Levels of Pain Conduction
Kidney	T8–L1	X (vagus)	T10–L1
Ureter	T10–L2	S2–S4	T10–L2
Bladder	T11–L2	S2–S4	T11–L12 (dome) S2–S4 (neck)
Prostate	T11–L2	S2–S4	T11–L2, S2–S4
Penis	LI & L2	S2–S4	S2–S4
Scrotum	NS	NS	S2–S4
Testes	T10–L2	NS	T10–L1

NS, not significant for nociceptive function.
From Malhotra V, Diwan S. Anesthesia and the renal and genitourinary systems. In: Miller RD, ed. *Anesthesia*, 5th ed. Philadelphia: Churchill Livingstone, 2000:1934–1959.

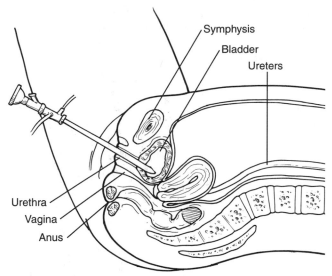

Figure 12-3   Cystoscope introduced into bladder, female anatomy. (Redrawn from Govan DE. *Roche manual of urologic procedures*. Hoffman-LaRoche, 1976.)

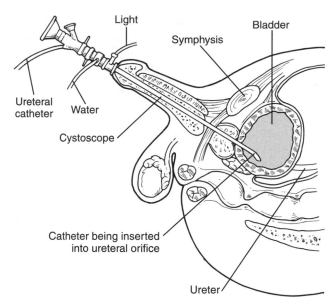

Figure 12-4   Cystoscope introduced into bladder via urethra, male anatomy. (Redrawn from Hardy JD. *Textbook of surgery*. Philadelphia: JB Lippincott, 1988.)

most feasible and reliable method of preventing muscle contractions during the procedure. General anesthesia may also be more practical for most patients because of the short duration of the procedure, which is typically performed on an outpatient basis.

Patients with spinal cord injury frequently experience bladder dysfunction, which predisposes them to urinary tract infections, pyelonephritis, nephrolithiasis, vesicoureteric reflux, and renal failure. These patients undergo frequent urologic procedures, including repeat cystoscopies. Patients with spinal cord lesions at or above the T4–T8 level (the level of the splanchnic outflow) are at risk for autonomic hyperreflexia, which is characterized by systemic hypertension and bradycardia. Autonomic hyperreflexia is manifested by acute paroxysms of sympathetic hyperactivity in response to cutaneous or visceral stimulation below the level of the spinal cord lesion. Loss of descending inhibition of reflex sympathetic nervous system activity over the splanchnic outflow tract results in generalized vasoconstriction below the level of the lesion and systemic hypertension. Subsequent stimulation of the carotid sinus results in reflex bradycardia and cutaneous vasodilation above the level of the lesion. Pallor, piloerection, somatic and visceral muscle contraction, and increased spasticity may be seen below the level of the lesion, while facial flushing, mydriasis, excessive sweating, and congestion of mucous membranes may be seen above the level of the lesion. The patient may complain of nasal congestion and a pounding headache. Severe, sustained hypertension can result in hemorrhagic or hypertensive strokes, seizures, retinal hemorrhages, arrhythmias, myocardial ischemia, and cardiac arrest.

Distension of a hollow viscus, such as the bladder or rectum, commonly precipitates autonomic hyperreflexia. Treatment includes removal of the inciting stimulus (e.g., bladder drainage or fecal disimpaction) and administration of peripheral vasodilating drugs such as sodium nitroprusside, nitroglycerin, or hydralazine. Regional or general anesthesia can be used in patients with high spinal cord lesions. Central neuraxial anesthesia can prevent autonomic hyperreflexia by blocking both limbs of the reflex arc. However, sparing of the sacral segments can sometimes occur with epidural anesthesia, resulting in incomplete block. If using general anesthesia, an adequate depth of anesthesia is required, as light anesthesia can lead to autonomic hyperreflexia.

TRANSURETHRAL RESECTION OF THE PROSTATE

Benign prostatic hypertrophy (BPH) is a nonmalignant enlargement of the prostate gland of men, typically developing after 50 years of age. The prostate surrounds the urethra at the base of the bladder, resulting in compression of the proximal urethra and obstruction to urine flow as the gland enlarges. Benign prostatic hypertrophy initially manifests as frequency, nocturia, and a sensation of incomplete emptying of the bladder. Urinary retention, hydronephrosis, uremia, and renal failure may occur as a result of untreated severe bladder outlet obstruction.

The symptoms of BPH can be attributed to a static component related to the excessive tissue growth and a dynamic component influenced by the tone of the smooth muscle in the prostate. Medical management is aimed at reducing these two components. The prostate gland is androgen-sensitive. Hence, androgen deprivation decreases the size of the prostate and the obstruction of the prostatic urethra, reducing the static component. Oral finasteride inhibits 5α-reductase and has been shown to be moderately effective in reducing the static component of BPH. This drug selectively inhibits the conversion of testosterone to dihydrotestosterone, which is necessary for growth of the prostate gland. Prostatic smooth muscle tone is influenced by alpha-adrenergic receptors present in the prostatic capsule and hyperplastic prostatic tissue. Alpha-adrenergic antagonists such as terazosin, doxazosin, and tamsulosin block adrenergic receptors in these tissues as well as in the bladder neck, decreasing the smooth muscle tone or dynamic component of BPH. While 5α-reductase inhibitors have minimal side-effects, alpha-adrenergic antagonists have vasodilating effects, which can lead to orthostatic hypotension.

Transurethral resection of the prostate (TURP) is one of the most commonly performed surgical procedures in men over the age of 60. Transurethral resection of the prostate is the primary treatment for symptomatic BPH in patients with prostate glands weighing less than 40–50 g. An alternative approach such as suprapubic, perineal, or retropubic prostatectomy is chosen if the prostate weighs more than 80 g. Patients with advanced prostatic carcinoma may also present for TURP to relieve symptomatic urinary obstruction. The procedure is typically preceded by cystoscopy to evaluate the size of the prostate gland and to rule out concomitant pathology such as bladder

tumor or stone. The operation is performed with the resectoscope, a specialized instrument having an electrode capable of both cutting and coagulating tissue (Figure 12-5). The hypertrophied tissue protruding into the prostatic urethra is then resected in small pieces called "chips." Bleeding is controlled with the coagulating current. Visibility is maintained by continuous irrigation, which distends the bladder and washes away blood and dissected prostatic tissue.

Major complications associated with TURP include bleeding, TURP syndrome, arrhythmias, and bladder perforation. Other potential complications include urinary retention, hypothermia, septicemia, and disseminated intravascular coagulation. Patients at increased risk for perioperative morbidity following TURP are those with large prostate glands (>45 g), resection times longer than 90 minutes, acute urinary retention, or age greater than 80 years.

The prostate gland contains a rich plexus of veins (Figure 12-6). Surgical resection opens the extensive network of venous sinuses in the prostate and potentially allows systemic absorption of the irrigating fluid. If the pressure of the irrigating fluid exceeds venous pressure, intravascular absorption of fluid may occur via these open sinuses. The amount of irrigant absorption is governed by the number and size of opened venous sinuses, the hydrostatic pressure of the irrigant (which is determined by the height of the irrigating fluid container above the surgical table), the length of the procedure, the venous pressure at the irrigant–blood interface, and the experience of the surgeon. Typically, 10–30 ml of fluid is absorbed per minute of resection time. There have been reports of absorption of up to 6–8 L of fluid during cases lasting up to 2 hours. Resections should ideally be limited to 1 hour or less, and should not exceed 2 hours because excessive intravascular absorption of the irrigating fluid may lead to cardiovascular and central nervous system (CNS) manifestations known as the TURP syndrome.

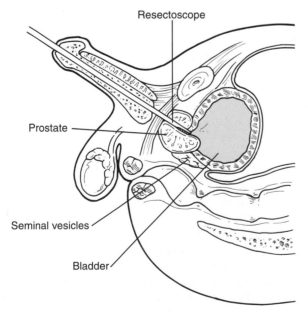

Figure 12-5   Transurethral resection of prostate using a resectoscope. (Redrawn from Govan DE. *Roche manual of urologic procedures*. Hoffman-LaRoche, 1976.)

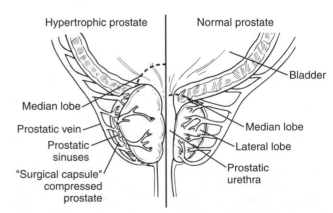

Figure 12-6   Anatomy of the normal and hypertrophic prostate gland. (Redrawn from Stoelting RK, Barash PG, Gallagher TJ. *Advances in anesthesia*. Chicago: Mosby/Year Book, 1986:379.)

Irrigating Solutions for Transurethral Resection of the Prostate

Solutes such as sorbitol, mannitol, glycine, urea, and glucose have been added to water to produce a solution with an osmolality closer to that of plasma (normal serum osmolality is 280–300 mosmol/L). Urea is no longer used because it passes freely into both the intracellular and extracellular spaces, resulting in elevated blood urea concentrations. Sorbitol is metabolized to fructose, which can cause severe hyperglycemia in diabetic patients. Sorbitol is also converted to lactate, resulting in metabolic acidosis proportionate to the amount of solution absorbed. Sorbitol can also induce an osmotic diuresis, resulting in dehydration and a hyperosmolar state. Glucose solutions share many of the problems associated with sorbitol. Absorption of large amounts of mannitol can cause marked intravascular volume expansion followed by osmotic diuresis with resultant dehydration and hyperosmolality.

Glycine is a nonessential amino acid that is thought to be a major inhibitory neurotransmitter, similar to gamma-aminobutyric acid (GABA), in the spinal cord, brain, and retina. Visual disturbances including transient blindness have been associated with the use of glycine-containing irrigation solutions during TURP. These visual disturbances were previously thought to result from cerebral edema secondary to hypervolemia and hyponatremia. However, visual impairment caused by a centrally acting mechanism, such as cerebral edema, manifests as loss of the blink reflex but preservation of light and accommodation reflexes. Blindness associated with hyperglycinemia, on the other hand, is accompanied by dilated pupils, preservation of the blink reflex, and absence of light and accommodation reflexes. Visual impairment typically resolves within 12–24 hours as plasma glycine levels approach normal.

Absorption of glycine may also result in CNS toxicity. Hyperammonemia resulting from oxidative deamination of glycine in the liver into ammonia and glyoxylic acid may cause CNS depression. Delayed awakening and encephalopathy in association with hyperammonemia following TURP, with the use of glycine-containing irrigation solutions, has been observed. Blood ammonia levels were noted to be as high as 834 μmol/L (normal 11–35 μmol/L) in these cases. Encephalopathy is said to occur when ammonia levels exceed 150 μmol/L. However, the relationship between glycine and ammonia levels does not seem to correlate, making the role of hyperammonemia in the TURP syndrome unclear.

Glycine may also compromise renal function. Hyperoxaluria due to metabolism of glycine to oxalate and glycolate places the patient at risk for calcium oxalate deposition in the kidneys. Adequate fluid intake should be maintained in the postoperative period to ameliorate this problem. The qualities of an ideal irrigant for TURP are listed in Box 12-3.

TURP Syndrome

TURP syndrome is characterized by circulatory fluid overload, water intoxication, and occasionally, toxicity from the solute in the irrigating fluid (Table 12-2). This syndrome may present intraoperatively or postoperatively as headache, nausea, restlessness, confusion, respiratory distress, arrhythmias, shock, seizures, and death. Neurologic manifestations are the result of cerebral edema caused by water intoxication and dilutional hyponatremia. Cardiovascular manifestations stem from volume overload and hyponatremia.

Acute hypervolemia due to rapid absorption of irrigating fluids can result in systemic hypertension and reflex bradycardia. Acute circulatory volume overload can cause pulmonary edema in the patient with impaired cardiac function. Pulmonary edema can also be caused by perioperative hyponatremia in association with systemic hypertension with a resultant water flux, along osmotic and hydrostatic pressure gradients, out of the intravascular fluid compartment and into the lungs. Hypovolemic shock and hypotension may ensue as a result of the intravascular fluid volume loss. Acute hyponatremia resulting from intravascular absorption of sodium-free irrigating fluids may cause CNS and electrocardiographic (ECG) changes (Table 12-3).

In the past, distilled water was used for bladder irrigation during TURP because it was nonconductive and it interfered least with visibility. However, intravascular absorption of large amounts of distilled water caused dilutional hyponatremia with resultant hemolysis of red blood cells and CNS symptoms. Electrolyte solutions

---

Box 12-3   Characteristics of an Ideal Irrigating Solution for Transurethral Resection of the Prostate

Isotonic
Nonhemolytic if absorbed
Nonelectrolytic (unable to conduct electrical current from electrocautery device)
Transparent (to allow clear visibility)
Nonmetabolized
Nontoxic
Rapidly excreted
Inexpensive

From Jensen V. The TURP syndrome. *Can J Anaesth* 1991;38:90.

Table 12-2   Manifestations of TURP Syndrome

Cardiopulmonary	Increased central venous pressure
	Hypertension
	Bradycardia
	Arrhythmias
	Pulmonary edema
	Hypoxemia
	Congestive heart failure
	Hypotension
	Myocardial ischemia/angina
	Cardiovascular collapse
Neurologic	
	Restlessness
	Nausea and vomiting
	Mental status changes
	Visual disturbances/blindness
	Seizures
	Coma
Hematologic	
	Hyponatremia
	Hypo-osmolality
	Hemolysis
	Metabolic acidosis
	Solute toxicity
	Hyperglycinemia (glycine)
	Hyperammonemia (glycine)
	Hyperglycemia (sorbitol)
Intravascular volume expansion (mannitol)	

Adapted from: Gravenstein D. Transurethral resection of the prostate (TURP) syndrome: a review of the pathophysiology and management. *Anesth Analg* 1997;84:438–446.

such as normal saline and Ringer's lactate, while better tolerated than distilled water when absorbed intravascularly, have the disadvantage of being highly ionized and able to conduct electrical currents, facilitating dispersion of high-frequency current from the resectoscope. Consequently, distilled water has been replaced

Table 12-3   Signs and Symptoms of Acute Hyponatremia

Serum Sodium Concentration (mEq/L)	Central Nervous System Changes	Electrocardiographic Changes
120	Restlessness Confusion	Possible widening of QRS
115	Nausea Somnolence	Widened QRS Elevated ST segment
110	Seizures Coma	Ventricular tachycardia Ventricular fibrillation

From Jensen V. The TURP syndrome. *Can J Anaesth* 1991;38:90.

with nonelectrolyte isosmotic or near isosmotic solutions for TURP.

While this has significantly reduced the incidence of hemolysis and severe CNS symptoms associated with cerebral edema due to extreme hypo-osmolality, the potential complications of fluid overload and hyponatremia remain. It is now believed that the TURP syndrome occurs if hyponatremia is accompanied by hypo-osmolality, and that CNS signs and symptoms may not manifest themselves if the osmolality remains normal. Because the blood–brain barrier is essentially impermeable to sodium but freely permeable to water, hypo-osmolality, rather than hyponatremia, appears to be the primary physiologic derangement leading to CNS dysfunction. Acute hypo-osmolality may cause cerebral edema and increased intracranial pressure with resultant hypertension and bradycardia.

However, the concentration of extracellular sodium must be in the physiologic range for normal neuronal function. When the serum sodium concentration falls below 110 mEq/L, loss of consciousness and seizures may ensue. Cardiovascular dysfunction secondary to the negative inotropic effects of hyponatremia such as arrhythmias, hypotension, and pulmonary edema may also occur, but is impossible to distinguish from signs and symptoms of fluid overload.

Treatment of TURP Syndrome

Treatment of TURP syndrome should be based on the severity of symptoms. In asymptomatic patients with normal or near normal serum osmolality, no intervention is required. Fluid restriction and a loop diuretic such as furosemide are usually sufficient for eliminating absorbed water. Hypertonic saline (3% sodium chloride solution) should be considered only in cases of symptomatic hyponatremia. Rapid correction of severe hyponatremia in the absence of symptoms can result in central pontine myelinolysis, or osmotic demyelination syndrome (a severe disorder characterized by pseudobulbar palsy and spastic quadriplegia caused by demyelination of corticospinal and corticobulbar tracts within the pons). The presence of symptoms is the most important factor determining morbidity and mortality from hyponatremia. In the symptomatic patient, serum osmolality should be monitored and corrected aggressively with hypertonic saline only until life-threatening symptoms resolve. Further correction of serum sodium concentrations should proceed at rate of approximately 8 mEq/L daily, as most cases of osmotic demyelination have occurred when the rate of correction exceeded 12 mEq/L daily. Hypertonic saline should not be administered at a rate exceeding 100 mL/hr to avoid exacerbation of circulatory fluid overload.

Anesthetic Technique

Although there is no evidence that general anesthesia carries a higher risk of perioperative morbidity and mortality than regional anesthesia, spinal anesthesia appears to be the anesthetic technique of choice for TURP, being used in more than 70% of these procedures in the United States. Spinal anesthesia allows the patient to remain awake, thus facilitating the early detection of TURP syndrome. In a patient who has had previous lumbar spine surgery, caudal epidural anesthesia is another option. An anesthetic level to T10 is required for adequate anesthesia. The more subtle signs of TURP syndrome may be masked under general anesthesia. In the awake patient, TURP syndrome may present as a classic triad of symptoms consisting of an increase in both systolic and diastolic pressures associated with an increase in pulse pressure, bradycardia, and a change in mental status.

Aside from allowing early diagnosis of TURP syndrome, there are other potential benefits of regional anesthesia. It allows the early recognition of bladder perforation and extravasation of irrigating fluid, a relatively common complication of TURP (with an estimated incidence of 1%). Perforation may result from insertion of the resectoscope through the bladder wall or from overdistension of the bladder with irrigating fluid. The majority of perforations are extraperitoneal. Awake patients may complain of nausea, diaphoresis, and pain in the periumbilical, inguinal, or suprapubic areas. The surgeon may also note an irregular return of irrigating fluid. Intraperitoneal extravasation of irrigating fluid resulting from a perforation through the wall of the bladder may produce generalized pain in the upper abdomen or referred pain from the diaphragm to the shoulder or precordial region as well as sudden unexplained hypotension (or hypertension). Extravasation of fluid into the retroperitoneum may produce back pain. While a T10 anesthetic level is required to block the pain associated with bladder distention during TURP, higher levels of spinal block may counter the advantage of regional anesthesia by abolishing abdominal and back pain. Regardless of the anesthetic technique employed, sudden hypotension or hypertension, especially in association with bradycardia (vagally mediated) is suggestive of bladder perforation.

Another advantage of regional anesthesia is the mitigation of intraoperative fluid overload resulting from the increased venous capacitance associated with sympathetic blockade. However, if the volume of irrigant absorption is large, dissipation of the block may acutely decrease venous capacity and result in circulatory overload. Regional anesthesia has also been shown to improve postoperative pain control compared with general anesthesia in patients undergoing TURP.

MINIMALLY INVASIVE TREATMENTS FOR BENIGN PROSTATIC HYPERTROPHY

The most common minimally invasive treatment of BPH is transurethral incision of the prostate. This technique is effective when the primary obstruction is located at the bladder neck and when the enlarged prostate weighs 30 g or less. Prostatic stents may be used in patients who are poor surgical risks.

A number of other techniques have been developed to avoid the morbidity of TURP. These involve either vaporization (electrocautery or laser) or thermocoagulation of the prostate (laser, microwave, radio frequency). The advantages of these procedures over TURP include shorter surgical time, no significant blood loss, and reduced risk of fluid absorption. Transurethral vaporization of the prostate (TUVP) is performed with a standard resectoscope and electrocautery. Visual laser ablation of the prostate (VLAP) is performed with Nd:YAG or Ho:YAG laser through a standard cystoscope. The procedure is very brief, usually 20 minutes or less, and requires that all operating room personnel and the patient wear protective glasses. Minimal blood loss and minimal fluid absorption nearly eliminate these two major complications of conventional TURP. Transurethral needle ablation of the prostate (TUNA) is a technique involving radiofrequency thermocoagulation. Transurethral microwave thermotherapy (TUMT) is performed with a catheter that has a microwave antenna attached to it. These procedures can be performed on an outpatient basis.

Medical management and minimally invasive surgical approaches have been developed to avoid intraoperative complications of surgery such as bleeding, hypervolemia or hypo-osmolality associated with systemic absorption of the irrigating fluid, and postoperative problems such as retrograde ejaculation, impotence, and urinary incontinence. However, TURP and open prostatectomy are the definitive treatments for BPH. Approximately one-third of all males who reach the age of 80 years will require a prostatectomy.

TRANSURETHRAL RESECTION OF BLADDER TUMORS

Bladder cancer is the second most common malignancy of the genitourinary tract, with a peak incidence in the sixth decade of life. Superficial transitional cell carcinoma is the most common bladder tumor and it occurs with a 3:1 male:female ratio. Several factors have been implicated in the etiology of this malignancy, including cigarette smoking, industrial carcinogens, and artificial sweeteners.

The diagnosis and treatment of bladder cancer is usually performed endoscopically. Transurethral resection of a bladder tumor can be performed with either regional or general anesthesia. If regional anesthesia is chosen, a T10 sensory level is required. If the tumor is located in close proximity to the obturator nerve, which courses along the lateral bladder wall and neck, general anesthesia with muscle paralysis will block the obturator reflex and is the preferred anesthetic technique. Transurethral resection of a bladder tumor is associated with a higher incidence of bladder perforation than is TURP. The bladder can be perforated with the endoscope either inadvertently or as a result of thigh adduction caused by electrocautery stimulation of the obturator nerve. Bladder perforation can also occur from overdistension, which can cause tears in areas of the bladder wall thinned by the resection.

EXTRACORPOREAL SHOCK WAVE LITHOTRIPSY

It is estimated that 12% of the population in the United States will experience renal stones at some point in their lifetime. Urolithiasis is three times more prevalent in men than in women with a peak incidence in the third to fourth decade of life. There are several predisposing factors in the pathogenesis of renal calculi (Table 12-4). Most renal stones are composed of calcium oxalate and the causes of hypercalcemia should be considered in these patients. The second most common type of renal stone, magnesium ammonium phosphate (struvite) stones, are associated with chronic urinary tract infections with urea-splitting organisms that produce ammonia. Uric acid stones are frequently

seen in patients with gout and are associated with persistently acidic urine that decreases the solubility of uric acid.

Stones in the renal pelvis are usually painless in the absence of infection or obstruction. Renal stones passing down the ureter, on the other hand, can produce severe intermittent flank pain that radiates down the abdomen along the course of the ureter to the groin and inner thigh. Associated fever, nausea, vomiting, and abdominal distension (secondary to ileus) may mimic an acute surgical abdomen. Urinalysis usually reveals gross or microscopic hematuria, unless there is complete obstruction. Although stones less than 4 mm in size generally pass spontaneously, 10–20% of stones require surgical treatment. Treatment of renal stones is based on the size of the stone, its location in the urinary tract, and its composition. Predisposing factors such as hyperparathyroidism, urinary tract infection, or gout should be corrected and adequate hydration should be maintained.

Since the introduction of extracorporeal shock wave lithotripsy (ESWL) in 1980, it has become the treatment of choice for disintegration of urinary stones in the kidney and upper two-thirds of the ureter. ESWL is a noninvasive alternative to percutaneous nephrolithotomy that is associated with low morbidity and can be performed on an outpatient basis. ESWL employs shock waves to disintegrate renal stones. All lithotripters have four basic components (Figure 12-7):
- An energy source, typically a spark plug
- A device to focus the shock wave, such as an ellipsoidal reflector or mirrors
- A device, fluoroscopy or ultrasound, to visualize and localize the stone in focus
- A coupling medium, either water or mineral oil.

Table 12-4   Composition and Etiology of Renal Calculi

Type of Stone	Incidence (%)	Radiographic Appearance	Etiology
Calcium oxalate	65	Opaque	Primary hyperparathyroidism Idiopathic hypercalciuria Hyperoxaluria Hyperuricosuria
Magnesium ammonium phosphate (struvite)	20	Opaque	Alkaline urine (usually due to chronic bacterial infection)
Calcium phosphate	7.5	Opaque	Renal tubular acidosis
Uric acid	5	Lucent	Acid urine Gout Hyperuricosuria
Cystine	1.5	Opaque	Cystinuria

From Coe FL, Parks, JH, Asplin, JR. The pathogenesis and treatment of kidney stones. *N Engl J Med* 1992;327:1141–1152.

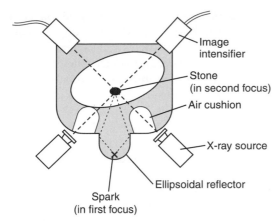

Figure 12-7   *Schematic representation of a lithotripsy unit. (Redrawn from Morgan GE Jr, Mikhail MS, Murray MJ. Anesthesia for genitourinary surgery. In: Clinical anesthesiology, 3rd ed. San Francisco: McGraw-Hill, 2002:692–707.)*

The original lithotripter, the Dornier HM-3, is still in clinical use and employs a warm water bath in a steel tub and a metal gantry chair to support the patient in the sitting position (Figure 12-8). The energy source is a spark-plug generator that creates an explosive discharge (beneath the patient in the first focus of the elliptical reflector) that transmits shock waves to the water. The high-energy shock waves are aimed by an ellipsoidal reflector at a focal point. Two fluoroscopes are oriented so that their beam paths intersect at the focal point above the ellipsoidal

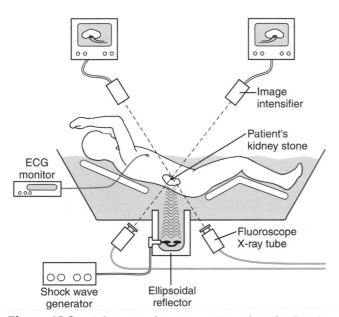

Figure 12-8   *Schematic of patient positioned in the Dornier HM-3 lithotriptor. (Redrawn from Hunter PT II. The physics and geometry pertinent to ESWL. In: Riehle RA Jr, Newman RC, eds. Principles of extracorporeal shock wave lithotripsy. New York: Churchill Livingstone, 1987:14.)*

reflector, and the patient is positioned in the tub so that the renal calculus is centered in these beam paths. Because body tissue has similar acoustic impedance to water, the shock waves travel through the body without dissipation or significant damage to tissue. However, the sudden change in acoustic impedance at the tissue–stone interface releases a blast of energy as the shock wave first encounters the stone and again as it exits the stone on the opposite side, resulting in fragmentation of the stone. Ureteral stents may be placed cystoscopically prior to the procedure to facilitate passage of stone fragments.

Any medium that dissipates the shock wave reduces the energy available to disintegrate the stone. If a nephrostomy or epidural catheter is in place, dressings and tape should be clear of the blast path. These media can absorb up to 80% of the shock wave energy, resulting in failure of lithotripsy.

Although shock waves pass through most tissues relatively unimpeded, some tissue injury does occur. Skin and flank ecchymoses or hematoma in the flank muscles may occur at the entry site of the shock wave. Soft tissue injury is more likely in thin patients, but usually resolves fairly quickly without sequelae. Hematuria is invariably present at the conclusion of the procedure as a result of shock wave-induced endothelial injury to the kidney and ureter. Clot retention can be prevented by maintaining adequate hydration perioperatively. More serious tissue injury can occur if the shock waves are improperly focused at air–tissue interfaces such as in the lung and intestine. Air trapped in alveoli presents an air–tissue interface that dissipates the shock wave energy with resultant alveolar rupture and hemoptysis. Pulmonary contusion is more likely in children or patients of small stature (height less than 48 in) because of the shorter distance of the lung bases from the kidneys. Styrofoam padding should be placed under the back in these patients to shield the lung bases from the shock waves. Stomach or bowel injury may cause abdominal distention, nausea, and vomiting. Inability to position the patient with lung and intestine away from the shock wave focus is a contraindication to ESWL.

Other contraindications include active urinary tract infection, a bleeding diathesis, and pregnancy. Antibiotic treatment for active urinary tract infections before ESWL will minimize septic complications. Coagulopathy increases the risk of perinephric or subcapsular renal hematoma. Even in the absence of a coagulopathy, a perinephric hematoma should be suspected if there is a significant decrease in the hematocrit postoperatively. Preoperative laboratory tests should include prothrombin time, partial thromboplastin time, platelet count, urinalysis, and, in women of childbearing potential, a pregnancy test.

Relative contraindications to ESWL include complete urinary tract obstruction distal to the stone, the presence of an orthopedic prosthesis, or aneurysm of the renal artery or aorta. While patients with small abdominal aortic aneurysms have been safely treated with ESWL following careful positioning, the risk of accidental rupture must be considered. In some centers, renal insufficiency and morbid obesity are also considered to be relative contraindications.

The presence of a cardiac pacemaker (with the exception of abdominally placed pacemakers) is no longer considered a contraindication to ESWL. Electrical interference from the spark gap generating the shock wave can potentially inhibit, reprogram, or damage the internal components of pacemakers, putting patients with these devices at risk for developing shock-wave-induced arrhythmias. In actuality, the incidence of major complications in pacemaker-dependent patients undergoing ESWL is rare. Nevertheless, the following precautions should be taken prior to performing ESWL on these patients:

- A preoperative cardiac evaluation to determine the type of pacemaker and its programmability
- A magnet or reprogramming device, and a programmer who can switch the pacemaker to a nondemand mode, available in the operating room
- An alternate means of pacing available in the operating room
- Positioning of the patient to keep the pacemaker clear of the shock wave path.

Treatment should begin with the lowest shock wave energy level, which is gradually increased while observing pacemaker function. Patients with automatic implanted cardiac defibrillator (AICD) devices also have been successfully treated with lithotripsy. However, AICDs should be shut off just prior to lithotripsy and reactivated immediately following treatment.

Shock waves are synchronized with the patient's ECG to decrease the incidence of arrhythmias during ESWL. The shock waves are usually delivered 20 msec after the R wave to correspond to the ventricular refractory period. Despite the synchronization of shock waves with the patient's ECG, shock-wave-induced cardiac arrhythmias (atrial and ventricular premature complexes, atrial fibrillation, and supraventricular and ventricular tachycardia) occur in 10–14% of patients. Because only a minimal amount of electrical energy generated by the lithotripter actually reaches the myocardium, the arrhythmias are most probably due to mechanical stresses on the conduction system by the shock waves, rather than to electrical currents. Arrhythmias typically resolve once the lithotripsy is stopped.

Water immersion during immersion lithotripsy produces significant effects on the cardiovascular and respiratory systems. The hydrostatic pressure of the water causes peripheral venous compression, resulting in an increase in central blood volume, with a subsequent increase in central venous and pulmonary artery pressures.

The increase in central venous and pulmonary artery pressures linearly correlates with the depth of immersion. Immersion to the clavicles can increase the central venous pressure by 10–14 cmH$_2$O. Despite the increase in venous return, immersion into a heated water bath may lead to transient hypotension as a result of vasodilatation. Increases in arterial blood pressure and a decrease in cardiac output secondary to increased systemic vascular resistance have also been observed in some patients. Patients with a history of congestive heart failure may decompensate if faced with a sudden increase in venous return and systemic vascular resistance. In patients with marginal cardiac reserve, minimal immersion so that only the entry site is covered in water, or a nonimmersion lithotripter, should be considered.

Respiratory effects of water immersion up to the clavicles may predispose the patient to ventilation-perfusion mismatch and hypoxemia. Extrinsic hydrostatic pressure on the upper abdomen and thorax can cause a 20 to 30 percent decrease in the vital capacity and functional residual capacity as well as an increase in the pulmonary blood flow. The increased work of breathing results in a shallow, rapid respiratory pattern. The use of intravenous sedation may potentiate the respiratory depressant effects of immersion (Table 12-5).

Temperature regulation can also be problematic during immersion lithotripsy. Heat transfer is facilitated by vasodilatation produced by anesthesia. Complications associated with hypothermia or hyperthermia can be avoided by maintaining the water temperature in the range of 35.8–37.5° C.

Newer, lower-energy lithotripter units (e.g., Siemens Lithostar, Dornier HM-4, Wolf Piezolith) have been developed to eliminate the water bath and the problems associated with immersion of the patient. These units require only a small amount of mineral oil on the skin to acoustically couple the patient to the energy source. The energy source is encased in a water-filled housing and comes

Table 12-5	Physiologic Effects of Immersion during Lithotripsy	
Cardiovascular	Increased	Central blood volume
		Central venous pressure
		Pulmonary artery pressure
Respiratory	Increased	Pulmonary blood flow
	Decreased	Vital capacity
	Decreased	Functional residual capacity
	Decreased	Tidal volume
	Increased	Respiratory rate

From Malhotra V, Diwan S. Anesthesia and the renal and genitourinary systems. In Miller RD, ed. *Anesthesia*, 5th ed. Philadelphia: Churchill Livingstone, 2000:1934-1959.

into contact with the patient via a plastic membrane. These lithotripter units generate shock waves electromagnetically or from piezoelectric elements. The lower energy of the shock wave minimizes the pain associated with the procedure.

Anesthetic Techniques for Extracorporeal Shock Wave Lithotripsy

The pain during lithotripsy occurs as a small amount of the shock wave energy is dissipated at the entry site at the skin surface and viscera. The pain is proportionate to the intensity of the shock wave. Lithotripter units that employ a water bath use high-intensity shock waves, which are painful and poorly tolerated without either regional or general anesthesia. The newer lithotripter units that are directly coupled to the patient use lower-intensity shock waves, which are less painful and easily tolerated with light sedation. Intravenous sedation and analgesia (e.g., low-dose propofol infusions with midazolam and opioid supplementation) usually provide sufficient anesthesia for treatment with these newer units.

General or regional anesthesia can be used for immersion lithotripsy. Continuous epidural anesthesia is commonly used for immersion lithotripsy. Epidural anesthesia facilitates patient positioning because the patient is awake and cooperative, thus decreasing the risk of bodily and peripheral nerve injuries. A T6 sensory level is required for adequate anesthesia. Loss of resistance to saline technique for identifying the epidural space may be preferable to loss of resistance to air. If loss of resistance to air is used, only the smallest amount of air necessary should be injected, as air in the epidural space will provide an air–tissue interface and cause dissipation of shock wave energy with potential injury to local tissue, including neural tissue. The epidural catheter must be taped away from the blast path so as not to dissipate the energy of the shock waves. Foam tape should not be used to secure the catheter for the same reason. Intravenous volume expansion may prevent profound postural hypotension associated with sympathetic blockade in conjunction with a sitting position and immersion in a warm water bath. Although spinal anesthesia has a more rapid onset than epidural anesthesia, it also has a higher incidence of hypotension and less control over the sensory level and duration of blockade. After the patient is properly positioned, supplemental oxygen by face mask or nasal cannula and light sedation may be given. A decrease in functional residual capacity with immersion mandates close monitoring of oxygen saturation.

The main disadvantage of regional anesthesia is the inability to control diaphragmatic movement. Excessive diaphragmatic excursion during spontaneous respiration can move the stone in and out of the shock wave focus, prolonging the procedure. Bradycardia associated with high sympathetic blockade also prolongs the procedure when the shock waves are synchronized to the ECG.

General endotracheal anesthesia provides the advantages of rapid induction of anesthesia and control of patient ventilation and movement. A muscle relaxant is often used to facilitate control of diaphragmatic movement. However, moving and positioning an unconscious patient increases the risk of positional injury. Intravenous volume expansion is again recommended prior to positioning and immersion in the water bath. Following the initial fluid loading, an additional 1000–2000 mL of lactated Ringer's solution is given during the procedure along with 10–20 mg of furosemide to maintain brisk urinary flow to help flush stone fragments and blood clots. Fluid management should be more cautious in patients with poor cardiac reserve.

PERCUTANEOUS ENDOUROLOGIC PROCEDURES

Percutaneous nephrostomy is commonly performed for the diagnosis and treatment of renal obstruction, stone extraction, biopsy of tumors, and ureteral stent placement. The procedure involves placement of a drainage catheter into the kidney, over a guidewire that is inserted into the renal collecting system under fluoroscopic guidance. This procedure requires the patient to be prone. Local anesthesia with intravenous sedation provides adequate analgesia unless the nephrostomy tract must be dilated. Passage of an endoscope through the nephrostomy tract or percutaneous nephrolithotomy (a procedure to remove renal stones too large to be treated with lithotripsy) requires serial dilation of the nephrostomy tract. Dilation of the nephrostomy tract is painful, necessitating either general or regional anesthesia.

Percutaneous nephroscopy procedures require continuous irrigation of fluid through the endoscope to prevent blood and debris from obscuring the field of view. Because electrocautery is rarely used during percutaneous endourologic procedures, 0.9% sodium chloride is used for irrigation. Extravasation of irrigation fluid into the retroperitoneal, intraperitoneal, intravascular, or pleural spaces is possible. The quantity of the irrigating fluid infused should be compared with the output of fluid into the suction and urinary catheters. Termination of the procedure should be considered if there is an unaccountable discrepancy in excess of 500 mL. Intravascular absorption of irrigation fluid during the procedure can result in electrolyte abnormalities and fluid overload with a clinical picture similar to TURP syndrome.

Although less invasive than open surgical procedures, serious complications can occur during percutaneous endourologic procedures. Trauma to the spleen, liver, or kidney can occur during insertion of the nephrostomy tube, requiring an emergency open surgical procedure. Colon injury may occur if a retrorenal colon overlies the lower pole of the kidney. Pleural injury can occur when the nephrostomy access is created above the 12th rib or if the kidney lies in a more cephalad position than normal, resulting in a pleural effusion or hydro-pneumothorax.

UROLOGIC LASER SURGERY

Lasers are being used increasingly for a wide variety of urologic problems including ureteral calculi, ureteral stricture, bladder neck contracture, BPH, interstitial cyst-itis, superficial carcinoma of the penis, bladder, ureter, and renal pelvis, and condyloma acuminatum of the external genitalia and urethra. The advantages of laser surgery over conventional surgical approaches include minimal blood loss and decreased postoperative pain. The various lasers available for clinical use each have specific indications and limitations.

The carbon dioxide laser produces intense heat with vaporization but cannot penetrate water and is capable of only minimal tissue penetration. Its use is primarily limited to treating cutaneous lesions of the external genitalia. The plume of smoke generated from the vaporization of condyloma acuminatum contains active human papilloma virus particles. During CO_2 laser therapy for genital lesions, a means of evacuating the smoke plume from the operating room should be available and all operating room personnel should wear protective laser masks to prevent inhalation of infectious particles.

The pulsed dye laser is used in laser lithotripsy for distal ureteral stones that are not amenable to ESWL. The pulsed dye laser generates pulsatile energy that is absorbed by the stone, causing its disintegration. The laser beam is carried over a bare wire passed through a rigid ureteroscope. There is potential for ureteral mucosal injury and perforation during this procedure. Patient movement should be avoided. If regional anesthesia is selected, a T8 sensory level should be achieved. Adequate intravenous hydration should be administered as hematuria is expected with this procedure.

The neodymium:yttrium–aluminum–garnet (Nd:YAG) laser produces deep tissue penetration via coagulation with minimal vaporization. This laser can penetrate water and urine with minimal absorption and uses a fiberoptic laser delivery system. The Nd:YAG laser has been used to treat lesions of the penis, urethra, bladder, ureters, and kidneys. However, its greatest potential in endourologic surgery may be in its use for laser prosta-tectomy. The advantages of laser prostatectomy over conventional TURP include minimal blood loss and minimal fluid absorption, virtually eliminating these major complications associated with conventional TURP procedures. Thus, laser prostatectomy is a promising alternative to conventional TURP in critically ill patients. Because bleeding is minimal during laser prostatectomy, copious irrigation is not necessary, minimizing bladder distension and allowing the use of caudal anesthesia in these patients.

The KTP-532 laser is a frequency-doubled Nd:YAG laser. It does not penetrate tissue as deeply as the Nd:YAG laser but it has a better cutting effect that is useful for the treatment of urethral strictures and bladder neck contractures. The argon laser can also penetrate water but is selectively absorbed by hemoglobin and melanin, making it useful for bladder procedures requiring coagulation of bleeding sites.

Appropriate eye protection should be worn by all operating room personnel during laser procedures, as both direct and reflected laser beams can cause eye injury. The part of the eye that is susceptible to injury is determined by the wavelength of the laser. Carbon dioxide laser beams can cause a corneal ulceration but energy is not transmitted to the retina. Because the argon, Nd:YAG, and KTP-532 lasers pass through the anterior chamber of the eye with minimal absorption, these lasers have potential for injury to the retina.

LAPAROSCOPIC UROLOGIC SURGERY

Laparoscopic surgery is minimally invasive and is associated with decreased postoperative pain, shorter hospital stays, and more rapid recovery than open surgical procedures. Laparoscopic urologic procedures include adrenalectomy, nephrectomy, nephroureterectomy, cystectomy, bladder suspension, hernia repair, varicocelectomy, and pelvic lymph node dissection. Pelvic lymph node dissection, which is used to stage prostate cancer, is the most commonly performed laparoscopic urologic procedure in adults. Laparoscopic pelvic lymph node dissection requires the use of a steep Trendelenburg position and rotation from side to side for surgical exposure. Hypothermia can result from copious fluid irrigation to remove clots from the pelvic fossa.

The usual cardiopulmonary alterations and complications associated with laparoscopy also apply to laparoscopic urologic procedures. However, laparoscopic urologic surgery presents an additional set of problems related to the retroperitoneal location of the urogenital system. Insufflation of the retroperitoneal space and its communications with the thorax and the subcutaneous tissue predispose these patients to subcutaneous emphysema, which may extend up to the head and neck. In severe cases pharyngeal swelling may occur as a result of submucous accumulation of CO_2. There is some evidence to suggest that CO_2 absorption is greater with extraperitoneal compared with intraperitoneal insufflation which, along with the lengthy nature of some laparoscopic urologic procedures such as cystectomy and nephrectomy, allows for sufficient absorption of CO_2 to result in acidemia. Ventilation must be monitored and adjusted as needed to maintain normocarbia.

Intraoperative oliguria despite adequate hydration has been associated with prolonged periods of pneumoperitoneum during laparoscopic nephrectomy. The oliguria is transient and resolves in the immediate postoperative period. The exact mechanism of this transient intraoperative oliguria is unclear but it may be due to decreased renal cortical blood flow and renal vein obstruction resulting from increased perirenal pressure associated with insufflation. Because intraoperative oliguria during prolonged laparoscopic procedures may not reflect intravascular volume depletion, overzealous fluid administration in this setting may lead to hypervolemia and congestive heart failure in susceptible patients.

OPEN UROLOGIC SURGICAL PROCEDURES

Open Prostate Surgery

Open procedures on the prostate gland include simple prostatectomy, radical prostatectomy, and retropubic exposure of the prostate for brachytherapy. Simple prostatectomy is performed for benign prostatic hypertrophy or adenoma that is too large to be resected transurethrally. The prostate gland is exposed through a retropubic approach and the anterior capsule is incised, exposing the central part of the prostate, which is then excised, leaving behind the peripheral prostate. In a suprapubic prostatectomy, the incision is made in the bladder and resection is performed from within the bladder.

Adenocarcinoma of the prostate is the most commonly diagnosed cancer in men and the second leading cause of cancer deaths in men older than 55 years of age. Localized prostate cancer is treated with either radiation therapy or radical prostatectomy. Radical prostatectomy involves a limited pelvic lymphadenectomy and *en bloc* removal of the entire prostate gland along with the bladder neck, the seminal vesicles and the ampullae of the vas deferens. The bladder neck remnant is anastomosed to the membranous urethra over an indwelling urethral catheter. The surgeon may request intravenous administration of indigo carmine dye for visualization of the ureters. This dye may cause a transient spurious decrease in oxygen saturation, hypertension, or a rare allergic reaction with bronchoconstriction and hypotension.

Massive blood loss may occur during control of the dorsal vein complex or if one of the branches of the hypogastric vein is inadvertently torn during pelvic lymphadenectomy. An arterial line is useful for continuous blood pressure monitoring and frequent blood draws. Central venous pressure monitoring to aid in the assessment of volume status may be indicated in patients with cardiopulmonary disease. Potential complications of this surgery include thromboembolism; hemorrhage; injuries to the obturator nerve, ureter, and rectum; urinary incontinence; and impotence. In more recent years, attention has been placed on preserving potency through techniques that spare nerves to the corpora cavernosa.

Radical prostatectomy is performed through either a retropubic or perineal approach depending on the surgeon's preference. Radical retropubic prostatectomy is performed via a low-midline abdominal incision with the patient in a supine hyperextended position (Figure 12-9) to facilitate exposure of the pelvis. The patient is positioned with the iliac crests over the break in the operating table, which is then extended, or the kidney rest is elevated. Elevation of the kidney rest may cause a decrease in blood pressure due to inferior vena cava compression. The operating table is then placed in Trendelenburg position until the legs and operative field are horizontal, which places the pelvis above the heart. Although venous air embolism due to a gravitational gradient between the prostatic veins and the heart has been reported; this appears to be a rare event.

Radical perineal prostatectomy is associated with less intraoperative blood loss, better exposure for the vesicourethral anastomosis, and shorter convalescence times. This approach requires the patient to be positioned in an exaggerated lithotomy position with slight flexion of the trunk and a Trendelenburg tilt that results in the sacrum and pelvis being tilted upward so that the perineum is parallel to the floor (Figure 12-10). This position forces the abdominal contents upon the diaphragm, which may cause respiratory embarrassment. The Trendelenburg position also induces venous distension of the upper body and neck. Prolonged Trendelenburg in combination with administration of large amounts of intravenous fluids can cause edema of the airway, tongue, and face, making airway management difficult should intubation be required during regional anesthesia.

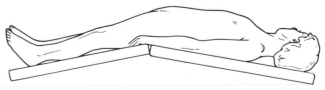

Figure 12-9   Hyperextended supine position. (Redrawn from Mikhail MS, Thangathurai D. Anesthetic considerations for genitourinary and renal surgery. In: Longnecker DE, Tinker JH, Morgan GE Jr, eds. *Principles and practice of anesthesiology*, 2nd ed. Portland: Mosby, 1998:1961–1987.)

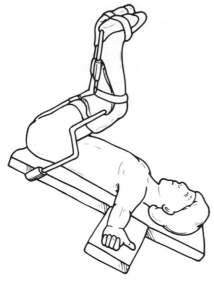

Figure 12-10   Exaggerated lithotomy position. (Redrawn from Mikhail MS, Thangathurai D. Anesthetic considerations for genitourinary and renal surgery. In: Longnecker DE, Tinker JH, Morgan GE Jr, eds. *Principles and practice of anesthesiology*, 2nd ed. Portland: Mosby, 1998:1961–1987.)

Regional (spinal, continuous spinal, continuous epidural), general, or a combined regional-general anesthetic technique is acceptable for open prostatectomy. Because of the extreme positioning for radical perineal prostatectomy, general or combined regional–general anesthesia may be preferable to regional anesthesia for patient comfort and airway management. If regional anesthesia is selected for open prostatectomy, a T8 block level is optimal. The benefits of regional anesthesia include decreased intraoperative blood loss and a lower incidence of thromboembolic complications. However, there is no difference in postoperative morbidity whether regional, combined regional–general, or general anesthesia is used. Postoperative pain can be controlled with patient controlled analgesia, epidural analgesia, intrathecal morphine, or a combination of ketorolac and rescue opiates.

Open Nephrectomy

Nephrectomies fall into three groups: simple, partial, and radical. A simple nephrectomy is the surgical excision of the kidney and only a small segment of the proximal ureter. Simple nephrectomy is performed for benign conditions such as chronic hydronephrosis, hypoplastic kidney, renovascular hypertension, and double collecting system. The procedure is generally performed via a dorsal approach with an incision extending from the 12th rib to the iliac crest along the lateral edge of the sacrospinalis muscle and quadratus lumborum muscle.

Partial nephrectomy is the surgical excision of the diseased segment of the kidney. It is typically performed for localized renal cell carcinomas and benign tumors

of the kidney such as angiomyolipomas, as well as for duplicated collecting systems. The flank approach is used for this operation. The incision is made over the 12th or 11th rib (or in between) and extended anteriorly.

Radical nephrectomy is the *en bloc* removal of the kidney, the ipsilateral adrenal gland, the surrounding perinephric fat, and Gerota's fascia, along with the proximal two-thirds of the ureter. This procedure includes paracaval or para-aortic lymphadenectomy. In adults, radical nephrectomy is most commonly performed for renal cell carcinoma (also known as hypernephroma), which accounts for approximately 3% of all adult malignancies. Renal cell carcinoma has a peak incidence between the 5th and 6th decades of life. Renal cell carcinoma is often associated with paraneoplastic syndromes such as erythrocytosis, hypercalcemia, hypertension, and nonmetastatic hepatic dysfunction. The classic triad of hematuria, flank pain, and a renal mass occurs in only 10% of patients. Unfortunately, the mass may reach a considerable size before symptoms become apparent.

Radical nephrectomy can be performed via a flank, anterior subcostal, transabdominal, or thoracoabdominal incision. If the flank approach is used, the patient is placed in the flexed lateral decubitus position with the operative side up and the kidney rest elevated beneath the 12th rib (Figure 12-11). The thoracoabdominal approach (Figure 12-12) is preferred for large tumors, especially if the tumor extends (as a thrombus) into the renal vein and inferior vena cava. The tumor thrombus may extend into the inferior vena cava but below the liver, up to the liver but below the diaphragm, or above the diaphragm and into the right atrium. If there is extensive tumor invasion into the inferior vena cava and right atrium, cardiopulmonary bypass and hypothermic circulatory arrest may be necessary. Acute blood loss and massive blood transfusion should be anticipated. Heparinization and hypothermia associated with cardiopulmonary bypass increase surgical blood loss. Arterial blood pressure monitoring and multiple large bore intravenous catheters are indicated. Central venous cannulation is used for pressure mon-

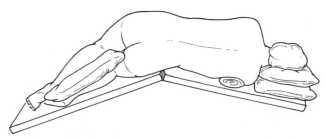

Figure 12-11   Flexed lateral decubitus position. (Redrawn from Mikhail MS, Thangathurai D. Anesthetic considerations for genitourinary and renal surgery. In: Longnecker DE, Tinker JH, Morgan GE Jr, eds. *Principles and practice of anesthesiology*, 2nd ed. Portland: Mosby, 1998:1961–1987.)

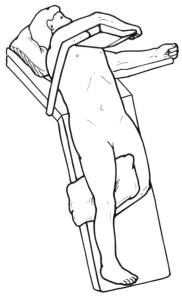

Figure 12-12 Modified hyperextended supine position for thoracoabdominal incisions. (Redrawn from Mikhail MS, Thangathurai D. Anesthetic considerations for genitourinary and renal surgery. In: Longnecker DE, Tinker JH, Morgan GE Jr, eds. *Principles and practice of anesthesiology*, 2nd ed. Portland: Mosby, 1998:1961–1987.)

itoring as well as for additional intravenous access. Central venous pressure will be high if there is venous obstruction from caval involvement of the tumor. Pulmonary artery catheterization may be indicated in patients with impaired left ventricular function, except in cases where the thrombus extends into the right atrium. Pulmonary embolization of the tumor may manifest as sudden arterial desaturation and profound hypotension or supraventricular arrhythmias. Intraoperative transesophageal echocardiography is useful in defining

the extent of the thrombus and in the hemodynamic management of patients with right atrial involvement.

Nephroureterectomy is a radical nephrectomy with resection of the ureter, including the ureteral orifice, and a cuff of the surrounding bladder wall. It is performed for transitional cell carcinoma of the renal collecting system or ureter, and is accompanied by a regional lymphadenectomy to aid in staging. The surgical approach is either transabdominal or extraperitoneal through an extended flank incision starting at the tip of the 11th rib and curving caudally along the lateral edge of the rectus abdominis muscle down to the pubic bone.

Open Cystectomy

Open cystectomies account for 15–20% of all urologic procedures and are categorized as simple, partial, or radical surgeries. Simple cystectomy involves the removal of the bladder only. It is performed for benign conditions such as contracted bladder, severe hemorrhagic cystitis, and radiation cystitis. The procedure is performed through a lower abdominal incision with the patient supine.

Partial cystectomy is the excision of only the diseased portion of the bladder. This procedure is reserved for invasive tumors located in the dome of the bladder of older patients who are too ill to safely undergo a major operation such as radical cystectomy. Cystoscopy is used to identify the site of pathology. The surgery is then performed through a lower abdominal incision with the patient supine. Spinal, continuous epidural, or general anesthesia has been used successfully for this procedure.

Radical cystectomy is the removal of the bladder and the distal ureters, as well as the prostate gland and seminal vesicles in men and the uterus, ovaries, and anterior vaginal wall in women (Figure 12-13). It is accompanied by a

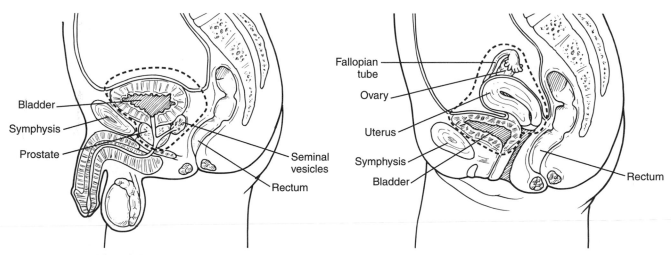

Figure 12-13 Anatomy of the pelvis, with tissue to be excised during a radical cystectomy outlined by the dashed line. **A**, male; **B**, female. (Redrawn from *Atlas of general surgery*. London: Butterworths, 1986.)

pelvic lymphadenectomy, which, along with cystoscopy and computed tomography or magnetic resonance imaging, aids in staging. Following cystectomy, a urinary diversion is created, usually as an ileal conduit or a colon conduit in which the ureters are implanted into a segment of bowel, which is brought through the abdominal wall as a stoma (Figure 12-14). Alternatively, bladder substitution (Figure 12-15) may be performed in which a segment of bowel is fashioned into a pouch into which the ureters are implanted. The dependent part of the pouch is then connected to the membranous urethra, avoiding a stoma.

Radical cystectomy is performed for the treatment of invasive transitional cell carcinoma of the bladder. Many of these patients may have coexisting cardiopulmonary disease, as transitional cell carcinoma of the bladder is associated with cigarette smoking. Some patients with bladder cancer may be treated with chemotherapy prior to surgery. The preoperative evaluation may be influenced by the chemotherapeutic agent used. Commonly used chemotherapeutic drugs include doxorubicin, methotrexate, vinblastine, and cisplatinum. Doxorubicin has cardiotoxic effects that may lead to impaired left ventricular function, methotrexate may cause hepatic toxicity, and both methotrexate and cisplatinum are associated with neurotoxicity and nephrotoxicity.

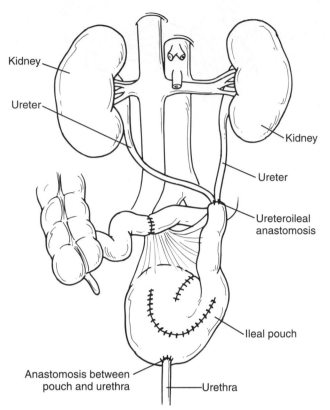

Figure 12-15 Bladder substitution. A segment of ileum is fashioned into a pouch and anastomosed to the urethra. The ureters are joined to the proximal, nondetubularized segment. (Redrawn from Gill HS, Freiha FS, Deem SA, Pearl RG. Urology. In: Jaffe RA, Samuels SI, eds. *Anesthesiologist's manual of surgical procedures*, 2nd ed. Philadelphia: Lippincott Williams & Wilkins, 1999:635–670.)

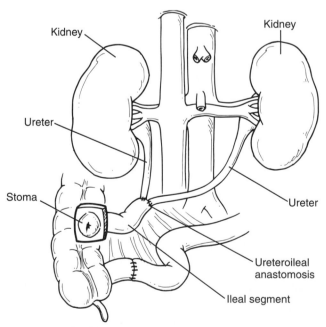

Figure 12-14 Ileal conduit. A segment of ileum is isolated from terminal ileum and continuity of the bowel is re-established with an end-to-end anastomosis. Ureters are joined to the proximal end of the ileal segment and the distal end is brought out to the skin as a stoma. (Redrawn from Gill HS, Freiha FS, Deem SA, Pearl RG. Urology. In: Jaffe RA, Samuels SI, eds. *Anesthesiologist's manual of surgical procedures*, 2nd ed. Philadelphia: Lippincott Williams & Wilkins, 1999:635–670.)

Radical cystectomy is a major operation and is usually performed through a midline incision that extends from the pubis to the xiphoid process. Fluid requirements are high, a result of preoperative bowel preparation, extensive intraperitoneal exposure, and significant blood loss. Blood transfusions are frequently necessary. Deliberate hypotension may reduce intraoperative blood loss and transfusion requirements in acceptable candidates. Relative contraindications for deliberate hypotension include cerebrovascular disease, cardiovascular disease, and severe pulmonary disease. Monitors should include an arterial line. Central venous pressure monitoring is advisable in patients with limited cardiac reserve and is useful as a guide to intravenous fluid administration, as urinary output as a measure of volume status is not available during the entire operation. A pulmonary artery catheter should be considered in patients with impaired ventricular function.

General anesthesia combined with a continuous thoracic epidural can facilitate induced hypotension, decrease intraoperative anesthetic requirements, and provide excellent postoperative analgesia. A potential drawback of epidural anesthesia is that unopposed parasympathetic activity due to sympathetic blockade may result in a contracted, hyperperistaltic bowel that makes a bladder substitution procedure technically difficult. A large dose of an anticholinergic agent such as glycopyrrolate (1 mg) or glucagon (1 mg) may mitigate this problem.

SUMMARY

Elderly patients with significant cardiovascular and pulmonary comorbidities frequently present for genitourinary surgery. Less invasive endoscopic surgical techniques have made it possible to include high-risk patients who may not have been considered to be surgical candidates in the past. A complete preoperative evaluation can help prevent perioperative complications and delays.

Segmental thoracolumbar and sacral innervation of the genitourinary system allows regional anesthesia to be used effectively for urologic surgeries. A T8 sensory level will provide adequate anesthesia and analgesia for surgery of the upper urinary system. However, the benefit of regional anesthesia in allowing early detection of bladder perforation may be lost if sensory blockade is higher than T10 during transurethral resection of bladder tumors and TURP, as pain symptoms may be abolished. While overall outcome appears to be similar when regional anesthesia is compared with general anesthesia for TURP, regional anesthesia may facilitate the diagnosis of TURP syndrome.

TURP syndrome manifests as a constellation of cardiopulmonary and neurologic symptoms associated with circulatory fluid overload, water intoxication, and toxicity from the solute in the irrigating fluid (particularly with the use of glycine-containing irrigation solutions). Fluid absorption is primarily determined by the hydrostatic pressure of the irrigating fluid (which depends on the height of the fluid bag) and the length of the resection. Neurologic symptoms reflect acute hypo-osmolality, with resultant cerebral edema and increased intracranial pressure, as well as neuronal dysfunction associated with hyponatremia. Treatment of TURP syndrome should be guided by the severity of symptoms. Over-aggressive correction of severe hyponatremia may result in central pontine myelinolysis. Once life-threatening symptoms resolve, correction of serum sodium concentrations should proceed more cautiously at a rate of 8–10 mEq/L daily.

Renal stones affect a significant proportion of the population of the United States. ESWL is the preferred treatment for urinary stones in the kidney and upper two-thirds of the ureter. Immersion lithotripsy produces predictable physiologic derangements of the cardiovascular and respiratory systems. Central venous and pulmonary artery pressures increase linearly with the depth of immersion. Immersion in water up to the clavicles can cause a decrease in the vital capacity and functional residual capacity as well as an increase in the pulmonary blood flow,

resulting in ventilation-perfusion mismatch and hypoxemia. Patients with limited cardiac reserve may experience congestive heart failure as a result of a sudden increase in venous return and systemic vascular resistance. Minimal immersion is recommended in susceptible patients. Newer lithotripter units have eliminated water immersion and the problems associated with it.

Major open urologic surgeries, in particular radical procedures for urologic malignancies, are associated with considerable blood loss, extensive incisions, and extremes of positioning. The need for blood transfusions and significant fluid requirements should be anticipated. Continuous epidural anesthesia provides excellent postoperative analgesia and should be considered, especially for radical nephrectomy or cystectomy. Proper positioning and close attention to protection of extremities and pressure points can help avoid iatrogenic nerve injuries.

SUGGESTED READING

Albin MS, Ritter RR, Reinhart R, *et al*. Venous air embolism during radical retropubic prostatectomy. *Anesth Analg* 1992; 74:151–153.

Azar I. Transurethral resection of prostate. In: Malhotra V (ed). *Anesthesia for renal and genitourinary surgery*. New York: McGraw-Hill, 1996:93–109.

Bromage PR, Bonsu AK, el-Faqih SR, Husain I. Influence of Dornier HM3 system on respiration during extracorporeal shock-wave lithotripsy. *Anesth Analg* 1989;68:363–367.

Cooper D, Wilkoff B, Masterson M, *et al*. Effects of extracorporeal shock wave lithotripsy on cardiac pacemakers and its safety in patients with implanted cardiac pacemakers. *Pacing Clin Electrophysiol* 1988;11:1607–1616.

Deem SA, Pearl RG, Gill HS, *et al*. Urology. In: Jaffe RA, Samuels SI, eds. *Anesthesiologist's manual of surgical procedures*, 2nd ed. Philadelphia: Lippincott Williams & Wilkins, 1999:635–670.

Drach GW, Weber C, Donovan JM. Treatment of pacemaker patients with extracorporeal shock wave lithotripsy: experience from 2 continents. *J Urol* 1990;143:895–896.

Gravenstein D. Transurethral resection of the prostate (TURP) syndrome: a review of the pathophysiology and management. *Anesth Analg* 1997;84:438–446.

Hoekstra PT, Kahnoski R, McCamish MA, *et al*. Transurethral prostatic resection syndrome – a new perspective: encephalopathy with associated hyperammonemia. *J Urol* 1983; 130: 704–707.

Kenyon HR. Perforation in transurethral operations: technic for immediate diagnosis and management of extravasations. *JAMA* 1950;142:798.

Lundergan DK. Practical laser safety. In: Smith JA Jr, Stein BS, Benson RC, eds. *Lasers in urologic surgery*, 2nd ed. Chicago: Year Book, 1989:165.

Malhotra V, Diwan S. Anesthesia and the renal and genitourinary systems. In: Miller RD, ed. *Anesthesia*, 5th ed. Philadelphia: Churchill Livingstone, 2000:1934–1959.

Mebust WK, Holtgrewe HL, Cockett AT, Peters PC. Transurethral prostatectomy: immediate and postoperative complications. A cooperative study of 13 participating institutions evaluating 3,885 patients. *J Urol* 1989;141:243-247.

Mikhail MS, Thangathurai D. Anesthetic considerations for genitourinary and renal surgery. In: Longnecker DE, Tinker JH, Morgan GE Jr, eds. *Principles and practice of anesthesiology*, 2nd ed. Portland: Mosby, 1998:1961-1987.

Monk TG, Weldon BC. The renal system and anesthesia for urologic surgery. In: Barash PG, Cullen BF, Stoelting RK, eds. *Clinical anesthesia*, 3rd ed. Philadelphia: Lippincott Williams & Wilkins, 1997:945-973.

Morgan GE Jr, Mikhail MS, Murray MJ. Anesthesia for genitourinary surgery. In: *Clinical anesthesiology*, 3rd ed. San Francisco: McGraw-Hill, 2002:692-707.

Roesch RP, Stoelting RK, Lingeman JE, *et al*. Ammonia toxicity resulting from glycine absorption during a transurethral resection of the prostate. *Anesthesiology* 1983;58:577-579.

Stoelting RK, Dierdorf SF. Renal diseases. In: *Anesthesia and co-existing disease*, 4th ed. Philadelphia: Churchill Livingstone, 2002:341-372.

Vassolas G, Roth RA, Venditti FJ Jr. Effect of extracorporeal shock wave lithotripsy on implantable cardioverter defibrillator. *Pacing Clin Electrophysiol* 1993;16:1245-1248.

Weber W, Back P, Wildgans H, *et al*. Anesthetic considerations in patients with cardiac pacemakers undergoing extracorporeal shock wave lithotripsy. *Anesth Analg* 1988;67:S251.

Weber W, Chaussy C, Madler C, *et al*. Cardiocirculatory changes during anesthesia for extracorporeal shock wave lithotripsy. *J Urol* 1984;4:246A.

Anesthesia for Hepatobiliary Surgery

PEDRO ALEJANDRO MENDEZ-TELLEZ

Case Study

A 48-year-old man with a history of chronic viral hepatitis B infection and mild cirrhosis presented with a 6-month history of weight loss, abdominal distention, and right upper quadrant pain. An abdominal computed tomography scan demonstrated the presence of a solid mass in the right lobe of the liver, hepatosplenomegaly and moderate ascites. On physical examination, the patient is malnourished and jaundiced. The platelet count is 45,000 mm^3 and the international normalized ratio is 2.5. He is scheduled for a partial hepatic resection.

ANATOMY OF THE LIVER AND THE BILIARY TRACT

The liver is the largest visceral organ. It weighs on average 1.2–1.5 kg. Anatomically, the liver is divided into the right and left lobes, which are separated by the falciform ligament. Surgically, the point of division between the right and left lobes is at the porta hepatis. The surgical right and left lobes are in turn divided into eight different segments, which guide the line of surgical resections.

Histologic Anatomy

The *hepatic lobule* is the basic histologic unit and the *acinus* is the functional unit of the liver. The hepatic lobule is a hexagonal unit with a centrilobular vein with converging cords of hepatocytes and sinusoids in a bicycle-spoke arrangement. At the periphery, the portal triads contain terminal bile canaliculi, portal venules, and hepatic arterioles, along with lymphatics and nerves. The functional unit of the liver, the acinus, is divided into three zones according to the distance from the portal triad.

Hepatocytes in zone 1, the periportal zone, are located closest to the triad. They receive blood with the highest oxygen content. These cells have the highest metabolic activity (i.e., protein synthesis). Transaminase levels are highest in this zone. Hepatocytes in zone 2, the mediolobular zone, receive blood with an oxygen content intermediate between that of zones 1 and 3. Hepatocytes in zone 3, the centrilobular zone, are located farthest away from the portal triad and receive the least oxygen. Many of the enzymes of biotransformation (i.e., NADPH-cytochrome P450 reductase) are in highest concentration in this zone. Hepatocytes in zone 3 are the most prone to ischemic and drug-induced injury.

Kupffer cells are macrophages of the reticuloendothelial system lining the hepatic sinuses. Kupffer cells play an important role. Their main function is the phagocytosis of particular matter, detoxification of endotoxin, and catabolism of lipids and glycoproteins among others.

The liver secretes 1–2 L of bile per day. Bile is stored in the gallbladder, where its volume is reduced and concentrated. Cholecystokinin, released by the mucosa of the proximal small bowel, stimulates gallbladder contraction while simultaneously relaxing the sphincter of Oddi.

HEPATIC BLOOD SUPPLY AND BLOOD FLOW

The liver receives a dual blood supply from the hepatic artery and the portal vein. Unlike other organs, the liver is highly dependent not only on the hepatic artery but also on the portal vein to meet its oxygen requirements. Blood from the liver is drained into the inferior vena cava by the hepatic veins.

Hepatic blood flow equals approximately 100 mL/min/100 g or approximately 25% of the cardiac output. The hepatic artery provides only 25–35% of the total hepatic blood flow and 40–50% of the hepatic oxygen requirements. The portal vein, which contains desaturated blood, supplies 65–75% of the total hepatic blood flow and 50–55% of the hepatic oxygen requirements (Table 13-1).

Total hepatic blood flow is directly proportional to the perfusion pressure and inversely related to the splanchnic vascular resistance. Portal blood flow is regulated mainly by the arterioles in the preportal splanchnic organs. Intrahepatic blood flow distribution is partially regulated by presinusoidal sphincters. Normal portal venous pressure is 7–10 mmHg. Intrasinusoidal pressure is determined by the tone of both the pre- and postsinusoidal sphincters and by the hepatic blood flow. Changes in venous vascular tone regulate both resistance and compliance and blood volume within the liver. Venous vascular tone is controlled mainly by the sympathetic innervation and mediated by alpha receptors.

Table 13-1 Hepatic Blood Flow	
Total hepatic blood flow	Sum of hepatic arterial and portal venous blood flows
	Equals 1.5 L/min or 25% of the cardiac output
Hepatic artery	Delivers arterialized blood at a rate of 350–525 mL/min or 25–35% of total hepatic blood flow
	Supplies 40–50% of the hepatic oxygen requirements
Portal vein	Supplies 65–75% of total hepatic blood flow (1 L/min)
	Delivers 50–60% of the liver's oxygen supply.
	Oxygen saturation is 60–75%

Hepatic flood flow is regulated by intrinsic factors, including metabolic and hepatic autoregulation, and the hepatic artery buffer response. Intrinsic regulatory factors include the sympathetic nervous system and several humoral factors.

Hepatic Blood Flow Autoregulation

Hepatic blood flow autoregulation refers to the ability of the hepatic artery to alter its resistance in response to changes in arterial pressure and portal blood flow to maintain total hepatic blood flow. There is a reciprocal response of the hepatic artery to reduction in portal venous perfusion. Changes in hepatic artery resistance compensate for changes in portal blood flow by a phenomenon referred to as the hepatic arterial buffer response. When portal venous flow decreases, hepatic arterial resistance decreases and hepatic arterial flow increases. Likewise, when portal venous flow increases, hepatic arterial resistance also increases and hepatic arterial blood flow decreases. This reciprocal relationship allows total hepatic blood flow and hepatic oxygen supply to be maintained despite changes in portal venous flow.

On the other hand, changes in hepatic arterial blood flow do not influence portal venous blood flow. Portal venous flow does not compensate for changes in hepatic arterial blood flow. Similarly, the hepatic arterial buffer response is altered by the fasted state, cirrhosis, volatile anesthetic agents, and other factors, including neural, humoral, and metabolic factors.

Hepatic Blood Flow in Pathologic States

Hepatic blood flow parallels mean arterial pressure. During a hypotensive episode, the hepatic artery flow increases up to a point. The maximal effect is a 140–160%

increase when the systolic arterial pressure decreases to 70–80 mm Hg. The administration of vasoactive drugs alters total hepatic blood flow by altering cardiac output and/or blood pressure. Norepinephrine, phenylephrine, and high doses of epinephrine reduce hepatic blood flow in animal models, despite increases in systemic arterial pressure. Stimulation of the sympathetic nervous system increases splanchnic vascular resistance decreasing hepatic blood flow and hepatic blood volume.

Intermittent positive pressure ventilation and positive end-expiratory pressure (PEEP) lead to increases in intrathoracic pressure and splanchnic vascular resistance and decreases in hepatic blood flow. Hypercapnia increases total hepatic blood flow likely secondary to an increase in portal venous blood flow rather than a decrease in hepatic arterial resistance. Hyperventilation and hypocapnia, on the other hand, lead to decreases in hepatic blood flow and increase in hepatic arterial resistance. Hypoxia, at least in the early stages, increases hepatic arterial resistance and decreases hepatic blood flow.

Intra-abdominal surgery and an elevated intra-abdominal pressure also decrease total hepatic blood flow. In cirrhotic patients, total hepatic blood flow is decreased despite a compensatory increase in total hepatic arterial blood flow. In patients with alcoholic or viral hepatitis, total hepatic blood flow is increased.

Hepatic Blood Flow During Anesthesia and Surgery

Either general inhalational or regional anesthesia decrease hepatic blood flow by 20–30% in the absence of surgical stimulation. Changes in hepatic blood flow are secondary to decreases in cardiac output and arterial pressure. Halothane causes a more significant decrease in hepatic blood flow than isoflurane, desflurane, or sevoflurane by impairing to a greater extent the autoregulatory mechanisms. Sympathetic activity in response to surgical stimulation reduces splanchnic circulation further. During upper abdominal surgery, total hepatic blood flow can decrease to 40% of control values.

FUNCTIONS OF THE LIVER

The liver plays a central role in the metabolism of protein, carbohydrate, and lipids. Other functions of the liver include bile production, bilirubin formation and excretion, iron and hormone metabolism, and blood coagulation, as well as drug and toxin metabolism (Box 13-1).

Box 13-1   Functions of the Liver

Energy metabolism
Protein synthesis and metabolism
Metabolism of plasma lipids and lipoproteins
Bilirubin metabolism
Bile acid metabolism
Bile formation
Blood coagulation
Iron storage and metabolism
Filtering functions
Metabolism of hormones, drugs and toxins

Energy Metabolism

The liver serves as an intermediary between the dietary sources of energy and the extrahepatic tissues that are the main users of energy. Glucose is stored in the liver as glycogen. Its storages are depleted within 24–48 hours of fasting. Prolonged starvation leads to the production of glucose by gluconeogenesis from lactate, pyruvate, glycerol, and the glucogenic amino acids.

Protein Synthesis

Protein synthesis is one of the major functions of the liver. Most of the proteins are synthesized by the hepatocytes. Albumin is produced at a rate of 10–15 g/day. It binds and transports drugs. Low serum albumin levels increase the concentration of free active drug. Other transport proteins such as lipoproteins, transferrin, ceruloplasmin, thyroid hormone-binding protein, and retinol-binding protein are also produced in the liver.

Other secretory proteins include several protease inhibitors, complement, serum amyloid A, C-reactive proteins and alpha-1-acid glycoprotein. Plasma cholinesterase is also produced by the liver with a half-life of 14 days. Plasma cholinesterase degrades succinylcholine, mivacurium, and ester local anesthetics. Decreased plasma cholinesterase levels may be found in patients with advanced liver disease.

Blood Coagulation

All coagulation factors, with the exception of factor VIII and von Willebrand protein are synthesized in the liver. Vitamin K is necessary for the synthesis of factors II, VII, IX, and X. Proteins C and S, which modulate the coagulation and fibrinolytic systems, are also vitamin-K-dependent. Advanced liver disease results in decreased protein synthesis and coagulopathy. Decreased protein synthesis may be compounded by malabsorption of vitamin K due to cholestasis. Thrombocytopenia secondary to hypersplenism may also occur.

PHARMACOLOGIC CONSIDERATIONS

The liver plays a significant role in drug metabolism. Pathways of drugs metabolism are often classified into two groups, phase I and phase II reactions. Phase I reactions include oxidation, reduction, and hydrolysis. Oxidative and reductive reactions alter and create new products that may retain some of the activity of the parent drugs and hydrolytic reactions cleave esters and amides. Phase II or conjugation reactions are reactions in which a drug or its metabolite is coupled to an endogenous substrate such as glucuronic acid (glucuronidation), acetic acid (acetylation), or sulfuric acid (sulfate conjugation), among others.

First Pass Effect

Certain drugs are removed from circulation as they initially pass through the liver. This *first-pass effect* determines the systemic availability of various drugs such as propranolol and warfarin. The presence of liver disease affects first-pass metabolism and alters the bioavailability of drugs.

Liver disease alters drug disposition in several ways. Liver disease may lead to changes in body composition with the production of ascites, altering the volume of distribution. Similarly, drug binding is altered by a decrease in serum albumin levels, the appearance of altered or defective plasma proteins, and the accumulation of several substances that compete with other drugs for the protein binding site.

Liver Disease and Drug Biotransformation

Hepatic oxidation and acetylation are impaired in presence of liver diseases. Phase II enzymatic pathways are nonmicrosomal, however, and are less affected in advanced liver disease. Glucuronidation is relatively well preserved until the late stages. Diazepam and chlordiazepoxide undergo oxidative biotransformation, so their clearance is impaired. On the other hand, since oxazepam and lorazepam undergo glucuronidation, their clearance is less affected in cirrhosis (Box 13-2).

PATHOPHYSIOLOGY OF LIVER AND BILIARY TRACT DISEASE

Acute Liver Diseases

Acute hepatocellular injury may be the result of infections, toxins, or drugs (ethanol, acetaminophen, aspirin, dantrolene, isoniazid, phenytoin, erythromycin, chlor-

---

Box 13-2   Mechanisms of Altered Drug Metabolism in Liver Disease

Changes in cardiac output
Altered hepatic blood flow
Reduced sinusoidal capillary perfusion
Portosystemic shunting
Altered enzymatic activity
• Induction
• Decreased enzyme activity
Altered volume of distribution
Changes in protein binding
Decreased hepatic cell mass
Impaired bile flow
Other mechanisms
• Malnutrition
• Decreased renal clearance

---

promazine, doxapram, indomethacin, verapamil, monoamine oxidase inhibitors, amitriptyline). Agents responsible for viral hepatitis include hepatitis virus types A, B C, D, and E, Epstein–Barr virus, cytomegalovirus, herpes simplex, echovirus, and Coxsackie virus (Table 13-2).

Chronic Liver Diseases

Chronic liver diseases are characterized by the progressive impairment of hepatic function and destruction of hepatic tissue. Cirrhosis represents the final common stage for such diseases. Several processes may result in chronic liver disease. Chronic active hepatitis may be the result of chronic viral infection, drug- or toxin-induced, or autoimmune. Alcoholic cirrhosis is the most common cause of portal cirrhosis. Biliary cirrhosis may be primary or secondary to chronic biliary obstruction. Other causes of cirrhosis include sclerosing cholangitis, cystic fibrosis, sarcoidosis, and inborn errors of metabolism such as hemochromatosis, Wilson's disease, and alpha-1-antitrypsin deficiency (Table 13-3).

The manifestations of chronic liver disease result from hepatocellular damage and portal hypertension. Findings include a hyperdynamic state with an increased cardiac output and a decreased systemic vascular resistance. Tissue perfusion is decreased as a result of systemic shunting. Pulmonary manifestations include aortopulmonary shunting, pulmonary hypertension, ventilation/perfusion mismatch, and impaired hypoxic pulmonary vasoconstriction. Renal blood flow tends to decrease. Hepatorenal syndrome may develop in those patients. Gastrointestinal bleeding, bone marrow depression, hypersplenism, and hemolysis may result in anemia and thrombocytopenia. Elevations in the prothrombin time

Table 13-2   Viral Hepatitis

	Hepatitis A	Hepatitis B	Hepatitis C	Hepatitis D	Hepatitis E
Virus	HAV	HBV	HCV	HDV	HEV
Viral marker	HAV RNA	HBV DNA DNA polymerase	HCV RNA	HDV RNA	Virus-like particles
Incubation (days)	14–49	28–160	15–160	28–180	14–60
Transmission	Fecal-oral				Fecal-oral
		Parenteral	Parenteral	Parenteral	
		Perinatal	? Perinatal	Perinatal	
	? Sexual	Sexual	? Sexual	Sexual	
Acute diagnosis	IgM anti-HAV	HBsAg	Anti-HCV (C33c, C223,NS5)	Anti-HDV	IgM/IgG anti- HEV
		IgM anti-HBc	HCV RNA	HDV RNA	
Acute mortality (%)	0.2	0.2–1.0	0.2	2–20	0.2
Mortality from fulminant hepatic failure (%)	30–40	50–60	85	(see HBV)	20
Progression to chronicity (%)	None	2–10	>20	2–70	None

HAV, hepatitis A virus; HbsAg, Hepatitis B virus surface antigen; HBV, hepatitis B virus; HCV, hepatitis C virus; HDV, hepatitis D virus; HEV, hepatitis E virus;

Table 13-3   Etiology of Chronic Liver Disease

Common causes	Hepatitis C
	Hepatitis B
	Alcoholic liver disease
	Cryptogenic
Uncommon causes	Autoimmune hepatitis
	Primary biliary cirrhosis
	Primary sclerosing cholangitis
	Hemochromatosis
	Wilson's disease
	Alpha-1-antitrypsin deficiency
	Granulomatous diseases
	Glycogen storage disease type IV
	Drug-induced liver disease
	Budd–Chiari disease and VOD of the liver

usually result from the depressed synthesis of vitamin-K-dependent coagulation factors (Table 13-4).

PREOPERATIVE EVALUATION AND PREPARATION

Preoperative Evaluation

Preoperative evaluation of patients with liver or biliary disease should include a complete medical history and physical examination. Past medical history should include exposure to drugs, toxins, infectious agents, and transfusions. During the physical examination, look for the presence of stigmata of chronic liver disease such as gynecomastia, jaundice, and spider nevi. The presence of a hyperdynamic circulation and a high cardiac output with a low peripheral vascular resistance, or the presence of the hepatopulmonary or hepatorenal syndromes, pulmonary hypertension, pleural effusions, and ascites will indicate the presence of chronic liver disease (Table 13-5).

The use of routine preoperative biochemical testing of liver function in an otherwise healthy patient is controversial. Laboratory studies in patients with pre-existing or suspected liver disease should include a complete blood count, coagulation studies, and serum chemistry, including serum electrolytes, creatinine, and urea nitrogen.

Preoperative Liver Function Testing

Common liver functions tests include transaminases, alkaline phosphatase, serum proteins and bilirubin, and prothrombin time (PT). Elevation of the serum aminotransferase enzymes, alanine aminotransferase (ALT) and aspartate aminotransferase (AST), usually indicates hepatocellular injury but can also indicate injury to organs other than the liver. Elevation of the enzymes alkaline phosphatase (ALP), gamma glutamyl transpeptidase (GGT), and leukocyte alkaline phosphatase (LAP)/5′-nucleotidase indicates a problem with bile formation and transport ("cholestatic enzymes"). Preoperative findings in patients with liver disease that are associated with an increased risk include malnutrition, marked coagulopathy, ascites, hypoalbuminemia, and hyperbilirubinemia.

Table 13-4   Abnormalities in Patients with Chronic Liver Disease

Neurological	Hepatic encephalopathy
	Portal-systemic myelopathy
	Central pontine myelinolysis
Cardiovascular	Hyperdynamic circulation
	Increased cardiac output
	Decreased systemic vascular resistance
	Relative hypotension
	Relative resistance to catecholamines
	Vasodilatation
	Increased total plasma volume
	Cardiomyopathy
	Decreased portal blood flow
Pulmonary	Intrapulmonary shunting
	Hepatopulmonary syndrome
	Pulmonary hypertension
	Ventilation perfusion mismatch
	Impaired hypoxic pulmonary vasoconstriction
Renal	Hepatorenal syndrome
Hematologic	Anemia
	Thrombocytopenia
	Impaired synthesis of factors II, V, VII and X
	Dysfibrinogenemia
	Enhanced fibrinolysis
	Decreased levels of anti-thrombin III
Metabolic	Hypoglycemia in fulminant liver failure
	Hyperglycemia due to impaired glucose tolerance
	Hyponatremia
	Hypokalemia and hypomagnesemia
	Respiratory and metabolic alkalosis
Endocrine	Activation of the renin–angiotensin–aldosterone axis
	Increased secretion of anti-diuretic hormone (ADH)
	Sick euthyroid syndrome
	Hyperestrogenism in males

Table 13-5   Evaluation of Patients with Cirrhosis

History	History of infectious or toxic hepatitis
	Alcohol consumption
	Blood transfusions
Physical examination	Jaundice
	Ascites
	Encephalopathy
	Nutritional status
	Cardiomyopathy
Laboratory testing	Complete blood count
	Serum electrolytes
	Arterial blood gases
	Liver function tests

Anesthetic Risk

The type and severity of liver disease are the main factors determining the anesthetic risk. The presence of other comorbid diseases will compound the risks associated with surgery and anesthesia in these patients.

Patients with acute viral hepatitis have an increased operative risk and perioperative mortality. Elective surgery during the acute episodes in such patients should be postponed until the liver function tests have returned to normal. The operative risk of patients with chronic hepatitis correlates with the severity of the disease. Patients with asymptomatic or mild chronic hepatitis seem to have minimal operative risk. In patients with symptomatic chronic active hepatitis surgical mortality is increased and elective surgery should be avoided. Asymptomatic carriers of the hepatitis B virus (HBV) surface antigen (HBsAg) are not at increased perioperative risk.

In patients with alcoholic hepatitis, elective surgery is associated a high mortality and is therefore contraindicated. The 30-day mortality may be as high as 50% in patients with severe alcoholic hepatitis. Elective surgery should be postponed until clinical resolution and the return of serum bilirubin levels to normal. Fatty liver may be the result of heavy alcohol consumption. It is characterized by hepatomegaly, mild transaminasemia, and an elevation of the alkaline phosphatases

Table 13-6 Child's Classification

	Class A	Class B	Class C
Albumin (g /dL)	>3.5	3.0–3.5	<3.0
Bilirubin (mg /dL)	<2.0	2.0–3.0	>3.0
Ascites	None	Controlled	Uncontrolled
Encephalopathy	None	Mild	Advanced
Nutritional status	Excellent	Good	Poor
Mortality	10%	30%	75%

and GGT levels. Elective surgery is not contraindicated in these patients. It is reasonable to postpone elective procedures until other alcohol-induced deficiencies are corrected.

Operative risk is increased in cirrhotic patients. Postoperative mortality rate is higher, as a result of sepsis, bleeding, renal failure, and hepatic failure. Preoperative factors associated with an increased operative risk include emergency surgery, upper abdominal procedures, hypoalbuminemia, prolonged PT and/or partial thromboplastin time (PTT), hyperbilirubinemia, anemia, ascites, encephalopathy, malnutrition, postoperative bleeding, and Child's classification.

Perioperative mortality in cirrhotics correlates with the severity of the cirrhosis. The most widely used classification of perioperative risk as related to hepatic function is that of Child and Turcotte (Table 13-6) and the Child–Pugh Score (Table 13-7). Child's classification is a good predictor of operative risk and mortality. In patients with Child's A cirrhosis, surgery can usually be performed without significant risk. The decision to perform surgery in patients with Child's class B or C cirrhosis should be considered very carefully (Table 13-8). The Child–Pugh score correlates with perioperative mortality in patients undergoing nonshunt surgery and in cirrhotic patients undergoing intra-abdominal procedures.

Table 13-7 Pugh Classification

	Points		
	1	2	3
Albumin (g/dL)	>3.5	3.0–3.5	<3.0
Bilirubin (mg/dL)	1.0–2.0	2–3	>3.0
(for primary biliary cirrhosis)	1.0–4.0	4.0–10.0	>10.0
Ascites	Absent	Slight	Advanced
Encephalopathy (Grade)	None	1.0–2.0	3.0–4.0
Prothrombin time (prolonged)	1.0–4.0	4.0–6.0	>6.0

Class A, 5–6 points; class B, 7–9 points; class C, 10–15 points.

Table 13-8 Child or Pugh Class and Operability

Class	Operability
A	No limitations
	Normal response to all operations
	Normal ability of liver to regenerate
B	Some limitations to liver function
	Altered response to all operations but good tolerance with preoperative preparation
	Limited ability of the liver to regenerate; large liver resections are contraindicated
C	Severe limitations to liver function
	Poor response to all operations regardless of operative efforts
	Liver resection is contraindicated

From Stone HH. Preoperative and postoperative care. *Surg Clin North Am* 1977;57:409–419.

Patients with obstructive jaundice are at increased surgical risk. Mortality ranges between 8% and 20%. Other factors associated with an increased mortality include a hematocrit below 30%, hyperbilirubinemia above 11 mg/dL, a malignant cause of obstruction, an elevated serum creatinine, and hypoalbuminemia.

Preoperative Preparation

Preoperative optimization may improve surgical risk in patients with moderate or advanced liver disease. Preoperative preparation for patients with severe liver dysfunction includes correction of coagulopathy, fluid volume status, electrolyte imbalance, and, whenever indicated and feasible, control of ascites; and reversal of renal dysfunction, encephalopathy, and malnutrition.

Coagulopathy

Homeostasis may be impaired in patients with liver disease because of inadequate vitamin-K-dependent factors, increased fibrinolytic activity, thrombocytopenia, and abnormal platelet function. A prolonged PT may be secondary to impaired hepatic synthesis of coagulation factors or impaired absorption of fat-soluble vitamin K. The administration of vitamin K will correct hypoprothrombinemia secondary to malnutrition or biliary obstruction but not that related to hepatocellular dysfunction. Fresh frozen plasma, cryoprecipitate, or platelet transfusion should be considered in patients with considerable liver dysfunction. Since hyperfibrinolysis may develop intraoperatively, antifibrinolytic agents, such as epsilon-aminocaproic acid or aprotinin, may decrease intraoperative transfusion requirements during liver transplantation, but their role in other surgical situations is unclear and there is always the potential for thrombotic complications.

Fluid and electrolyte imbalances are common in patients with liver disease. Ascites is the result of portal hypertension, hypoalbuminemia, leakage of hepatic lymph, hyperaldosteronism, and a hyperreninemic state leading to sodium retention. If possible, preoperative control of the ascites is recommended. Salt restriction, spironolactone, and a loop diuretic are commonly used. In refractory cases, or those patients with tense ascites, a large-volume paracentesis may be indicated. For patients with refractory ascites, a transjugular intrahepatic portosystemic shunt may be indicated. Electrolyte abnormalities include hyponatremia, as a result of impaired free water clearance, and a hypokalemic alkalosis. Chronic hyponatremia is generally well tolerated. On the other hand, deficits in potassium, phosphate, and magnesium should be corrected.

Renal dysfunction is common in patients with advanced liver disease. It is important to distinguish the etiology. Patients may present with prerenal renal failure, acute tubular necrosis, or the hepatorenal syndrome. Any potentially nephrotoxic drugs should be avoided or used with great caution.

Hepatic encephalopathy can be precipitated by gastrointestinal hemorrhage, high protein intake, constipation, progressive liver disease, azotemia, hypokalemic alkalosis, infection and sepsis, and hypoxia. Elective surgery should be postponed until clinically overt encephalopathy is corrected. Management of encephalopathy includes avoidance of precipitating factors, protein intake restriction, and the administration of oral or rectal lactulose, oral neomycin, and/or metronidazole.

Patients with advanced liver disease suffer from severe malnutrition, which may adversely affect survival. Preoperative nutritional support may improve nutritional status, hypoalbuminemia, and the Child's score and, potentially, may decrease the postoperative mortality rate in patients with advanced cirrhosis.

Premedication

Routine premedications should include those drugs required to control the underlying state. Other medications, such as hypnotics and opioids, should be withheld or their dose should be decreased and titrated to effect. Patient with advanced liver disease have or should be considered to have a full stomach. Preparation for induction of anesthesia should include the administration of sodium citrate, metoclopramide, and an H_2-receptor antagonist.

INTRAOPERATIVE CARE

Monitoring

Intraoperative monitoring for patients with advanced liver disease should be dictated by the surgical procedure. In addition to standard monitoring, arterial cannulation will facilitate blood pressure monitoring and blood sampling, particularly for those patients undergoing major surgical procedures. A central venous catheter or a pulmonary artery catheter will guide intraoperative fluid therapy and optimization of cardiac performance, hemodynamics, and hepatic oxygen supply. Urine output should be closely monitored. Monitoring of blood coagulation, hemoglobin and oxygen saturation, and acid–base and electrolyte balance must be considered for patients undergoing extensive procedures.

Induction and Maintenance of Anesthesia

Anesthetic management should be aimed at preserving hepatic blood flow and maintaining hepatic oxygen supply. Inadequate hepatic oxygen supply will occur whenever oxygen-carrying capacity is low (because of hypoxemia or anemia) or when cardiac performance is inadequate. Regional anesthesia may be considered whenever possible and in the absence of a coagulopathy. For patients requiring general anesthesia, a rapid sequence induction or even an awake intubation may be necessary to prevent aspiration.

The ability of the liver to metabolize and clear certain drugs is impaired in patients with advanced liver disease. Drug selection should be based on their pharmacokinetic and pharmacodynamic profile and on their effects on hepatic blood flow. For instance, diazepam and midazolam, which are mostly metabolized by oxidative mechanisms, have significantly increased half-lives. Lorazepam, which is cleared by glucuronidation, has a normal half-life. Drugs that bind to albumin, such as barbiturates, should be titrated carefully, since hypoalbuminemia will increase their active free fraction. The volume of distribution may be increased in patients with advanced liver disease. A larger initial dose may be required to achieve a desired effect. Administering larger doses, however, will prolong their effect because of the impaired hepatic blood flow, metabolism, and clearance.

All anesthetics, particularly inhaled agents, will decrease total hepatic blood flow to a variable degree and in a dose-dependent fashion. Halothane should be avoided since it decreases hepatic blood flow to a greater extent. Because of its sympathomimetic effects, nitrous oxide may further decrease total hepatic blood flow, making its use undesirable. Opioids have an impaired clearance in patients with advanced liver disease. These agents can be used safely, keeping in mind their pharmacokinetic and pharmacodynamic profile. Opioids may induce spasm of the sphincter of Oddi. Volatile agents attenuate the effect of opioids on the sphincter of Oddi. Spasm may be relieved by atropine, naloxone, or glucagon. Neuromuscular blocking agents may also be used safely, so long as they are titrated and closely monitored to the desired effect. Using atracurium or cisatracurium seems to be advantageous, since their metabolism and elimination is independent of hepatic or renal function.

Adequate renal function should be maintained. Close monitoring of urine output, intravascular volume, and hemodynamics may prevent the development of renal dysfunction. Ventilator management should be aimed to avoid unwanted increases in intrathoracic pressure, which impairs venous return, cardiac output, and hepatic blood flow. Hypoxemia and hypocapnia should also be avoided since they also decrease total hepatic blood flow. Correction of intraoperative coagulopathy includes the administration of platelets, fresh frozen plasma, and cryoprecipitate.

POSTOPERATIVE CARE AND COMPLICATIONS

Postoperative Hepatic Dysfunction

Postoperative hepatic dysfunction is common; it may be a direct consequence of anesthesia and surgery or it may reflect progression of a pre-existing liver disorder that is exacerbated by perioperative events (Box 13-3). It ranges from a mild elevation in liver enzymes to overt fulminant hepatic failure. The diagnosis of anesthesia-induced liver dysfunction is usually one of exclusion. Fortunately, the great majority of cases resolve within a few days.

Box 13-3   Etiology of Postoperative Liver Dysfunction

Hepatic oxygen deprivation
- Hypoxia
- Hypotension and low cardiac output
- Decreased hepatic blood flow

Viral hepatitis
Chronic hepatitis
Fulminant hepatic failure
Drug-induced
Blood transfusion
Infection/sepsis

Halothane-Induced Hepatitis

There are two types of halothane-induced liver dysfunction; the first is due to hepatotoxic lipoperoxidases generated during reductive metabolism of halothane in a hypoxic environment. The more fulminant form is due to an immunologic phenomenon whereby an oxidative metabolite of halothane, trifluoroacetyl chloride, binds to hepatocytes, creating a neoantigenic structure to which antibodies may be generated.

The diagnosis of halothane-induced hepatic dysfunction is one of exclusion. The presentation is variable, ranging from a mild elevation in serum transaminase levels, fever, or jaundice to fulminant hepatic failure and death. Predisposing factors include previous halothane exposure, obesity, advanced age, and female gender. It is very rare in pediatric patients.

Postoperative Jaundice

Postoperative jaundice can be the result of one or any combination of three causes:
- Overproduction and overload of bilirubin from perioperative blood transfusion, resorption of hematomas, or hemolysis
- Hepatocellular injury secondary to postoperative viral hepatitis, aggravation of pre-existing liver disease, exposure to drugs or toxin, or, more likely, inadequate hepatic blood flow or oxygen supply
- Extrahepatic biliary obstruction may be secondary to gallstones, strictures or pancreatitis. Intrahepatic cholestasis may be due to drugs or sepsis.

SUMMARY

Patients with advanced liver disease have an increased surgical risk. The anesthetic management of such patients requires an understanding of normal hepatic physiology and the pathophysiology of liver disease. Preoperative evaluation of patients with liver disease includes a history, physical examination, and the evaluation of laboratory and other radiological tests. Important issues to be addressed during the preoperative evaluation are the type of liver disease (acute or chronic) and the degree of impairment of liver function. Prediction of surgical risk is based on the degree of liver dysfunction, the type of surgery and the preoperative clinical status of the patient. Factors contributing to perioperative morbidity and mortality include the deleterious effect of anesthesia and surgery on hepatic blood flow and hepatic function, altered drug pharmacokinetics, abnormal hemostasis, postoperative liver dysfunction, and the development of encephalopathy and multiple organ system dysfunction. Elective surgery should be postponed in patients with decompensated cirrhosis and acute hepatitis.

SUGGESTED READING

Gelman S. General anesthesia and hepatic circulation. *Can J Physiol Pharmacol* 1987;65:1762–1779.

Gopalswamy N, Mehta V, Barde CJ. Risks of intra-abdominal non-shunt surgery in cirrhotics. *Dig Dis* 1998;16: 225–231.

Pratt DS, Kaplan MM. Evaluation of abnormal liver-enzyme results in asymptomatic patients. *N Engl J Med* 2000;342: 1266–1271.

Stone HH. Preoperative and postoperative care. *Surg Clin North Am* 1977;57:409–419.

Ziser A, Plevak DJ. Morbidity and mortality in cirrhotic patients undergoing anesthesia and surgery. *Curr Opin Anesthesiol* 2001;14:707–711.

CHAPTER 14

Anesthesia for Transplant Surgery

JOSÉ M. RODRÍGUEZ-PAZ

INTRODUCTION

During the last decade, as a result of advances in the management of the end-stage organ failure, surgical techniques, and immunosuppressant therapies, the number of suitable candidates for transplant surgery has increased. Because of the severity of the organ failure, the comorbid conditions of the recipients and the pathophysiological changes that occur during surgery, the anesthesiologist should have a complete understanding of the pharmacological, pathophysiological, and anesthetic demands that occur during the perioperative period in these critically ill patients.

This chapter will review the perioperative pathophysiological changes, preoperative considerations, and specific anesthetic management of the most commonly performed transplant procedures (liver, kidney, lungs, and heart). In addition, the management of the donors (both cadaveric and living related) and of the transplanted patient undergoing nontransplant surgery will be reviewed.

ANESTHESIA MANAGEMENT OF THE ORGAN DONOR

Management of organ donors (both living and cadaveric) requires perioperative management goals of optimizing organ retrieval, maintaining viability of the organ, and successful transplantation of the organ(s).

The principle of donor management is aimed at minimizing end-organ damage by maintaining oxygen delivery to peripheral tissues by keeping an adequate mean arterial pressure (over 60 mmHg) and arterial oxygen saturation (P_aO_2) with the lowest F_iO_2 possible. Also, it is very important to maintain the body temperature between 35–37° C, urine output over 1–2 mL/kg/hr and the hematocrit above 25% while minimizing blood transfusions, and aggressively treating any metabolic disarrangement while avoiding high doses of vasopressors and inotropes. Part of the management of these patients includes minimizing the cold organ ischemia time (time from clamping of the donor aorta to time of re-establishment of arterial flow in the recipient), since the shorter this time the more successful the transplantation.

Prior to the transplant procedure, the recipient and the donor will undergo blood crossmatch and histocompatibility assays.

Cadaveric Donation

During 2001, approximately 6,100 brain-dead donors underwent organ harvesting, with a total of 17,000 recovered organs. Although the majority of procurements are performed on brain-dead donors, the number of organ donations obtained from non-heart-beating donors is increasing (up to 20% of cadaveric donations in some areas).

Once brain death has been established, if the patient meets criteria for organ donation, quick organization of a coordinated team including the different surgical teams, anesthesiologists, anesthesia technicians, operating room nurses, transplant coordinators, and intensive care unit teams is fundamental for successful transplantation.

It is very important to understand that brain death is associated with multiple metabolic and physiological derangements. These include elevated intracranial pressure with autonomic dysfunction, dysrhythmias, hemodynamic instability, neuroendocrine dysfunction (especially hyperglycemia and catecholamine release) and loss of body temperature regulation.

The first part of the donation includes the dissection of all the organs to be harvested. Once the dissection is completed, the donor receives a full heparinization dose

(25,000 units) and then the surgeons proceed to cannulate and cross-clamp the aorta and add preservative solutions to the harvested organs (generally University of Wisconsin Solution; Table 14-1).

Generally, the kidneys are the first organs to be removed, followed by the liver and heart, which are dissected simultaneously. If the lungs are harvested, ventilation needs to be continued until the lungs are flushed with preservative solution and the trachea is clamped. Remember to make sure that the time of death is certified before going to the operating room.

The anesthesiologist's tasks include keeping an adequate volume status (if blood is transfused, cytomegalovirus-matched blood needs to be given), correction of any metabolic imbalances and maintaining hemodynamic and respiratory support. Dopamine (2–5 µg/kg/min) is the inotrope of choice for its effects on end-organ perfusion, although vasopressin (0.5–15 U/hr) is gaining popularity. Phenylephrine is normally avoided secondary to its specific effect on decreasing splanchnic blood flow. Volatile anesthetics are used to control blood pressure and neuromuscular blocking agents to control any motor activity. Emergency drugs and infusion pumps, warming devices, and a defibrillator should be readily available in the operating room. In cases of non-heart-beating donors, the anesthetic care is minimal and time is of essence to procure the organs.

To sum up, these patients should be managed like any critically ill patient in the operating room, including invasive monitoring, correction of any pathophysiological derangements, and aggressive maintenance of organ viability.

Table 14-1   Constituents of the Most Commonly Used Organ Preservative Solution

Content (mmol/L)	University of Wisconsin (Belzer's solution)	Celsior	HTK
Glucose	–	–	–
Mannitol	100	80	–
Glutamate	–	60	30
Phosphate buffer	25	–	–
Bicarbonate buffer	–	–	–
Histidine buffer	–	30	180
Colloid; HES	50 g	–	–
Na	30	100	15
K	120	15	10
Mg	5	13	4
Ca	–	0.25	0.015
pH	7.4	7.3	7.2
Osmolarity	320	360	310
Use/disadvantage	Standard for liver, kidney, and pancreas transplantation – high price and viscosity		For cardiac transplant

HES, hydroxyethyl starch; HTK, histidine–tryptophan–ketoglutarate solution.

Living Related Donation

An increasing number of living related and unrelated donations have occurred during the last few years. The number of living donors is, as of 2001, higher than the number of cadaveric donors but corresponds only to one-fourth of the total organs donated. The majority of donated organs from living donors correspond to kidney, liver, and lung lobes.

In principle, the majority of the donors are healthy, but a complete assessment of their history with a physical examination, as well as the function of the organ to be donated is very important in order to rule out any potential complications after the donation. Anesthetic care in this setting should not be any different than the anesthesia management for resection of diseased organs in any other patient. Particular attention needs to be paid to pain control (especially to the use of regional techniques) and the avoidance of damage to the organ to be harvested. The overall rate of intra- and postoperative complications is minimal if careful anesthesia and surgical care is given to these patients.

ANESTHESIA MANAGEMENT FOR LIVER TRANSPLANT

Orthotopic liver transplantation (OLT) is the curative procedure for end-stage liver disease (ESLD). In 2001 more than 5,000 liver transplants were performed in the United States. Because of improved surgical and anesthesia techniques, intensive care and new immunosuppressant therapies, survival rates of 75% at 3 years are common.

Preoperative Considerations

Patients undergoing liver transplantation present with different levels of severity of their ESLD. The great majority of patients present with viral hepatitis (most commonly hepatitis C) or alcoholic liver disease. The list of liver diseases associated with ESLD is extensive but commonly includes primary biliary cirrhosis, primary sclerosing cholangitis, cryptogenic cirrhosis, hepatocellular carcinoma, drug-related hepatotoxicity (most commonly acetaminophen), and alpha-1-antitrypsin deficiency.

Contraindications for transplant include: systemic malignancy (unless in remission for 5 years), sepsis or infections resistant to treatment, severe lung disease, hepatoma larger than 6 cm, severe pulmonary hypertension (the transplant should be canceled if the pulmonary vascular resistance is greater than 250 dyn/sec/cm^5 and/or the mean pulmonary artery pressure is greater that 50 mmHg), and advanced cardiac disease.

The details and specific physiology of ESLD is beyond the scope of this chapter but the preoperative evaluation of patients undergoing liver transplant has to be done while taking in consideration what effects hepatic dysfunction has in multiple organ systems (Box 14-1).

Because of the high incidence of preoperative hepatic encephalopathy, some of these patients will present with increased intracranial pressure (ICP) due to cerebral edema. Standard treatment of cerebral edema includes the use of steroids, mannitol, barbiturates, and hyperventilation. The use of ICP monitors during the perioperative period is controversial and the data available supporting its use is limited, even for the increased ICP that can occur during reperfusion. Hypertonic saline, used in other scenarios of cerebral edema, needs to be used cautiously because most of these patients present with hyponatremia and rapid corrections increase the risk of developing central pontine myelinolysis.

Box 14-1   Pathophysiology of End-stage Liver Disease: Anesthetic Considerations

Central Nervous System: Hepatic encephalopathy (fulminant acute hepatic failure) and edema (impaired ammonia metabolism)

Pulmonary: Hypoxemia due to shunting, ↓ functional residual capacity, pleural effusions, abnormal hypoxic pulmonary vasoconstriction, and hepatopulmonary syndrome (liver dysfunction, intrapulmonary vasodilatation and hypoxemia refractory to high F_iO_2), orthodeoxia (↓ P_aO_2 >3 mmHg on standing from supine)

Cardiac: Hyperdynamic state due to arteriovenous shunting and decreased systemic vascular resistance (secondary to ↓ response to catecholamines); ↓ cardiac contractility (alcohol)

Renal: Water ↑ due to ↑ antidiuretic hormone, ↑ aldosterone, ↓ albumin (ascites, altered drug pharmacokinetics), inability to concentrate urine, hepatorenal syndrome (severe prerenal oliguria, Na$_{URINE}$ ≤10 mEq/l and azotemia), hypovolemia; ↓ sodium (if Na <120 liver transplantation should be deferred), ↓ Ca^{2+}, ↓ Mg^{2+}

Gastrointestinal: Previous abdominal surgery, portocaval surgery, intra-abdominal infections, and ascites may cause the procedure to be more technically difficult.

Hemostasis: Coagulopathy secondary to ↓ clotting factors synthesis (I, II, V, VII, IX and X), ↓ synthesis of plasminogen activator inhibitor, and ↓ plasminogen activator hepatic clearance; thrombocytopenia (hypersplenism), disseminated intravascular coagulation, and fibrinolysis

Metabolism: Hypoglycemia (secondary to loss of glycogenesis).

Fulminant acute hepatic failure requires emergency liver transplantation since it carries an extremely high mortality (90%); however, the 1-year survival after transplant is more than 70%. Because of the severity of the presentation in fulminant hepatic failure, most of these patients are admitted to the intensive care unit and are receiving treatment for cerebral edema, renal failure, and coagulopathy. In most cases they require supportive measures to correct for multiple organ dysfunction (mechanical ventilation, renal replacement therapy, and hemodynamic support). In some institutions, these patients may be undergoing experimental modes of hepatic replacement therapy (artificial liver). An additional consideration is that, because of lack of available grafts, during the 1990s, half of the candidates for liver transplantation were in intensive care units and almost 30% were receiving life support.

Lines and Monitoring

It is very important to establish good intravenous access. Typically, the recipient should have at least three or four large-bore intravenous lines, preferably at least one 8.5 French sheath introducer (either peripherally or centrally). One or two of the large-bore intravenous lines are used with a rapid infusing system and the venovenous bypass (VVBP) if needed, and a central line (introducer) is reserved for the pulmonary artery catheter. Also, if VVBP is used, a femoral venous line is inserted to monitor pressures below the clamp.

It is essential to use strict aseptic techniques during line placement in order to avoid infection during the postoperative period. Also, it is a standard of practice to avoid the use of heparin for the flush solutions so as not to interfere with the patient's coagulation and the use of the thromboelastogram.

Besides standard noninvasive monitors (electrocardiogram, pulse oxymetry, blood pressure cuff, capnography) an arterial line (preferably radial), temperature probe (preferably rectal), cerebral blood flow monitor (although its value during the procedure is controversial), and pulmonary artery catheter should be placed. Transesophageal echocardiography (TEE) is becoming routine in many centers. Even although the role of ICP monitoring is still controversial, as mentioned, many anesthesiologists will request the placement of one for the more severe cases of encephalopathy. Most monitors except for noninvasive routine monitors can be inserted after induction except for those patients with comorbid conditions that require more aggressive monitoring prior to induction.

Another popular monitor used during OLT is the thromboelastogram. It allows a more accurate way of checking the recipient's coagulation status during the procedure. The analysis of the graphic obtained by this technique allows a qualitative interpretation of coagulation and its appropriate correction. The review of this technique is beyond the scope of this chapter.

Anesthesia Setup

The anesthesia cart should be well equipped and frequently restocked. Besides the anesthesia drugs (see discussion below), the following medications should be ready: phenylephrine, epinephrine, norepinephrine, ephedrine, nitroprusside, nitroglycerine, calcium chloride, sodium bicarbonate, insulin, furosemide, mannitol, lidocaine, and dextrose. Antifibrinolytic medications, antibiotics, steroids (usually methylprednisolone 500 mg), and immunosuppressant medications (discuss with the surgical team) should be available. Multiple infusion pumps should be readily available.

It is very important to contact the blood bank to set up enough blood products, including platelets and cryoprecipitate. These blood products should be either in the room or readily available, and should include 15 units of packed red blood cells and 15 units of fresh frozen plasma. Plasmalyte, a crystalloid with composition close to that of plasma, is the fluid of choice for the majority of liver transplant centers and should be available.

Warming devices, including thermal blankets, convective devices, and rapid infusing fluid warmers, are mandatory to avoid hypothermia. Aggressive correction of hypothermia is needed in order to avoid exacerbation of metabolic derangements (acidosis), electrolyte abnormalities, impaired oxygen delivery, and a worsening coagulopathy.

Anesthesia Management

The anesthetic management of a liver transplantation is a very complex task that requires an understanding not only of both the technical aspects and the needs of the patient but also of the surgical technique. Also it is fundamental to establish good communication with the surgical team and other professionals involved (blood bank, anesthesia technicians, etc.). It is important to determine the time for the recipient to enter the operating room and be ready for surgery, since the graft must be transplanted into the recipient within 12–18 hours of procurement to minimize the cold ischemia time.

Liver transplantation has been traditionally divided in three phases, each with specific anesthesia management considerations:

Pre-anhepatic or Recipient Hepatectomy
This portion of the procedure includes the hepatectomy, the resection of the gallbladder, hepatic veins, and inferior vena cava and if needed the establishment of access for VVBP (most commonly left femoral and portal vein to upper body venous access).

During this phase, the main concerns that the anesthesiologist will face include: bleeding from dissection and hepatectomy, portal hypertension, thrombocytopenia, and coagulopathy (fibrinolysis is not usually an issue during this period). Also, it is not uncommon that the liver transplant recipient presents during this phase with hemodynamic instability secondary to bleeding, drainage of large volume of ascites, and/or vascular compression. Hence, maintenance of intravascular volume by using fluids or blood products is very common. The amount of blood products required for liver transplantation varies, but the blood bank needs to be ready to provide large amounts of blood products (including red blood cells, fresh plasma, cryoprecipitate, and platelets). In addition, hypothermia, hyperglycemia, hypoxemia, and oliguria are not uncommon during this phase.

Anhepatic

This phase starts with the cross-clamping of the portal vein/vena cava and ends before the release of the vascular clamps. Typically the surgeons start by establishing the anastomosis from the graft's suprahepatic vena cava to the recipient's vena cava, followed by the reconstruction of infrahepatic vena cava and portal vein. Flushing of preservation fluid and removal of air from the graft concludes this phase. If a "piggyback technique" is used, the clamp is placed across the hepatic veins where they join the vena cava, thus minimizing the obstruction to flow. Although this technique is commonly used during living-related transplants, a growing number of surgeons prefer this technique for standard OLT.

The main consideration that the anesthesiologist needs to address, during this phase, is the effect that clamping the vena cava has on venous return. Depending upon the degree of venous obstruction (complete or partial clamp, a piggyback surgical technique, or VVBP) the hemodynamic changes may be different for each recipient.

Furthermore, during this stage the anesthesiologist will face metabolic derangements. These include metabolic acidosis (especially if VVBP is not used), hypocalcemia from transfusion (citrate), coagulopathy/fibrinolysis/bleeding, decreased ionized magnesium, hypothermia, and renal dysfunction. Hyperkalemia from acidosis and organ fluid preservation is very common. Avoidance of aggressive correction of hypokalemia, unless the potassium is less than 3 mmol/L, correction of acidosis and flushing of the graft with cold solution (normal saline) prior to revascularization will minimize hyperkalemia.

Postanhepatic

The last phase of the OLT includes reperfusion of the graft, release of the inferior vena cava clamp or separation from VVBP, reperfusion of the allograft, and completion of the hepatic artery anastomosis. The procedure concludes with the removal of the graft's gallbladder, and the bile duct anastomosis, and closure.

The reperfusion of the allograft is one of the most critical steps of the procedure. Throughout this period, the anesthesiologist should be aware of the possibility of hyperkalemia from reperfusion, metabolic acidosis, and the reperfusion syndrome (Box 14-2). Moreover, bleeding, fibrinolysis, cardiovascular instability (mainly severe hypotension requiring vasopressors), oliguria/renal dysfunction, hypothermia, and decreased calcium and magnesium are common. Early aggressive correction of these derangements is fundamental to avoid severe cardiovascular collapse and instability. Recognition of any early complications (dysfunction of graft, bleeding, severe metabolic derangements) while still in the operating room is essential to have an optimal outcome.

The use of premedication, short-acting benzodiazepines or opioids, will depend on the patient's medical status and anxiety. Since benzodiazepines are metabolized by the liver and their free fraction increases in the presence of hypoalbuminemia; these drugs should be administered cautiously.

Generally, liver transplantation is done under general anesthesia. However, in some centers, and depending upon the level of the patient's coagulopathy, regional techniques may be used. In any case, the drugs used during the perioperative period should depend on the assumption of altered pharmacokinetics that is associated with ESLD. Drugs that are metabolized independent of liver function – such as succinylcholine, esmolol, remifentanil, atracurium, cisatracurium – can be safely used in liver transplantation. On the other hand, drugs that rely on liver metabolism – such as benzodiazepines (cytochrome oxidase metabolism), lidocaine, and many neuromuscular relaxants – need to be careful monitored during the procedure. Since conjugation is normally

---

Box 14-2   Reperfusion Syndrome

Definition: Drop in mean arterial pressure of 30% or more that lasts more than 1 minute and occurs immediately after reperfusion of the graft (<5 min)

Electrocardiographic changes: Commonly T-wave changes and widening of QRS interval

Incidence: Decreased with flushing of graft prior to releasing clamp

Etiology: Unclear – $\uparrow K^+$, $\downarrow pH$, $\downarrow T^0$, inflammatory mediators from reperfusion injury, emboli, right heart dysfunction/pulmonary hypertension

Treatment: Flushing of the graft prior to reperfusion, correcting metabolic/electrolyte derangements (especially hyperkalemia – intraoperative dialysis may be necessary), keep patient warm, pretreatment with calcium, hemodynamic support (volume, vasopressors), aprotinin (?)

relatively preserved, drugs that depend on this route of biotransformation (i.e., opioids, propofol) may be better tolerated. Although in ESLD there is a reduction in the production of pseudocholinesterase, succinylcholine can be used safely in a single intubating dose.

Most of these patients require rapid sequence induction secondary to full stomach (ascites, patients coming from home, nausea and vomiting secondary to their ESLD, and/or possible history of upper gastrointestinal bleeding secondary to esophageal varices). For maintenance of anesthesia an inhalational agent and opioids along with a neuromuscular relaxant are typically used.

Although all volatile anesthetics can affect hepatic flow secondary to their potent negative inotropic effect (especially halothane and enflurane), isoflurane is commonly used during OLT. Desflurane, because of its potential to cause a smaller decrease in splanchnic blood flow and oxidative metabolism than other agents, is an attractive option during liver transplantation. Nitrous oxide is normally avoided, especially if VVBP is used.

Mannitol is an osmotic diuretic used during liver transplantation and other organ transplants. There is limited evidence that suggests beneficial effects of osmotic diuretics in the outcome of liver transplantation. However, mannitol is commonly used before the recirculation of the new graft because of its properties as a free radical scavenger, as well as to increase urine production.

In the presence of coagulopathy, the goal should be to maintain an international normalized ratio of 1.5 or less, keeping the platelet count above 50,000/mm^3, and using cryoprecipitate to keep the fibrinogen level above 100 mg/dL.

The choice of analgesia is limited mainly to the use of opioids, although regional techniques can be used in selected patients (i.e., neuroaxial blockade). The choice of opioids is left up to the preference of the anesthesiologist, although fentanyl (either boluses or infusion) and hydromorphone are generally the most commonly used, while methadone is another valid option.

Positioning the patient is very important during the procedure since the arms may be tucked along the side of the body and various forms of retractors are used to facilitate exposure. The anesthesiologist has to be aware of peripheral nerve damage, scalp necrosis, and tissue damage during the procedure and carefully monitor the pressure points.

The use of VVBP is not widely accepted and still controversial in some centers (see Clinical Caveat, below). VVBP may reduce most of the complications associated with venous cross-clamping, including decreased venous return with better hemodynamics, acidosis, decreased renal function secondary to decrease perfusion pressure to the kidneys, intestinal swelling, and potentially decreased blood loss. In contrast, if VVBP is not used, there may be a more significant reduction of venous return with marked hypotension. Essentially, the bypass is performed via a centrifugal pump without any heparin. Thrombosis is avoided by keeping flows at least at 1-1.5 L/min.

If renal failure develops during the perioperative period, especially in the setting of intraoperative oliguria/anuria and severe hyperkalemia, continuous hemofiltration is indicated and additional venous access may be needed.

Clinical Caveat: Venovenous Bypass

Need for perfusionist
Need for extravenous access
Inadvertent decannulation or line clotting
Thromboembolism/pulmonary embolism
Air embolism
Increased fibrinolysis and potential increased blood loss
Pump failure
Vascular injury
No evidence of beneficial effect on outcome

Once the graft is reperfused the anesthesiologist should recognize the signs that indicate a working graft, including reversal of coagulopathy, gradual resolution of acidosis, bile production, fibrinogen production, normalization of drug pharmacokinetics, increasing levels of glucose, and improvement in body temperature. After venous revascularization of the allograft and during the immediate postoperative period, a common practice is to keep the central venous pressure below 10 mmHg to avoid congestion of the new graft.

Postoperative Considerations

These patients require intensive medical care in the immediate postoperative period. Most patients are transported intubated and sedated to the intensive care unit and if they follow an uncomplicated course will spend 24-48 hours in the intensive care unit. Some patients may follow fast-track pathways if they are hemodynamically stable and meet criteria for early extubation, as long as the graft is functional. During the immediate postoperative period and in some cases for several weeks these patients continue to have the typical hyperdynamic state of the ESLD patient, which will eventually resolve.

The most common complications that occur after transplant include neurological (25-80%), infections, biliary stenosis and leaks, graft malfunction or nonfunction requiring retransplant (5-15%), vascular thrombosis (most commonly hepatic artery thrombosis, which may require a postoperative Doppler ultrasound to confirm flows), and respiratory failure secondary to volume over-load. The most feared complication is primary graft non-function. It has an increased morbidity and mortality and the patient will require a new graft in 2–3 days. Other complications include central pontine myelinolysis, coagulopathy and bleeding, acute lung injury, and renal dysfunction that may require renal replacement therapies.

ANESTHESIA MANAGEMENT FOR KIDNEY TRANSPLANT

Kidney transplantation is the most common type of transplant surgery in the United States. During 2001, more than half of the transplants performed in the United States were kidney transplants, with a total number of 14,000. Some 35% of the grafts were obtained from living donors.

Kidney transplantation represents the ultimate mode of renal replacement therapy and cure of end-stage renal disease (ESRD). The great majority of kidney transplant recipients were receiving some form of renal replacement therapy at the time of transplant, so kidney transplantation improves not only the life expectancy of ESRD patients but also their quality of life. In general, 85–95% of kidney transplants are successful and up to 80% of the grafts survived more than 5–10 years, being especially successful in cases with a living donor.

Because a considerable percentage of patients with ESRD have difficult-to-control diabetes type 1, combined kidney–pancreas transplantation has become an alternative in some institutions, to the point that in 2001 approximately 2,500 of these operations were performed in the United States.

Even although kidney transplantation is technically less demanding and complex than the other transplants described in this chapter, it still deserves a full understanding of the pathophysiology of the disease and knowledge of the anesthesia requirements of these patients.

Preoperative Considerations

Similar to any other transplant, the preoperative evaluation of the transplant candidates includes a multidisciplinary team approach including nephrologists, transplant surgeons, and anesthesiologists. The list of causes of ESRD is very extensive but the most common etiologies that lead to ESRD include glomerulonephritis, diabetes mellitus, hypertension, and polycystic kidney disease. In common with other transplants, contraindications include an active oncologic process, infections, and severe comorbid diseases. Age is less of a contraindication than in other forms of transplantation.

A complete medical history needs to be obtained and a physical examination performed. It is very important to know whether the patient produces any amount of urine, the type of renal replacement therapy, the frequency of dialysis, and the last time that the patient received dialysis. Prior to the transplant, it is necessary to obtain laboratory results (especially electrolytes, hemoglobin, acid–base status, and blood glucose if the patient is diabetic). The majority of these patients, independent of age, have different degrees of cardiovascular disease, including hypertension, coronary artery disease, and congestive heart failure. Therefore, many of these patients, especially those with poorly controlled hypertension and diabetes, should have a complete cardiac evaluation, including noninvasive tests, prior to transplant. Commonly, these patients present with different degrees of hyperkalemia. Another common finding in these patients is the presence of chronic anemia, which in some cases can be severe. Transfusions are normally avoided, so as to not create HLA antibodies; the mainstream approach to anemia is the preoperative administration of erythropoietin. Other aspects of the pathophysiology of patients with ESRD are included in Box 14-3.

Box 14-3 Pathophysiology of End-stage Renal Disease

Electrolyte/Metabolism: $\uparrow\uparrow K^+$, $\uparrow PO_4^-$ (if aggressively treated – difficulty weaning, central nervous system dysfunction, susceptibility to muscle relaxants), metabolic acidosis, $\downarrow HCO_3^-$, $\downarrow Na^+$, azotemia, $\uparrow Mg^{2+}$ (muscle weakness, increased sensitivity to muscle relaxants), $\downarrow Ca^{2+}$, hypoalbuminemia (protein malnutrition and protein loss during peritoneal dialysis)

Fluid balance: Volume overload, hypovolemia post-dialysis

Central Nervous System: Acute encephalopathy (blood urea nitrogen >120 mg/dL), neuropathy

Cardiovascular: Hypertension (primary or secondary to hyperreninemia), ischemic heart disease, congestive heart disease, increased cardiac output secondary to anemia, hyperlipidemia, uremic pericarditis

Respiratory: $\uparrow$ Minute volume to compensate for chronic metabolic acidosis

Hematopoiesis: Anemia (secondary to $\downarrow$ levels of erythropoietin, hemodialysis, $\downarrow$ iron absorption), thrombocytopenia (secondary to uremic bone marrow depression)

Coagulation: Platelet dysfunction secondary to uremia ($\downarrow$ endothelial release of von Willebrand factor–factor VIII complex), thrombocytopenia, $\downarrow$ antithrombin III, heparin used during hemodialysis

Lines and Monitoring

Standard monitoring is used for kidney transplantation. Except for patients with comorbid conditions that require more aggressive monitoring, an arterial line is rarely indicated. Central venous pressure monitoring, although commonly used to monitor intravascular volume status, probably gives limited information on the volume status since most of these patients have abnormal cardiac compliance.

The patient should have adequate intravenous access for the procedure. The anesthesiologist should avoid gaining intravascular access or placing noninvasive blood pressure monitoring on the arm where the dialysis access is located (i.e., arteriovenous fistula). Generally, one or two 16-gauge intravenous lines are sufficient. Depending on the time that these patients have been on hemodialysis and the number of places used for access, they may have very poor peripheral intravenous access.

Anesthesia Setup

Although the level of anesthesia care is less aggressive than with other transplants, and less preparation is needed, there is a basic setup that any kidney transplantation requires. In general, other than the standard warming devices no warming equipment is needed.

Besides the standard anesthesia drugs, the anesthesia cart should include furosemide, heparin, mannitol, insulin, calcium chloride, sodium bicarbonate, and the immunosuppressant medications (generally methylprednisolone, azathioprine, OKT3, and tacrolimus). The replacement fluid generally used for kidney transplantation is normal saline whereas lactated Ringer's solution and Plasmalyte are avoided because of their potassium content.

Anesthesia Management

The procedure is carried out through an incision in either lower quadrant. The graft is placed in the extraperitoneal iliac fossa and the ureter is anastomosed to the native bladder. Then the vascular anastomoses are performed with the external iliac vein first, followed by the iliac vein.

Any premedication, induction agent, or anesthetic can be safely used, as long as the pharmacokinetics of these drugs in patients with ESRD is understood. Many drugs depend on the kidneys for their elimination and transformation. Some drugs like gallamine, digoxin, or antibiotics like beta-lactams, vancomycin, or aminoglycosides depend totally on the kidney for their elimination. Anticholinergic and cholinergic drugs, some steroid-based neuromuscular agents, phosphodiesterase inhibitors, and the commonly used antifibrinolytics depend partially on renal elimina-

tion. In addition, some drugs commonly used during the transplant (morphine, meperidine, diazepam and midazolam, pancuronium, and vecuronium) have active metabolites that are eliminated by the kidneys. Because of the altered pharmacokinetics of renal failure, propofol seems the agent of choice for induction. Although any muscle relaxant can be used, vecuronium, rocuronium, and cisatracurium are the agents of choice.

Most kidney transplants are performed with limited time to prepare the patient, so the patients are considered to have a full stomach, especially in patients with diabetes, in whom gastroparesis is a common occurrence. Accordingly, rapid sequence induction is recommended. Succinylcholine can be used provided the potassium level is less than 5.5 mEq/L; rocuronium is a safe alternative. For maintenance, most of the modern inhalational agents can be safely used, although these drugs have the potential for decreasing blood flow to the cortex of the kidney. A balanced technique, including an opioid, is preferable to avoid marked hypotension.

The main goal for the kidney transplantation is to maintain euvolemia and adequate perfusion to the new graft. The incidence of primary nonfunctional grafts is less than 15% in most studies with short ischemic time and adequate volume resuscitation. In the past, the use of albumin was common practice but, based on the current available literature, it is not now recommended.

Another common practice, although the literature to support it is not strong, is to promote diuresis by giving mannitol and furosemide intravenously prior to completion of the anastomoses, to reduce the incidence of acute tubular necrosis. In addition, another common practice, the so-called "renal dose dopamine," has no place during kidney transplantation. The available evidence suggests that, except for increasing cardiac output in those patients with decreased cardiac function, the lower doses of dopamine have no effect on promoting diuresis or changing the outcome during acute tubular necrosis.

If pancreatic transplantation is performed at the same time as kidney transplantation, the pancreas is transplanted after the kidney. The procedure increases the intraoperative time to an average of 4-8 hours when the transplant is performed through a midline incision. Alternatively, it can be performed through a low transverse incision, depending upon where the anastomosis is completed – either to the ileum (via a duodenal stump) or to the bladder (pancreaticoduodenal cystostomy). Commonly the reperfusion of the new pancreas increases blood loss. In these patients, it is necessary to start an insulin infusion prior to surgery to adjust blood glucose levels to keep them, preferably, less than 120 mg/dL.

Since the metabolic acidosis present during kidney transplantation is due mainly to bicarbonate losses (although a moderate anion gap acidosis, secondary to sulphates and phosphates, may be present), extubation can be safely done at the end of surgery. In some cases it may be necessary to administer bicarbonate to compensate for the metabolic acidosis and to facilitate extubation. It is advisable to always document what the function of the arteriovenous fistula is both during surgery and after transport of the patient to the recovery area.

Postoperative Considerations

Commonly, these patients are extubated at the end of the case and are transported to a monitored bed for recovery and close follow-up of the potential complications.

The most common complications are cardiovascular, with either hypotension or, more commonly, hypertension and its associated complications (such as anastomotic bleeding, stroke, myocardial ischemia). These patients are also at risk of postoperative pulmonary complications secondary to the increased work of breathing to compensate for metabolic acidosis, pulmonary edema secondary to hypervolemia and low oncotic pressure (hypoalbuminemia), and atelectasis.

It is not unusual for the graft to show signs of dysfunction secondary to prolonged warm ischemia time (longer than 1 hr) and/or cold ischemia time (longer than 18 hr). The graft may not regulate electrolyte, water, or acid–base balance for up to 24 hours, so it is very important to carefully monitor electrolyte (especially potassium) and water levels.

Other complications include graft dysfunction (either primary – up to 60% in cadaveric donors – or secondary, most commonly to prerenal causes), rejection, infection, and new-onset diabetes, which will affect graft survival and the recipient's mortality and morbidity.

ANESTHESIA MANAGEMENT FOR HEART TRANSPLANT

The first human heart transplant was performed in the mid 1960s. During 2001, 2,200 heart transplants were performed in the United States. Approximately 85-90% of patients who receive a heart will survive the first year and up to 75% will be alive at least 3 years after the transplant.

The main indication for heart transplant is the treatment of irreversible chronic heart failure (end-stage heart disease; Box 14-4). The definition of end-stage heart disease includes those patients with New York Heart Association (NYHA) class III and IV symptoms of cardiac failure on maximal medical therapy and a prognosis of 1-year survival of less than 75%. The etiology of end-stage heart disease includes ischemic cardiomyopathy, idiopathic, alcoholic, or viral cardiomyopathy, valvular disease, congenital, and previous transplantation. Severe

---

Box 14-4   Pathophysiology of End-stage Heart Disease

Systolic dysfunction: Frank–Starling curve shifted down and to the right: requiring ↑ preload to maintain cardiac output

Congestive heart failure: Orthopnea, dyspnea, and reduced exercise tolerance are mainly due to pulmonary venous congestion secondary to left ventricular failure

Right-sided failure: Hepatic congestion with signs of hepatic dysfunction (coagulopathy), jugular distention, and significant peripheral edema.

Compensatory mechanisms to maintain cardiac output include renin–angiotensin–aldosterone system with increase in sodium levels and therefore water levels (if sodium levels are below 130, patients have worse survival), vasopressin system, and increase in heart rate and vasoconstriction via autonomic nervous system (high levels of catecholamines); ↑ catecholamines → downregulation of expression of adrenoreceptors with ↓ responsiveness to adrenergic agonist.

Low circulatory states: Mild renal dysfunction, hepatic dysfunction

---

pulmonary hypertension, age older than 70 (although transplant in older patients have been done successfully), irreversible hepatic, renal, or pulmonary disease (especially emphysema), documented cerebrovascular disease, and severe peripheral vascular disease are potential contraindications for transplant.

Preoperative Considerations

Potential cardiac transplant recipients may present with a wide range of severity of their disease. Initial evaluation of the potential recipient will include an echocardiogram, cardiac catheterization to check for coronary artery disease, pulmonary vascular resistance and valvular disease, biopsy, and exercise tolerance tests to determine maximal oxygen consumption (<10 mL/kg/min is associated with poor survival). All the data from these studies must be present in the chart for review by the anesthesiologist.

As with any other transplant candidate, a complete history and physical examination must be obtained. The patient's past medical history allows the anesthesiologist to identify other comorbid conditions that determine any other organ dysfunction. It is especially important to obtain a history of any previous intrathoracic surgery and aprotinin use, renal, lung and hepatic function, and coagulation status. A significant percentage of these patients will have ventricular assist devices and/or other implantable devices (implantable cardioverter defibrillator and pacemakers).

Lines and Monitors

For standard heart transplantation, the most common lines include: two large bore intravenous lines (14-gauge) and a right internal jugular central line, preferably an 8.5 French introducer (the left internal jugular is preferred to leave the right side for future heart biopsies). Pulmonary artery catheters are not normally used because of the resection of the artery during the procedure.

Besides the standard monitors used for cardiac surgery, including arterial line, rectal and nasopharyngeal temperature probes, a TEE probe is commonly used. As is the standard for all other transplants, strict aseptic technique during line placement is fundamental to avoid infection during the postoperative period.

In cases of repeated sternotomy, it is advisable to place transcutaneous pacing pads on the patient. Some patients who present for transplant have implantable devices, and attention needs to be paid to coordinating the different phases of the procedure to the function of these devices.

Anesthesia Setup

The setup for any cardiac transplant case should be similar to that of any other standard cardiac anesthesia case. Common medications that should be readily available include (both infusions and boluses): dopamine, isoproterenol, nitroprusside, epinephrine, vasopressin, dobutamine, nitroglycerine, insulin, furosemide, mannitol, calcium chloride, and milrinone. Epsilon-aminocaproic acid is commonly used as an antifibrinolytic but aprotinin is indicated for reoperations, even although it could be used in all cases. Steroids and antibiotics should be available. Easy access to nitric oxide is mandatory in case of severe right heart dysfunction secondary to pulmonary hypertension after transplantation.

As with any cardiac procedure, blood products should be either in the room or readily available. Also, besides the use of the cardiopulmonary bypass (CPB) machine, blood warmers and other warming devices should be ready for the case. In addition, working pacemakers should be checked and ready to use during, and especially after CPB.

Anesthesia Management

A dedicated heart transplant team should be readily available for the transplant. Good communication between the transplant coordinators, cardiac surgeons, and anesthesiologists is fundamental for a smooth and safe procedure. It is crucial for a successful heart transplant to establish good coordination with the different teams so cross-clamp time can be kept under 4 hours.

The procedure is done through a median sternotomy, followed by a pericardiotomy. Following exposure of the heart, the vena cava and aorta are cannulated following standard cardiac surgical procedures, and then the aorta is cross-clamped. Standard CPB is started after the cross-clamp is placed. Then the pulmonary artery and aorta are transected (at this point, if a pulmonary catheter is inserted it needs to be pulled back) and the heart is removed. The donor heart is attached to the recipient though suture lines at the native pulmonary veins in the left and right atrium. The next step involves reattachment of the aorta and pulmonary artery. Ischemic time ends with the removal of the cross-clamp. After careful de-airing, the graft is separated from CPB following the usual procedures.

Cardiac surgeons need to be present during induction in case of cardiac arrest. Induction should not take place until the surgical team reports that the graft is in good condition. Slow circulatory times are expected for most drugs because of decreased cardiac function. A common method of induction includes a technique with high-dose opioids (frequently fentanyl 5–20 µg/kg) with etomidate (0.3 mg/kg). Succinylcholine and pancuronium, at standard doses, are preferred for neuromuscular blockade. Midazolam can also be used during induction or as premedication. For the majority of these patients (especially if coming from home), full-stomach precautions are employed.

As discussed during the explanation of the pathophysiology of end-stage heart disease, these patients are very sensitive to a decrease in preload, contractility, and heart rate, so careful attention is necessary to maintain adequate cardiac function, although these patients are accustomed to low systemic blood pressures. In any case, volume and in most cases inotropic medications need to be used or increased during induction (the same care needs to be applied if an intra aortic balloon pump or ventricular assisted device is in place). The use of drugs that increase afterload, such as phenylephrine, may cause profound decreases in cardiac output.

Intraoperative coagulopathy is not unusual, especially in patients who have already had cardiothoracic procedures prior to transplant. Important steps to correct it include correction of surgical bleeding, platelets (preferably single donor), fresh frozen plasma, cryoprecipitate, and antifibrinolytics.

Maintenance of anesthesia during dissection, CPB, and separation from CPB does not differ from regular cardiac anesthesia management. After the graft is implanted, the denervated heart initially presents with junctional rhythm secondary to the lack of innervation to the atrial sinus, so isoproterenol or external pacing may be needed to achieve an adequate heart rate (usually

>90–100 beats/min). This lack of innervation makes the graft more dependent on preload to maintain adequate cardiac output. Because of the lack of vagal innervation of the graft, atropine and neostigmine do not affect the heart rate. Also, it is not uncommon to see two different P waves on the electrocardiogram secondary to the presence of unresected native heart tissue. In case of right ventricular failure, different approaches may be taken but, commonly, one or more of the drugs or maneuvers listed in Box 14-5 are used.

It is not unusual for these patients to present with oliguria during the transplantation. The use of diuretics (mannitol and furosemide), although widely practiced, remains controversial, since the majority of studies have failed to show any positive effect of diuretic therapy on outcome. Secondary to the use of corticosteroids and because of the level of stress, these patients are prone to develop hyperglycemia, which needs to be treated aggressively.

Steroids are normally given prior to the removal of the cross-clamp. Azathioprine may be given before or after the separation from CPB. Like any other long procedure, careful attention needs to be paid to the patient's positioning to avoid nerve or tissue damage.

Box 14-5 Management of Acute Pulmonary Hypertension/Right Ventricular Dysfunction

AVOIDANCE OF PULMONARY VASOCONSTRICTION

Avoid hypercapnia, overventilation, hypoxia and acidosis, release of catecholamine secondary to light anesthesia and pain

TREATMENT OF PULMONARY VASOCONSTRICTION

Sodium nitroprusside
Prostaglandin E_1 at 0.02–0.1 μg/kg/min
Adenosine infusion (start at 50 μg/kg/min)
Volatile anesthetics
Nitric oxide (20–40 ppm)
Isoproterenol (secondary to its pulmonary vasodilatory effects) at 0.01–0.1 μg/kg/min
Nitroglycerine

INOTROPE THERAPY

Epinephrine
Dobutamine
Milrinone at 0.125–0.375 μg/kg/min

UNRESPONSIVE HEART FAILURE

Metaraminol (0.5–2 mg)
Right ventricular assisted device
Cardiopulmonary bypass

Postoperative Considerations

The specific management of the critically ill post-transplant patient goes beyond the scope of this chapter. All these patients should go to an intensive care unit with medical personnel accustomed to the management of cardiac surgery patients.

The primary cause of death during the postoperative period is infection, followed by acute rejection. Other common complications in the immediate postoperative period include: right heart dysfunction (<10%), dysrhythmias (5–10%), bleeding (2–5%) and hyperacute rejection (<1%). Rejection is commonly seen between the time of transplant and 3 months post-transplant. The post-transplant echocardiogram with rejection shows typical findings of diastolic dysfunction. In hyperacute rejection, due to a profound immunologic response against the new graft, cytotoxic antibodies are directed against the donor coronary arteries, causing an acute thrombosis of the coronary arteries with ischemic heart failure that is generally unresponsive to therapy.

Long-term problems associated with heart transplantation include allograft coronary artery disease (accelerated atherosclerosis) and hypertension. The prevalence of accelerated atherosclerotic disease is 10–20% at 1 year and usually affects small vessels. Normally, patients do not have anginal symptoms.

ANESTHESIA MANAGEMENT FOR LUNG TRANSPLANT

Lung transplantation is a very complex surgical procedure with a complicated perioperative management, and requires a dedicated and experienced team of surgeons, cardiothoracic anesthesiologists, pulmonologists, intensivists, nurses and transplant coordinators.

Lung transplantation is the recommended treatment for end-stage lung failure (Box 14-6). The most common causes of lung failure include chronic obstructive pulmonary disease (COPD), including emphysema (45% of all lung transplants), suppurative lung disease (cystic fibrosis or bronchiectasis), pulmonary fibrosis, and irreversible pulmonary hypertension. Absolute contraindications include severe extrapulmonary organ dysfunction, acute critical illness, cancer, sepsis, and inability to walk with a poor rehabilitation potential. Preoperative colonization with panresistant bacteria, commonly seen in cystic fibrosis patients, and mechanical ventilation preoperatively (excluding noninvasive) are considered to be relative contraindications.

During 2001 approximately 1,050 patients underwent single- or double-lung transplantation in the United States.

Box 14-6 Pathophysiology of End-stage Lung Disease

Respiratory: $\dot{V}/\dot{Q}$ mismatch; resting or exercise hypoxemia; hypercarbia; ↑ secretions; chronic pulmonary infection; pulmonary fibrosis with decreased lung diffusion, ↓ forced expiratory volume in 1 sec (FEV_1), and vital capacity (pulmonary fibrosis); possibility of left recurrent laryngeal nerve paralysis secondary to enlarged pulmonary artery
Cardiovascular: Evidence of severe pulmonary hypertension with right ventricular dysfunction and signs of failure; mean pulmonary artery pressures >55 mmHg with ↓ cardiac output; possibility of right to left shunts in case of severe pulmonary hypertension.
Neurological: Thromboembolic episodes (right to left shunt) – avoid injection of air in the intravenous line
Musculoskeletal: Muscular wasting with cachexia
Hematological: Polycythemia secondary to hypoxemia
Endocrine: Chronic steroids in cases of chronic obstructive pulmonary disease

The most common type of lung transplantation is the single-lung transplant, followed by bilateral or sequential lung transplantation (generally reserved for patients with cystic fibrosis or bronchiectasis). Heart–lung transplantation is less commonly performed (only for Eisenmenger's syndrome and irreparable cardiac defects), since the right ventricular dysfunction generally improves after lung transplant. Lobe transplantation from a living donor is becoming more accepted in some centers.

Although results vary from institution to institution, the fact is that survival rates have improved only slightly during the last 10 years. The median survival is 3.7 years, with a 3-year survival rate of 42% and a perioperative mortality of 10% in some series.

Preoperative Considerations

These patients have severe functional limitations due to their respiratory disease and in general have to be less than 65 years of age (younger for bilateral lung or heart–lung transplant) and free of any other comorbid conditions.

These patients undergo extensive workup prior to transplantation. This includes cardiac studies (echocardiogram, exercise tolerance tests, pulmonary artery pressures), respiratory functional studies (pulmonary function tests), and ventilation/perfusion scans. These tests permit the anesthesiologists and surgeons to establish the patient's functional status, the need for CPB intraoperatively and the ability to tolerate lung isolation. The primary cause of end-stage lung disease will determine the need for intraoperative CPB. For example, in COPD oxygenation is not usually a problem and CPB may not be needed, while in the case of interstitial lung disease more marked problems with oxygenation may occur. Severe primary pulmonary hypertension with mean pulmonary pressures greater than 40 mmHg and pulmonary vascular resistance higher than 250 dyn/sec/cm⁵ meets criteria for CPB. However, CPB should be avoided if at all possible, as the complications associated with it (inflammatory response, vascular complications, fibrinolysis, etc.) worsen outcome. Moreover, the available evidence in the literature suggests that outcome may be improved if CPB is not used during lung transplantation.

Lines and Monitoring

It is recommended that there is adequate venous access for the case. This consists of at least two big peripheral intravenous lines (14 G or an 8.5 Fr introducer) and a central line in either the left or right side (8.5 Fr would be preferable to facilitate the placement of a pulmonary artery catheter). Besides the standard monitors, a radial artery line and a pulmonary artery catheter are also inserted. In some high-risk patients, and in preparation for emergency CPB, some anesthesiologists prefer to cannulate the femoral artery also. It is recommended for most cases, especially if pulmonary hypertension is an issue, to place a TEE probe to follow right ventricular function. Also, in most cases a double-lumen tube is placed for lung isolation – it is important to have access to a bronchoscope to verify tube positioning. All the procedures need to be performed under strict sterile technique with full drapes, gloves, and gown.

Anesthesia Setup

Lung transplantation involves a very complex perioperative management and good preparation is fundamental for a successful outcome. Besides the monitors and lines needed for the procedure, a stocked cart should include the common drugs normally used for any thoracic, cardiac, or transplant case. The following infusions should be readily available in infusion pumps: dopamine, nitroprusside, nitroglycerin, phenylephrine, vasopressin, epinephrine, and milrinone. Prostaglandin E_1 (0.1–0.4 µg/kg/min) should be ordered from the pharmacy but not mixed until ready to use. Nitric oxide should also be readily available. In addition, mannitol, diuretics, adequate antibiotics (especially in case of cystic fibrosis with pseudomonas infection), antifibrinolytics (aprotinin), bronchodilators, and immunosuppressant agents (cyclosporine, prednisone, and azathioprine, with the use of a cytolytic agent) should be available.

Most cases are performed with one-lung ventilation, so double-lumen tubes of different sizes and bronchial blockers should be in the room. A rapid infusion system for intravenous fluids should also be to hand, as should be the CPB machine and the perfusionist, in case it is necessary to go on bypass urgently. As with liver transplantation, sufficient blood products should be either in the operating room or readily available.

Anesthesia Management

Lung transplantation is one of the most challenging procedures that anesthesiologists face. The procedure can be long and demand both rapid assessment and intervention in often life-threatening situations. The management of these patients requires an understanding not only of the pathophysiology and perioperative considerations of end-stage lung failure but also of patients with heart disease and of the technical aspects of the surgical procedure, lung isolation, the pathophysiology of CPB, mechanical ventilation, pulmonary hypertension, and acute right ventricular failure.

The surgical procedure involves a single thoracotomy, or clamshell thoracotomy for double-lung transplantation, followed by the resection of the native lung(s) and clamping of the pulmonary aorta. At this point, and prior to clamping of the pulmonary artery if CPB is needed, the surgeons will continue with the standard cannulation for CPB. After reinsertion of the graft(s) and completion of the different anastomoses (starting with the airways), the pulmonary artery is unclamped (after reinflation of the lungs) and the surgeons proceed with the closure.

If a single thoracotomy is performed, the patient will be placed in lateral decubitus, as opposed to the supine position for the clamshell incision, so protection of the patient's limbs, head, and body are very important. Although, in general, lung transplantation can be a long procedure (>10 hr), the cold ischemia time for the graft should not exceed 6–8 hours.

Because benzodiazepines and opioids may produce respiratory depression in a patient who is already hypercarbic, with a potential further increase in pulmonary artery pressures, their use for sedation must be judicious. Induction is carried out using standard cardiac induction techniques with a hypnotic and opioids, a long-acting muscle relaxant, and, always, a surgeon present in the room. In deciding which agents to use, bear in mind that a significant percentage of procedures are canceled after the patient has been induced because of problems with the graft. The use of ketamine is preferred by some thoracic anesthesiologists because of its stable effects on the respiratory system and minimal effects on the cardiovascular system. Since the recipients are given only a few hours' notice of the transplant they should be considered to have a full stomach and a rapid sequence induction should be performed.

Most of these patients are on oxygen at home, so it is very important to continue oxygen therapy throughout induction. Those patients on vasodilator therapy for pulmonary hypertension should have the therapy continued during the case.

After induction, initial tracheal intubation is commonly carried out using a double-lumen tube or a bronchial blocker and a standard technique. Positive-pressure ventilation needs to be applied very carefully, since it can cause dynamic hyperinflation secondary to air trapping and decreased venous return. In most patients, protective ventilatory strategies with low tidal volume, high frequencies, and longer than usual I:E ratios may help. In severe cases, some centers have successfully used high-frequency jet ventilation, although this is still controversial.

In addition, once one-lung ventilation is instituted, these patients frequently develop hypoxemia, which in some cases can be severe. The approach to this situation should be the same as in any regular thoracic case with intraoperative lung isolation. Common maneuvers include increasing F_iO_2, adjusting the ventilator, adding continuous positive airway pressure to the non-dependent lung, and positive end-expiratory pressure (PEEP) to the dependent lung. In some cases the surgeons may need to partially clamp the pulmonary artery to improve $\dot{V}/\dot{Q}$ match. (Do not forget to pull back the pulmonary artery catheter!) Clamping the pulmonary artery may cause a sudden increase in pulmonary artery pressure, worsening or causing acute right ventricular failure, so in some cases there is no other option but to start CPB. Hence, constant communication with the surgeons is very important. These patients require frequent suctioning, especially in the case of cystic fibrosis or bronchiectasis, so a sterile closed suction circuit is advisable.

Maintenance of anesthesia depends on the recipient's status, type of operation, and primary disease. In the cases performed without CPB, the combination of opioids, a volatile agent, or an intravenous agent and a long-acting muscle relaxant is adequate. When CPB is used, management and separation from CPB should be the same as in any other cardiac procedure carried out under CPB.

It must be borne in mind that these patients require an adequate intravascular volume, since decreased venous return may impair right ventricular performance. Because it is common for the graft to present with edema after reperfusion (resection of lymphatic drainage, use of CPB, and massive inflammatory response), surgeons try to keep the patient as dry as possible by restricting the amount of fluid administered. The best management is controversial but avoidance of significant hypovolemia and hypotension in the setting of right ventricular dysfunction is very important. Occasionally, inotropic support is also needed to improve right ventricular function.

Immunosuppressants are given normally at the beginning of the case and steroids are administered prior to reperfusion (in a double transplant, give steroids with the reperfusion of each graft).

Very common problems seen during lung transplantation are the presence of severe graft edema, especially if prolonged ischemia or CPB has been used, and right ventricular dysfunction has occurred. The approach to the first problem is complex but includes adjusting the ventilator to optimize oxygenation, frequent suction and applying PEEP. Also, in case of single-lung transplantation, it is not unusual to find a significant difference in compliance between the native lung and the graft, particularly if the recipient has emphysema. In this case, and if the standard maneuvers do not improve the clinical picture, it may be necessary to leave the double-lumen tube and apply differential ventilation using two ventilators. Always keep in mind that plateau pressures after the new graft is in place should not exceed 30–35 cmH2O and that a fresh bronchial/tracheal anastomosis may not tolerate high peak pressures, so both peak inspiratory pressures and PEEP need to be applied carefully. The overall goal after reperfusion should be to achieve adequate gas exchange with as low a F_iO_2 as possible to maintain oxygen saturation over 90%, and to follow closely any signs of right ventricular dysfunction. The approach to acute right ventricular dysfunction is outlined in Box 14-5.

Analgesia for the procedure and for the postoperative period can be achieved with use of opioids. However, some centers routinely use thoracic epidurals, even in cases in which CPB may be used. In general, a reasonable approach, if epidural analgesia is considered, would be to place the epidural in the intensive care unit once coagulopathy secondary to the use of CPB has been corrected.

At the end of the case, if possible, it is recommended that the double-lumen tube is changed to a single tube. (Remember to use an endotracheal tube big enough to facilitate repeated bronchoscopy.)

Postoperative Considerations

All these patients are transported to the intensive care unit for their postoperative management, with different levels of support, ranging from minimal to considerable degrees of support, including a right ventricular assisted device, nitric oxide, and, in some cases, extracorporeal membrane oxygenation. All patients are transported intubated and sedated. As in any other complex cases, the patient can be awakened and extubated once all physiological parameters have achieved the desired target.

The most common postoperative complications include: bleeding (5%), pulmonary interstitial edema secondary to the removal of the lymphatic drainage (20%), which can evolve into primary graft failure (15%), airways complications (<15%), infection, especially pulmonary (30–40%, more common than with other organ transplants), and rejection (divided between hyperacute [rare], acute [75% at 10–21 days], and chronic).

ANESTHESIA MANAGEMENT OF PATIENTS WITH A TRANSPLANTED ORGAN

In the United States in 2001 more than 24,000 transplants were performed. In some cases, these patients will need either reinterventions related to their transplant or surgery not related to the original transplant, both electively or as an emergency. Frequently, these procedures are carried out in institutions where transplants are not done routinely, so it is important for the anesthesiologist to become familiar with the specific problems arising in the management of these patients.

The management of transplanted patients requires a good understanding of the altered physiology of the transplanted graft and its influence on the rest of the system, the pharmacology of the immunosuppressant medications, and associated risks that these patients pose (infection and rejection).

One of the most common considerations when managing these patients is the interaction of the immunosuppressants with the drugs used during the perioperative period. In short, what most immunosuppressants do is to alter the normal function of the immune response by either affecting the activation and proliferation of T-cells (cyclosporine A, tacrolimus, and sirolimus), blocking the production of inflammatory mediators and lymphocytes (steroids), or blocking the proliferation of lymphocytes by affecting their nucleic acid synthesis (azathioprine, mycophenolate mofetil, and mizoribine). In some institutions an antilymphocyte antibody (OKT3) is added to the immunosuppressant regime. The understanding of the pharmacology of these drugs and their side effects is very important to determine how to handle them perioperatively. In Box 14-7, all the known side effects and interactions relevant during the perioperative period are listed. Besides the changes in drug level due to interactions with other medications, always keep in mind that significant fluid shifts can change the volume of distribution of these drugs and their plasma levels.

Although it is important to continue all these medications during the perioperative period, this is particularly important in the case of cyclosporine and tacrolimus. It is also true in the case of lung transplantation, unless there is a specific contraindication (e.g., infection). Always contact a transplant surgeon if any question arises during the perioperative period.

The preoperative evaluation of the transplanted patient should include an assessment of the function of the graft and of other organ systems through laboratory results, history, physical examination, and any invasive studies, since the presence of rejection or infection is associated with higher rates of perioperative morbidity and mortality. It should always be considered that the

Box 14-7 Immunosuppressant Medications – Considerations for the Anesthesiologist

CYCLOSPORINE A AND TACROLIMUS

Narrow therapeutic window
Side effects:
- Nephrotoxicity by reducing afferent glomerular arteriolar flow
- Hypertension (cyclosporine A)
- Hypercholesterolemia
- Tacrolimus can cause tremor, seizures and coma
- Diabetes (tacrolimus)
- Hyperkalemia
- Hypomagnesemia.

Drugs that affect blood level: phenobarbital ($\downarrow$ level), calcium channel blockers and metoclopramide ($\uparrow$ cyclosporine A)

Drugs affected by cyclosporine: $\uparrow$ pentobarbital, fentanyl, vecuronium, pancuronium, and atracurium

Drugs that can worsen nephrotoxicity: catecholamines, cimetidine, ranitidine, nonsteroidal anti-inflammatory drugs, vancomycin, gentamicin

MYCOPHENOLATE MOFETIL

Side effects: Anemia, leukopenia, and thrombocytopenia

OKT3 (MONOCLONAL ANTIBODIES DIRECTED AGAINST CD-3 ANTIGEN OF HUMAN T LYMPHOCYTES)

Side effects: Leukopenia, anaphylaxis, and fever

STEROIDS

Side effects: Diabetes, hypertension, neurotoxicity, adrenal axis suppression, bone mass loss

ANTI-THYMOCYTE GLOBULIN

Narrow therapeutic window
Side effects: Similar to OKT3

AZATHIOPRINE

Side effects: Anemia, leukopenia, thrombocytopenia
Increases bone marrow toxicity with angiotensin-converting enzyme inhibitors

---

dependent than normal hearts on preload to maintain adequate cardiac output, so hypovolemia should always be avoided. In this case, neuroaxial blockade may cause further decrease of preload due to sympathectomy and cause decreased cardiac output. Moreover, some of the cardiovascular drugs normally used during the perioperative period either do not work or have paradoxical effects. Most of the indirectly acting cardiac drugs do not cause an increase in heart rate (e.g., anticholinergic drugs, ephedrine), catecholamine response is altered (e.g., epinephrine and norepinephrine have an augmented inotropic effect, dopamine acts by release of norepinephrine and has less inotropic effect), and pancuronium and neostigmine do not cause an increase in heart rate. Of all the available cardioactive drugs, isoproterenol and dobutamine have the best inotropic profile on denervated hearts.

In order to avoid risk of infection, it is very important to maintain strict sterility during any procedure. It is prudent to use only invasive monitoring in those cases in which significant fluid shifts will occur or in any major procedure. In any transplanted patient, the risk of aspiration is always present. This is especially true in patients who have undergone lung transplantation, in whom cough reflexes may be abolished below the tracheal anastomosis.

Nonsteroidal anti-inflammatory drugs should not be used during the perioperative period to avoid a further detrimental effect on the kidneys. Regional techniques, especially neuroaxial blockade, can be useful for postoperative analgesia as long as there is no contraindication (i.e., thrombocytopenia secondary to immunosuppressants).

Lastly, a relatively common clinical scenario that may be encountered by anesthesiologists is the transplanted pregnant patient who presents for labor and delivery. Any of the techniques used in obstetric anesthesiology can be safely used but the risks of pre-eclampsia, prematurity and low birthweight of the newborn are increased. In heart-transplanted patients, tocolytic beta-agonists may not be safe and other alternatives need to be used (i.e., magnesium).

allograft, after transplant, may not totally recover normal function. Therefore, the degree of organ dysfunction and physiological changes to the new organ need to be considered when decided which drugs to use for anesthetic management.

There is no benefit of general anesthesia over regional anesthesia. Both are appropriate for these patients, as long as you understand the pathophysiology of the denervated graft. For example, transplanted hearts, because of the lack of sympathetic or parasympathetic enervation, do not have normal vagal tone; therefore they are more

SUMMARY

During the last decade both the number and complexity of transplants performed have increased significantly. Also, the number of surgical procedures performed on transplanted patients has increased. Because of the intensity of these procedures, the severity of the disease, the existing organ failure, and the comorbid conditions that these patients present during the perioperative period, anesthesiologists are faced with a growing number of challenges. These challenges require a good understanding of all the pharmacological and pathophysiological changes that occur during the perioperative management of these frequently critically ill patients. An understanding of the physiology of these patients and the pharmacology of the new immunosuppressant therapies is essential to manage these patients safely.

In the near future, transplants of other organs and new techniques are likely to increase. Likewise, the restrictions limiting the number of suitable candidates for transplantation surgery are likely to increase, thus providing for more critically ill patients in the operating room. Because of this increasing degree of complexity some of these transplant procedures will require dedicated teams with specific knowledge of the challenges associated with the organs transplanted, especially heart, lung, and liver. However, even in those centers without transplant programs, anesthesiologists will have to take care of patients with transplanted organs. This chapter has reviewed some of these challenges and the fundamentals associated with transplant anesthesia.

SUGGESTED READING

Braunfeld M. Anesthesia for liver transplantation. *ASA Refresher Courses Anesthesiol* 2001;29:83-96.

Carton EG, Rettke SR, Plevak DJ, *et al.* Perioperative care of the liver transplant patient: part 1. *Anesth Analg* 1994;78:120-133.

Carton EG, Rettke SR, Plevak DJ, *et al.* Perioperative care of the liver transplant patient: part 2. *Anesth Analg* 1994;78: 382-399.

Dickstein ML. Anesthesia for heart transplantation. *Semin Cardiothorac Vasc Anesth* 1998;2:131-139.

Jaffe RA, Samuels SI, eds. *Anesthesiologist's manual of surgical procedures*, 2nd ed. Philadelphia: Lippincott, Williams & Wilkins, 1999.

Koehntop DE, Beebe DS, Belani KG. Perioperative anesthetic management of the kidney-pancreas transplant patient. *Curr Opin Anaesthesiol* 2000;13:341-347.

McRae KM. Pulmonary transplantation. *Curr Opin Anaesthesiol* 2000;13:53-59.

Mathew MC, Wendon JA. Perioperative management of liver transplantation patients. *Curr Opin Crit Care* 2001;7: 275-280.

Myles PS. Aspects of anesthesia for lung transplantation. *Semin Cardiothorac Vasc Anesth* 1998;2:140-154.

Sprung J, Kapural L, Bourke DL, O'Hara JF. Anesthesia for kidney transplant surgery. *Anesthesiol Clin North Am* 2000;18: 919-951.

Toivonen HJ. Anaesthesia for patients with a transplanted organ. *Acta Anaesthesiol Scand* 2000;44:812-833.

Anesthesia for Orthopedic Surgery

MICHAEL F. MULROY

LILA A. SUEDA

INTRODUCTION

Anesthesia for orthopedic surgery includes the same considerations as for other surgical procedures, specifically the need for muscle relaxation, hemodynamic stability, lack of awareness, and analgesia during and after the procedure. In addition to these overall considerations, orthopedic patients have specific aspects to their care that influence the choice of anesthetics (Box 15-1).

First, orthopedic surgery is among the most painful that is performed, and the need for residual postoperative analgesia is critical in this group. The pain can last for several days, as in knee surgery, and may limit patients' recovery and rehabilitation. These challenges call for innovative approaches. Intravenous opioids are traditional but do not completely relieve the extensive pain with major orthopedic procedures, especially the additional pain associated with motion.

Another major consideration is that frequently these patients are either suffering an acute traumatic injury or more likely have chronic debilitating disease that makes it difficult for them to be moved to the operating table or into positions for the performance of surgery or regional techniques. Intraoperatively, positioning is also frequently a challenge. Some of these patients have defor-

mities due to chronic arthritis problems, which may require attention to padding and protection. They may also not be able to assume certain positions, and thus the operating configuration must be altered.

A third consideration is that these procedures frequently produce significant blood loss, and any modification of the anesthetic technique to reduce blood loss will benefit the patient population. Another aspect is that orthopedic procedures frequently require muscle relaxation.

GENERAL OR REGIONAL ANESTHESIA?

While regional anesthesia techniques may be desirable intraoperatively and postoperatively, there are limitations in this patient population. First, many of these procedures require active physical therapy and rehabilitation in the postoperative period, which requires active movement on the part of the patients. Thus a motor block associated with an analgesic technique may limit the patient's rehabilitation. More importantly, many of these patients receive systemic anticoagulation to prevent venous thrombosis and pulmonary embolism, which were previously frequent causes of morbidity in orthopedic surgery. While modern thromboprophylactic regimens are extremely effective, they also increase the risk of bleeding associated with regional anesthesia techniques, particularly in central neuraxial techniques. The use of epidural analgesia in the postoperative period is limited by this, as well as by the need to avoid orthostatic hypotension and motor blockade.

Despite all these considerations, there is an extensive role for regional anesthesia during the performance of orthopedic surgery. Multiple specific examples will be discussed. Specifically, one of the advantages is that neuraxial techniques have been shown to reduce blood loss with some surgical procedures. More importantly,

Box 15-1 Special Considerations for Orthopedic Procedures

May be necessitated for trauma
Requires manipulation of extremities, joints
Often painful
Immobilization may predispose to deep venous thrombosis
Elective procedures frequently performed on elderly debilitated patients
Potential for blood loss
Requires muscle relaxation
Necessitates postoperative analgesia, immobilization
Often requires anticoagulation/thromboprophylaxis
Usually have pre-existing disease such as rheumatoid arthritis with limited mobility, positioning issues

Table 15-2 Regional Versus General Anesthesia

General	Regional
Easy to administer	Intraoperative muscle relaxation
Allows variability during procedure	Mental stability in elderly??
Allows variable muscle relaxation	Potential for postoperative analgesia for rehabilitation
Some risks of cardiovascular depression, postoperative nausea	Decreased blood loss
	Risk of neurologic injury

peripheral nerve blocks are highly effective in providing good muscle relaxation during surgery and excellent pain relief for a prolonged period postoperatively. The use of continuous indwelling peripheral nerve catheters can greatly enhance this analgesia and prolong it for an indefinite duration. Peripheral nerve catheters have the advantages of not producing orthostatic hypotension nor the potential of neuraxial hematoma. Multiple series have been reported of various solutions and infusion rates, which all appear to provide excellent prolonged postoperative analgesia (Table 15-1).

Of course, the usual contraindications to regional techniques apply, such as untreated systemic sepsis, local infection at the site of injection, or severe coagulopathy.

Table 15-1 Continuous Peripheral Nerve Catheters: Published Solutions and Rates

Location	Solution	Infusion Rate
Interscalene	Bupivacaine 0.15%	5 mL/h
	Bupivacaine 0.25%	0.25 mg/kg/hr
	Ropivacaine 0.2%	5-10 mL/h
Axillary	Bupivacaine 0.25%	3-5 mL/h
	Bupivacaine 0.25%	0.25 mg/kg/hr
	Ropivacaine 0.1%	0.125 mg/kg/hr
Femoral	Lidocaine 1%, morphine 30 μg/mL, clonidine 2 μg/mL	0.1 mL/kg/hr
	Bupivacaine 0.125%, sufentanil 0.1 μg/mL, clonidine 1 μg/L	10 mL/hr
	0.2% Ropivacaine	12 mL/hr
Psoas	Bupivacaine 0.125%	6-10 mL/hr
	Bupivacaine 0.25% with epinephrine 1:200,000	1-2 mL/kg every 8 hr prn

On the other hand, general anesthesia works well for these patients, especially in the face of acute trauma. In this situation, blood loss has frequently occurred and the institution of neuraxial blockade can precipitate sudden and dramatic hypotension. General anesthesia is usually easy to initiate, although orthopedic patients are more likely to have limitations of neck or jaw motion, which can make endotracheal intubation more challenging. Care must be taken to include a significant amount of opioids to provide a transition to postoperative analgesia, especially in the patient who has developed tolerance because of chronic use or dependence on analgesics. In the following sections, it will be assumed that general anesthesia may well be the technique of choice in the presence of acute traumatic injuries and in the face of specific patient preference, but the majority of this discussion in the following sections will focus on the potential use of regional techniques for orthopedic procedures because of their specific advantages (Table 15-2). This chapter will not discuss specifics of regional anesthesia techniques, as these are described in great detail with extensive illustrations in many excellent texts.

UPPER EXTREMITY SURGERY

Procedures performed on the shoulder, arm, and hand are amenable to regional techniques, and these techniques provide an excellent transition to postoperative analgesia in the outpatient setting. Regional techniques are facilitated by the anatomy of the brachial plexus. The nerve roots to the entire arm lie in a single plane (between the anterior and middle scalene muscles) that is readily identified and filled with single injections of local anesthetic.

Shoulder

There are a wide variety of procedures performed on the shoulder, ranging from simple exploratory arthroscopy of the joint to resection of the distal clavicle and more extensive acromioplasties and repairs of the rotator cuff mechanism. While all of these can be performed under general anesthesia, the use of an interscalene block provides adequate anesthesia for the majority of these procedures. A classic interscalene block will also provide anesthesia of the lower cervical plexus, which will include the sensory branches to the shoulder and the upper arm. This distribution of anesthesia is sufficient for shoulder arthroscopy with the occasional exceptional absence of anesthesia in the area of the posterior ports on the back. Anesthesia is generally adequate for all procedures unless the surgeons specifically require muscle relaxation of the pectoralis muscles for the Bankart surgical repair. In this case, supplemental general anesthesia and muscle relaxation may be required.

If an interscalene block is performed, lidocaine is an excellent drug for intraoperative anesthesia. If prolonged analgesia is desired, a longer-acting agent should be chosen. Mepivacaine will provide 6–8 hours of analgesia, while bupivacaine and ropivacaine can provide motor block for approximately 10 hours and sensory analgesia for 12–14 hours. This may be ideal for patients having rotator cuff repair who are sent home from surgery. It will provide at least some analgesia for the first half day.

If prolonged analgesia is desired, continuous catheters can be inserted using either the classic interscalene approach or newer approaches through the intrasternocleidomastoid approach, or even from the posterior approach past the transverse process of C6. Fixation of the catheter through the skin is always the major challenge with this technique, since routine motion of the neck will frequently cause standard catheters to work their way out. Tunneling the catheter under the skin and allowing it to emerge several centimeters away from the initial point of entry can prolong catheter longevity. Delivery of dilute solutions of local anesthetic by a fixed rate elastomeric bulb infusion device (Figure 15-1) or

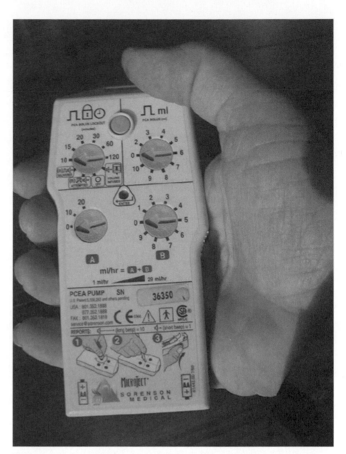

Figure 15-2 Battery-powered portable infusion pump for continuous peripheral nerve infusions. The pump can be programmed to deliver a constant infusion plus incremental supplemental boluses.

a battery-powered variable infusion pump with a "patient-control" option (Figure 15-2) provides an indefinite period of prolonged analgesia with minimal motor blockade.

The most frequent side effect of interscalene block is the paralysis of the ipsilateral diaphragm, which occurs 100% of the time. This is usually not a problem in the young, healthy patient, but should be a consideration in anyone with respiratory impairment. Improperly performed interscalene blocks can also result in epidural or spinal anesthesia, or even spinal cord injury. Injection into the vertebral artery or large veins in the neck is also possible and requires frequent aspiration and injections of small increments of local anesthetic. Nevertheless, these techniques are relatively safe and effective for most procedures around the shoulder.

Arm

Anesthesia in the arm also can be provided by brachial plexus blockade. The pattern of distribution varies with the level of blockade. The interscalene technique

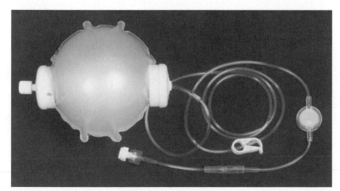

Figure 15-1 Elastomeric infusion pump for continuous peripheral nerve blocks or wound infusions. Local anesthetic is injected into the elastic bulb and delivered through a filter and fixed resistance to provide a constant hourly output.

described above provides excellent anesthesia of the shoulder, upper arm, and particularly the radial side of the arm, but frequently misses the nerve roots providing sensory anesthesia to the ulnar side of the arm. In this situation, more distal blockade at the supraclavicular or infraclavicular level will provide more reliable anesthesia of the three trunks (and thus all the terminal nerves) of the brachial plexus. The infraclavicular technique is particularly well suited to the insertion of indwelling catheters, since fixation of the catheter to the skin surface above the pectoralis muscle is usually associated with less movement and dislodgement in the postoperative period. Pneumothorax is the main risk associated with performance of the block at this level, and may be less with the infraclavicular approach.

More distal blockade of the plexus can be performed in the axilla. The drawback of axillary blockade is that several of the nerves have already departed the neurovascular bundle at this point and require separate injections. Specifically, the musculocutaneous nerve needs to be anesthetized by a separate injection into the coracobrachialis muscle, and the brachial cutaneous and antebrachial cutaneous nerves need to be anesthetized by subcutaneous injection in the axilla. With these supplemental injections axillary blockade will provide anesthesia sufficient even for the elbow. Simple injection of the three main nerves surrounding the artery (radial, median, and ulnar) will provide excellent anesthesia for surgery of the hand itself but will not provide reliable surface anesthesia for the forearm.

Hand Surgery

As mentioned, simple axillary blockade will anesthetize all three of the major nerves to the hand. These branches can also be blocked at the level of the wrist where the three nerves are relatively superficial and easily identified by bony or tendon landmarks. Carpal tunnel surgery, one of the most frequently performed procedures, can be done with simple local anesthesia over the wrist itself, as long as some supplemental analgesia is given to reduce the discomfort of the injections. Surgery on the fingers can be performed by blockade of the digital nerves. All these peripheral nerve blocks require some "soak time" for the local anesthetic to reach peak effectiveness and thus may necessitate some delay before starting surgery after placing the block.

SPINE SURGERY

Realignment of the thoracic or lumbar spine to correct congenital abnormalities or compression fractures caused by trauma or malignancy are some of the most challenging orthopedic procedures. The approach is difficult and blood loss is often extensive. The necessity of avoiding neurologic injury is paramount and requires careful attention to technique. The majority of these procedures are performed under general anesthesia, although epidural catheters can be inserted to provide postoperative pain relief following some of these very extensive procedures (Table 15-3). Because of the blood loss associated with many of these operations, hypotensive anesthetic techniques are frequently employed. These require a delicate balance between reducing the blood loss and providing adequate cerebral and neural circulation during these often-prolonged operations.

In the face of extensive distortion and realignment of the spinal cord, neurologic evaluation intraoperatively is often dictated. This presents a particular challenge to the anesthesiologist. It is usually accomplished by the performance of either sophisticated neurological monitoring or a "wake up test," or a combination of the two. Neurological monitoring can be performed by the use of somatosensory evoked potential monitoring. This requires placement of electrodes in the lower extremities with monitoring of the transmitting signal at the brain-stem level. Disruption of the signals is usually indicative of loss of function in the dorsal horn entry zones of the spinal column and requires readjustment of the orthopedic manipulation or of the perfusion. The ventral part of the spinal cord mediates motor function and is more difficult to monitor, frequently necessitating the use of the "wake up" test to evaluate motor function from the ventral horns. This requires the

Table 15-3	Regional Anesthesia Techniques for Orthopedic Surgery
Spine surgery	Epidural for postop analgesia
Shoulder	Interscalene
Arm	Infraclavicular
Hand	Axillary
Femur	Spinal
	Epidural
	Femoral nerve block
	Psoas compartment block
Knee	Spinal
	Epidural
	Combined sciatic and femoral
Ankle	Spinal
	Epidural
	Combined sciatic and femoral
	Popliteal fossa block
Foot	Spinal
	Epidural
	Popliteal fossa block
	Combined sciatic and femoral
	Ankle block

anesthesiologist to lighten the anesthesia and reverse the muscle relaxation to the point where the patient can respond to verbal commands to move the extremities to document persistent function of these neural tracks.

Extensive blood loss requires innovative approaches. As mentioned, hypotensive anesthesia is the simplest to employ. Active hemodilution by removing some of the patient's own blood at the beginning of the procedure is another way of reducing the total red cell loss. Because of all these factors, spine surgery represents one of the more challenging areas of orthopedic surgery for the anesthesiologist.

LOWER EXTREMITY SURGERY

The anesthetic choice for lower extremity orthopedic surgery includes general anesthesia and regional anesthetic techniques, which encompass spinal and epidural anesthesia as well as peripheral nerve blocks. Each anesthetic technique has its relative benefits and risks and overall major morbidity and mortality is low with either technique. Therefore, patient as well as surgical factors need to be considered in the anesthetic selection to maximize the advantages while minimizing the disadvantages.

Hip Surgery

Surgical procedures on the hip are many and include elective total hip arthroplasty for degenerative joint disease or rheumatoid arthritis, and acute procedures such as hip pinning or internal fixation for hip fractures in often elderly patients with coexisting diseases. Anesthetic choice often depends on the nature of the procedure (elective versus emergency), patient factors, and the presence of coexisting diseases or anticoagulation status, as well as surgical factors such as need for positioning. Regional anesthetic techniques convey advantages for patients undergoing hip surgery. Regional anesthesia allows for prompt postoperative recovery, enhanced postoperative analgesia, decreased incidence of postoperative nausea and vomiting, decreased frequency of venous thrombosis and pulmonary embolism, the potential for decreased hospitalization and inpatient costs, and increased alertness. Appropriate choices of anesthesia in patients undergoing hip surgery include general, spinal, epidural, and combined lumbar and sacral plexus block.

Central Neuraxial Blocks

Anesthesia for hip surgery can be performed effectively with central neuraxial blockade (i.e. spinal anesthesia or epidural anesthesia). Spinal anesthesia can be performed as a single shot or continuously through a catheter inserted in the subarachnoid space to effectively block the lumbar and sacral plexus. Spinal anesthesia offers the advantage of being technically easy to perform with a rapid onset of anesthesia and analgesia. Systemic toxicity is minimized as less local anesthetic is used with this approach.

Patients can often be positioned for the surgery with the hip to be operated on nondependent and a hypobaric solution such as 0.1% tetracaine injected into the subarachnoid space. Standard premixed hyperbaric solutions, such as 0.75% bupivacaine in dextrose, are frequently used. Hyperbaric solutions often spread to the midthoracic levels, leading to potential side effects such as hypotension and bradycardia, impaired ventilatory mechanics, and hypothermia. A more localized distribution (almost a unilateral spinal) can be attained by leaving the patient with the operative side dependent for 15-20 minutes, but this is time-consuming.

The use of isobaric solutions (0.5% bupivacaine) will usually not produce as high a block level as hyperbaric solutions, but this technique is less predictable. In an effort to control block height and to avoid the sudden onset of sympathetic block, which may be particularly dangerous in patients with aortic stenosis or volume depletion, continuous spinal anesthesia might be an alternative to single injection spinals. Alternatively, lower doses of bupivacaine potentiated by small doses of fentanyl have been shown to be effective.

Lumbar epidural anesthesia is also an attractive choice, particularly if the length of the surgical procedure is unknown or if bilateral total hip arthroplasty is planned. Epidural anesthesia also affords the anesthesiologist the ability to provide for postoperative analgesia. In elderly patients undergoing surgical treatment of traumatic hip fracture, postoperative epidural infusion with bupivacaine and fentanyl produces lower visual analog scale scores and a reduction in the incidence of perioperative myocardial ischemia.

Peripheral Nerve Blocks

Peripheral nerve blocks may play an important role as the primary anesthetic for patients undergoing hip surgery or reduction of hip fractures. Hip surgery requires anesthesia of the lumbar plexus, which is formed in the psoas muscle from the anterior rami of the L1-L4 spinal nerves, and can be accomplished by a psoas compartment block. Complete anesthesia requires anesthesia of the sacral plexus as well, which is formed from the anterior rami of the L4-L5 lumbar nerves and the S1-S3 sacral nerves. Both femoral nerve block alone and psoas compartment block have been shown to reduce acute pain due to hip fractures, and can be useful prior to surgery in allowing positioning of the patient or facilitating performance of spinal, epidural, or general anesthesia.

Complete lumbosacral blockade can be used for the surgery itself. These blocks are more complex to administer but have the advantage of avoiding the hypotension seen with neuraxial blockade, which is often aggravated by the pre-existing blood loss associated with hip fracture in the elderly. When compared to general anesthesia alone, general anesthesia combined with a single injection lumbar plexus block provides effective analgesia for total hip arthroplasty while reducing intra- and postoperative opioid requirements as well as decreasing blood loss.

Additionally, peripheral nerve blocks may confer advantages by providing continued analgesia well into the postoperative period, facilitating rehabilitation and possibly allowing for quicker discharge times. Continuous psoas compartment block for postoperative analgesia after total hip arthroplasty provides optimal analgesia with fewer side effects compared to epidural or systemic opioid analgesia.

General Anesthesia and Regional Anesthesia Outcomes

Total hip arthroplasty can be associated with significant blood loss, deep vein thrombosis with pulmonary embolism, alterations in the cardiopulmonary status, and alterations in mental status. Furthermore, percutaneous pinning or open reduction internal fixation of hip fractures is often performed in elderly patients with coexisting cardiopulmonary disease. Meta-analysis of randomized control trials comparing regional anesthesia and general anesthesia for traumatic hip surgery reveals that the risk of deep vein thrombosis is lower for regional anesthesia; although there is no consistent effect on mortality at 1 month. For this operation, there is no superiority of regional anesthesia for lowering intraoperative blood loss.

A more recent meta-analysis of randomized trials of general versus regional anesthesia for hip fracture surgery showed a significant advantage for regional anesthesia over general anesthesia in terms of the incidence of deep vein thrombosis and fatal pulmonary embolism, and survival at 1 month, whereas general anesthesia conferred no significant advantages.

Knee Surgery

The three most common surgical procedures involving the knee are knee arthroscopy, repair of the anterior cruciate ligament, and total knee arthroplasty. While general anesthesia is an option for all these procedures, regional anesthesia is an ideal choice for surgery on the knee. Spinal anesthesia, epidural anesthesia, and peripheral nerve blocks (i.e. femoral and sciatic nerve blocks) are options as they provide excellent anesthesia as well as having the potential to provide for excellent postoperative analgesia.

Outpatient Knee Arthroscopy

Knee arthroscopy can be performed with local, general, spinal, or epidural anesthesia. Local infiltration of the portal sites usually needs to be combined with some intravenous sedation and is adequate for 80–90% of patients. It does not provide substantial motor relaxation, and thus may not be satisfactory for some surgeons who need to manipulate the knee to visualize the various compartments. General anesthesia can provide adequate analgesia and relaxation, but obviously removes the patient's ability to view the findings on the monitor and does require a longer recovery period and the provision of some analgesia, such as filling the joint with bupivacaine and infiltrating the portals.

A combination of sciatic and femoral nerve blocks has also been used, but this requires a longer onset time than general anesthesia and may leave the patient with a numb extremity at the time of discharge (or a prolonged recovery until the numbness is gone).

Neuraxial blockade is another alternative. Spinal anesthesia is simple and rapid in onset, but has been regarded with suspicion because of the syndrome of transient neurologic signs (TNS) after lidocaine spinal anesthesia in 15–30% of patients in this setting. Bupivacaine causes this syndrome rarely but is associated with longer discharge times, even in 5 mg doses. Most recently, low dose lidocaine (20–25 mg combined with fentanyl) has shown some promise in providing rapid discharge and a low incidence of TNS, but further study is needed. Epidural anesthesia with 2-chloroprocaine has been used effectively for this procedure and is associated with discharge times equivalent to general anesthesia with propofol.

Although each of these methods works well in various settings, the use of the regional techniques has been shown to improve efficiency (recovery and discharge times) in the outpatient setting.

Outpatient Anterior Cruciate Ligament Reconstruction

Arthroscopically assisted reconstruction of the anterior cruciate ligament is a common orthopedic surgical procedure. Until recently, the majority of these procedures were performed on an inpatient basis. Because of improvements in postoperative analgesia, particularly the use of regional anesthetic techniques, anterior cruciate ligament reconstruction is now most often performed as an outpatient procedure. This is more palatable to most patients and is also cost-efficient for the institutions, with cost savings of approximately $2,900 per case.

Once again, the choices for anesthesia include general anesthesia and regional anesthesia, including spinal or epidural anesthesia or the use of peripheral nerve blocks (i.e. femoral and sciatic nerve blocks). Again, all work well, and provide equivalent discharge times. The major problem with this procedure is not the surgical anesthesia but the postoperative analgesia necessary to make a patient sufficiently comfortable to go home, especially after patellar tendon autograft repair.

Most institutions employ a multimodal approach, which includes local infiltration of the portals, injection of bupivacaine in the joint, use of cryotherapy (continuous cold water or ice application to the joint), and systemic nonsteroidal anti-inflammatory drugs plus oral opioids. A femoral nerve block is also very effective in reducing pain in the first 24 hours – 25 mL of 0.25% bupivacaine will provide 22–24 hours of analgesia in most patients. The only substantial side effect is the possibility of instability due to quadriceps weakness. This analgesia can be prolonged by the use of continuous infusions through a femoral or psoas compartment catheter.

Total Knee Arthroplasty

This is one of the most painful orthopedic procedures performed on a frequent basis, and is becoming increasingly frequent as the epidemic of obesity expands in the United States. Regional anesthetic techniques have been shown to be superior to general anesthesia for patients undergoing total knee arthroplasty in terms of providing analgesia in the postoperative period. Effective pain control has been shown to improve early rehabilitation. Additionally, a statistically significant decrease, compared with general anesthesia, has been shown in the incidence of deep vein thrombosis with regional anesthesia.

While anesthesia for total knee arthroplasty can be provided with general, spinal, or epidural anesthesia, or with peripheral nerve blocks, such as femoral and/or sciatic nerve blocks, postoperative analgesia is optimized and rehabilitation is facilitated by the performance of regional anesthetic techniques rather than with intravenous patient-controlled analgesia. Single-injection femoral nerve techniques can significantly reduce morphine requirements in the first 12 hours and provide analgesia for as long as 18 hours. Continuous techniques can prolong this relief indefinitely. They have been shown to provide better analgesia than intravenous patient-controlled analgesia, and fewer side effects than epidural infusions. In the European experience, they also have been shown to shorten rehabilitation time and expedite hospital discharge, although further study is needed to see if these findings will apply to the American model of rapid rehabilitation and discharge with multimodal therapy.

Ankle and Foot Surgery

The peripheral nature of the ankle and foot makes regional anesthesia an attractive choice for surgical procedures involving these sites. Regional anesthesia is effective, safe, and can provide effective postoperative analgesia while minimizing the complications associated with general or central neuraxial blockade. The ankle and foot are innervated by five nerves: the saphenous nerve, which is a branch of the femoral nerve, in addition to the deep peroneal, posterior tibial, superficial peroneal, and sural nerves, which are branches of the sciatic nerve. The major trunks of the sciatic and femoral nerves can be blocked or their terminal branches can be blocked. This can be accomplished with peripheral nerve blocks or with spinal anesthesia. Epidural anesthesia may not produce adequate anesthesia for ankle or foot surgery because of sacral sparing.

Commonly performed procedures on the ankle and foot include open reduction internal fixation of ankle fractures, Achilles tendon repair, and transmetatarsal amputations. Transmetatarsal blocks provide reliable anesthesia for distal operations involving the toes. However, procedures on more proximal parts of the ankle and foot or procedures involving the use of a proximal calf tourniquet require blockade of the major nerve trunks and are amenable to popliteal fossa and saphenous nerve blocks.

Popliteal Fossa Block

The posterior approach is the classic approach to performing a popliteal fossa block and, if combined with a saphenous nerve block, provides anesthesia of all the areas below the knee. This block can also be performed in the supine position using a lateral approach. Success seems to be enhanced by obtaining two motor responses (one from each branch of the sciatic) with a nerve stimulator. Both these approaches provide excellent anesthesia of the ankle and foot, and also allow insertion of a continuous catheter for postoperative analgesic infusions. Use of such infusions with a portable pump has allowed patients to be discharged home with no pain or very little pain 72 hours after surgery, with dramatic reductions in opioid use and in sleep disturbance.

Ankle Block

An ankle block is an attractive choice for surgical procedures involving the metatarsal bones and phalanges or the bones of the midfoot (navicular, cuboid, and cuneiform bones). It is simple and provides predictable anesthesia for mid- and forefoot surgery. The five nerves supplying the foot are the superficial peroneal, deep peroneal, posterior tibial, saphenous, and sural nerves. These nerves can be blocked by five separate injections depending on the location of the surgical procedure. Ankle blocks alleviate the risks of general or spinal anesthesia and can provide optimal postoperative analgesia if a long-acting local anesthetic is used.

Case Study

A 62-year-old woman is scheduled for a right knee replacement. She is moderately obese, at a weight of 122 kg, height 5'5". Past medical history includes mild hypertension and occasional exertional angina, treated with metoprolol and nitroglycerin prn. She denies sleep apnea but has esophageal reflux that awakens her from sleep once a week.

- What anesthetic technique would you recommend for surgery?
- Would the use of perioperative coumadin or low-molecular-weight heparin affect your decision?
- You are concerned about postoperative analgesia – what alternatives would you discuss with the patient?
  - Intravenous patient-controlled analgesia with opioids?
  - Epidural infusion?
  - Femoral nerve catheter?
  - Psoas compartment catheter?

SUGGESTED READING

Ben-David B, DeMeo PJ, Lucyk C, Solosko D. A comparison of minidose lidocaine–fentanyl spinal anesthesia and local anesthesia/propofol infusion for outpatient knee arthroscopy. *Anesth Analg* 2001;93:319–325.

Brown AR, Weiss R, Greenberg C, *et al*. Interscalene block for shoulder arthroscopy: comparison with general anesthesia. *Arthroscopy* 1993:9:295–300.

Capdevila X, Barthelet Y, Biboulet P, *et al*. Effects of perioperative analgesic technique on the surgical outcome and duration of rehabilitation after major knee surgery. *Anesthesiology* 1999;91:8–15.

Hadzic A, Vloka JD. A comparison of the posterior versus lateral approaches to the block of the sciatic nerve in the popliteal fossa. *Anesthesiology* 1998:88:1480–1486.

Ilfeld BM, Moery T, Enneking F. Continuous infraclavicular brachial plexus block for postoperative pain control at home. *Anesthesiology* 2002:96:1297–1304.

Klein SM, Grant SA, Greengrass RA, *et al*. Interscalene brachial plexus block with a continuous catheter insertion system and a disposable infusion pump. *Anesth Analg* 2000:91:1473–1478.

Mulroy MF, Larkin KL, Hodgson PS, *et al*. A comparison of spinal, epidural, and general anesthesia for outpatient knee arthroscopy. *Anesth Analg* 2000:91:860–864.

Mulroy MF, Larkin KL, Batra MS, *et al*. Femoral nerve block with 0.25% or 0.5% bupivacaine improves postoperative analgesia following outpatient arthroscopic anterior cruciate ligament repair. *Reg Anesth Pain Med* 2001:26:24–29.

Rawal N, Alvin R, Axelsson K, *et al*. Patient-controlled regional analgesia (PCRA) at home. *Anesthesiology* 2002:96:1290–1296.

Singelyn FJ, Deyaert M, Joris D, *et al*. Effects of intravenous patient-controlled analgesia with morphine, continuous epidural analgesia, and continuous three-in-one block on postoperative pain and knee rehabilitation after unilateral total knee arthroplasty. *Anesth Analg* 1998;87:88–92.

Urwin SC, Parker MJ, Griffiths R. General versus regional anaesthesia for hip fracture surgery: a meta-analysis of randomized trials. *Br J Anaesth* 2000;84:450–355.

Valanne JV, Korhonen AM, Jokela RM, *et al*. Selective spinal anesthesia: a comparison of hyperbaric bupivacaine 4 mg versus 6 mg for outpatient knee arthroscopy. *Anesth Analg* 2001;93:1377–1379.

Wedel DJ, ed. *Orthopedic anesthesia*. New York: Churchill Livingstone, 1993.

CHAPTER 16

Anesthesia for the Trauma and Burn Patient

DAVID M. ROSENFELD

MELISSA R. ROSENFELD

EPIDEMIOLOGY OF TRAUMA

Introduction

Traumatic injury is the fourth leading cause of death in the United States, trailing only heart disease, cancer, and cerebrovascular disease. It is also the leading cause of death under the age of 40. The National Safety Council identified 92,200 deaths in 1998, which represents a fatal injury every 6 minutes. A disabling injury occurs every 2 seconds in the United States. Motor vehicle accidents are the leading cause of accidental death, totaling 38% of fatalities, followed by falls, gunshot wounds, and pedestrian accidents. The distribution of fatalities is bimodal, with a disturbing peak at age 20 due primarily to men who die from motor vehicle accidents or gunshot wounds. The second peak occurs at age 80, when falls, and motor vehicle accidents in elderly populations, become more common (Figures 16-1 and 16-2).

Trauma Centers

Total deaths from trauma related injuries are generally on the decline. The highest recorded total was 116,385 in 1969, and the lowest was 86,777 in 1992. Much of this decline is attributed to improved vehicle, occupational, and home safety; and the organization of trauma centers with improved techniques in trauma care. The organization of level 1 centers across the United States is determined predominantly by acuity, patient volume, and available personnel. Many trauma centers in the US are

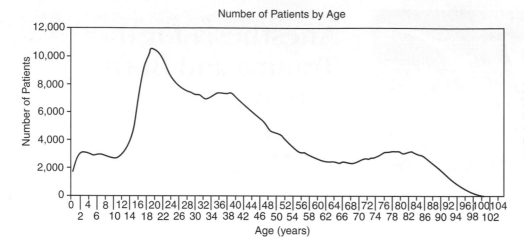

Figure 16-1   National Trauma Data Bank 2002 – number of trauma patients at each age. n = 430, 557. (Redrawn from American College of Surgeons. *National Trauma Data Bank Report 2002*.)

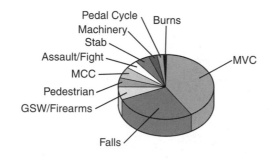

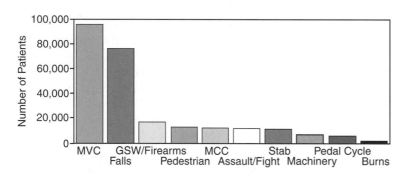

Figure 16-2   National Trauma Data Bank 2002 – proportional distribution of patients, grouped by mechanism of injury. n = 250,995. GSW, gunshot wounds; MCC, motor cycle crashes; MVC, motor vehicle crashes. (Redrawn from American College of Surgeons. *National Trauma Data Bank Report 2002*.)

facing financial crisis, and consolidation of level 1 care to fewer centers is commonplace in large urban areas. The anesthesiologist performs an instrumental role in delivery of trauma care from initial evaluation, to the operating room, and subsequent management in the intensive care unit.

Initial Evaluation

Initial evaluation of the trauma patient may take place in the field, the emergency room, or, rarely, in the operating suite. Care was standardized by the advent of Advanced Trauma Life Support (ATLS), developed by the American College of Surgeons, whose first protocol appeared in 1980. Ideally, trauma evaluation includes highly coordinated evaluation by an emergency physician and/or

surgeon, an anesthesiologist, specialized nursing, and a radiographer with portable capability. Neurosurgical and orthopedic personnel should be within a reasonable response time. The primary goal of the anesthesiologist is to preserve central nervous system function, maintain adequate respiratory gas exchange, and achieve circulatory homeostasis.

According to ATLS protocol, initial evaluation should include three components: rapid overview, primary survey, and secondary survey (Figure 16-3).

- *Rapid Overview*: This phase should take seconds and should determine if the patient is stable, unstable, dead, or dying imminently.
- *Primary Survey*: More detailed evaluation of physiologic function crucial to survival. This is where airway,

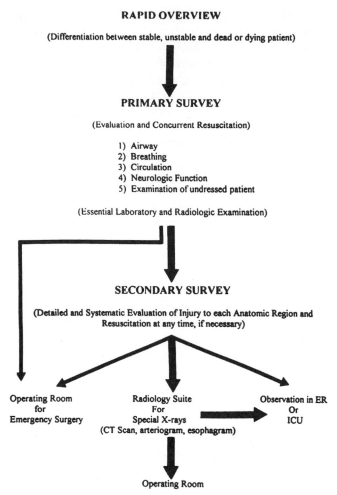

RAPID OVERVIEW

(Differentiation between stable, unstable and dead or dying patient)

⬇

PRIMARY SURVEY

(Evaluation and Concurrent Resuscitation)

1) Airway
2) Breathing
3) Circulation
4) Neurologic Function
5) Examination of undressed patient

(Essential Laboratory and Radiologic Examination)

⬇

SECONDARY SURVEY

(Detailed and Systematic Evaluation of Injury to each Anatomic Region and Resuscitation at any time, if necessary)

| Operating Room for Emergency Surgery | Radiology Suite For Special X-rays (CT Scan, arteriogram, esophagram) | Observation in ER Or ICU |

Operating Room

Figure 16-3   Clinical sequence followed during initial management of the major trauma patient. (From Capan LM, Miller SM. Trauma and burns. In: Barash PG, Cullen BF, Stoelting RK. *Clinical anesthesia*, 3rd ed. Philadelphia: Lippincott-Raven, 1997:1173–1204.)

Table 16-1 Glasgow Coma Scale	
Eye Opening	
Spontaneous	4
To Voice	3
To Pain	2
None	1
Verbal Responses	
Oriented	5
Confused	4
Inappropriate	3
Incomprehensible	2
None	1
Motor Response	
Obeys Commands	6
Localizes Pain	5
Withdraws (pain)	4
Flexion (pain)	3
Extension (pain)	2
None	1

mate 35% mortality. Other scales include the Trauma Index, the Injury Severity Score (ISS), and the CRAMS Scale.

AIRWAY MANAGEMENT

The anesthesiologist plays an integral role in early management of trauma patients to secure the airway and act as a consultant for other emergency personnel. Evaluation requires diagnosis of soft tissue trauma, assessment of potential or active obstruction, and prediction of possible exacerbation of injury by airway intervention.

Hypoxia

Hypoxia in a trauma setting is frequently the result of airway obstruction, apnea, thoracic injuries, and low circulatory flow states. The presence of cyanosis can be difficult to detect in those who are anemic, hypovolemic, or of dark pigmentation. Combativeness in the trauma suite is often the result of hypoxemia. Pulse oximetry is mandatory to assess oxygenation, and arterial blood gas analysis should be utilized early if there is any uncertainty. Supplemental oxygen should be administered, and definitive airway intervention undertaken if there is any concern of inadequate tissue oxygenation.

Airway obstruction is often due to laceration, bleeding, secretions, foreign body, fracture, or tissue laxity in an unconsciousness patient. Initial interventions include supplemental oxygen, a chin lift with jaw thrust, clearing of the oropharynx, and an oral or nasal airway. Ventilation should be supported if necessary using a self-inflating bag, cricoid pressure, and cervical spine immobilization.

breathing, and circulation are critical. If there is compromise of any of these vital functions, corrective measures should commence immediately. Assessment of disability through a focused neurological examination occurs at this time.

• *Secondary Survey*: Detailed and systematic evaluation of each anatomic region. Disposition determined. Information from the patient or others regarding underlying health conditions.

Many trauma scoring systems are in use throughout the world. The Glasgow Coma Scale (GCS), introduced by Teasdale and Jennett in 1974 (Table 16-1), assesses level of consciousness and is the most commonly used neurological scoring system. The strength of the GCS lies in its consistency between different observers and its ability to assess neurological status and clinical outcome. A score of 13 or higher represents a mild brain injury with good prognosis, a score of 9–12 correlates to moderate injury, and below 8 indicates severe injury, which carries an approxi-

Definitive Airway Management

Definitive control of the airway is vital to protect the patient from pulmonary aspiration and airway obstruction, and to maintain alveolar gas exchange during resuscitation. The absolute immediate indications for intubation include a GCS of less than 9, profound shock, airway obstruction, a combative patient requiring sedation, chest trauma with hypoventilation, hypoxia, and cardiac arrest. When the decision to intubate is made, the role of oral or nasal airways is limited to maintaining airway patency temporarily until an endotracheal tube can be placed. A cervical spine fracture must be assumed in a trauma patient even if there is limited evidence of injury above the clavicles. A cross-table lateral radiograph of C1–C7, with an odontoid view, and 'swimmers view', can identify up to 91% of cervical fractures. Standard cervical radiographs cannot completely rule out ligamentous injury, and flexion and extension views under fluoroscopy may be necessary to clear the cervical spine if the examination is unreliable. Computed tomography (CT) has improved sensitivity versus plain radiography and may further define anatomy. Cervical collars are necessary but do not provide complete immobilization and may cause skin breakdown with prolonged use.

Aspiration Risk

A full stomach is assumed in any trauma patient, and the urgency of securing the airway often precludes pharmacologic treatment of gastric pH. If time permits, the use of nonparticulate antacid may buffer gastric pH, and metoclopramide expedites gastric emptying. H₂-blockers will reduce gastric acidity, although may take up to 45 minutes to be effective. Emphasis should be placed on safe and rapid procurement of a definitive airway, versus pharmacologic aspiration reduction. Denitrogenation of the lungs with administration of 100% oxygen should be accomplished. Properly applied cricoid pressure (Sellick maneuver), with in-line stabilization of the cervical spine, decreases the risk of pulmonary aspiration (Figures 16-4 and 16-5). The laryngeal mask airway may be used as a bridge during difficult intubation prior to fiberoptic attempt or tracheotomy. Cricoid pressure should be maintained to reduce aspiration risk. A fiberoptic scope may be passed through a laryngeal mask airway, which helps to identify the vocal cords and maintains mask ventilation. Rapid sequence intubation with a hypnotic agent and muscle relaxant is the preferred technique in a stable patient without significant oral, maxillofacial, or cervical spine injury.

Pharmacology

The choice of hypnotic agent for intubation is dependent on the patient's hemodynamic status. Propofol or thiopental is acceptable in euvolemic patients where myocardial depression and vasodilation are usually well tolerated. Etomidate and ketamine are preferred with moderate to severe hypovolemia. The use of a muscle relaxant is dependent on the clinical situation. Succinylcholine is an obvious choice because of its rapid onset of action but should be avoided in patients with burns or spinal cord injury more than 24 hours after the injury because of the potential for a massive hyperkalemic response. Rocuronium (1–1.5 mg/kg) provides intubating conditions in 60–90 seconds and can be administered if succinylcholine is contraindicated. For further discussion

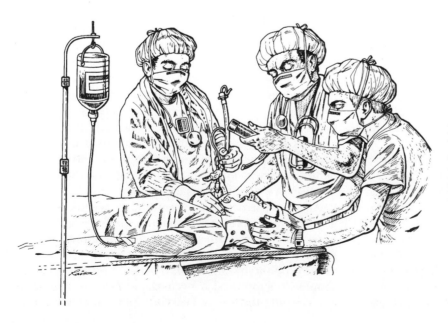

Figure 16-4   Emergency intubation technique using cricoid pressure, with in-line stabilization. (From Stene JK. Anesthesia for the critically ill trauma patient. In: Siegel JA. *Trauma emergency surgery and critical care*. New York: Churchill Livingstone, 1987:843–862.)

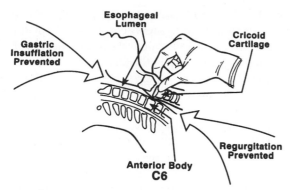

Figure 16-5   Cricoid pressure. (From Cicala RS, Grande CM, Steve JK *et al*. Emergency and elective airway management for trauma patients. In: Grande CM, ed. *Trauma anesthesia and critical care*. St Louis: Mosby, 1993.)

of these agents please refer to the section on induction of anesthesia

DIFFICULT AIRWAY

Trauma patients may present with difficulty establishing a definitive airway independent of the mechanism of injury. As for any patient, evaluation of the airway should focus on the Mallampati score, mouth opening, thyromental distance, neck anatomy, and dental condition. Awake laryngoscopy, or fiberoptic intubation with spontaneous respiration, should be undertaken with topicalization if a difficult airway is suspected. These techniques must be balanced against the risk of increasing intracranial or intraocular pressure in patients who may buck or cough. Surgical tracheostomy is always a viable option in a difficult airway with multiple severe injuries, or if primary airway trauma exists.

DIRECT AIRWAY INJURY

Primary airway injury may be the result of blunt or penetrating trauma and can be seen from the nasopharynx down to the bronchi. Clinicians should assess for multiple foci of injury since persistent dysfunction may be seen after identification and correction of the initial issue.

Pharyngeal Injury

Soft tissue edema, laceration, hemorrhage, hematoma, or debris in the oropharyngeal cavity should be ruled out in any blunt or penetrating trauma above the clavicles. Dental injury or a foreign body may lead to acute obstruction and complicate management. Progression of tissue edema or hematoma formation is a concern in the first 12 hours after soft tissue injury and prophylactic intubation should be performed if there is uncertainty. More exten-

sive damage, especially to the esophagus, should also be considered in the initial evaluation process.

Facial Fractures

Airway management in the presence of maxillofacial fracture depends on the presenting condition and the underlying injury. The majority of patients with an isolated facial fracture do not require emergency airway intervention, and surgery may often be delayed until edema subsides and comprehensive radiographic studies are obtained. The presence of an airway-compromising fracture or facial injury in a patient with other life threatening injury will require definitive airway management prior to precise diagnosis. The decision to proceed with rapid sequence induction, awake intubation, or tracheostomy depends on the suspected injury and impending airway compromise at presentation.

Mandibular fractures occur most often at the ramus. If there is bilateral involvement of the articulation of the condyle of the temporomandibular joint, mouth opening may be inhibited as a result of mechanical jaw locking. Zygomatic fracture may further affect the temporomandibular joint, especially after a blow to the side of the head, when fracture fragments may impinge on the joint, resulting in jaw locking. In these situations the jaw will not open in response to muscle relaxation. Recognition of this prior to intervention is key to avoid an emergency cricothyroidotomy. These mechanical problems should be separated from inability to open the mouth because of pain, which may be treated with titration of short-acting opioids, allowing improved evaluation and management decisions.

LeFort fractures

These represent the most severe of facial fractures. The *LeFort I fracture* is a horizontal fracture of the maxilla. Characteristics include fracture above the floor of the nose involving the lower third of the septum with mobilization of the palate, maxillary alveolar process, pterygoid process, and part of the palatine bones. Airway management is improved because the fracture mobilizes the upper jaw and allows more maneuvering of the laryngoscope blade. A *LeFort II fracture* is pyramidal, beginning at the upper margin of the anterior nasal aperture and involving the orbit, the lacrimal bone, and the zygomaticomaxillary suture. The *LeFort III fracture* involves the lateral orbit and extends to the temporal bone. These fractures rarely appear in the classic form and are often found in a variety of combinations.

In LeFort II and III fractures, airway management is complicated by disruption of the mid-face posteriorly, which encroaches on the pharynx, resulting in airway compromise. The presence of a *basilar skull fracture* is seen in LeFort II and III fractures and represents a contraindication

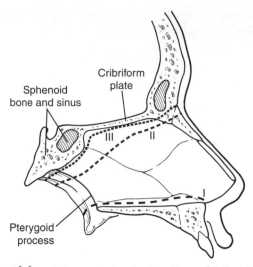

Figure 16-6   Anteroposterior fracture lines of LeFort I, LeFort II, LeFort III injuries. Note that in the LeFort III fracture the pterygoid process, the only facial buttress posteriorly, is injured from its base, allowing the entire midface to shift posteriorly. In this injury the cribriform plate may also be fractured. (Redrawn from Capan LM, Miller SM, Glickman R. Management of facial injuries. In: Capan LM, Miller SM, Turndorf H, eds. *Trauma anesthesia and intensive care*. Philadelphia: JB Lippincott, 1991:383.)

to nasotracheal intubation. Rhinorrhea is not an absolute indicator of a basilar skull fracture. Other signs that the anesthesiologist should be able to identify include periorbital or mastoid ecchymosis and hemotympanum (Figure 16-6).

Laryngeal Trauma

Laryngotracheal trauma is typically seen in motor vehicle accidents in which the head is extended and the larynx is exposed. Other mechanisms include 'clothes-line' injury in motorcycle accidents, strangulation, or contact sport trauma. Open laryngeal trauma may be associated with severe major vessel hemorrhage, hematoma, or edema. Findings in closed laryngeal injury may be subtle and include tenderness, subcutaneous emphysema, respiratory distress, stridor, dysphagia, hoarseness, and hemoptysis. Airway management depends on the stability of the patient and the degree of respiratory compromise. In a stable patient with minimal respiratory insufficiency, radiographs of the chest and cervical spine, and a CT examination of the neck are used to determine the extent of injury. Fiberoptic pharyngoscopy may be performed by an otolaryngologist to examine the anatomy and, if damage is minor, subsequent anesthesia may be performed with routine orotracheal intubation. If time permits, patients should be taken to the operating room, with an otolaryngologist present and scrubbed, prior to any attempt to secure the airway.

Controversy exists when the airway is unstable or if there is mucosal disruption, edema, hemorrhage, or a laryngeal skeletal fracture. Awake laryngoscopy with topicalization, or fiberoptic bronchoscopy using a small diameter tube, both in a spontaneously breathing patient, are nonsurgical options. The threshold for tracheostomy under local anesthesia is quite low with unstable laryngeal trauma and should be performed in any circumstance where the airway is uncertain. In difficult-to-sedate or combative patients, a low-solubility volatile anesthetic or careful intravenous titration of a hypnotic agent may be used while tracheotomy is performed. Certainly, aspiration of gastric contents is a concern; therefore the anesthetic should be titrated to the lowest level that allows patient cooperation while maintaining airway protective reflexes.

MANAGEMENT OF VENTILATION

When the airway has been secured attention should focus on ventilation and oxygenation. Nearly all critically injured patients require assisted or mechanical ventilation. A nonrebreathing self-inflating bag/mask device is used in spontaneously breathing patients and may be attached to an endotracheal tube in intubated patients. When injury severity is less acute and the airway is intact, oxygen delivery via nasal cannula or open mask is adequate as long as the patient is alert, with protective reflexes. When intubated, positive pressure ventilation should be instituted once tube position is verified by the presence of end-tidal CO_2, bilateral chest rise, and auscultation. Arterial blood gases can aid in determining the adequacy of ventilation and oxygenation.

Tension pneumothorax and flail chest are immediately life-threatening conditions that must be identified and addressed quickly. Tension pneumothorax occurs when air enters the pleural space through a one-way valve either in the lung or the chest wall. Air enters the thorax on inspiration but is unable to escape, resulting in collapse of the ipsilateral lung, tracheal deviation away from the affected side, distended neck veins, severe hypotension, tachycardia, and tachypnea. These signs may initially be subtle; therefore a chest radiograph is obtained if the diagnosis is in question. Positive pressure ventilation can convert an unrecognized open pneumothorax to a tension pneumothorax. If the patient is unstable or x-ray is not immediately available, and there is clinical suspicion, insertion of a 14-gauge needle in the midclavicular line between the second and third ribs is performed to decompress the chest. Placement of a chest tube remains the definitive intervention.

The presence of fractures in at least three consecutive ribs, with a sternal fracture or costochondral separation, is suggestive of a flail chest. Paradoxical chest wall movement with respiration is seen and, combined with radiographs, may confirm the diagnosis. Associated pulmonary contusion and hemothorax can worsen the respiratory insufficiency caused by the paradoxical chest motion (Figure 16-7).

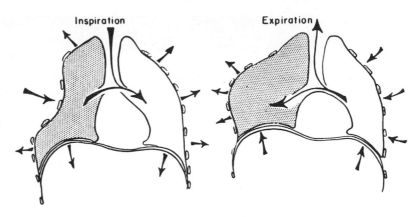

Figure 16-7 Paradoxic motion (inspiration and expiration) of the chest wall in flail chest injuries results in inefficient ventilation. (From Wilkins EW. Noncardiovascular thoracic injuries: chest wall, bronchus, lung, esophagus, and diaphragm. In: Burke JF, Boyd RJ, McCabe CJ, eds. *Trauma management: early management of visceral, nervous system, and musculoskeletal injuries.* St Louis: Mosby/Year Book, 1988.)

Box 16-1   Criteria for Intubation

P_aO_2 < 70 mm Hg with oxygen supplementation
P_aCO_2 > 50 mmHg
pH < 7.25
Tachypnea > 30/min
Vital capacity < 15 mL/kg
Negative inspiratory force < −20 cmH$_2$O

Careful and frequent reassessment of these patients is required to rule out significant ventilatory insufficiency, but a flail chest is not *per se* an indication for mechanical ventilation. Inappropriate use of mechanical ventilation may actually increase the risk of pulmonary complications, and morbidity, in these patients. Adequate analgesia may postpone or negate the need for mechanical ventilation by decreasing splinting and respiratory effort. Thoracic epidural analgesia is an excellent option to improve ventilation while reducing the respiratory depression of parenteral opioids. A coagulation profile should be measured prior to epidural placement. Clinical observation, sequential arterial blood gas analysis, and assessment of vital capacity and inspiratory force determine the need for endotracheal intubation (Box 16-1).

MANAGEMENT OF CIRCULATION AND SHOCK

Hypotension in the trauma patient is most often the result of hemorrhage and hypovolemia. Other etiologies include pericardial tamponade, cardiac contusion, pre-existing coronary disease, tension pneumothorax, and spinal cord injury.

Hemodynamic variables are the key to initial evaluation of volume status. Examination of heart rate, blood pressure, pulse pressure, urine output, respiratory rate, and mental status in the absence of head injury are the simplest and most reliable parameters used to determine circulatory status. Systemic response to hemorrhage include increased plasma renin production, antidiuretic hormone secretion, and catecholamine activity, which results in tachycardia and arteriolar vasoconstriction. These mechanisms serve to maintain blood pressure until there is a 30–40% reduction in blood volume. Therefore, a patient may be severely hypovolemic yet have normal blood pressure. Once approximately 40% blood loss is exceeded compensatory mechanisms may fail and hypovolemic shock ensues. Persistent poor perfusion results in organ ischemia, loss of membrane integrity, and progressive intracellular hypoxia. Developed by the American College of Surgeons, Table 16-2 is a helpful guideline to estimate blood loss using selected physiologic variables.

Intravenous Access

Immediate establishment of large-bore intravenous cannulae is mandatory. At least two 14- or 16-gauge intravenous lines should be placed ideally above and below the diaphragm in severe injuries to provide volume in the event of superior or inferior vena caval injury. Placement of invasive monitors has a limited role during initial resuscitation and should not delay supportive treatment. Internal jugular, subclavian, or femoral vein catheters provide excellent access, especially in situations of massive blood loss where peripheral cannulation is difficult. *Central venous pressure* monitoring in the operating room is also an advantage to help estimate overall volume status. Invasive *arterial monitoring* should be placed as soon as possible in situations of ongoing blood loss, or hemodynamic instability. *Pulmonary artery catheters* are rarely indicated in immediate resuscitation of the trauma patient. Subsequent placement of this monitor is useful in myocardial injury, sepsis, or severe hemodynamic instability, where measurement of cardiac filling pressures, cardiac output, and mixed venous oxygen saturation may alter management.

Table 16-2   Advanced Trauma Life Support Classification of Hemorrhagic Shock*

	Class I	Class II	Class III	Class IV
Blood loss (mL)	≤750	750–1500	1500–2000	≥2000
Blood loss (% blood volume)	≤15	15–30	30–40	≥40
Pulse rate (per min)	<100	>100	>120	≥140
Blood pressure	Normal	Normal	Decreased	Decreased
Pulse pressure	Normal or increased	Decreased	Decreased	Decreased
Capillary refill test	Normal	Positive	Positive	Positive
Respiratory rate (breaths/min)	14–20	20–30	30–40	<35
Urine output (mL/hr)	≥30	20–30	5–15	Negligible
CNS mental status	Slightly anxious	Mildly anxious	Anxious and confused	Confused, lethargic
Fluid replacement (3:1 rule)	Crystalloid	Crystalloid	Crystalloid + blood	Crystalloid + blood

* For a 70 kg male patient; based on initial presentation.
CNS, central nervous system.
Adapted from American College of Surgeons Committee on Trauma. Shock. *Advanced trauma and life support course for physicians.* Chicago: American College of Surgeons, 1993.

Selection of Fluid

Controversy remains regarding whether administration of crystalloid or colloid in the early phases of resuscitation is preferable; clearly there is no consensus. Many clinicians believe that colloid has no obvious advantage in the acute setting, with little justification for the added expense. Initial fluid resuscitation should begin with a balanced salt solution such as Ringer's lactate, while the patient's blood is being typed and crossmatched. Normal saline in very large volumes is associated with excessive chloride load and may exacerbate intracellular acidosis. There are encouraging studies using hypertonic salt solutions alone or in combination with colloid, although their use is not widespread at present.

Generally, the infusion of 2,000 mL of Ringer's lactate over 15 minutes should restore normal vital signs in patients who have lost 10–20% of their blood volume. If normalization is transient, then the possibility of 20–40% or greater blood loss exists. No improvement with initial crystalloid bolus occurs when hemorrhage exceeds 40% of total blood volume. In this situation blood, colloid and crystalloid should be administered to replenish the intravascular and interstitial compartments rapidly and efficiently. Of the available colloids, 5% albumin and hydroxyethyl starches are most commonly used. Starch solutions should be limited to 20 mL/kg because of concerns about transient bleeding dysfunction.

Successful fluid replenishment is indicated by a decreasing pulse rate below 100 beats/minute, a pulse pressure greater than 30 mmHg, urine output greater than 1 mL/kg/hr, improvement of mental status, and minimal metabolic acidosis.

Oxygen Delivery

Determination of serum hematocrit levels should be carried out immediately on arrival and frequently thereafter if bleeding is suspected. Interpretation of serum hematocrit must take into consideration the presence or absence of fluid resuscitation prior to its determination. Serum hematocrit may be falsely elevated prior to adequate fluid resuscitation despite significant ongoing hemorrhage, emphasizing the importance of postresuscitation measurement.

In situations of obvious severe hemorrhage, red cell therapy should be initiated to maintain optimal oxygen carrying capacity. Type O negative packed cells are administered if the situation will not allow time for type-specific blood. In cases where 50–75% of the patient's red cell volume has been replaced with type O negative whole blood, continued administration is recommended to avoid intravascular hemolysis from anti-A or anti-B antibodies if type-specific blood is given. It is always preferable to administer at least type-specific blood to avoid this situation. Next in the order of preference is typed and screened cells, in which serum is screened for major blood group antibodies (requires 15 minutes to perform). A full cross-match takes 45 minutes and involves mixing donor cells with recipient serum to rule out any antigen–antibody reactions.

The exact threshold for transfusion depends on the presence or absence of ongoing blood loss, patient age, and comorbidities, including major cardiac or vascular disease. The elderly and those with major cardiovascular disease should be maintained at or above 30%, while the young and healthy may tolerate levels as low as 20%, as long as hemostasis is maintained.

Coagulation

When several blood volumes have been replaced, dilutional thrombocytopenia and low clotting factor levels are seen. Replacement should be guided by appropriate laboratory evaluation. Platelets are generally required for platelet counts below 50,000 with clinical evidence of microvascular bleeding. Fresh frozen plasma is administered for irregularities of the prothrombin time (PT) or partial thromboplastin time (PTT), when they achieve 1.5 times normal values. Cryoprecipitate, which contains factor VIII, fibrinogen, fibronectin, and factor XIII, is indicated to correct isolated coagulation deficiencies or fibrinogen levels below 80–100 mg/dL. With massive ongoing transfusion and evidence of microvascular bleeding, factor replacement may be initiated prior to the availability of clotting studies. Calcium replacement is indicated when ionized calcium levels decrease secondary to citrate chelation, or when hypotension occurs despite adequate volume replacement.

MANAGEMENT OF ACID–BASE AND ELECTROLYTE STATUS

Acidemia

The most common acid–base disorder encountered in the trauma patient is acidemia of either metabolic or respiratory etiology. *Respiratory acidosis* is common in hypoventilatory states seen in diminished level of consciousness, atelectasis, pneumothorax, and pulmonary contusion. Establishment of a definitive airway and mechanical ventilation of sufficient minute volume should improve a respiratory acidosis.

Metabolic acidosis (pH <7.35, HCO_3 <21 mEq) is frequently the result of low cardiac output associated with hypovolemia and hemorrhage. Exceptions include direct cardiac contusion, tamponade, or tension pneumothorax, which may compromise cardiac output with relatively intact intravascular volume. Other considerations are alcoholic lactic acidosis or ketoacidosis, diabetic ketoacidosis, and carbon monoxide in thermal injuries. Differentiation between these etiologies requires measurement of serum lactate, urine ketone levels, blood glucose, and monitoring of intravascular volume. Severity of acidemia is assessed using arterial blood gases, serum bicarbonate, and the *base deficit*. At a base deficit of −10 mEq, cardiovascular effects become evident, including dysrhythmias, decreased contractility, increased pulmonary vascular resistance, hypotension, and resistance to exogenous catecholamines. A level of −14 mEq or greater indicates severe hypovolemia. High serum lactate suggests anaerobic activity and lactic acidosis; however, these levels improve slowly after correction of pH.

The definitive treatment for metabolic acidosis requires correction of the underlying etiology. Initial steps include rectifying hypoxemia, expansion of intravascular volume, improving oxygen carrying capacity, and maximizing cardiac performance.

There is considerable debate regarding the use of sodium bicarbonate in severe cases of metabolic acidosis refractory to initial corrective measures. The traditional approach is to administer sodium bicarbonate when pH falls below 7.2. This is based on the concept that alkalinization will improve systemic hemodynamics, and response to catecholamines. There is little convincing data supporting the use of sodium bicarbonate to improve lactic acidosis, and no study has shown improvement in clinical outcome. In experimental animals sodium bicarbonate transiently increases systemic blood pressure and pH, although intracellular pH is not improved. Acidemia may even be worsened by enzymatic conversion of sodium bicarbonate, raising P_aCO_2 levels. Mechanical ventilation and adequate pulmonary blood flow is vital to remove this increased P_aCO_2, and sodium bicarbonate should be used with extreme caution in nonventilated patients. A leftward shift in the oxyhemoglobin dissociation curve decreasing tissue oxygen unloading is a potential detrimental effect of sodium bicarbonate, and may worsen hypoxemia. Hypernatremia, resulting in a hyperosmolar state, and hypokalemia are other harmful effects of sodium bicarbonate administration.

Despite available data, sodium bicarbonate is still widely used as a temporizing measure until correction of the underlying etiology is accomplished. Calculating the whole body base deficit (body weight/kg × 0.3 × base deficit) may guide therapy. Half of the deficit is corrected initially and is followed by a repeat blood gas.

Electrolytes

Disorders of potassium are common in trauma patients. *Hypokalemia* occurs when metabolic or respiratory alkalosis (usually iatrogenically induced during resuscitation) causes potassium shift into the cell in exchange for hydrogen ions; and/or when endogenous catecholamines released in response to shock activate the Na^+/K^+ pump transporting potassium into cells. *Hyperkalemia* may be seen in association with dysrhythmias in situations of hypovolemic shock with metabolic acidosis and should be treated aggressively during resuscitation. Hyperkalemia is also a theoretic concern in massive transfusion, although potassium readily enters red cells when they warm to body temperature. Further management of electrolytes should focus on normalization of glucose, calcium, and magnesium levels, especially with multiple transfusions.

ANESTHESIA FOR TRAUMATIC INJURY

Following arrival in the operating room, monitors should be placed depending on patient injury, hemodynamic status, and comorbid conditions. General anesthesia is usually the technique, with regional approaches reserved for isolated peripheral extremity injuries. The goal of general anesthesia is adequate maintenance of ventilation and oxygenation, cardiovascular stability, control of intracranial hypertension, acid–base/electrolyte normalization, and prevention of hypothermia and coagulopathy.

Induction of Anesthesia

A rapid sequence induction using thiopental or propofol, with succinylcholine, is often employed in a stable patient. Careful titration with volume loading may be required to minimize cardiovascular side effects. There is no consensus regarding the ideal induction agent for an unstable patient. Ketamine and etomidate are both acceptable when used appropriately. Ketamine maintains blood pressure via indirect sympathetic stimulation but may cause paradoxical hypotension in the chronically hypotensive patient who is catecholamine-depleted. Ketamine should be avoided in closed head injury because of its ability to raise intracranial pressure (ICP). Etomidate possesses the greatest cardiovascular stability of all the induction agents secondary to its lack of effect on the sympathetic nervous system and autonomic reflexes. Induction results in minimal decreased heart rate, blood pressure, and systemic vascular resistance.

Succinylcholine (1–1.5 mg/kg) is the muscle relaxant of choice for the rapid-onset muscle paralysis required for laryngoscopy and intubation. Onset is less than 60 seconds and duration of action is limited to 5–10 minutes in most cases. Succinylcholine is associated with complications such as hyperkalemia, arrhythmias, increased intracranial and intraocular pressure, and malignant hyperthermia. It is now felt that succinylcholine is safe for patients with open eye injuries but should be avoided for 24 hours or longer following spinal cord or burn injuries. Rocuronium (1–1.5 mg/kg) is an excellent nondepolarizing alternative to succinylcholine in terms of onset, creating intubating conditions in 60–90 seconds, but has a duration of action similar to vecuronium (use with caution in patients with a difficult airway).

Maintenance of Anesthesia

Anesthesia is maintained using a combination of oxygen, volatile agent, nondepolarizing muscle relaxant, and short-acting opioids. Inhalational agents include isoflurane, sevoflurane, and desflurane. All volatile agents produce dose-related decreases in blood pressure from alterations in vascular tone and/or cardiac output. The agent chosen should be titrated to maintain mean arterial pressure and cerebral perfusion pressure. Nitrous oxide should be added very selectively and avoided in any case where pneumothorax, pneumocephaly, or gas-filled bowel loops are present. Fentanyl and sufentanil are the most commonly used narcotics in trauma patients and have minimal effect on cardiac output. In situations of ongoing hypotension, a high-dose narcotic technique using titrated benzodiazepine, minimal volatile agent, and inotropic and vasopressor support may be required.

Hypothermia is a frequent complication of trauma surgery, and is associated with increased mortality. Consequences of hypothermia include cardiac dysrhythmias, left shift of the oxyhemoglobin dissociation curve, platelet dysfunction, impaired renal function, and poor wound healing. Prevention requires warming of intravenous and irrigation fluids, humidifying gasses, warming the operating room, and employing radiant heaters.

Emergence from anesthesia depends on the physical condition prior to surgery, and the extent and outcome of the operation. Many severely injured trauma patients require postoperative intubation and prolonged intensive care. Pulmonary edema, adult respiratory distress syndrome, sepsis, and multisystem organ failure are frequent postoperative complications. When extubated in the operating room, the patient should be awake and breathing spontaneously, have adequate cough reflexes, and respond appropriately to commands.

MANAGEMENT OF SPECIFIC INJURIES

Head Injury

Classification

The pathologic classification of traumatic brain injury (TBI) is divided into two categories: primary and secondary injury. *Primary injury* is defined as damage occurring at the moment of trauma from biomechanical forces applied to the skull. Examples are fracture, brain contusion, laceration, diffuse axonal injury, and vascular injury. *Secondary injury* is an insult to the brain after initial injury, which may eventually lead to severe disability or death. Causes of this phenomenon include intracranial hemorrhage, increased ICP, hypoxemia, hypercarbia, hypotension, and infection. Acute management of TBI is focused on prevention and treatment of secondary injury. The brain's extremely high oxygen consumption, high blood flow, and significant oxygen extraction render cerebral tissue extremely vulnerable to ischemia during periods of hypotension. Hemorrhage into the cranium rarely results in sustained hypotension independently, and low blood pressure in the setting of severe head injury is usually the result of concomitant intra-abdominal, chest, or extremity trauma.

Diagnosis

Diagnosis of TBI is based on clinical and radiographic findings. A rapid baseline neurologic assessment is performed including level of consciousness, pupillary response, brain-stem reflexes, lateralizing signs, and global motor activity. Initial assessment should ideally take place prior to the administration of any muscle relaxants, opioids, sedatives, or hypnotics. The face and scalp should be examined for evidence of fracture or laceration. The Glasgow Coma Scale is a clinical classification of injury and is shown in Table 16-1. Eye opening, motor response, and verbal communication are used to determine severity of injury, assess for triage, follow clinical progression, and predict outcome.

In a patient with altered consciousness, hypoxia and shock should be identified and addressed as a first priority. When these parameters are restored and mental depression continues, TBI should be assumed and managed accordingly. Clinical signs of TBI and increased ICP, in addition to the GCS, include dilation of pupils or sluggish or absent pupillary responses. Severe intracranial hypertension may precipitate reflex arterial hypertension, bradycardia, and respiratory irregularities (Cushing's triad). Electrocardiographic abnormalities and ventricular arrhythmias have also been reported. Noncontrast CT scanning is the cornerstone of TBI imaging, with magnetic resonance providing little advantage in the acute setting. Findings include bony fracture, midline shift, distortion of ventricles, effacement of sulci, and the presence of epidural, subdural, or intraparenchymal hemorrhage. Generalized diffuse swelling and edema may be seen and usually represent severe nonsurgical injuries. Prognosis of patients with TBI is a function of the admission GCS score, the initial cranial CT scan, the age of the patient, and the extent of secondary injury.

Pathophysiology of Traumatic Brain Injury

Immediately following TBI there is initial reduction in cerebral blood flow (CBF), which is often inadequate to meet the brain's metabolic needs. Reduction in CBF, accompanied by increased ICP, creates a fertile environment for widespread secondary injury. Reduction in CBF appears to be a direct response to impact not related to, although aggravated by, systemic hypotension. CBF often normalizes 24 hours after injury. Cerebral arteriovenous oxygen content difference is abnormally high in the first few hours after injury, and then progressively decreases.

With decreased intracranial compliance and increased ICP, the homeostatic mechanism of autoregulation often fails in as many as 50% of patients. This is more likely to occur in severe injury, although it may also be seen in mild to moderate injury. With impaired autoregulation, significant systemic hypotension or hypertension can worsen secondary injury. Hypotension decreases cerebral perfusion pressure and may lead to ischemia.

Conversely, hypertension may precipitate vasogenic edema which can further increase ICP and compromise CBF. In contrast to autoregulation, vascular reactivity to P_aCO_2 is usually preserved and, if absent, is a poor prognostic sign indicative of complete vasomotor paralysis.

Traumatic brain injury often results in significant brain swelling, edema, hematoma formation, and increase in brain volume. Subsequent increases in ICP will worsen secondary injury, and even lead to herniation and death. This underscores the importance of aggressive treatment of ICP. In general the swollen brain is caused by an increase in cerebral blood volume (CBV) in the early stages after trauma, or by increases in brain tissue water in later stages.

Coagulation abnormalities are common after TBI. The brain is rich in thromboplastin, which, when released as a result of injury, can lead to disseminated intravascular coagulation and intracerebral hemorrhage. The association of *hyperglycemia* with poor neurologic outcome is well documented and evidence suggests that it worsens ischemic insult to the brain. Maintenance of normoglycemia prevents the development of lactic acidosis and subsequent injury to neurons.

Treatment of Intracranial Hypertension

The treatment for intracranial hypertension (ICP > 20 mmHg) requires a combination of ventilatory, pharmacologic, and surgical approaches. Several recommendations have developed regarding ICP monitoring in anesthetic management. One recommendation is to employ ICP monitoring when the GCS is less than 8 with an abnormal CT scan, in severe TBI with a normal CT scan if the age is greater than 40, or if systolic blood pressure is less than 90 mmHg. ICP monitoring is not generally indicated in mild or moderate injury.

Maintenance of oxygen partial pressure above 60 mmHg prevents cerebral vasodilation. P_aO_2 should therefore be maintained well above this level using appropriate F_iO_2 to ensure adequate tissue delivery. There is controversy regarding the use of hyperventilation in intubated TBI patients for brain protection. Hyperventilation results in decreased CBF, CBV, and ICP at P_aCO_2 levels to 25–30 mmHg, and may be a life saving maneuver in cases of severe intracranial hypertension. Despite its effectiveness in acute reduction of ICP, the resultant decreased CBF may worsen ischemia, especially in patients with reduced CBF or cerebral vasospasm. Arbitrary hyperventilation in absence of severe intracranial hypertension is not recommended for these reasons. Hyperventilation will lose its ability to decrease ICP in approximately 24 hours, and small subsequent increases in P_aCO_2 can lead to dramatic increases in CBF, CBV, and ICP.

Mannitol is an osmotic diuretic that reduces intracranial volume by drawing water from brain tissue and cerebrospinal fluid. Recent studies suggest that water is drawn primarily from areas adjacent to sites of injury. A dose of 0.25–1.0 g/kg is administered over 15 minutes, and a brisk diuresis ensues, relaxing brain tissue and decreasing ICP. The loop diuretic furosemide has a beneficial effect on ICP by dehydrating the brain and reducing cerebrospinal fluid formation. Adequate sedation will decrease metabolism, CBF, CBV, and possibly ICP. Nondepolarizing muscle relaxant decreases resistance to ventilation, and improves venous drainage. Head elevation to 30° in a neutral position will also improve venous outflow. Barbiturates may have a role by reducing metabolism and CBF, although their use has not been shown to improve outcome in TBI patients. Intravenous corticosteroids have no proven role in TBI.

Types of Brain Injury

Acute epidural hematoma is an uncommon finding in TBI patients and clearly represents a surgical emergency. Disruption of the middle meningeal vessels and dural separation from the skull is usually associated with an underlying skull fracture. Rapid increases in ICP can be seen with progressive hematoma, which may result in transtentorial herniation of the brain. Physical examination findings include nausea and vomiting, ipsilateral pupillary dilation, contralateral hemiparesis, or even decerebration. The classic finding on CT scan is a biconvex or lenticular-shaped lesion adjacent to the skull. Mortality is 5–43% in this injury and depends on the level of consciousness at presentation. Emergent craniotomy and evacuation is the definitive treatment.

Acute subdural hematoma is a more common injury, seen in as many as 22% of severe TBI. Tearing of the bridging vessels from acceleration–deceleration injuries or by accumulation of blood around a parenchymal laceration is seen. There is often significant parenchymal damage with a subdural hematoma, making this lesion more lethal than an epidural, carrying mortality rates of 50% or higher. Clinical presentation depends on the severity of the brain injury at the time of impact and rate of hematoma growth. Signs and symptoms range from minimal neurological deficits to a comatose state. Motor deficits and anisocoria are most common. On CT scan the classic appearance is a high-density crescentic lesion deforming the surface of the brain. Rapid surgical evacuation via wide craniotomy or burr hole is indicated. Severe edema causing herniation through the craniotomy site may occur because of increased CBV and vasoparalysis. This situation carries an exceptionally high mortality rate.

Acute intracerebral hematoma and contusions are most common in patients between 21 and 40 years of age. The majority of these occur when the moving head strikes a fixed object. They can also be seen from blows to the head where a depressed fracture causes underlying hematoma or contusion. Clinical presentation may vary from lucid to comatose states. CT findings vary from homogeneous well-delineated areas of high-density to heterogeneous, poorly defined, mixed-density lesions surrounded by a low-density zone signifying edema.

Penetrating injuries are the result of projectile invasion such as knives, bullets, and pointed instruments that produce local damage but minimal rotational or angular movement. Rapid assessment involves immediate evaluation of the overall medical condition and neurological status, examination of entrance and exit wounds, and a lateral skull radiograph to determine the presence and location of the penetrating object. CT is crucial to determine the missile tract and to rule out areas of hemorrhage. Operative goals include debridement of the penetrating tract, evacuation of hematoma, hemostasis, removal of fragments if possible, and complete dural and scalp closure.

General Anesthesia in Traumatic Brain Injury

The goal of intubation in TBI is to preserve systemic oxygenation and CO_2 elimination, prevent aspiration of gastric contents, maintain hemodynamics, minimize increases in ICP, and avoid aggravation of cervical spine injury. Cervical spine injury is seen in as many as 10% of severe TBI patients, so in-line stabilization is required during laryngoscopy. Blind nasal intubation may secure the airway without pharmacologic agents but carries a small risk of intracranial placement in patients with maxillary or basal skull fractures. Cardiopulmonary stability should not be compromised during intubation in an effort to reduce CBF, cerebral blood volume, metabolism, or ICP.

Both thiopental and etomidate dose-dependently reduce metabolism, CBF, and ICP. Etomidate is generally the safer agent because of its superior maintenance of blood pressure in hypovolemic patients. The total dose of induction agent should be reduced regardless of the agent in situations where hypotension is suspected. Intravenous lidocaine will blunt sympathetic responses to intubation and limit increases in ICP. Midazolam decreases CBF, does not increase ICP, and will provide satisfactory hemodynamic stability when given in small doses. Propofol reduces ICP and CBF in TBI; however, hypotension may be poorly tolerated in hypovolemic patients. The role of muscle relaxants is to facilitate rapid and effective laryngeal exposure. After acute TBI, succinylcholine is appropriate despite its association with small, transient increases in ICP.

Prompt restoration and maintenance of arterial blood pressure is essential. Improvement of intravascular volume is the mainstay of treatment, although the use of vasopressors will improve perfusion pressure prior to adequate volume resuscitation. No single fluid has been shown to be the ideal replacement. Hypotonic solutions, including Ringer's lactate, are more likely to increase brain water content than normal saline. Studies of experimental TBI have demonstrated that infusion of colloid solutions were associated with lower brain water accumulation than infusion of crystalloid solutions. In experimental animal models the use of hypertonic (3.0% or 7.5%) saline is associated with lower ICP than isotonic or slightly hypotonic compositions, and may improve outcome.

Intraoperative management should include standard American Society of Anesthesiologists monitoring with invasive arterial catheterization. Central venous or pulmonary artery catheterization may address uncertainty about intravascular volume and cardiac performance. Historic recommendations to restrict fluid appear outdated and unsupported by clinical evidence, and aggressive hemodynamic support with larger volumes of fluid appears not to worsen outcome. In head-injured patients undergoing non-neurosurgical procedures, ICP monitoring may be required. Acute intracranial hypertension should be treated immediately.

Anesthesia is usually maintained with combinations of barbiturate, benzodiazepine, narcotic, N_2O, and volatile anesthetic. Volatile agents are associated with increased CBF and ICP and should therefore be limited to less than 1 MAC. Isoflurane, sevoflurane, and desflurane are the most common agents used. Nitrous oxide should be avoided in cases of pneumocephalus or pneumothorax. The synthetic opioids are generally well tolerated. Long-acting narcotics should generally be avoided when postoperative neurological evaluation is needed. Of the nondepolarizing agents, vecuronium and rocuronium have few hemodynamic side effects and do not impact CBF or ICP.

Oxygen partial pressure should be maintained at a minimum of 60 mmHg, and mild hyperoxia (PO_2 to 100–250 mmHg) may improve cerebral oxygenation during correction of hypotension or ICP. In patients with respiratory compromise, mechanical ventilatory intervention should be used despite the potential for increase in ICP. Treatment of systemic hypertension with vasodilators may induce unacceptable cerebral vasodilation, and barbiturates, narcotics, or labetalol can reduce blood pressure with less risk. Vasoconstrictors should be used for transient hypotension to maintain cerebral perfusion pressure until the etiology is corrected. Once the dura is opened, ICP quickly reaches zero. Hypertension should be controlled at this stage because a sudden increase in cerebral perfusion pressure may abruptly increase CBF.

At the conclusion of emergency brain surgery, most patients are not awakened or extubated unless preoperative mental status was normal or has rapidly declined because of expanding hematoma. If awakening is the goal, then long-acting narcotics, benzodiazepines, and hypnotics should be discontinued prior to emergence. If the patient is to remain intubated, adequate sedation, analgesia, and even muscle relaxation should be used for transportation to the intensive care unit with full monitoring in place.

Spinal Cord Injury

Assessment

All trauma patients are presumed to have a spinal cord injury until proven otherwise. Cervical injuries are associated with head trauma, thoracic fractures with chest trauma, and lumbar fracture with abdominal and long bone fractures. The cornerstone of initial evaluation of spine trauma is to diagnose instability and determine the extent of neurologic injury. In the conscious patient a history of motor vehicle crash, industrial accident, athletic injury, fall, penetrating trauma with neurologic loss below a certain spinal level, or pain and tenderness at the location of a specific vertebra strongly suggest spinal injury.

As in any trauma, the initial evaluation should identify signs of respiratory insufficiency, airway obstruction, chest, or facial injury. Serial neurologic evaluation should assess cord function above and below the level of injury. If cervical injury is suspected, evidence of compromise of the fifth cervical segment should be sought. Function of the biceps, deltoid, and brachioradialis is tested for evidence of weakness or paralysis and, if these muscle groups are flaccid, then partial diaphragmatic paralysis exists. A complete lesion at C4 or above will require mechanical ventilation as a result of complete diaphragm paralysis. Loss of intercostal function in high or mid-thoracic injuries may inhibit cough reflexes and hinder natural airway protection. There is a remote chance of recovery after complete cord injuries, although incomplete lesions may have varying degrees of functional restoration.

Initial radiographic evaluation requires a cross-table lateral view of the cervical spine, which may detect 70% of all lesions. A 'swimmer's' view may aid in visualization of C6, C7, and T1, and an open-mouth odontoid view can improve detection of C1–C2 fractures. A CT scan is the most reliable modality and will have 100% sensitivity to detect fracture when combined with three-view plain radiographs. Cervical radiography may appear normal in unstable soft tissue injuries and, if clinical suspicion warrants, flexion–extension views under fluoroscopy may be obtained to identify dislocation missed by conventional views. Immobilization of the injured spine is of unquestionable importance, and is achieved using inline stabilization with cervical collar. A careful log-rolling maneuver should be employed to protect the thoracic and lumbar spine.

Airway Management

Respiratory failure is the most common cause of death in acute cervical cord injury. A cervical collar with pine board should be used at all times, and overall movement of the patient should be limited. Awake fiberoptic intubation with good airway topicalization is ideal to limit cervical movement, although blind nasal intubation may be used in the absence of facial or basilar skull fracture. In emergency situations direct rapid-sequence laryngoscopy with cricoid pressure should be used, using in-line traction and minimal flexion and extension of the neck.

Operative Management

Surgical intervention for spinal trauma depends on the extent of neurologic injury and radiographic appearance of displacement or instability. Positioning in the operating suite is of critical importance in patients with cord injuries or those with instability without cord compromise. Careful precautions must be taken to avoid further injury to the central nervous system, especially when turning patients prone. Cervical spine injuries are most often treated with anterior open reduction and fusion. Lateral traction of the carotid artery may compromise blood flow to the brain, and retraction on the esophagus and trachea may result in laryngeal edema or recurrent laryngeal nerve injury. Thoracolumbar dislocations are typically repaired from a posterior approach.

Spinal Shock and Spinal Cord Protection

Spinal shock is an acute response to transection of the cord and results in cessation of cord function below the level of the injury. This phenomenon may last from several days to as long as 3 months. Flaccid paralysis, loss of somatic and visceral sensation, and loss of vasopressor reflexes are commonly seen. Hemodynamic threatening bradycardia may occur if the injury inhibits the cardioaccelerator fibers at T1–T4, and vagal episodes during airway instrumentation are dangerous. Atropine or isoproterenol may be used to treat severe bradycardia. The condition of marked loss of sympathetic tone in the periphery below the level of injury, and absent cardioaccelerator activity, is a set-up for severe hypotension without a tachycardic response. This highlights the importance of adequate fluid resuscitation combined with potent vasoconstrictors and cardiac chronotropic support. Invasive monitors should be placed for mid- to high cervical lesions to follow filling pressures and cardiac output. Vasodilation from profound sympathectomy disrupts temperature regulation and aggressive warming techniques are therefore mandatory.

The goal of general anesthesia is preservation of spinal cord blood flow through maintaining mean arterial pressure and intravascular volume. A combined opioid and low-dose volatile anesthetic technique will help to preserve spinal cord perfusion pressure. Pulmonary management should be targeted at avoiding prolonged hyperventilation, which may diminish spinal cord perfusion. Neurophysiologic monitoring using somatosensory evoked potentials (SSEPs), and motor-evoked potentials (MEPs), may be employed to detect cord ischemia. Less common is the use of a wake-up test to assess neurologic dysfunction intraoperatively.

Methylprednisone is used in large doses in an attempt to improve outcome from cord injuries and decrease secondary injury. A bolus of 30 mg/kg within 8 hours of injury, followed by an infusion of 5.4 mg/kg/hr, is used for 24 hours. This may only provide small benefit, although no significant increase in complication rates has been shown with high-dose corticosteroids.

Respiratory Function

Respiratory dysfunction occurs in nearly all spinal cord injuries. The need for assisted ventilation depends on the level of injury, where lesions above C4 result in diaphragmatic paralysis and universally require mechanical ventilation. Lower cervical lesions encounter reduction in tidal volume and vital capacity, because of impaired intercostal/abdominal muscle function, and paradoxical respirations. These patients require emergency mechanical ventilation less frequently. Airway protection, cough reflex, accessory muscle use, and expiratory reserve improve as the lesion descends the cord to T7.

Pulmonary edema may develop from a catecholamine surge that increases pulmonary blood flow, and transudation of fluid across capillary beds. Aspiration of gastric contents, atelectasis, and bronchospasm are also considerations in situations of hypoxia.

Succinylcholine and Autonomic Hyperreflexia

Massive potassium release, a result of proliferation of extrajunctional acetylcholine receptors, has been documented as a cause of cardiac arrest in paralyzed patients who receive induction doses of succinylcholine. The use of this muscle relaxant is considered safe in the first 24 hours after injury, although it should not be used after this window. Nondepolarizing relaxants are considered safe in spinal cord injury patients.

Thoracic Trauma

Thoracic trauma can be thought of as either blunt or penetrating. Gunshot wounds are likely to create widespread damage due to high velocity on impact causing diffuse tissue injury. Stab wounds are less complex, with damage confined to areas underlying the point of contact. Most blunt injuries are the result of the direct impact and the momentum of structures within the thoracic cavity exerting shearing forces on underlying viscera.

Pneumothorax

Open pneumothorax is a consequence of penetration of the chest wall and lung by sharp objects, including rib fragments. A large defect in the chest wall effectively equalizes intrapleural pressure with the atmosphere, and a 'sucking' chest wound is a fairly obvious clinical observation. Immediate treatment is to occlude the defect until a chest tube can be placed.

Tension pneumothorax is observed when air enters the pleural cavity and cannot escape. It may result from blunt or penetrating trauma, or when mechanical ventilation is initiated. In conscious patients breath sounds are markedly reduced, the trachea is deviated, and cyanosis and cardiovascular collapse can follow. During general anesthesia, a dramatic decrease in respiratory compliance with hemodynamic collapse will alert the clinician. Nitrous oxide should be discontinued immediately, as it accentuates the size of the pneumothorax. Often this condition is mistaken for pericardial tamponade, myocardial infarction, or hypovolemic shock. Valuable time should not be wasted obtaining radiographs, and immediate treatment with a large-bore needle placed in the second intercostal space in the midclavicular line will decompress the lung.

Flail Chest

Paradoxical movement in the anterolateral chest wall may result from multiple rib fractures after blunt trauma. On inspiration, the injured segment encroaches on the lung, leading to impairment of ventilation and oxygenation. This injury is rarely isolated and is often an ominous sign indicating severe damage to underlying thoracic and abdominal organs. The condition is often unnoticed and may be overshadowed by more overt injuries. Rib fractures and parenchymal damage to the lung may be missed on early radiographs, and progressive hypoxia is often a presenting sign. The chest is stabilized using sandbags and pillows until a definitive treatment plan can be determined. Intubation is guided by patient condition and is discussed earlier in this chapter.

Traumatic Hemothorax

Massive hemothorax is defined as the rapid accumulation of more than 1500 mL of blood in the chest cavity. Life-threatening hemorrhage is often seen with penetrating injury or rupture of major intrathoracic vessels from blunt trauma. Hemorrhage from the great vessels is usually devastating, allowing only 15% of patients to reach a medical facility alive. Diagnosis is made by knowledge of the mechanism of injury and by clinical examination of the chest. Initial chest radiographs may be misleading. Massive hemothorax is suspected when hypovolemic shock is associated with diminished breath sounds. A chest tube should be inserted and, if initial return is greater than 1500 mL of blood, thoracotomy will be required for further management of blood loss and identification of injury.

Thoracic Aortic Injury

A history of high impact trauma to the chest should alert the clinician to the possibility of thoracic aortic injury. The presence of first and second rib fractures is suggestive, since these injuries only appear with high-impact deceleration. Patients may complain of 'ripping' chest pain radiating to the back, and a widened mediastinum, blurred aortic knob, left pleural or apical cap, or deviation of the trachea is seen on initial chest radiograph. The most common location of injury is just distal to the left subclavian artery or in the ascending aorta. The mortality rate with aortic rupture is 80–90% and most patients die within 60 minutes. The degree of hemodynamic stability on presentation depends on the extent of the injury and the rapidity of blood loss. The definitive diagnostic study is an arch aortogram and contrast-enhanced CT scan. Transthoracic echocardiography (TTE), or transesophageal echo (TEE), are also useful in the early diagnosis of aortic injuries. Because of the obvious potential for massive blood loss, large-bore intravenous access and rapid infusion devices are mandatory. During anesthesia, extremes in blood pressure are avoided. Cardiopulmonary bypass with a double-lumen endotracheal tube may be utilized during surgical repair, depending on the location and severity of trauma.

Tracheobronchial Injuries

Most patients with severe tracheal injuries die at the scene of the accident. Of surviving patients, most present with dyspnea, cough, hemoptysis, subcutaneous emphysema, and cyanosis. Often other associated injuries such as tension pneumothorax, cervical spine fracture, and esophageal, cardiac, or diaphragmatic laceration are seen. Approximately 80% of injuries occur within 2.5 cm of the carina. All patients require diagnostic bronchoscopy as soon as they are stable. Small tracheal wounds may be treated with intubation, placing the cuff below the site of the wound, although surgical repair is often indicated. More distal injury may require a double-lumen endotracheal tube, and fiberoptic technique is useful to better position a tube. Tracheostomy should always be considered, especially when there is obvious damage to the larynx or cervical trachea or when endotracheal intubation is unsuccessful.

Diaphragmatic Injury

Patients with diaphragmatic injury often present with respiratory distress and associated rib fractures or flail chest. A diaphragmatic injury may permit migration of abdominal contents into the chest, where they may compress the lung and impair gas exchange. Cardiac compression resulting in dysrhythmias is also seen. Herniation of bowel contents does not always occur immediately, and unexplained changes in pulmonary compliance, incarceration, or obstruction may be a presenting sign. Chest radiography demonstrating bowel in the thorax, or the presence of a nasogastric tube above the level of the diaphragm, aids in the diagnosis. Pulmonary aspiration is a risk, and surgical repair should be pursued as patient condition permits.

Cardiac Tamponade

Disruption of the cardiac vessels from blunt or penetrating trauma may result in pericardial tamponade. Accumulation of 100–200 mL of fluid in the pericardium may create an outflow obstruction, limiting diastolic filling and stroke volume. In hypotensive patients with injuries around the neck, precordium, or upper abdomen, tamponade should be considered. The classic triad of distended neck veins, hypotension, and muffled heart sounds (Beck's triad) is often absent. A decline in systolic blood pressure of 10 mmHg or more on inspiration (pulsus paradoxus) may be noted, although it is often difficult to detect. The electrocardiogram may be normal or have nonspecific ST-segment or T-wave abnormalities. If a central venous or pulmonary artery catheter is in place, equalization of chamber pressures and pronounced systolic x-descent is seen.

Rapid use of TTE is the gold standard for diagnosis, although pericardiocentesis should be undertaken as a temporizing measure if rapid deterioration is observed. A 16- or 18-gauge metal needle is inserted at the xiphoid 35° towards the left shoulder and removal of 30–60 mL of blood may result in dramatic improvement. Reaccumulation is often rapid and surgical correction should be carried out as soon as possible.

Patients with tamponade have limited diastolic filling, so anesthetic management should focus on maintaining a high heart rate, minimizing myocardial depression, and avoiding decreases in systemic vascular resistance.

Cardiac Contusions

Cardiac contusion is often unrecognized because the symptoms are vague and nonspecific. Clinical signs include angina-like pain unresponsive to nitrates, dysrhythmias, and left- or right-sided heart failure manifested as hypotension. ST or T-wave changes, axis shift, and bundle branch block are common. Cardiac enzymes are of some clinical value and should be obtained. Two-dimensional TTE is the most reliable diagnostic modality. Segmental wall motion abnormalities, increased wall thickness, septal shift, pericardial effusion, and myocardial hematoma are often observed. Patients with these injuries should be handled similarly to those with myocardial infarction, with the exception of anticoagulation.

Abdominal Trauma

Significant blunt trauma to the abdomen frequently presents as hypotension. Injury to the aorta, or other large vessel, is less common in blunt trauma, though frequently seen in penetrating injuries. Ultrasound is evolving as a rapid and accurate method to evaluate blunt abdominal trauma. Abdominal distention is sometimes an unreliable sign, since large volumes of blood may accumulate before distention is observed. CT is the most accurate modality to identify surgical injury. When surgical injury presents, or clinical suspicion suggests abdominal pathology, exploratory laparotomy is indicated. Airway, breathing, and circulation should be managed as any major traumatic injury with potential for large blood loss. Monitoring, access, and approach to anesthesia, depends on severity of suspected injury and hemodynamics.

Direct Eye Injury

Management of emergency anesthesia for an open eye injury requires the clinician to balance the need to prevent aspiration of gastric contents and to avoid damaging increases in intraocular pressure. Early administration of an H_2 blocker and metoclopramide will decrease gastric acidity and offer some aspiration protection. Rapid-sequence induction is chosen using propofol or thiopental, succinylcholine, lidocaine, and a short-onset narcotic to blunt airway responses and minimize increase in intraocular pressure. Such increases with succinylcholine are usually transient, and it is now considered safe for patients with open eye injury. High-dose rocuronium actually decreases intraocular pressure and may be used for rapid sequence induction when a difficult airway is not a factor. Maintenance of anesthesia should be directed towards prevention of patient movement, amnesia, analgesia, and hemodynamic stability. Muscle relaxation is advantageous to help prevent unexpected patient movement during crucial surgical intervals.

On emergence, the dilemma of preventing coughing and bucking while extubating the patient in the awake state with intact airway reflexes is difficult. Lidocaine and moderate doses of a short acting narcotic are helpful to prevent globe-threatening increases in intraocular pressure on emergence.

Orthopedic Trauma

Pelvic Fractures

Motor vehicle accidents and crush injuries represent the cause of nearly all pelvic fractures. The extreme forces required to fracture these bones leads to a high incidence of concomitant injury. Associated injuries include colorectal disruption, genitourinary damage, major vascular laceration, and compromise of neural tissue. Significant hemorrhage is frequent, especially in posterior ring or open-book fractures, and transfusion is often required. Arterial injury may cause uncontrollable hemorrhage, and arterial embolization of the hypogastric vessels may be life-saving. Blood at the urethral meatus precludes the placement of a Foley catheter and a percutaneous technique is required for bladder catheterization. Surgical treatment includes the use of MAST stabilization, external fixation, or less common, open surgery to repair bony and vascular injury. Heavy blood loss should be expected.

Extremity Fractures

Fracture of long bones require extreme force and may result in significant internal bleeding: in excess of 2 liters of blood may be lost in a severe femoral shaft fracture. Assessment includes visual inspection for asymmetry, palpation of distal pulses, recognition of skin distention, and identification of pain location. Pain, pulselessness, paresthesias, and pallor indicate a potential arterial injury. Angiography is often indicated.

Regardless of whether a fracture is open or closed, surgical repair should be performed as soon as possible. Delay in treatment increases the risk of deep vein thrombosis, pulmonary or fat embolism, infection, and sepsis. Open fractures should be repaired in less than 6 hours to decrease the high incidence of sepsis. Severe pain in an affected extremity, or calf pain on dorsiflexion, should raise suspicion of compartment syndrome. Compartment pressures exceeding 40 cm H_2O require immediate surgery to prevent limb loss and permanent nerve injury.

General anesthesia is indicated for most acute orthopedic injuries, although regional anesthesia or a combined general–regional technique may be used. Sudden hypotension, with associated decrease in end-tidal carbon dioxide, is consistent with pulmonary or fat embolism, a potentially devastating complication of orthopedic injury. Intraoperative treatment is generally supportive.

MANAGEMENT OF THE BURNED PATIENT

Introduction

The skin serves many functions including preventing fluid loss, protecting against infection, maintaining body temperature, receiving sensory stimuli, producing vitamin D, and determining an individual's identity. Consequently, management of burn patients remains extremely challenging and is best approached by a multidisciplinary team involving the anesthesiologist, surgeon, intensivist, nurse, and respiratory therapist.

Thermal injuries affect over 2 million people annually, with 4% being admitted to hospitals and 0.5% dying as a result. It is helpful to determine the severity of burns in order to assign an appropriate level of care. Major burns are full-thickness injury involving over 10% of the total body surface area (TBSA), partial-thickness burns of over 25% TBSA in an adult or 20% TBSA at the extremes of age. Injury involving the face, hands, feet or perineum, or burns in patients with serious pre-existing medical conditions, are also considered to be major. Electrical or chemical burns, those with coexisting inhalational or traumatic injuries, and injury suspected to be the result of abuse or neglect are also indications for burn unit admission.

Determining burn size

Survival from burn injury is strongly related to age, burn size, and the presence or absence of inhalational injury. The burn size is classified according to TBSA and tissue depth. The extent is important in initial triage and in determining fluid requirements, drug doses, and outcome. The well-known "rule of nines" accurately assesses the surface area involved in thermal injury in adults. For children up to the age of about 12, the head represents a greater proportion of surface area, so this rule is modified accordingly (Table 16-3).

First-degree burns are pink and dry, without blisters, and involve primarily the epidermis. Common causes are overexposure to sunlight or brief scalding from hot

Table 16-3 'Rule of Nines' for Calculating Percentage of Body Burned (% TBSA)

	Child	Adult
Head/neck	18	9
Arm	9	9
Anterior trunk	18	18
Posterior trunk	18	18
Leg (groin to toe)	14	18

TBSA, total body surface area.
From Goodwin CW, Finkelstein JL, Madden MR. Burns. In: Schwartz SI. *Principles of surgery*. New York: McGraw-Hill, 1994:230.

liquids. A *second-degree*, or *partial-thickness* burn, involves the epidermis and dermis. The skin is painful, erythematous, moist, blistering, and blanches to the touch. A *full-thickness burn* appears white, is insensate, and does not blanch. Thrombosed veins may sometimes be seen through this devitalized tissue, which is referred to as eschar. Fluid losses, and metabolic effects of deep dermal burns, are equivalent to full-thickness burns (Table 16-4).

Special Circumstances: Electrical and Chemical Burns

Electrical burns require special consideration secondary to associated cardiac morbidity. Electrical injury manifests in a variety of forms ranging from cardiopulmonary arrest with minimal tissue damage to devastating electrocution and vaporization of major body parts. Tissue is burned from the flow of alternating or direct current. Alternating current produces tonic muscle contraction, resulting in an inability to release the source of electricity. Alternating current is also associated with a high incidence of cardiac arrest and coma. Cardiopulmonary arrest is most common in high-voltage electrical injuries and is treated with resuscitation according to the American Heart Association Advanced Cardiac Life Support (ACLS) guidelines. These patients should be observed on telemetry for at least 48 hours beyond the last arrhythmia, as repeat arrhythmias may recur. Of note, lightning injury usually causes immediate cardiopulmonary arrest due to apnea caused by electrical paralysis of the brain-stem respiratory center. Survivors frequently have recurrent arrhythmias and infarction patterns.

There is a high incidence of renal failure following electrical injury. Rarely, electrical current causes intestinal perforation, pancreatic or gallbladder necrosis, and hepatic injury. The treating physician must have a high index of suspicion for these occult injuries.

While electrical and chemical injuries have unique importance, the most common mechanism of burn injury remains fire. Fires occurring in a closed space

Table 16-4   Diagnosis of Burn Wound Depth

| | Second-degree Burns | | |
First-degree Burns	Superficial	Deep Dermal	Third-degree Burns
Cause			
Sun	Hot liquids	Hot liquids	Flame
Minor flash	Flashes of flame	Flashes of flame	Immersion scalds
	Brief exposure to dilute chemicals	Prolonged exposure to dilute chemicals	High-voltage electricity
			Exposure to concentrated chemicals
			Contact with hot objects
Color			
Pink	Pink to bright red	Dark red or mottled yellow-white	Pearly white or charred
			Translucent and parchment-like
Surface			
Dry or small blisters	Variably sized, usually large bullas	Smaller bullas, often ruptured	Dry with adherent nonviable epidermis
	Copious exudate	Slightly moist	Thrombosed vessels may be visible
Sensation			
Painful	Painful	Decreased pinprick sensation	Anesthetic
		Intact deep pressure sensation	Deep pressure sensation
Texture			
Soft with minimal edema and later superficial exfoliation	Thickened by edema but pliable	Moderate edema with decreased elasticity	Inelastic and leathery
Healing			
2–3 days	5–21 days	3 weeks	None – grafting required

From Goodwin CW, Finkelstein JL, Madden MR. Burns. In: Schwartz SI. *Principles of surgery*. New York: McGraw-Hill, 1994:231.

should alert the physician to the potential for airway injury, which must be thoroughly investigated.

Airway Complications

Three distinct syndromes of inhalational injury can occur and are distinguished according to clinical features and the time since injury. *Early complications* occurring in the first 24 hours include airway obstruction, pulmonary edema, carbon monoxide, and cyanide toxicity. *Delayed injury* is seen 2–5 days following the burn and manifests as the acute respiratory distress syndrome (ARDS). *Late damage* in subsequent weeks presents as pneumonia, atelectasis, and pulmonary emboli.

Early Inhalational Injuries

The presence of soot around the face, singed nasal hairs and eyebrows, coughing, hoarseness, or stridor should raise suspicion of an inhalational injury if the mechanism is appropriate. Breathing superheated air, or steam, even briefly, leads to massive edema and rapid airway obstruction. Obstruction is often due to macroglossia, epiglottitis, and/or laryngotracheal bronchitis. Airway edema may even ensue in mild inhalational injuries. The extent of damage can be assessed by direct laryngoscopy or fiberoptic nasopharyngoscopy. Alternatively, flow–volume curves have been shown to correlate with the degree of edema observed by fiberoptic bronchoscopy. These curves show a variable extrathoracic inspiratory obstruction in the setting of mild edema, and a fixed extrathoracic obstruction with more severe narrowing of the airway.

Inhalational injury may confer up to a tenfold increase in mortality for the burned patient. Early recognition and securing of the airway is life-saving. In the normal airway, tracheal intubation is usually achieved using a rapid sequence induction. There is a general consensus that succinylcholine is safe in the first 24 hours after a burn, prior to the proliferation of extrajunctional acetylcholine receptors. Should succinylcholine be used after the first 24 hours, rapid hyperkalemia may ensue, resulting in cardiac arrest. This effect may persist until a year after the last burn is healed, although the exact time course is unclear. There is no contraindication to nondepolarizing muscle relaxants in thermal injury.

Awake fiberoptic intubation is often the safest technique in a burn patient with distorted facial anatomy, who may present difficult mask ventilation. The airway should be promptly secured when impending obstruction from edema is suspected. Again, awake fiberoptic intubation may be the safest option. The optimal location for performing a prophylactic intubation is the operating room where the anesthesiologist has skilled assistants, an expanded collection of airway equipment, and an improved environment for performing a surgical airway if necessary. Spontaneous ventilation helps maintain adequate oxygenation if mask ventilation proves difficult. The fiberoptic bronchoscope, Bullard laryngoscope, and intubation via a laryngeal mask airway have all been used successfully. While a primary surgical airway may be appropriate if the upper airway is badly damaged, it is associated with greater morbidity and should be considered as a last resort. The incidence of infectious complications from tracheostomy through burned skin is extremely high. Even with delayed tracheostomy, long-term complications occur in 28% of patients and include tracheal stenosis, tracheoesophageal fistula, and tracheoarterial fistula. Tracheostomy after successful neck skin grafting decreases the infection risk.

After the airway is secured, and following initial resuscitation, bronchoscopy is performed to delineate the extent of injury. The endotracheal tube is maintained until after the third post-burn day in order to allow for resolution of upper airway edema. The clinician should be watchful for evidence of more significant lung injury in these patients.

Delayed and Late Inhalational Injuries

Some 85% of patients with large-airway injury seen on bronchoscopy also have clinically significant pulmonary parenchymal damage. Initial chest radiographs and P_aO_2 are often normal. These injuries result from distal propagation of incomplete products of combustion to the terminal bronchioles at the time of the fire. The structural lining cells are damaged and commonly slough, obstructing small airways. Vascular endothelial cells adjacent to the alveoli may also be injured, allowing loss of intravascular fluid. Resulting pneumonia, atelectasis, and pulmonary edema may not appear until 4–7 days after the injury. Once this occurs the subsequent mortality is approximately 60%. Treatment ranges from suctioning, incentive spirometry, and humidified oxygen-enriched air, to mechanical ventilation with positive end-expiratory pressure. Prophylactic steroids and antibiotics have not been shown to improve outcome.

Carbon Monoxide Poisoning

Carbon monoxide, a product of the incomplete combustion of wood, gasoline, and coal is the major cause of hypoxia and asphyxia in fire-related deaths in urban environments. Carbon monoxide is a colorless, odorless, and tasteless gas with 300 times as great an affinity for hemoglobin as oxygen. The resulting compound, carboxyhemoglobin, has a diminished oxygen carrying capacity and a lessened ability to release oxygen to tissue. A left shift in the oxyhemoglobin dissociation curve is observed.

Carboxyhemoglobin is a cause of tissue hypoxia and metabolic acidosis. The suspicion of carbon monoxide poisoning is raised by an appropriate mechanism such as a closed-space fire. Dyspnea, mental obtundation, oxygen saturation of 85% with a normal or high P_aO_2, and an elevated mixed-venous oxygen saturation is common. One should note that although the P_aO_2 may remain normal, the total blood oxygen content is decreased according to the equation:

$$O_2 \text{ content} = (\text{Hemoglobin} \times 1.34 \times O_2 \text{ sat}) + (0.003 \times P_aO_2).$$

The diagnosis can be confirmed by co-oximetry, which reveals the true oxygen saturation and the percentage of carbon monoxide present in arterial blood. Carboxyhemoglobin concentrations over 60% are usually associated with coma and death (Table 16-5).

Prolonged carbon monoxide exposure is associated with profound myocardial depression that is unresponsive to fluids and inotropic support. Shock, acidosis, and death usually ensue. The pathognomonic cherry-red skin of this type of poisoning is rarely evident in burn patients.

Optimal treatment of carbon monoxide poisoning consists of 100% oxygen administered by tight-fitting face mask or endotracheal tube and mechanical ventilation if the patient has altered mental status. The half-life of carbon monoxide is reduced from 240 minutes to 40 minutes by increasing oxygen concentrations from 21% to 100%. Hyperbaric oxygen treatment can further decrease this time, although it has not been conclusively shown to improve survival (Table 16-6).

Patients may have persistent neuropsychiatric sequelae, and as many as 10% develop a syndrome of gait disturbances, mental deterioration, and urinary incontinence around the second week after injury. Some 10% of these individuals have neurologic deficits at 3-year follow-up. Brain CT in these patients shows bilateral areas of decreased density in the globus pallidus, which are also seen after other anoxic events. Hyperbaric oxygen has

Table 16-5 Symptoms of CO Toxicity as a function of the Blood Carboxyhemoglobin (COHb) Level

Blood COHb	Level Symptoms
<15–20	Headache, dizziness, and occasional confusion
20–40	Nausea, vomiting, disorientation, and visual impairment
40–60	Agitation, combativeness, hallucination, coma, and shock
>60	Death

From Capan LM, Miller SM. Trauma and burns. In: Barash PG, Cullen BF, Stoelting RK. *Clinical anesthesia*, 3rd ed. Philadelphia: Lippincott-Raven, 1997:1187.

Table 16-6 Effect of Increasing Oxygen Administration on Carbon Monoxide Elimination

O$_2$ Pressure (atm)	Half-life (min)
0.21	240
1.0	40
3.0	25

From Goodwin CW, Finkelstein JL, Madden MR. Burns. In: Schwartz SI. *Principles of surgery*. New York: NcGraw-Hill, 1994:241.

not been shown to alter the development of this tragic late consequence of smoke inhalation.

Cyanide toxicity

Plastics found in laminates can cause cyanide toxicity when burned and inhaled. Cyanide molecules undergo one of three possible reactions (Figure 16-8). When combined with cytochrome oxidase cyanide, toxicity occurs, as this portion of the electron transport chain is blocked and oxidative phosphorylation cannot occur. This prevents mitochondrial oxygen consumption and results in cell death. At 50 ppm cyanide, a patient experiences headache, dizziness, tachycardia, and tachypnea. Above 100 ppm cyanide, lethargy, seizures, and respiratory failure occur. Metabolic acidosis, cardiac dysrhythmias, increased mixed venous oxygen saturation, and pulmonary shunting are expected. Treatment consists of 100% oxygen delivered by face-mask, or mechanical ventilation. Pharmacologic treatment is aimed at pushing the reaction toward the formation of either methemoglobin, with resulting thiocyanate production, or cyanocobalamin, and away from the interaction of cyanide with cytochrome oxidase. Although methemoglobin does not transport oxygen, patients tolerate levels of up to 40%. Thus, treatments include sodium thiosulfate (150 mg/kg over 15 min) or 3% sodium nitrate (5 mg/kg over 5 min), which convert hemoglobin to methemoglobin. Hydroxocobalamin combines with cyanide to form cyanocobalamin or vitamin B$_{12}$. Thiocyanate is cleared via the kidneys, and toxicity may occur in patients with renal failure.

Fluid Replacement

Hypovolemic, or burn shock may occur immediately following injury. Normal and burned tissues have

CN- + methemoglobin → cyanomethemoglobin
CN- + thiosulfate → thiocyanate
CN- + cytochrome oxidase → cyanide toxicity

Figure 16-8 Cyanide molecule reactions in cyanide toxicity.

increased microvascular permeability in the first 12–24 hours, resulting in leakage of protein-rich fluid from the intravascular to the interstitial compartment. Subsequent tissue edema persists for at least 24 hours in nonburned tissues and over 72 hours in badly burned tissues. These fluid shifts, combined with decreased cardiac output due to circulating humoral factors, reduced responsiveness to circulating catecholamines, and decreased coronary blood flow, all contribute to the hypotension seen in the early postburn period.

The increased systemic vascular resistance may not adequately counteract these changes. Patients with low cardiac output, high systemic vascular resistance, and significant metabolic acidosis have reduced survival.

The late postburn period, occurring after 24–48 hours, is characterized by cytokine release with resultant increased cardiac output, reduced systemic vascular resistance, and increase in the metabolic rate, as is seen in the systemic inflammatory response syndrome. This picture is clinically similar to sepsis; however, no infectious agent can be identified from the blood and it is important not to treat with antibiotics.

Adequate fluid resuscitation can normalize cardiac output by 18–24 hours postinjury. Many formulas exist to calculate fluid requirements for patients during the initial resuscitation after a thermal injury. It is controversial whether any formula is superior, or whether colloid has advantages over crystalloid for fluid replacement. However, there is general consensus that fluid requirements are greater than expected, especially in children. Some advocate administering the calculated fluids to children under 4 years old in addition to their maintenance requirements. Crystalloids have the advantage of being simple, inexpensive, and provide an equivalent outcome when compared clinically to colloids. Hypertonic saline is sometimes used, although its safety has not been demonstrated.

The *Parkland Formula* for volume replacement is a simple calculation based on the TBSA burned. This formula requires 4 ml/kg/%TBSA burned, with one-half given in the first 8 hours and the remainder over the ensuing 16 hours. Good urine output should follow adequate fluid replacement (minimum 0.5 mL/kg/hr), as the kidney is the most poorly perfused organ in burn shock and its blood flow only increases after other vital organ perfusion is adequately achieved. Therefore, good renal function, with urine output as a crude indicator, is an overall indicator of adequate volume replacement and perfusion.

Renal failure may also occur due to the liberation of myoglobin from injured muscle. Without brisk urine flow, myoglobin is both directly toxic and precipitates in renal tubules, leading to acute tubular necrosis. Adding insult to injury, elevated levels of catecholamines, angiotensin, and vasopressin contribute to renal arterial vasoconstriction. The potential development of sepsis further promotes renal dysfunction. Prevention of acute renal failure requires vigorous fluid replacement, alkalinization of urine with bicarbonate, and brisk diuresis using loop diuretics such as furosemide. Mannitol may also have a role as a free radical scavenger. The mortality from acute renal failure in the burns patient is 73–100%.

Burn injuries rarely require fluid replacement with blood products. In the first 48 hours primarily noncellular fluid is translocated to the interstitium, causing a rise in hematocrit counterbalanced by resuscitative efforts. With the resulting normodilution, red cell transfusion is rarely necessary. Most patients with major burns eventually develop anemia due to multiple operations, phlebotomy, and chronic wound bleeding. Another suggested cause of anemia is a shortened erythrocyte half-life. Most patients without significant cardiovascular comorbidity tolerate this state and respond to iron supplementation. Thrombocytopenia is also common during the resuscitation period, although platelet counts return to normal by the end of the first week. Platelet replacement is rarely indicated for bleeding unless massive hemorrhage has occurred. Clotting factors are both diluted and consumed in the post burn period, because of fluid replacement and direct injury to blood vessels, which activates the intrinsic clotting pathway. Disseminated intravascular coagulation is a rare complication seen in deep and extensive burns. In the weeks after a major burn, patients are hypercoagulable as a result of elevated protein C, protein S, and antithrombin III levels. Prophylaxis is usually administered to prevent deep venous thrombosis and pulmonary embolism.

Standard monitors and a Foley catheter are adequate during the resuscitation of most burn patients; however, vital signs alone may remain normal in the face of severe hypovolemia. It may be technically difficult to use routine monitors such as electrocardiographic pads, so other devices, including needle electrodes, can be secured to the skin with a stapler. Invasive monitoring is appropriate in patients with cardiovascular disease, at extremes of age, or who are unresponsive to volume replacement and require inotropic support.

Pharmacology

It has been shown that burned patients have increased plasma protein binding of bases, including neuromuscular blockers. This may be due to hepatic dysfunction precipitating an increase in alpha-1-acid glycoprotein levels. This phenomenon, combined with upregulation in the number of junctional acetylcholine receptors, explains the increased doses of nondepolarizer muscle relaxants required. Reversal agents should be used liberally and titrated with the aid of a peripheral nerve stimulator.

Succinylcholine, when given 24–48 hours after a burn, can cause lethal hyperkalemia. Depolarization of upregulated extrajunctional acetylcholine receptors in burned tissue causes excessive muscle contraction and efflux of intracellular potassium relative to the size of the burn. Potassium levels as high as 10 mEq/L have been documented. This effect has been shown to persist for more than a year after the last burn has healed.

Anesthesia for the Burned Patient

The burned patient will undergo many surgical procedures and anesthetics. Full-thickness injuries will require extensive grafting in order to heal. Definitive treatment of partial-thickness burns involves removal of the eschar, which acts as a culture medium for bacterial growth. Surgical repair can be accomplished using full-thickness grafts, frequently taken from the groin or axilla, or split-thickness grafts from any viable site. Cosmetics, durability, and tissue bulk are improved with full-thickness grafts, although donor locations are limited. Regardless of the approach, early (within 7–10 days) excision of the eschar, and grafting, provides a decrease in infectious complications, leading to reduced hospitalization and earlier initiation of physical therapy.

The anesthetic technique should provide sedation, amnesia, analgesia, and hemodynamic stability. Airway concerns are discussed elsewhere in this chapter. Generally, balanced anesthesia using oxygen, narcotic, muscle relaxation, and volatile agent is employed. Significant blood loss should be anticipated and specific attention must be given to adequate ventilation, oxygenation, clearance of secretions, and renal preservation. With extremity burns, a tourniquet may be used to minimize blood loss.

Normothermia in the burned patient is approximately 38.5° C, which is due to resetting of the hypothalamic thermal regulatory center and postburn hypermetabolism. Hypothermia causes increased physiologic stress, decreased drug metabolism, increased bleeding complications, and poor wound healing. The room temperature should be raised to avoid an excessive cooling gradient; and heating blankets, fluid warmers, and humidified gases can all be employed to prevent hypothermia. Hemodynamic lability during early resuscitation is predictive of a more difficult intraoperative course. Additional hemodynamic monitoring is recommended in this scenario. High peak airway pressures can be anticipated during mechanical ventilation as a result of restrictive disease of the chest wall from contracting eschar, bronchospasm, pulmonary secretions, and possible pneumonia.

SUMMARY

Trauma and burns are leading causes of morbidity and mortality in the Unites States and the most common mechanism of death in young people. The anesthesiologist is frequently one of the first clinicians to evaluate and treat severe traumatic injuries. Successful initial evaluation, airway management, resuscitation, and specific organ preservation are all critical to patient survival in the first days after insult. While some controversies remain unresolved, such as the optimal fluids and formulas for resuscitation, improvements in prehospital care, standardization of ACLS protocols, expansion of transfusion medicine, and advances in diagnostic and therapeutic modalities have greatly improved survival in these difficult patients.

SUGGESTED READING

American College of Surgeons Committee on Trauma. Shock. *Advanced trauma and life support course for physicians*. Chicago: American College of Surgeons, 1993.

American College of Surgeons. *National Trauma Data Bank: Report 2002*. Available on-line at: http://www.facs.org/trauma/ntdb.html.

Avellino AM, Lam AM, Winn HR. Management of acute head injury. In: Albin MS. *Textbook of neuroanesthesia*. New York: McGraw-Hill, 1997:1137–1176.

Bendo AA, Kass IS, Hartung J, Cotrell JE. Anesthesia for neurosurgery. In: Barash PG, Cullen BF, Stoelting RK. *Clinical anesthesia*, 3rd ed. Philadelphia: Lippincott-Raven, 1997:699–746.

Biaz BB, Smok JT, Finucane BT, Abrams KJ. Thoracic trauma. In: Kaplan JA, Slinger, PD. *Thoracic anesthesia*, 3rd ed. Philadelphia: Churchill Livingstone, 2003:315–326.

Capan LM, Miller SM, Glickman R. Management of facial injuries. In: Capan LM, Miller SM, Turndorf H. *Trauma: anesthesia and intensive care*. Philadelphia: JB Lippincott, 1991:383.

Capan LM, Miller SM. Trauma and burns. In: Barash PG, Cullen BF, Stoelting RK. *Clinical anesthesia*, 3rd ed. Philadelphia: Lippincott-Raven, 1997:1173–1204.

Cicala RS, Grande CM, Stene JK, Behringer EC. Emergency and elective airway management for trauma patients. In: Grande CM. *Textbook of trauma anesthesia and critical care*. St Louis: CV Mosby, 1993:344–380.

Drummond JC, Patel PM. Neurosurgical anesthesia. In: Miller RD. *Anesthesia*, 5th ed. New York: Churchill Livingstone, 2000:1895–1934.

Fouche Y, Tarantino DP. Anesthesia considerations in chest trauma. *Chest Surg Clin North Am* 1997;7:227–238.

Goodwin CW, Finklestein JL, Madden MR. Burns. In: Schwartz SI. *Principles of surgery*. New York: McGraw-Hill, 1994:225–277.

Gotta AW. Maxillofacial trauma. In: Grande CM. *Textbook of trauma anesthesia and critical care*. St Louis: CV Mosby, 1993:529–539

Grande CM, Baskett PJF, Donchin Y, et al. Trauma anesthesia for disasters: anything, anytime, anywhere. *Crit Care Clin* 1991;7:1.

Hanowell LH. Perioperative management of thoracoabdominal trauma. In: Grande CM. *Textbook of trauma anesthesia and critical care*. St Louis: CV Mosby, 1993:559–582.

Hartman GS. Burns. In: Yao FF. *Anesthesiology: problem-oriented patient management*. Philadelphia: Lippincott-Raven, 1998:898–918.

Lee LA, Sharar SR, Lam AM. Perioperative head injury management in the multiply injured trauma patient. *Int Anesthesiol Clin* 2002;40:31–52.

Mackenzie CF, Geisler FH. Management of acute cervical spinal cord injury. In: Albin MS. *Textbook of neuroanesthesia*. New York: McGraw-Hill, 1997:1083–1136

MacLennan H, Heimbach DM, Cullen BF. Anesthesia for major thermal injury. *Anesthesiology* 1998;89:749–769.

Marshall LF. Head injury: recent past, present, and future. *Neurosurgery* 2000;47:546–561.

Morgan GE, Mikhail MS. *Clinical anesthesiology*, 2nd ed. Stamford, CT: Appleton & Lange, 1996: chs 5, 26, 29, 30, 41.

Nichols BJ, Cullen BF. Anesthesia for trauma. *J Clin Anesth* 1988;1:115–129.

O'Connor PJ, Russell JD, Moriarty DC. Anesthetic implications of laryngeal trauma. *Anesth Analg* 1998;87:1283–1284.

Prough DS, Mathru M. Acid base, fluids, and electrolytes. In: Barash PG, Cullen BF, Stoelting RK. *Clinical anesthesia*, 3rd ed. Philadelphia: Lippincott-Raven, 1997:157–188.

Stene JK, Grande CM. Anesthesia for trauma. In: Miller RD. *Anesthesia*, 5th ed. New York: Churchill Livingstone, 2000:2157–2172.

Stene JK. Anesthesia for the critically ill trauma patient. In: Siegel JA. *Trauma emergency surgery and critical care*. New York: Churchill Livingstone, 1987:843–862.

Wedel DJ, Horlocker TT. Orthopedic surgery. In: Barash PG, Cullen BF, Stoelting RK. *Clinical anesthesia*, 3rd ed. Philadelphia: Lippincott-Raven, 1997:1025–1038.

Wilkins EW. Noncardiovascular thoracic injuries: chest wall, bronchus, lung, esophagus, and diaphragm. In: Burke JF, Boyd RJ, McCabe CJ. *Trauma management: early management of visceral, nervous system, and musculoskeletal injuries*. St Louis: Mosby/Year Book, 1988:140–152.

CHAPTER 17

Anesthesia for Ophthalmic Surgery

M.S. BATRA

INTRODUCTION

Anesthesiology as a specialty is relatively new and its evolution is a testimonial to the vision and perseverance of pioneers in the field. History shows that anesthesia was developed by surgeons, as there were no anesthesiologists in the early part of its development. It did not take very long to recognize, however, that the provision of good and safe anesthetic care required another physician who was well versed in the disciplines that were essential to that practice. The very foundations of anesthesiology include knowledge of regional anatomy, physiology, pharmacology, physical principles, and internal medicine relevant to the perioperative period. Anesthesia, general or regional, as an anesthetic modality is best conducted by an anesthesiologist trained in the field.

There is no better representation of this concept than in the area of neuraxial anesthesia. Anesthesiologists are uniquely qualified to provide that care as they have mastered the art and science of that modality. Physicians spe-

cializing in neurosciences may be more qualified in the understanding and treatment of neurological anatomy, physiology, and disorders but they are not qualified when it comes to the subject of neuraxial anesthesia.

Ophthalmologists have traditionally delivered ophthalmic anesthesia because anesthesiologists have failed to embrace that field as part of our domain. The anatomical concepts are simple and the technical aspects can be learned very quickly. The principles of perioperative care are no different and the side effects and some of the complications require our expertise to modify the outcome. However, as we embark on this endeavor, it behoves us to exercise due diligence. We must learn and demonstrate that such practice will enhance patient care as it has in other areas of our specialty. It is imperative that we acquire a thorough knowledge of some of the unique features of the anatomy of the eye, its vascular supply, neural connections, and the surrounding structures, in and around the orbit. In addition, we need to understand the essential and relevant physiological functions and pharmacological principles that are peculiar to the eye.

ESSENTIAL ANATOMY FOR OPHTHALMIC ANESTHESIA

The globe is somewhat oblong and the axial length (from the anteriormost surface of the cornea to the posterior pole of the globe) is normally about 22–24 mm. Knowledge of this parameter is essential prior to embarking on an approach that curves the needle behind the globe (e.g. retrobulbar or intraconal block). This length is longer in myopic patients and places them at higher risk of globe perforation during peribulbar/retrobulbar needle placements. The sclera, the outermost layer of the eye, is a tough structure primarily made up of collagen and elastic fibers. The thickness of the sclera varies around the globe; it measures around 1 mm in its thickest parts.

Myopic eyes typically have a thinner sclera. Unfortunately, it is easy to penetrate these thin parts with a misdirected needle and the results naturally are catastrophic.

The cornea, forming a smaller sphere than the rest of the globe, is a delicate and transparent membrane. It is about 1 mm thick with thinning in the central region. The transparent cornea is kept moist by tears and the blinking action. During surgery, active blinking being absent, the delicate cornea becomes quite vulnerable. The epithelium of the cornea is somewhat resistant to chemicals but also can be damaged easily. Various agents, including local anesthetics, affect repair of the damaged cornea. Excessive use of topical agents should therefore be avoided. Nourishment for the outer layers of the cornea comes from the tears and the inner layers from the aqueous humor. This liquid is an ultrafiltrate of plasma, secreted by the ciliary body, and is absorbed via the trabeculae into the canal of Schlemm. This is the site of surgery to improve drainage during glaucoma.

The ciliary body consists of the posterior muscular part, the pars plana, and the anterior part, the pars plicata. The latter secretes aqueous humor whereas the former provides an avenue for the various surgical approaches to the vitreous and the retina.

The four ribbon-shaped extraocular recti muscles (superior, medial, inferior, and lateral) diverge from their posterior attachment to the fibrous ring, the annulus, and attach to the corresponding surfaces of the globe near the equator. An intermuscular fascia connects their margins to each other. This anatomical configuration leads to the formation of a cone-like structure in the retrobulbar area. Injection into this cone is classically termed intraconal or retrobulbar and outside the cone, extraconal or peribulbar in nature. It has long been recognized, but not well appreciated, that the intermuscular fascia bridging the recti is a somewhat incomplete structure allowing drugs and solutions to pass between the extraconal and intraconal compartments. Most of the muscles receive their innervation on the inner surface and therefore the onset of neural blockade is much more rapid when local anesthetic is deposited inside the cone.

The superior, medial, and inferior recti and inferior oblique muscles are supplied by the oculomotor nerve (III cranial nerve), while the lateral rectus receives its supply from the abducens nerve (VI cranial nerve). The superior oblique muscle, supplied by the trochlear nerve (IV cranial nerve), receives its innervation over the outer and lateral surface. The sensory innervation to most of the eye structures (cornea, sclera, iris, ciliary body, lens capsule, etc.) is in the ciliary nerves that traverse the small ciliary ganglion situated on the lateral side of the optic nerve inside the cone. Placement of local anesthetic close to these nerves (an intraconal approach), once again produces a very rapid neural blockade. Deposition of drugs and agents outside the cone (the various periconal and sub-Tenon's approaches) produce a sensory-

motor block that is slow in onset and not always complete. The delay and incompleteness is simply based on anatomical distances and tissue barriers that exist in some patients. The fact that the drugs eventually get there in most instances is also significant, in that the partitions are not complete. Such barriers exist even within the cone, as perfect placement of solution can on occasion fail to block all the nerves.

There are two other innervations around the eye that are worth considering. It is not well appreciated that the branches of the ophthalmic division of the trigeminal nerve (V cranial nerve) innervate the conjunctiva, covering the anterior aspect of the sclera. Most surgical incisions, however, are made through this membrane and typically antibiotics and other drugs are injected into the subconjunctival space. This tissue and surrounding area are highly sensitive and local anesthetic frequently fails to reach the nerves supplying this layer following an intraconal injection. These nerves can be blocked separately with small volumes of local anesthetics placed very superficially at the supraorbital and infraorbital nerves, or simply by topical instillation.

The other structures of importance are the eyelids, which need to be immobile (not blinking) during surgery on a patient who is awake. The blinking activity (which is often exaggerated because of anxiety) is a function of the orbicularis oculi muscle (innervation derived from the facial nerve – VII cranial nerve). The ocular branches of this nerve are generally spared following an intraconal injection, necessitating a separate block. Interestingly, both the conjunctiva and the orbicularis oculi are variably blocked following extraconal and sub-Tenon's injections. The degree and completeness of the block of these structures seems to depend upon the amount of local anesthetic and solution injected. One way to effect a block of these tissues during an intraconal injection is to inject some of the solution during the needle withdrawal phase, depositing local anesthetic in the periconal region.

External to the extraocular muscles is a fascial plane called the Tenon's capsule. This is a relatively dense layer enveloping the globe and extraocular muscles. It extends from the limbus to the optic nerve. All the muscles penetrate this capsule, with the recti muscles typically entering just behind the equator. The capsule anterior to the muscular penetrations is called the anterior portion and extends to the limbus. The posterior portion, behind the muscular penetrations, is thin and closely apposes the sclera with no discernible sub-Tenon's space. The anterior Tenon's capsule and sclera are separated by the intermuscular septum (the fascia between the recti). This capsule and the intermuscular septum fuse to form one fascial layer about 3 mm from the limbus, which then fuses with conjunctiva next to the limbus.

A conjunctival incision about 5 mm from the limbus allows passage through Tenon's capsule and the intermuscular septum separately to reach the sub-Tenon's or episcleral region. This, being closer to the equator, also allows easier reach towards the posterior aspect of the globe. An injection in this narrow space allows the solution to spread circumferentially and posteriorly to affect the nerves within the cone. Depending upon the volume and agents injected, adequate diffusion will produce anesthesia of the conjunctiva and the orbicularis oculi muscles as well. This is not always the case, as the failure rate is higher with extraconal injections (classical peribulbar or sub-Tenon's blunt cannula) than with the intraconal approach.

The part of the orbit behind the globe narrows towards its apex, where vital structures (optic nerve, ophthalmic artery, etc.) are packed in a narrow space. Needle advancement into this area is fraught with danger as these delicate conduits/fibers can get easily damaged by direct needle trauma or by external compression from injected solutions.

The optic nerve in the orbit is typically surrounded by the intracranial meninges and the intracranial subarachnoid space communicates with the narrow orbital extension allowing passage of drugs centrally if a needle accidentally penetrates the optic nerve coverings. Fortunately the optic nerve travels in the medial part of the orbit and joins the posterior part of the globe about 3 mm medial to its posterior pole. Therefore, a retrobulbar injection should approach the cone from its inferolateral aspect and the tip of the needle must never cross the midpupillary plane (in a neutral gaze).

The globe, being a sphere, has an equator. Knowing the approximate location of this dimension is very important while performing eye blocks. During neutral gaze, the equator lies parallel to the coronal plane of the body, whereas the anterior window of its housing, the orbital opening, lies at a tangential plane to the plane of the equator. The orbital opening slants backwards as it slopes laterally. The significance of this slant is that, in the lateral part, the equator of the globe is at, slightly behind, or slightly in front of the lateral orbital rim. This unique anatomical feature makes it an ideal site for introduction of a needle directed towards the posterior aspect of the globe (Figure 17-1).

THE OCULOCARDIAC REFLEX

Slowing of the heart via vagal stimulation secondary to various stimuli (that travel through the ciliary and trigeminal nerves) around the globe is the hallmark of this phenomenon. Pressure over the eyeball or traction on the extraocular muscles are common causes. The reflex can be modified by anticholinergics and abolished by blocking the afferent pathways following various bulbar blocks.

REGIONAL VERSUS GENERAL ANESTHESIA

The salient issues regarding the choice of a regional or general anesthetic for ophthalmic surgery are summarized in Table 17-1.

LOCAL ANESTHETIC PHARMACOLOGY – SALIENT ASPECTS

Topical Local Anesthetics

Topically applied local anesthetics have a rapid onset of action (less than 20 sec). Most agents produce a stinging sensation on instillation followed by corneoconjunctival anesthesia. The stinging can be reduced by diluting the first few drops with balanced salt solution before proceeding with the full strength. Contrary to common belief, the duration of most local anesthetics (even longer-acting agents such as tetracaine) is quite brief (10–15 min). This is due to washout by tears and other irrigating solutions used during surgery. The effects of cocaine are somewhat longer but the agent is ultimately toxic to corneal epithelium. Other long-acting agents also produce corneal toxicity with prolonged usage.

Common topical agents in use today are:

- *Lidocaine*: 4%, isotonic, least toxic to corneal epithelium, moderate stinging
- *Proparacaine*: 0.5%, ester-linked agent, less stinging, intermediate corneal toxicity
- *Tetracaine*: 0.5%, somewhat slower onset, causes more stinging. Otherwise it is a good agent.

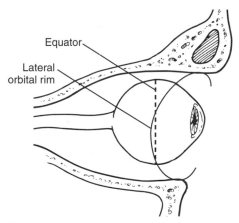

Figure 17-1   The orbital opening viewed from the side. The outward slant shows that the lateral aspect is posterior, relative to the other margins. Note that the equator of the globe is at or near the rim in this area. A needle entering the orbit at its inferolateral angle is immediately beyond the equator, protecting the globe from perforation.

Equator

Lateral
orbital rim

Table 17-1   Advantages and Disadvantages of Regional and General Anesthesia for Ophthalmic Surgery

Issue	Regional Anesthesia	General Anesthesia
Surgical conditions	Adequate for most procedures	Adequate for all procedures
Complexity	Simple	Complicated, with many steps
Oculocardiac reflex	Blocked	Intact and frequently active
Hemodynamic stability	Very stable	Can be unstable without special steps
Airway	No control required	Control required, with all the potential drawbacks
Recovery	Fast	Long
Baseline mental state	Maintained	Slow to return
Nausea/vomiting	Absent	High incidence
Postoperative analgesia	Usually prolonged	None
Significant retrobulbar hemorrhage	Possible but uncommon	Absent
Globe perforation	Possible but rare	Absent
Damage to extraocular muscles	Possible	Absent
Other perioperative complications	None	Possible and not uncommon
Turnover time	Minimal	Variable and can be long
Cost	Minimal	Higher

Common Injectable Local Anesthetics

Common injectable local anesthetics in use today are:
- *Lidocaine*: Commonly used in combination with bupivacaine where the ultimate concentration of lidocaine is 1% and that of bupivacaine 0.375%. The surgical anesthesia with this mixture is primarily produced by lidocaine, with some enhancement provided by the longer-acting bupivacaine. The latter agent, however, is responsible for prolonged postoperative analgesia. If lidocaine is used alone, a concentration of 2% is preferred for a longer duration.
- *Bupivacaine*: An excellent agent for surgical anesthesia. A concentration of 0.5% is adequate for sensory and motor blockade of long duration. A higher concentration, 0.75%, has the potential for producing central neural toxicity when the drug finds its way intracranially via the meningeal coverings of the optic nerve.

Other agents, such as *mepivacaine* for intermediate duration and *etidocaine* or *ropivacaine* for long duration, are excellent substitutes.

It is important to remember that injection of local anesthetics directly into the extraocular or eyelid muscles can produce myotoxicity with permanent weakness. The muscles are especially vulnerable to longer-acting agents.

Hyaluronidase is an excellent agent to enhance local anesthetic spread around the eyeball. When added to most local anesthetic mixtures in a concentration of 7.5–15 units/mL it speeds the onset of action and improves the quality of both sensory and motor block.

This property seems to be peculiar to its ophthalmic application.

Addition of *epinephrine* to enhance neural blockade and prolong duration of anesthesia has been employed in regional anesthesia in many of its applications. Unfortunately, the vascular supply to the globe is via the retinal artery, which is an end-artery. Epinephrine in this situation may produce vasoconstriction, which can have adverse effects on already compromised vision. Use of epinephrine as a general rule, therefore, is not recommended for ophthalmic regional anesthesia.

REGIONAL ANESTHESIA

Retrobulbar (Intraconal) Block

Regional anesthesia, as an extension of topical anesthesia, was introduced into clinical medicine in 1884 by Knapp (an ophthalmologist). He injected cocaine into the retrobulbar area to enucleate an eye. Atkinson, introducing many safety features, including the use of procaine and epinephrine, modified the technique of retrobulbar block. The block remains in use today because of its extremely rapid onset and near-complete ocular anesthesia (sensory, motor, and autonomic) with the use of a minimal volume of local anesthetic mixture. The technique is associated with a few serious complications that have led to the development of alternative techniques. These complications are rare and proponents of the continued use of the retrobulbar block stress the importance of absolutely meticulous execution by practitioners well versed in regional anatomy.

The injection is typically given at the junction of the lateral third and medial two-thirds of the infraorbital rim. The needle can be introduced percutaneously or through the conjunctiva (which can be topically anesthetized prior to injection). The position of the globe should be in neutral gaze (looking straight ahead) and a 38 mm 25–27-gauge flat-grind (Atkinson's) needle is directed posteriorly and medially towards a point behind the center of the pupil. Immediately after passing the infraorbital rim the needle is deflected cephalad in a semicircular motion to traverse around the globe and penetrate the musculofascial cone. It is important to point the needle bevel towards the globe for it to slide over the sclera in case of contact, and the tip of the needle must not cross the midpupillary point to protect the optic nerve and its meningeal coverings (Figure 17-2). When the needle contacts the musculofascial cone the eye deflects in a downward and outward direction and falls into neutral position upon penetration of the cone. Excessive movement of the globe and undue resistance during slow-needle advancement signals eyeball contact and the needle should be immediately withdrawn.

Hamilton has suggested a modification of the classical technique. This approach calls for the needle to be introduced further laterally, at the junction of the inferior and the lateral orbital rim (Figure 17-3). The advancing needle passes through a relatively avascular area in the orbit, between the lateral and the inferior rectus muscles. This will also avoid damaging the inferior rectus and inferior oblique muscles.

The volume of local anesthetic required is generally small, approximately 3 mL. It may be necessary to inject up to 5 mL in younger patients.

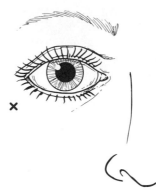

Figure 17-3   Point of entry (X) for a retrobulbar block (modified approach).

Peribulbar (Periconal) Block

Davis and Mandel first introduced the peribulbar block into practice in 1986. The impetus for the introduction of this alternative technique was from a desire to reduce the serious complications associated with the use of the traditional retrobulbar (intraconal) technique. They advocated two posterior injections at a depth of 35 mm, one above and the other below the globe (Figure 17-4). The volume of solution injected is considerably larger (usually around 10 mL) than the retrobulbar approach and is characterized by the following advantages:

- The incidence of serious complications is lower.
- Anesthesia of the facial nerve develops from diffusion of local anesthetic to the lid muscles, obviating the need to block that nerve separately.
- Conjunctival anesthesia is superior, as innervation to this tissue comes from branches of the ophthalmic division of the trigeminal nerve that are traveling in the extraconal space.

However, there are several disadvantages:

- The onset is slow (may take up to 30 min for complete spread).
- The failure rate is very high, requiring supplementation after a lengthy delay.
- Associated with unsightly chemosis.
- Incidence of extraocular muscle damage is greater.
- Serious complications (globe perforation, orbital hemorrhage, retinal artery spasm, etc.) still occur.

Various modifications have been introduced since its initial introduction. Bloomberg promoted a single injection to a depth of 20 mm (less than an inch), of 8–10 mL in the inferotemporal region, directed towards the orbital floor, with a success rate of 95%. Others have not been able to achieve similar success rates. Most modifications still rely on two injections. Hamilton suggests the use of injections in the least vascular areas, one adjacent to the lower end of the temporal orbital rim and the other medial to the inner canthus. He advocates the use of short, fine needles

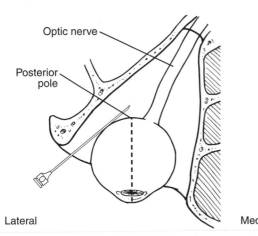

Optic nerve

Posterior pole

Lateral   Medial

Figure 17-2   After penetrating the muscular cone during a retrobulbar injection, the needle tip must not project beyond the midpoint of the pupil (in neutral gaze). This precaution is necessary to avoid injury as well as entry into the submeningeal spaces surrounding the optic nerve.

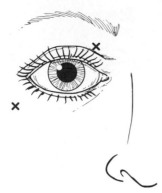

Figure 17-4 Points of entry (X) for a peribulbar block (classic two-injection technique).

(25–27-gauge and no longer than 25 mm, or about 1 in) that are introduced parallel to the orbital walls.

Sub-Tenon's Anesthesia

Several innovations have been introduced over the years with the goal of totally avoiding the use of a needle that can potentially produce major problems. The most significant among them is the deposition of local anesthetic into the sub-Tenon's space via a blunt cannula that is introduced through a small opening in the conjunctiva made under topical anesthesia. Greenbaum in the United States and Stevens in the United Kingdom independently introduced their technique of a sub-Tenon's block in 1992. Greenbaum used a very small volume of 2 mL, claiming total success in a small group of 50 patients. Others have not been able to achieve such good results and the degree of motor block has been found to be directly proportional to the volume of local anesthetic injected. The best results have been associated with the use of 4–5 mL of a local anesthetic mixture, which is often uncomfortable in awake patients. Complications (predominantly hemorrhage, chemosis, and damage to important venous channels) continue to occur with variable frequency and patients often need intraoperative sedation.

New and Innovative Approaches

Regional anesthesia as a primary modality during ophthalmic surgery is more suited to shorter procedures. The main reason is that surgical anesthesia from most blocks lasts a finite period of time. This is because most practitioners have stopped using long-acting local anesthetics in high concentrations (e.g. 0.75% bupivacaine), as central intracranial spread, albeit uncommon, has produced catastrophic results. Most surgical blocks last about 1.5–2 hours even when bupivacaine is added to the mixture, as its concentration is usually not greater than 0.375%. This produces good analgesia but not surgical anesthesia. The other local anesthetics most commonly used, and responsible for the surgical block, are lidocaine or mepivacaine.

To extend the block beyond a limited period, Jonas and colleagues have recently introduced a catheter technique. They employed a 28-gauge spinal microcatheter that was commercially available (in Europe) and would easily pass through an 0.8 mm (outer diameter), 38 mm long retrobulbar needle, and placed in the intraconal region. They were able to intermittently inject through the catheter to extend surgical anesthesia as well as provide postoperative analgesia until the next morning. This approach definitely warrants further study, as:

- Somewhat longer procedures can thus be managed with regional anesthesia
- Prolonged postoperative analgesia can be effected
- Some of the postoperative problems (e.g., prolonged nausea due to ocular pain) can be avoided.

Other workers have reported similar limited work with the peribulbar (Bernard and Hommeril) and sub-Tenon's (Behndig) approach.

TOPICAL ANESTHESIA

It is interesting to note that, when local anesthetics were first introduced into medical practice, the initial application was in the field of ophthalmology. Cocaine enjoyed that enviable role for a while but eventually it was found to be too toxic to the cornea, and its absorption following large doses produced systemic toxicity. It also became quickly apparent that topical application provided patient comfort for only a limited number of procedures. Surgical conditions with injectable regional anesthesia were found to be far superior and what was not possible with injectable techniques could be easily managed with general anesthesia.

However, serious complications associated with the injectable techniques, albeit rare, have provided an impetus for the resurgence of topical anesthesia. The newer agents are less toxic, locally and systemically, and improvements in the technical aspects of cataract removal have made this mode of anesthesia the norm in many centers.

It is noteworthy that topical application of local anesthetics provides only corneoconjunctival anesthesia. Other limitations include:

- No anesthesia of the deeper structures (e.g. iris, ciliary apparatus, lens capsule, etc.).
- The globe is not immobile, as the extraocular muscles are unaffected.
- The blinking of eyelids is active, as the orbicularis oculi is not blocked.
- Vision remains intact, making it difficult for the patient to look into the bright light during the procedure.
- Lack of complete anesthesia necessitates patient selection and sedation which may be problematic.

Surgically, some modifications in the technique are also required that are not always easy for the surgeons to adopt. Needless to say, many ophthalmologists are using the technique successfully with conscious sedation.

COMPLICATIONS OF INJECTABLE BLOCK TECHNIQUES

Complications are rare but can be very serious. Significant ones are:

- Retrobulbar hemorrhage
- Spread to brain-stem areas
- Globe perforation
- Damage to the optic nerve
- Oculocardiac reflex

Bleeding in the area behind the eye is not that uncommon, but significant hemorrhage that might affect visual function is rare. Damage to the veins is associated with hematoma formation, and gentle pressure following injection limits its development. The occurrence of this adverse event is perhaps frequent yet of minimal significance. When bleeding occurs rapidly it usually signifies arterial trauma, and tension behind the globe can build up quickly. This latter complication is relatively rare and close monitoring and prompt decompression will ameliorate the problem. Surgery may have to be postponed if the orbital pressure remains high. This can occur with any injection technique.

Central spread to the brain stem is a very rare complication that can develop rather quickly, within about 2 min or may be delayed by as much as 15 minutes. It can manifest in a myriad of ways and the development of symptoms or signs other than ipsilateral ocular effects should alert one to its possibility. The clinical manifestations could include changes in level of consciousness, a variety of neural signs and symptoms (pupillary dilation on the side opposite to where the block is being attempted, generalized muscular hypotonia, etc.), and unusual cardiorespiratory events. The untoward effects generally last about 2–4 hours, or longer when longer-acting local anesthetics are used. The likely mechanism for this complication is injection into the coverings of the optic nerve, which provide a direct pathway to intracranial spaces and hence to areas of the central nervous system. Recovery from this complication is complete as a rule, provided the condition is recognized in time and supportive treatment is provided until recovery. This complication is unique to retrobulbar injection and therefore deep penetration, more than 31 mm beyond the infraorbital rim, is not recommended.

Globe perforation is not a frequent complication but probably occurs with greater frequency than perceived. The degree of needle trauma to the globe can vary in severity from scleral penetration only to entry and exit out of the globe. The injury to the eye will depend upon the nature of the perforation. A knowledge of the axial length prior to injection, due diligence during needle advancement, and not injecting when resistance or pain is encountered are paramount towards prevention of this complication. It is perhaps important to consider that injury to the globe can occur with minimal penetration into the orbit, if the needle is misdirected. Acute angulation towards the globe early during advancement can lead to scleral contact. Larger and blunter needles may lead to greater trauma. It is worth remembering that the sclera is not uniform in its thickness especially in elongated globe with axial length greater than 25 mm. Moreover, myopic eyes have a much thinner sclera.

The optic nerve can be damaged either directly by the needle or by pressure from a rapidly forming hematoma that produces vascular compromise. During the execution of an ocular block, the needle should never cross the mid-pupillary point and the length of the needle in the orbit must not exceed 31 mm. A 38 mm needle (the common length available) should never be buried into the orbit.

Bradycardia associated with stimulation of the oculocardiac reflex should be an extremely rare occurrence during the execution of an eye block. Strong vagal stimulation follows traction of extraocular muscles or when undue pressure is applied over the globe. This can occur even when the patient is deeply sedated or under general anesthesia. While blocking the eye such manipulations are generally not necessary; therefore the bradyarrhythmias encountered are usually due to a vasovagal phenomenon in an anxious or uncomfortable patient. Proper sedation and painless conditions while performing the block will prevent this complication.

GENERAL ANESTHESIA

It is not in the scope of this chapter to review general anesthesia in great detail. Salient and important considerations during its application in ophthalmic surgery are as follows.

- Intraocular pressure can increase quickly and measures should be taken to minimize its occurrence. Factors that cause the pressure to increase acutely include: hypoxia, hypercarbia, pressure on the globe, succinylcholine, ketamine, laryngoscopy, coughing, and other situations associated with the Valsalva maneuver.
- Use of nitrous oxide should be avoided when the surgeon plans to leave an air bubble in the eye following surgeries such as vitrectomy.
- The oculocardiac reflex should be prevented or treated promptly with anticholinergics.
- Nausea and vomiting are common and protracted after ophthalmic surgery under general anesthesia.

Appropriate measures (including eye blocks) should be taken to minimize this unpleasant condition.

- Use of a laryngeal mask for airway management should be considered as it obviates airway manipulations and stimulations that can be detrimental to a patient undergoing eye surgery. This holds true at induction and at the end of anesthesia.

SUMMARY

It is readily apparent that anesthetic care for ophthalmic surgery requires a thorough knowledge of pertinent regional anatomy, physiology, and pharmacology. Regional anesthesia is a highly effective and safe modality for most ophthalmic surgical procedures. Complications are uncommon and largely avoidable with meticulous technique. Regional anesthesia offers many advantages, as the patients are generally older, suffer from many other ailments and most surgical procedures are performed in an ambulatory setting. The choice of regional technique should largely be based on the experience of the individual administering the block. In a given patient, when regional anesthetic is not appropriate, general anesthesia can be administered safely.

Case Study

An anxious 79-year-old patient presents for extracapsular cataract extraction and implantation of an intraocular lens. Significant medical problems include a complete heart block, for which the patient has a sequential pacemaker in place, chronic obstructive pulmonary disease, type II diabetes, and protracted nausea and vomiting following general anesthesia in the past. She uses an inhaler frequently and takes metformin for her diabetes. She appears to be totally pacemaker-dependent, S_pO_2 on room air is 92% and her fasting blood sugar is 178 mg/dL. Her ocular axial length is 26 mm.

- What special preoperative measures are required?
- What would be the anesthetic modality of choice?
- How should her diabetes be managed?
- How should her anxiety be managed perioperatively?

SUGGESTED READING

Atkinson WS. Retrobulbar injection of anesthetic within the muscular cone (cone injection). *Arch Ophthalmol* 1936; 16:494.

Atkinson WS. The development of ophthalmic anesthesia: the Sanford R. Gifford Lecture. *Am J Ophthalmol* 1961; 51:1-14.

Bloomberg LB. Anterior periocular anesthesia: five years experience. *J Cataract Refract Surg* 1991;17:508-511.

Davis DB II, Mandel MR. Posterior peribulbar anesthesia: an alternative to retrobulbar anesthesia. *J Cataract Refract Surg* 1986;12:182-184.

Freidman DS, Bass EB, Lubomski LH, *et al*. Synthesis of the literature on the effectiveness of regional anesthesia for cataract surgery. *Ophthalmology* 2001;108:519-529.

Greenbaum S. Parabulbar anesthesia. *Am J Ophthalmol* 1992; 114:776.

Grizzard WS. Ophthalmic anesthesia. In: Reinecke RD, ed. *Ophthalmology annual*. New York: Raven Press, 1989: 265-294.

Hamilton RC, Gimbel HV, Strunin L. Regional anaesthesia for 12,000 cataract extractions and intraocular lens implantation procedures. *Can J Anaesth* 1988; 35: 615-623.

Jonas JB, Jager M, Hemmerling TM. Continuous retrobulbar anesthesia for scleral buckling surgery using an ultra-fine spinal anesthesia catheter. *Can J Anesth* 2002;49: 487-489.

Konstantatos A. Anticoagulation and cataract surgery: a review of the current literature. *Anaesth Intensive Care* 2001;29: 11-18.

Koornneef L. The architecture of the musculo-fibrous apparatus in the human orbit. *Acta Morphol Neerl-Scand* 1977;15: 35-64.

Nicoll JM, Treuren B, Acharya PA, *et al*. Retrobulbar anesthesia: the role of hyaluronidase. *Anesth Analg* 1986;65: 1324-1328.

Stevens JD. A new local anaesthesia technique for cataract extraction by one quadrant sub-Tenon's infiltration. *Br J Ophthalmol* 1992;76:670-674.

CHAPTER 18

Anesthesia for Ear, Nose, and Throat Surgery

LAUREN C. BERKOW

INTRODUCTION

The wide variety of patient populations and types of surgical procedures in ear, nose, and throat (ENT) surgery can provide a challenge to the anesthesiologist. A large subgroup of these procedures involve infants and children, some of whom may present with complicated congenital syndromes. Adult patients presenting for ENT procedures may have coexisting medical conditions requiring evaluation.

Any patient scheduled for an ENT procedure may potentially be a difficult mask ventilation or intubation. A high degree of suspicion, thorough airway evaluation, and proper advance planning are vital in order to provide safe and efficient anesthesia. Even if a difficult airway is not suspected, it is safest to proceed with intubation with the ENT surgeon present in the operating room.

The ultimate goal during anesthesia for ENT surgery is to provide a safe balance between ideal surgical conditions and the safety of the patient. Anesthesia should provide a safe intubation as well as a timely and smooth extubation of the patient.

PEDIATRIC EAR, NOSE, AND THROAT PROCEDURES

Ear, nose, and throat procedures are among the more common surgical procedures performed on the pediatric population. Many of these procedures are performed on healthy children in an outpatient setting, while others may involve children with significant medical issues or congenital anomalies.

Some significant differences exist between the airway anatomy of the pediatric and adult populations (Table 18-1). These differences may have a significant impact on how the pediatric airway is managed. In addition, certain anomalies, such as cleft lip and palate, papillomas, and laryngomalacia, are much more commonly encountered in the pediatric population. Certain pediatric congenital syndromes are associated with difficulties in ventilation and intubation, and special preparations should be undertaken in these patients (Table 18-2).

Most children presenting for routine ENT procedures should have a complete history and physical examination, in particular focusing on symptoms such as snoring, airway obstruction, stridor, and recent symptoms of a upper respiratory infection. Many of these patients have chronic upper respiratory infections, so it should be at the discretion of the anesthesiologist as to whether symptomatology is significant enough to postpone the procedure. Whether a child with an ongoing upper respiratory infection should undergo anesthesia is still controversial. Often these children will continue to have recurrent infections until the problem is surgically corrected.

Current Controversies: When to Cancel a Pediatric Patient with Upper Respiratory Symptoms

Proceed if:	Cancel if:
Lungs clear, no wheezing or rhonchi	Presence of wheezing, decreased lung sounds
Absence of fever or chills	Presence of fever or chills
Patient not clinically toxic appearing	Patient toxic appearing
Emergent surgery	Purulent nasal discharge (controversial)

Tonsillectomy and Adenoidectomy

These two procedures are often performed simultaneously. Young children with recurrent tonsillitis or tonsillar hyperplasia are candidates for this procedure. Enlargement of adenoid tissue can lead to nasopharyngeal obstruction or chronic infection. Patients with enlarged tonsils and/or adenoids may develop airway obstruction, leading to sleep apnea. This may be mild, presenting only during sleep, or significant enough that the child develops airway obstruction while awake. Significant sleep apnea can lead to chronic hypoxemia and hypercarbia, which over time can lead to right ventricular hypertrophy and pulmonary hypertension. Fortunately, these sequelae are often reversible after surgical repair. In patients with severe obstructive sleep apnea, intravenous induction should be considered, since inhalational induction may lead to significant obstruction and an inability to ventilate.

The goals of anesthesia during tonsillectomy and adenoidectomy are adequate anesthesia and analgesia as well as optimal surgical conditions. Oral RAE tubes are often used, providing better oral access for the surgeons and easier placement of their retractors. Compared to a standard endotracheal tube, the oral RAE tube is curved at a 90° angle towards the patient's chin. The tube can be secured to the chin as opposed to the upper lip, allowing better surgical preparation and access to the mouth and nose. Intravenous access is required for these procedures and is often achieved after inhalational induction. Premedication may be used as needed to make the experience more pleasant for the child but should be used cautiously or avoided if sleep apnea or airway obstruction is present. Intravenous placement prior to induction of anesthesia may also be considered in sleep apnea patients. Allowing a parent to remain in the operating room until inhalational induction is completed may be helpful and improve cooperation of the child.

Standard monitors, including blood pressure, electrocardiogram, pulse oximetry, and end-tidal carbon dioxide monitoring, plus a precordial stethoscope, are routinely employed. The esophageal stethoscope is particularly important as the airway will be shared with the surgeon and the endotracheal tube can become dislodged, kinked, or clotted with blood or secretions during the procedure.

Table 18-1   Differences Between the Adult and Pediatric Airway

	Adult Airway	Pediatric Airway
Larynx	More caudad	More cephalad, slanted downward
Vocal cords	Perpendicular to trachea	Angled to axis of trachea
Narrowest part of airway	Glottis	Cricoid cartilage
Location of glottis	C5–C6	C3–C4 or higher
Epiglottis	Shorter, wider	Longer, more rigid, U-shaped

Children have large tongues compared to the size of their mouths, as well as more prominent tonsils and adenoids, making vocal cord visualization potentially more difficult.

Table 18-2   Pediatric Congenital Syndromes Associated with Difficult Ventilation/Intubation

Pierre Robin syndrome	Micrognathia, glossoptosis (large obstructing tongue), cleft palate; difficult intubation; often develop sleep apnea; often require tracheostomy or mandibular osteotomy at an early age
Treacher Collins syndrome (mandibulofacial dysostosis)	Mandibular hypoplasia, malar hypoplasia; 30% have cleft palate; also often very difficult intubation
Goldenhar syndrome (hemifacial microsomia)	Maxillary, mandibular, and malar hypoplasia, temporal-mandibular joint malformation; may have associated cervical spine malformations; very difficult intubation

Emergence from anesthesia after tonsillectomy should be smooth and fairly rapid, and the child should be awake and alert prior to removal of the endotracheal tube. The stomach should be emptied prior to emergence to reduce the risk of aspiration as well as of postoperative emesis. These patients are often placed in the lateral position after extubation to prevent blood from entering the pharynx. Potential complications after extubation include laryngospasm, airway obstruction, aspiration, and vomiting (often due to blood in the airway or stomach). Delayed complications include bleeding, pharyngeal edema, pain, emesis, and pulmonary edema if preoperative airway obstruction was significant or long-standing.

Ear Surgery

Pediatric patients commonly present for myringotomy and tube placement as a result of recurrent otitis media. These procedures are fairly short, often done in the outpatient setting, and can usually be performed under mask anesthesia with or without intravenous placement. These patients often have chronic associated upper respiratory infections. Premedication is usually avoided because of the short duration of the procedure. If the procedure is performed without an intravenous line, intranasal fentanyl (2 μg/kg) can be used for intraoperative and postoperative pain management.

Tympanoplasty and mastoidectomy may also be performed in children. These procedures are longer in duration, usually requiring endotracheal intubation and intravenous placement. Facial nerve monitoring may be employed by the surgeons, prohibiting the use of skeletal muscle relaxants.

Drug Interactions: Nitrous Oxide

Use should be avoided in ear surgery
Can cause an increase in negative pressure in the middle ear
Associated with postoperative nausea and vomiting after ear procedures

Cleft Lip and Cleft Palate Repair

Cleft lip and palate may occur alone or in association with a variety of congenital syndromes, some of which are listed in Table 18-2. Some of these syndromes may be associated with difficult ventilation or intubation, although an isolated cleft palate may also lead to difficult intubation or ventilation. Airway obstruction or laryngospasm may occur during induction. Cleft lip repair is usually performed around the age of 1-2 months, while cleft palate

repair is performed around the age of 1 year to promote normal speech development. These patients are at risk of aspiration and pneumonia because of their inability to feed normally. Nasal trumpets or tongue stitches may be placed during the repair to prevent postoperative airway obstruction.

Induction of anesthesia is usually performed by mask inhalation, followed by intravenous placement and muscle paralysis after ventilation is secured. Routine monitors, as described previously, are employed, including a precordial stethoscope. Oral RAE tubes are often used for these procedures to allow the surgeon easier access to the oropharynx. Beware of the endotracheal tube becoming dislodged or kinked during the procedure.

Local anesthetics containing epinephrine may be infused into the surgical site during the procedure, which can lead to hypertension or arrhythmias due to systemic absorption. Pharyngeal packs are used intraoperatively, which can lead to postoperative airway obstruction if they are not removed prior to extubation. Postoperative pharyngeal edema can also lead to laryngospasm and airway obstruction. Extubation should be performed when the patient is fully awake and alert.

ADULT EAR, NOSE, AND THROAT PROCEDURES

Parotid Surgery

Parotid surgery is usually performed for benign or malignant tumors. Large tumors may lead to decreased jaw mobility or mouth opening, potentially causing difficulty in intubation. Because of the relationship between the parotid gland and the facial nerve, intraoperative nerve monitoring is usually necessary, often requiring the absence of muscle paralysis during the procedure. The anesthesia technique must be modified to allow smooth operating conditions without muscle relaxation. Even with close monitoring of the facial nerve, damage or sacrifice of the branches may occur, resulting in postoperative facial droop.

The patient is often turned 90-180° away from the anesthesiologist in order to provide better access for the surgeons. When placing monitors and securing the endotracheal tube, it is important to keep this in mind.

Thyroidectomy

Thyroidectomy may be performed for benign or malignant tumors. Patients with large goiters or recurrent laryngeal nerve involvement may present preoperatively with stridor or hoarseness. Thyroid tumors of any size may make vocal cord visualization challenging, and it is important to discuss the plan for intubation with the

ENT surgeon prior to proceeding if a difficult airway is suspected. In a patient with a suspected difficult airway or significant stridor, the most conservative approach is an awake intubation. Patients with benign thyroid disease should be euthyroid prior to undergoing surgery. Preoperative evaluation should rule out signs and symptoms of either significant hyperthyroidism or hypothyroidism. If surgery is undertaken as an emergency, beta-blockers and iodides should be used to treat the tachycardia and dysrhythmias seen with uncontrolled hyperthyroidism.

While blood loss and postoperative pain are usually minimal after these procedures, there is the potential for intraoperative or postoperative bleeding. Bleeding postoperatively can potentially lead to life-threatening airway obstruction. Other potential complications that can lead to postoperative hoarseness or obstruction include recurrent laryngeal nerve injury, severe hypocalcemia due to loss or damage to parathyroid gland tissue, and tracheomalacia. Tracheomalacia can occur after the removal of a large goiter or mass as a result of collapse of weakened tracheal rings. Patients should be monitored postoperatively for signs and symptoms of thyroid storm. While thyroid storm is relatively uncommon in patients made euthyroid prior to surgery, it can be life-threatening.

Clinical Caveats: Thyroid Storm

Due to release of thyroid hormones in a patient with hyperthyroidism

Signs and symptoms include tachycardia and dysrhythmias, increased temperature, altered consciousness

Should be treated and controlled prior to surgery whenever possible

May occur postoperatively as a result of intraoperative manipulation of the thyroid gland

Treatment includes beta-blockers to control heart rate, iodides to block the synthesis and release of thyroid hormones

Monitoring on an intensive care unit is indicated for these patients until stabilized

---

Surgery for Head and Neck Tumors

Preoperative evaluation of these patients should focus on the airway examination and on coexisting diseases. Head and neck cancers are often associated with chronic smoking and alcohol consumption, requiring a careful assessment of potential medical conditions such as coronary and respiratory disease. Depending on the size and location of the tumor, patients may have dysphagia, hoarseness, or stridor. Dehydration and malnutrition may also be present, potentially causing anemia or electrolyte abnormalities.

Types of surgery for these patients vary from direct laryngoscopy and biopsy to aggressive resection of the tumor (total laryngectomy, radical neck dissection). Depending on the nature and location of the tumor, the procedure may include tracheostomy or creation of a laryngeal stoma. Tracheostomy made be performed either at the beginning or end of the procedure, or even prior to anesthesia if significant obstruction exists.

Careful evaluation of the airway is also necessary, and an intubation plan should be outlined with the ENT surgeon prior to anesthesia. These patients are often difficult to mask ventilate and intubate, so an awake intubation or intubation by the ENT surgeon may be the preferred route. Tumors may limit mouth opening or vocal cord visualization, and patients with hoarseness or stridor may develop complete airway obstruction after induction of anesthesia. Preoperative sedation should be avoided in patients with airway obstruction, and administration of an antisialogogue may be appropriate if awake intubation is planned. Preoperative radiation therapy may limit neck mobility, and tissue edema due to the tumor may limit mask ventilation and intubation. Depending on the surgical site, a nasally placed endotracheal tube may be preferred.

Blood loss can be significant during these sometimes lengthy procedures, so invasive monitoring is often indicated, especially in a patient with significant comorbidities. Central venous monitoring, if indicated, should be placed in a location that will not interfere with the surgical field, often the subclavian or femoral route. The operating table may be turned 90° or 180° away from the anesthesiologist, limiting intraoperative access to the patient.

Intraoperatively, blood pressure should be monitored closely, as hypertension may increase intraoperative blood loss. Nerve monitoring may be required, especially if the procedure includes radical neck dissection, which may preclude the use of muscle relaxants. Venous air embolism is a potential risk if air is allowed to enter an open neck vein. Vasoconstrictive agents should be avoided if a flap reconstruction is performed, and volume status should be adequate in order to maintain blood flow to the flap.

If a tracheostomy or stoma is not performed, extubation at the conclusion of the procedure should depend on the difficulty of intubation, the patient's underlying medical status, and the length of the procedure. If significant swelling exists because of the nature or length of the procedure, or difficulty with reintubation is suspected, the patient should remain intubated and be taken to an intensive care setting. Newly performed tracheostomies or stomas are often monitored in the intensive care unit postoperatively.

Nasal Surgery

The two most commonly performed procedures in this category are nasoseptoplasty and endoscopic sinus surgery. Nasoseptoplasty may be performed for anatomic or cosmetic reasons, and may be done on an outpatient basis. These patients are usually otherwise healthy and often benefit from preoperative sedation. Anesthesia can vary from intravenous sedation to general anesthesia depending on the patient and the extent of the procedure. Blood loss during endoscopic surgery is usually minimal, although it may be difficult to quantify because of the large amounts of irrigation used. Local anesthetics, often containing epinephrine or cocaine, are used to provide both anesthesia and vasoconstriction to the nasal tissues. Careful hemodynamic monitoring is required during injection of these substances. The addition of vasoconstrictors to local anesthetics decreases blood loss as well as local anesthetic absorption. The anesthesiologist should be aware of the total administered dose as well as the toxic dose of the agents used. Cocaine uniquely provides both anesthesia and vasoconstriction and is well absorbed from mucosal tissues. It is often provided in a colored solution to prevent accidental administration.

Airway Surgery

Unlike many other surgical scenarios, this type of surgery requires the anesthesiologist to share the airway with the surgeon. Close communication between the two teams is critical to provide a safe operative environment for both the patient and the operating room staff.

Tracheostomy

Tracheostomy may be performed either electively or as an emergency. Elective tracheostomy is usually performed on chronically mechanically ventilated patients that cannot be weaned. These procedures may be performed either percutaneously at the bedside or through an open technique in the operating room. Patients undergoing percutaneous tracheostomy at the bedside should be carefully chosen, and an ENT surgeon is required, as well as an anesthesia team to provide deep sedation and fiberoptic guidance (Box 18-1).

More commonly, patients are brought to the operating room for open tracheostomy. Other underlying medical conditions should be stabilized prior to the procedure to allow for safe transport to and from the operating room. Anesthesia should include muscle relaxation and adequate sedation and analgesia, via either an inhalational or an intravenous technique. Routine monitoring as well as any invasive monitoring already in place should be maintained during the procedure and during transport. End-tidal carbon dioxide monitoring is crucial during the procedure to ensure a patent airway.

Drug Interactions: Cocaine and Epinephrine

Potential risk of arrhythmias, especially if inhaled anesthetics used (heart sensitized to catecholamines)

Block norephinephrine reuptake →avoid medications that act synergistically:
- Methyldopa
- Monoamine oxidase inhibitors
- Reserpine
- Tricyclic antidepressants
- Guanethidine

Cocaine metabolized by pseudocholinesterase; effect may be prolonged if:
- Pseudocholinesterase deficiency
- Echothiophate use (glaucoma)
- Physostigmine or neostigmine use (myasthenia gravis)

Use of epinephrine and cocaine together may exacerbate arrhythmias, prolong toxic effects

Maximum safe dose of cocaine 3–4 mg/kg

Box 18-1   Percutaneous Tracheostomy

Patients must be chosen carefully:
- Stable vital signs, able to tolerate sedating medications
- Normal neck anatomy, no prior neck or airway surgery
- Normal body habitus
- Absence of coagulopathy, normal platelet count

Procedure performed at bedside with ENT surgeons and anesthesia personnel

Sedation administered; local anesthetic administered by surgeon

Fiberoptic scope placed by anesthesia personnel into trachea through endotracheal tube

Wire placed through skin into trachea under direct vision, dilators passed over wire to enlarge tract for tracheostomy tube

Endotracheal tube removed after tracheostomy tube placement confirmed

Quick procedure, no electrocautery used; does not require a formal neck incision

Does require fiberoptic expertise and training in use of percutaneous tracheostomy kit

The endotracheal tube should not be completely removed from the airway until correct placement of the tracheostomy is confirmed. Electrocautery should not be used directly on the trachea because of the risk of airway fire. Postoperative monitoring of the new tracheostomy in an intensive care unit should be strongly considered if the patient was not previously located in an intensive care unit setting.

Laser Surgery

Laser surgery may be used to treat conditions such as laryngeal papillomas, tracheal webs or scarring, subglottic stenosis, or ENT neoplasms. The laser beam allows intense energy to be focused on to a specific target. Tissue can be precisely dissected and coagulated with the laser, resulting in minimal blood loss. The amount of smoke and debris produced depends on the type of laser used.

Anesthesia for these procedures can be performed in a variety of ways, and will depend on the expected length of the procedure and the location of the target. While all endotracheal tubes are flammable, special endotracheal tubes have been developed that may be more resistant to ignition (Box 18-2). Which tube is "safest" remains controversial. To further prevent combustion, it is recommended that the cuff be filled with saline instead of air. The saline may be colored to allow faster identification of cuff rupture. The lowest acceptable inspired oxygen level should be used, and nitrous oxide should be avoided. Air or helium can be used to lower the inspired oxygen concentration. Inhaled anesthetics or intravenous agents such as propofol can be used. Neuromuscular blockade is often helpful to limit motion of airway structures. Postoperative laryngospasm is a potential complication due to swelling or debris in the airway. Other hazards include potential laser injury to blood vessels or other structures as well as to operating room personnel.

Other options that avoid endotracheal intubation include mask ventilation with intermittent apnea during laser use, jet ventilation through a bronchoscope, or hyperventilation followed by intermittent extubation and reintubation. All these techniques require close monitoring of pulse oximetry and inspired oxygen levels.

Box 18-2 Special Endotracheal Tubes for Laser Surgery

Stainless steel endotracheal tube
Foil-wrapped polyvinyl chloride (PVC) tube
Red rubber endotracheal tube
Silicone tube with laser-resistant coating

Special precautions must be taken to protect both the patient and the operating room staff. Appropriate eye protection should be worn by all personnel, and signs should be posted to alert others that laser is in use. The patient's eyes should be covered with either a shield or opaque wet cloth to protect them from injury. Smoke and debris should be suctioned from the surgical site to prevent contamination into the atmosphere. Fire due to laser use can occur, both in the operating field and on the surgical drapes, and constant vigilance should be maintained. Misdirected laser energy can cause injury to either the patient or operating room staff.

Clinical Caveats: Treatment of an Airway Fire

1. Turn off all gas flow, especially nitrous oxide; disconnect endotracheal tube from circuit
2. Remove the endotracheal tube and extinguish any flaming material
3. Ventilate patient by mask with 100% oxygen
4. Perform bronchoscopy and esophagoscopy to assess damage and remove any debris
5. Reintubate patient or perform tracheostomy if necessary

Patient may require prolonged ventilation if there is extensive damage

Bronchial lavage and intravenous steroids may be helpful to reduce inflammation

---

Panendoscopy

Panendoscopy usually combines bronchoscopy, esophagoscopy, and direct laryngoscopy, usually for diagnosis and potential treatment of airway tumors. Patients presenting for this procedure may have significant obstructive symptoms and a potentially difficult intubation or mask ventilation may be anticipated, in which case preoperative sedation should be avoided. The anesthetic plan should be drawn up in conjunction with the ENT surgeon, and will depend on the patient's anatomy and the projected length of the procedure. Often the airway will be given to the surgeons after induction, and an endotracheal tube may be placed by them or intermittent mask ventilation may be used. Preoperative administration of an antisialogogue such as glycopyrrolate or atropine may improve operative and intubating conditions. Muscle relaxation may facilitate placement of rigid surgical scopes as well as decreasing mobility of airway structures during the procedure. Extubation should be performed with the patient fully awake and with intact airway reflexes.

EAR, NOSE, AND THROAT EMERGENCIES

Airway Trauma

Management of airway trauma may begin in the emergency room or the operating room, depending on the severity of trauma. Anesthesia personnel may be requested to assist in management of the airway in the emergency room. Management of these patients may also be complicated by hemodynamic instability, associated injuries, or intoxication. All trauma patients should be considered a "full stomach" with the potential for aspiration of stomach contents or blood occurring during or after the trauma.

The extent of airway or facial injury may be difficult to ascertain on examination, and the possibility of an associated head injury or cervical spine injury should be considered. Bruising around the eyes or blood or cerebrospinal fluid leaking from the ear may be associated with the presence of a basilar skull fracture, and nasotracheal intubation should be avoided in these patients. Neck stabilization should be maintained during intubation until a cervical spine injury is ruled out. Awake intubation is the safest approach, if tolerated by the patient.

If induction of anesthesia or deep sedation is planned prior to intubation, the possibility of increased intracranial pressure should be considered. Ketamine should be avoided, and the patient should be hyperventilated prior to intubation to prevent any worsening of intracranial pressure. Inhalational anesthetics, opioids, and muscle relaxants have minimal affects on intracranial pressure.

Patients with mandibular or maxillary (LeFort) fractures often present a challenge to the anesthesiologist (Figure 18-1). These fractures may be associated with a basilar skull fracture or nasal fractures, prohibiting nasotracheal intubation. Jaw instability or blood in the airway may make intubation difficult, and access to the oral cavity by the surgeons may necessitate tracheostomy. Muscular damage may cause masseter muscle spasm (trismus), forcing the mouth closed. This spasm may or may not resolve after induction of anesthesia and muscle relaxation.

Foreign Body Aspiration

While foreign body aspiration can occur at any age, it is much more common in children. Foreign bodies can become lodged in the trachea, esophagus, or bronchial tree, leading to dysphagia, dyspnea, or partial or complete airway obstruction. The urgency of removal will depend on the extent of obstruction, although all objects should be removed in a timely fashion because of the risk of migration, infection, or further injury. The majority of objects lodge in the right main stem bronchus. Patients

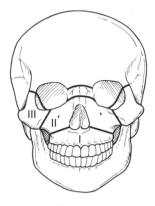

LeFort I: Fracture of maxilla above floor of nose, through lower third of pterygoid plate; palate mobilized

LeFort II: Pyramidal fracture through upper nose extending to medial wall of orbit

LeFort III: Midface fracture paralleling base of skull; facial bones separated from cranium. Cribriform plate may be fractured; zygomatic arch fracture; facial concavity often present

Figure 18-1   Types of LeFort fracture. Nasotracheal intubation is contraindicated in LeFort III fracture.

often present with a full stomach, further complicating airway management. Depending on the time of last oral intake and the degree of obstruction, either an intravenous or inhalational induction may be performed. An intravenous induction may be preferred if difficulty is anticipated with mask ventilation. Bronchoscopy and/or esophagoscopy is performed under anesthesia to remove the foreign body. Postoperative intensive care monitoring may be required, depending on the extent of the damage caused by the object.

Intravenous anesthesia is often used for these procedures as the airway is shared with the surgeons, and a variety of techniques may be used – mask ventilation with intermittent apnea, intubation with extubation during bronchoscopy, jet ventilation through the bronchoscope. The use of spontaneous versus controlled ventilation remains controversial, as is the use of muscle paralysis during these procedures. A continuous infusion of a short-acting paralytic such as succinylcholine or mivacurium can provide a motionless field for the surgeons as well as rapid emergence and extubation.

Close monitoring of oxygen saturation levels is essential, as these patients may have significant atelectasis, leading to rapid oxygen desaturation. Bronchodilators, steroid therapy, and racemic epinephrine may help not only to prevent but also to treat wheezing and airway edema after foreign body removal.

Postoperatively, potential complications include wheezing and airway edema as well as bronchospasm and/or laryngospasm. Extubation at completion of the procedure will depend on the difficulty of extraction as well as the extent of injury, and may be delayed until edema resolves.

Bleeding Tonsil

Postoperative bleeding after tonsillectomy can occur acutely within 24 hours of surgery or up to 10 days after surgery as the surgical scar retracts. Acute bleeding tends to be more serious and brisk than delayed bleeding. Patients are usually hypovolemic and potentially anemic, and should be considered to have a full stomach. Resuscitation should be undertaken prior to operative intervention to avoid further instability during anesthetic induction. Adequate intravenous access should be established in the operating room, if not already in place, and blood products should be available. Significant airway edema may make mask ventilation difficult or impossible. Intubation may be difficult because of blood in the airway, and the ENT surgeon should be present during induction and intubation. A rapid sequence induction and intubation with cricoid pressure should be performed, followed by evacuation of the stomach with an orogastric tube. The patient should be extubated when fully awake and alert with intact airway reflexes.

Epiglottitis/Croup

Epiglottitis is an inflammation of the supraglottic area, most commonly due to infection by *Hemophilus influenzae* bacteria, although cases due to group A streptococci have been reported. It usually occurs in children aged 3–8, and has a rapid onset, often leading to acute airway obstruction. Cases of epiglottitis are fairly rare today, although they still occur. Supraglottic edema leads to stridor and respiratory distress.

Treatment involves securing the airway, followed by antibiotics and extubation once the edema resolves. An inhalational induction may be preferred because of the significant stridor in these patients. Although sevoflurane has replaced halothane in many instances for inhalational induction of anesthesia, halothane may be a better choice in these patients because of the possibility of reaching a deeper level of anesthesia. If a deep plane of anesthesia can be achieved while maintaining the airway, these patients can be intubated without the use of muscle relaxants, avoiding the risk of airway collapse.

Croup is a viral infection that causes subglottic inflammation. It usually has a more gradual onset than epiglottitis, although patients can still develop acute airway obstruction. It most commonly affects children under age 3. Patients often present with a barking-type cough and hoarseness. Treatment is supportive, often involving humidified oxygen, steroids, and racemic epinephrine.

Children presenting with either of these conditions should be hydrated and watched closely for signs of airway obstruction. Cases requiring airway management should be brought to the operating room and treated as acute airway obstruction. Airway obstruction can occur quickly, and may require nasotracheal intubation or tracheostomy.

Clinical Caveats: Differential Diagnosis of Epiglottitis Versus Croup

Epiglottitis	Croup
Older children (3–8 years)	Younger children (<3 years)
Supraglottic obstruction	Subglottic obstruction
Bacterial origin, less common	Viral origin, more common
Sudden onset	More insidious onset
High fever, dysphagia, drooling	Low-grade fever, barking cough
Child sitting up, leaning forward	Child hoarse, lethargic
Airway intervention common	Airway intervention rarer

Acute Airway Obstruction

Acute airway obstruction should always be considered a true emergency, and these patients should be brought urgently to the operating room whenever possible for management, accompanied by a physician skilled in airway management (anesthesiologist, surgeon, or both). Stressful procedures (blood draws, x-rays, diagnostic procedures) should be deferred if possible until the airway is secured. The goal is to establish a patent airway distal to the obstruction. In a rapidly deteriorating patient, cricothyroidotomy may be a life-saving maneuver. A catheter, small endotracheal tube, or tracheostomy tube is placed through the cricothyroid membrane to establish an airway. It is important to remember that this is a temporary airway and should be converted to a formal tracheostomy once the patient is stabilized.

Obstruction may be due to foreign body aspiration, infection, tumor, trauma, congenital anomaly, or a disease process. Management will depend on the location of the obstruction as well as on the severity of symptoms. Obstruction at or below the vocal cords may require tracheostomy. Induction of anesthesia may result in complete loss of the airway or hemodynamic instability in a trauma patient; however, instrumentation of the airway prior to sedation may worsen the obstruction in an anxious patient. Intubation via the nasal route may bypass some types of obstruction. Contraindications to nasal intubation include nasal fractures or tumors, basilar skull fracture, or coagulopathy.

If intubation is planned, some type of sedation will usually be required, although paralysis should be avoided unless absolutely necessary. The most experienced physician in the room should attempt intubation, and a variety of intubating tools should be available, as well as a tracheostomy kit. A surgeon should be present who is able to immediately perform a tracheostomy if necessary. After intubation, the patient should be monitored in an intensive care setting, and extubation should be performed in a controlled manner after the obstruction is completely resolved.

SPECIAL CONSIDERATIONS

Difficult Airway Management

Any patient presenting for ENT surgery may be an anticipated or unanticipated difficult airway. Any patient who is difficult or impossible to ventilate or intubate falls into this category. Some of these patients will have a known history of difficult airway management, but many will be experiencing anesthesia for the first time.

Several steps should be taken to prevent complications when anesthetizing these patients. The ENT surgeon should always be present during induction and intubation, and a variety of rigid intubating scopes and a light source should be available. A plan for induction and ventilation should be established with surgical input prior to bringing the patient into the room, as well as backup plans in case the first plan is unsuccessful. An awake intubation or awake tracheostomy may be the safest way to secure the airway. Should induction of anesthesia precede attempts at intubation, be prepared for loss of the airway at any time, and anticipate potential difficulties with mask ventilation (Box 18-3).

No one single technique is preferred for management of a difficult airway, and the technique chosen should be tailored to the individual patient. A variety of intubating aids exist for the difficult airway. Extubation after the procedure must be carefully evaluated, and extubation in a controlled monitored setting with the ENT surgeon at the bedside may be the safest course, especially if airway edema is suspected. Intraoperative administration of corticosteroids may prevent or treat edema.

Postoperative airway complications may be more prevalent in patients undergoing ENT procedures, especially if difficulty in airway management was encountered. Airway edema can develop from multiple intubation attempts or surgical manipulation of airway structures. Edema may present immediately postoperatively or several hours later. Bleeding into the airway or adjacent to the

---

Box 18-3   Tools for Intubation of a Difficult Airway

Fiberoptic scope: For nasal or oral intubation, in an awake or anesthetized patient
Eschmann stylette: Can be placed into trachea blindly or when only the tip of cords is seen and the tube advanced over it
Laryngeal Mask Airway (LMA): Placed blindly into pharynx for ventilation when mask ventilation difficult or unsuccessful; fiberoptic scope can be placed through it to intubate trachea
Intubating LMA: Placed like LMA; endotracheal tube passed through it either blindly or with fiberoptic guidance, LMA then removed
Bullard intubating scope: Laryngoscope blade with fiberoptic attachment and light source; tube passed along side of blade under direct vision
Light wand/Trachlight: Lighted stylette placed inside endotracheal tube, placed blindly; light appears in trachea and tube is advanced into trachea
ENT rigid scopes (Hollinger, Dedo): Rigid scopes with light source, allow visualization of vocal cords in patients with difficult anatomy; Eschmann stylette needed to place endotracheal tube (scope too narrow)

---

airway can cause compression or laryngospasm and may require emergency reintubation.

Postoperative Nausea and Vomiting

Nausea and vomiting is one of the most common postoperative complications after ENT surgery. It is especially prevalent after procedures involving the ear or nose. Postoperative nausea and vomiting can lead to prolonged recovery room stays as well as unplanned hospital admission. Emesis is triggered both centrally through the chemoreceptor trigger zone and peripherally through blood products and secretions in the gastrointestinal tract and the labyrinth apparatus in the ear. Patients undergoing maxillary or mandibular procedures may require wiring of the jaw, further complicating the management of postoperative emesis and increasing the risk of aspiration.

Emptying the stomach intraoperatively and immediately prior to extubation can decrease gastric distention, lessening the potential for postoperative emesis. Minimal use of opioids whenever possible can also lower the incidence of postoperative nausea. Infiltration of local anesthesia or regional blocks can be used to minimize the need for narcotic administration. Avoidance of nitrous oxide and use of anesthetic agents less likely to promote emesis may also be beneficial. Propofol-based anesthetics have been associated with a significant decrease in postoperative nausea and vomiting. A variety of antiemetic agents exist that can be given intraoperatively to reduce the incidence of nausea and vomiting.

Clinical Caveats: Post-operative Nausea and Vomiting

PROEMETIC AGENTS	ANTIEMETIC AGENTS
Nitrous oxide	Propofol
Inhalational anesthetics	Metoclopramide
Ketamine	Histamine blockers (ranitidine)
Etomidate	Serotonin blockers (ondansetron)
Opiates	Ketorolac

SUMMARY

Patients of all ages commonly present for ENT surgery, including infants and small children. Patients must be evaluated preoperatively for significant medical conditions, including the presence of a difficult airway, which may complicate their management. A plan for intubation and extubation should be created in advance with input from the ENT surgeon. The clinician should be prepared for the possibility of intraoperative and postoperative complications that may occur due to manipulation of the airway. The anesthesiologist should be aware of new procedures such as percutaneous tracheostomy, new airway devices, and airway algorithms that continue to be developed and updated. The ultimate goal in successful care of patients presenting for ENT surgery is safe airway management while providing adequate surgical conditions.

Case Study

A 64-year-old man is scheduled for tongue biopsy, possible resection and radical neck dissection. Past medical history is significant for daily alcohol use, hypertension, and smoking (2 packs per day). He has noticed significant weight loss over the past few months and has some difficulty swallowing and occasional hoarseness. Airway examination demonstrates poor dentition, a large tongue, and inability to visualize the uvula.
- Is any further preoperative work-up necessary?
- How will you manage the airway?
- What anesthetic technique will you use, and what might you avoid?
- Will you extubate this patient? Why/why not?

SUGGESTED READING

Brown BR, ed. *Anesthesia and ENT surgery. Contemporary Anesthesia Practice 9.* Philadelphia: Davis, 1987.

Dougherty T, Nguyen D. Anesthetic management of the patient scheduled for head and neck cancer surgery. *J Clin Anesth* 1994;6:74-82.

Gotta A, Ferrari L, Sullivan C. Anesthesia for ENT surgery. In: Barash PG, Cullen BF, Stoelting RK, eds. *Clinical anesthesia*, 3rd ed. Philadelphia: Lippincott-Raven, 1997: 929-943.

Practice guidelines for management of the difficult airway. *Anesthesiology* 1993;78:597-602.

Practice guidelines for management of the difficult airway. An updated report by the American Society of Anesthesiologists task force on management of the difficult airway. *Anesthesiology* 2003; 98: 1269-1277.

Rampil I. Anesthetic considerations for laser surgery. *Anesth Analg* 1992;74:424-435.

Verghese ST, Hannallah RS. Pediatric otolaryngologic emergencies. *Anesthesiol Clin North Am* 2001;19:237-256.

Anesthesia for Plastic Surgery

BRANDON LUCAS VILLARREAL

INTRODUCTION

With our aging American population it is predicted that over the next two decades the number of surgical procedures performed will double to approximately 40 million operations annually. Included in this surgical growth will be procedures performed by plastic surgeons that will provide our nation's consumers with a physically pleasant and youthful appearance to accompany their personal vitality. As the location of plastic surgery procedures has shifted from hospitals to free-standing surgery centers, and directly into surgical offices, the anesthetizing location has presented the anesthesiologist with a number of unique challenges.

With the innovation of noninvasive cardiovascular monitors, pulse oximetry, capnometry, laryngeal mask airways of varying sizes, short-acting anesthetics, and improved medications for postoperative nausea and pain control, anesthesiologists today possess the capacity to provide a safe and cost-efficient anesthetic to an often self-paying consumer who expects a minimum of physical and emotional discomfort and personal inconvenience. This chapter will highlight the unique characteristics that encompass the fascinating discipline of anesthesia for plastic and cosmetic surgery.

OFFICE-BASED ANESTHESIA FOR PLASTIC SURGERY

Plastic surgeons perform operative procedures in their offices because it is convenient, cost-effective, and minimally invasive. With the safe practice of monitored anesthesia care and the introduction of both tumescent lidocaine and the laryngeal mask airway into anesthetic practice, both anesthetic and surgical morbidity and mortality have been minimized.

In addition it is profitable for them to do so, particularly in their own offices where they control cost structures and can spread their variable costs (supplies, pharmaceuticals, and linen) over a multitude of patients, having predictably consistent procedures performed in their office settings on a daily basis – i.e., they are cost-efficient because their procedures are predictable and they are capable of achieving a greater degree of productivity (Box 19-1).

Cosmetic surgery performed in office locations includes face and brow lifts, blepharoplasty, liposuction, breast augmentation, otoplasty, rhinoplasty, facial laser resurfacing, and abdominoplasty. In the 1980s these procedures were usually performed in hospitals but began appearing in free-standing surgery centers. With the evolution of managed care over the past 20 years, and the economic realities imposed on the highly competitive surgical cosmetic industry, many plastic surgeons began performing operations in their offices.

Office-based anesthesia for plastic surgery has flourished, in part because of the innovation of short-acting anesthetics such as propofol, alfentanil, remifentanil, versed, ketamine, and sevoflurane; as well as the advent of the laryngeal mask airway, pulse oximetry, capnometry, portable invasive and noninvasive cardiovascular monitoring devices, and charcoal filters to scavenge anesthetic gases. Patients are discharged home earlier and, with the advent of the newer antiemetics and analgesics, are relatively free from nausea and pain.

Office-based anesthesia poses many unique challenges to the anesthesiologist. With the exception of a few states, such as California and Florida, most states do not regulate office locations for plastic surgery procedures. This presents the anesthesiologist with the highly important task of defining and implementing those operational characteristics that insure the safety of anesthesia delivery. Moreover, the system must have the operational consistency necessary to acquire expertise in managing such off-site locations to preserve the quality of care delivered and enforce the safety precautions that already exist in regulated free-standing surgery centers and inpatient hospital operating rooms.

Of paramount concern, and certainly always to be anticipated by the diligent anesthesiologist, is the surgical, medical, or anesthetic mishap that might endanger the life of a patient receiving anesthesia for plastic surgery. Office locations must be properly equipped to deliver oxygen, provide a source of continuous suction, possess the medications to successfully resuscitate a patient, maintain a properly functioning portable defibrillator, and have readily available emergency airway tools to maintain oxygenation and ventilation, as well as sedatives, hypnotics, and analgesics to provide uninterrupted monitored anesthesia care or general anesthesia.

Perhaps the greatest controversy in office-based anesthesia for plastic surgery is patient selection. In the 1980s free-standing surgery centers became a less expensive alternative to hospital services. Initially, only American Society of Anesthesiologists (ASA) category I patients were thought to be candidates to undergo anesthesia in an

off-site location (outside the setting of a hospital operating room). By the mid-1990s ASA III patients with chronic stable medical conditions began appearing in free-standing surgery centers. Clearly, as surgeons and anesthesiologists acquire the managerial experience and clinical expertise to care for patients with chronic stable disease, such patients will ultimately begin appearing in plastic surgery office-based anesthesia practices, particularly as our population ages and people live longer, healthier lives.

Patients who are obese, those possessing unstable cardiorespiratory disease, those incapable of voluntary control of movement on command, and those unable to communicate with the anesthesiologist are not good candidates for anesthesia in an office-based plastic surgery practice. Laboratory evaluation and preoperative assessment must be performed by an anesthesiologist who acquires a history and physical examination and then determines the appropriate laboratory and/or additional investigations required to produce an anesthetic plan.

MONITORED ANESTHESIA CARE AND PLASTIC SURGERY PROCEDURES

Sedation, as defined by the American Society of Anesthesiologists Practice Guidelines for Sedation and Analgesia by Non-Anesthesiologists is a continuum that spans minimal sedation/analgesia (anxiolysis), moderate sedation/analgesia (conscious sedation), deep sedation/analgesia, and general anesthesia. Preoperative, intraoperative, and postoperative care is delivered by an anesthesiologist in a diligent manner, anticipating the variability (and unpredictability) of patient's response to the administration of hypnotics, amnestics, and analgesics; and one who is trained to manage a patient's airway and impaired cardiorespiratory consequences in the unresponsive and/or completely unconscious patient during plastic surgery procedures. It is imperative to anticipate a patient's unpredictable response to monitored anesthesia care and to possess the airway and cardioresuscitative tools and medications, as well as the knowledge, to successfully rescue a patient from both cardiorespiratory compromise and loss of airway reflexes.

There is a clinically discernible distinction between anxiolysis, conscious sedation, deep sedation, and general anesthesia. Basically, the patient may be on a continuum that spans on the one end being sedated with intact airway reflexes and communicating comfortably, and at the other a complete loss of consciousness in which the airway is completely supported and managed by the anesthesiologist to maintain oxygenation and ventilation.

Many patients undergoing plastic and cosmetic surgery procedures do so with short-acting intravenous medications that provide amnesia, analgesia, anxiolysis, cardiorespiratory stability, and a conducive operating environment that allows the surgeon to focus on their technical tasks while providing the patient with a psychologically comfortable and nonpainful operative experience. It is imperative that the anesthesiologist safely provides patients with the anesthetic experience they anticipate, which includes feeling no pain and being unaware of their environment, yet maintaining a patient who is cooperative and whose airway is protected while comfortably breathing (Box 19-2).

All plastic surgery procedures commonly performed in the United States may be performed with ultra-short (remifentanil) and short-acting (alfentanil, propofol) intravenous anesthetics and the local infiltration of highly dilute concentrations of lidocaine (tumescent lidocaine) in the communicating and cooperative patient. Tumescent lidocaine revolutionized lipoplasty procedures that contour body shape and many other plastic and cosmetic procedures. Following the operative procedure under monitored anesthesia care there is a minimum of side effects, often characterized by dysphoria, dizziness, delayed emergence, nausea and vomiting, and cardiorespiratory depression. Ideally, the postoperative course is without agitation (a characteristic of hypoxia, hypercarbia, local anesthetic toxicity, and hypotension resulting in decreased brain perfusion) and patients are pain free and ready for discharge home or to an overnight suite when they are able to stand upright, swallow water, and void without assistance.

The pharmacokinetics of intravenous sedation are dose-dependent. There is an ideal therapeutic range that achieves an ideal response (pharmacodynamics) to the effect of a medication at specific receptor sites. When the plasma drug concentration is below the ideal plasma drug concentration, analgesia, amnesia, and anxiolysis are not achieved and the patient may be agitated or may move uncontrollably; on the other hand, if the plasma drug concentration is too high the patient may be oversedated and at risk of hypoxia, hypercarbia, hypotension, and loss of the protective airway reflexes.

Until recently, the elimination half-life was the predominant pharmacokinetic parameter used to predict the duration of action of a drug. Unfortunately, medications do follow a single-compartment model of elimination; therefore the concept of the context-sensitive half-time was developed, which describes the time required for the plasma drug concentration to decline by 50% following either a bolus or continuous infusion. Both distribution and metabolism of drug disposition are taken into consideration, and computer-assisted modeling simulates the multicompartmental model of drug disposition. Assuming a normal cardiac output, well spaced, small boluses of medications will most probably produce the desired level of sedation. If cardiac output is compromised, initial doses of medications are not redistributed as rapidly and their effects are prolonged and additive with additional doses.

LIPOSUCTION

Liposuction (lipoplasty) is the most common plastic surgery procedure performed in the United States. It was first introduced at the meeting of the American Society for Aesthetic Plastic Surgery in 1980 and the first article on liposuction appeared in *Plastic and Reconstructive Surgery* in 1981. Since its early beginnings it has undergone a multitude of innovative changes. Today, it is a procedure that creates shape, an attractive silhouette, and a pleasing contour over very specific body parts, particularly the thighs and buttocks, although it may be performed over many body regions.

Box 19-2 Goals of Monitored Anesthetic Care During Plastic Surgery Procedures

Achieve analgesia, amnesia, and anxiolysis
Achieve a protected airway with a communicating, cooperative, and spontaneously breathing patient
Achieve a state of complete relaxation in a comfortable, nonmoving patient who responds to commands
Address and attempt to achieve both the patient's and surgeon's expectations while delivering a safe and comfortable operating environment

Clinical Caveat: Liposuction/Lipoplasty

Liposuction is an esthetic procedure to shape and esthetically contour specific body parts. It is not a procedure to surgically correct obesity – the patient should have a body mass index not exceeding 32.5 to be an ideal candidate for lipoplasty.

In the early 1980s liposuction was performed "dry" (without "wetting" solutions) under general anesthesia with a 10 mm cannula attached to a dilatation and curettage suction canister. Approximately 1,500 mL of aspirate (without infiltrate) containing blood and adipose tissue were suctioned from the patient's subcutaneous space; often, the patient received up to several units of autologous or donor-specific blood as well as isotonic crystalloid to replace the third-space losses that occurred following a "dry" lipoplasty.

Under "dry" conditions 20–45% of the aspirate contained blood from torn "feeder" vessels, which bled profusely both intraoperatively and postoperatively. Pathophysiologically, lipoplasty is an extensive burn underneath the skin surface and patients were and still are today (though certainly less so) at risk of developing intravascular dehydration (requiring aggressive fluid resuscitation regimens), manifested as both intraoperative and postoperative hypotension secondary to third-space losses.

In the mid-1980s Fodor advocated the "superwet" technique (a ratio of infiltrate to total aspirate of 1:1), and Klein introduced the "tumescent" technique (a ratio of infiltrate to total aspirate of 2–7:1), so that only 1% of the aspirate contained blood. These techniques revolutionized lipoplasty, as they allowed a greater volume of aspirate to be suctioned without pain and the threat of ongoing hemorrhage, as well as allowing lipoplasty to be performed in an outpatient surgery center and/or the surgeon's office with the patient being discharged home without the disorientation or sedation from opioid analgesics following the procedure.

There are a multitude of "wetting" solutions, although they generally consist of 30 mL of 1% lidocaine and 1 mL of epinephrine 1:1,000 in 1 L of lactated Ringer's solution. Klein's tumescent technique is performed in the surgeon's office under monitored anesthesia care; the patient is comfortably sedated with minimal doses of versed and fentanyl and is typically without pain during the procedure because of the local anesthetic affect of lidocaine. The added epinephrine vasoconstricts the bleeding feeder vessels to significantly control both intraoperative and postoperative hemorrhage.

The additional advantage of the tumescent technique is that it eliminates the need to administer intravenous fluid; instead, intravascular fluid replacement is achieved by using the principle of hypodermoclysis, which is the absorption of subcutaneously administered fluid into the vascular compartment. These patients are at risk of hypervolemia and pulmonary edema if the total intraoperative fluid administered (both intravenously and subcutaneously) exceeds the patient's vascular capacity. Patients planning to have 4 L or more of aspirate removed are routinely monitored with a Foley catheter with the expectation that they will void more than 0.5–1.0 mL/kg/hr intraoperatively and postoperatively, and are diligently assessed for pulmonary edema.

The precise physiology of hypodermoclysis during and following lipoplasty is unknown; therefore, how the anesthesiologist replaces third-space losses is not scientifically established. It is been observed that 70% of the infiltrate remains in the subcutaneous space after liposuction and, despite fluid egress through the incisions postoperatively, large fluid volumes eventually enter the intravascular space during the first 24 hours following lipoplasty. There is a correlation between the total intraoperative (both infiltrate and intravenous) fluid administered and the rate of urine output in the recovery room. Clearly, when the amount of aspirate exceeds 4 L (which is considered to be a large-volume aspirate) it is imperative that the anesthesiologist and surgeon employ due diligence in diagnosing the patient who is fluid-overloaded even when not displaying overt clinical signs of pulmonary edema, such as mild dyspnea, tachypnea, and hypertension.

Current Controversy: Intraoperative and Postoperative Fluid Administration

The physiology of hypodermoclysis is not scientifically known

About 70% of the infiltrate injected subcutaneously is not removed in the aspirate; therefore the patient is at risk for pulmonary edema when aspirate volume exceeds 4 L

The patient is at risk for hypovolemia and hypotension during small-volume aspirates (<4 L), because it is scientifically unknown how to replace both insensible and ongoing losses intraoperatively

Lidocaine and epinephrine are very important components of the subcutaneous "wetting" infiltrate. Epinephrine should not exceed an upper limit of 10 mg for the entire procedure. When diluted in 1 L of isotonic lactated Ringer's solution, 1 mL of epinephrine (1:1,000) has a final concentration of 1:1,000,000. With this regimen epinephrine toxicity, manifested as tachycardia and hypertension, has not been reported. The administration of less than 10 mg of epinephrine, even in large-volume aspirates (15 L) has been shown to be safe.

The administration of 30 mL of 1% lidocaine in 1 L of isotonic fluid is very dilute, so its absorption is quite slow and peak plasma levels occur 12 hours following administration. Thus it is theoretically possible to deliver large doses of lidocaine during a lipoplasty procedure, usually around 35–55 mg/kg, without reaching toxic plasma levels.

Typically, clinical analgesia is achieved for up to 18 hours postoperatively and plasma blood levels are detectable for up to 24 hours following lipoplasty.

It is imperative that the anesthesiologist observes the patient for lidocaine toxicity, as manifested by lightheadedness, tinnitus, and a numb tongue. More severe signs include seizures, unconsciousness, and respiratory arrest, and when the plasma concentration of lidocaine reaches 25 μg/mL, cardiac arrest may occur.

Typically the patient undergoing lipoplasty will have 2 L of aspirate removed while undergoing either suction or ultrasound-assisted lipoplasty; under such circumstances the dose of epinephrine will usually not exceed 3 mg and the total dose of lidocaine administered is usually no more than 25–35 mg/kg of ideal bodyweight. Lidocaine and epinephrine toxicity are always an anesthetic priority to consider, particularly when large-volume aspirates exceeding 4 L are planned.

Acidosis and hypercarbia may occur as a result of lidocaine toxicity, which will increase cerebral perfusion and decrease lidocaine protein binding, both of which increase central nervous system lidocaine levels. On the other hand, it is known that the seizure threshold of lidocaine (and other local anesthetics) is increased by the administration of barbiturates and benzodiazepines during conscious and deep sedation. The administration of epinephrine in the infiltrate will reduce the systemic absorption of lidocaine. Lidocaine, like all local anesthetics, will block the cardiac conduction system via a dose-dependent block of sodium channels.

Drug Interaction: Sedative, Hypnotics, Analgesics and Lidocaine

During liposuction under monitored anesthesia care with intravenous sedation, patients undergoing tumescent lipoplasty are carefully observed for level of consciousness and respiratory efforts. If they become lightheaded or unconscious the anesthesiologist considers as a possible etiology not only lidocaine toxicity but also oversedation. If patients are underventilating they will become hypercarbic and central nervous system acidosis will increase the potency of lidocaine within the central nervous system. Therefore it is important to observe, and if necessary communicate with, patients to ascertain their level of consciousness.

Perioperatively, the patient should discontinue the use of birth control pills prior to surgery, as birth control pills are a known risk factor for deep vein thrombosis. Most patients are ASA I and II patients with medically minor and stable illnesses; they do not exceed their ideal body weight by more than 30% nor do they have unstable cardiac or respiratory disease. A patient with sleep apnea who is to undergo monitored anesthesia care with deep sedation is not an ideal candidate for liposuction. As stated earlier, fluid replacement is more "art" than "science" during these procedures, and the patient is at risk for hypovolemic shock at one extreme and pulmonary edema at the other, particularly when performing large-volume aspirations.

Lidocaine has a dose limit (as defined by the Food and Drug Administration) of 7 mg/kg. Extremely dilute lidocaine (0.1%) is injected subcutaneously and, as long as doses (of dilute lidocaine) do not exceed 55 mg/kg, mean lidocaine plasma levels will not exceed the cardiotoxic threshold of 5 μg/ml. It is postulated that deaths attributed to lidocaine toxicity are the result of terminal asystole from progressive local anesthetic depression of intracardiac conduction and ventricular contractility. It is estimated that the liver's maximum clearance capacity is 250 mg of lidocaine per hour, which ultimately becomes the limiting factor in the disposition of lidocaine; therefore patients with hepatic disease are not ideal candidates for large-volume liposuction.

Liposuction is neither a technically easy procedure to perform nor a benign procedure to undergo. Up until the mid-1990s the public media portrayed lipoplasty as a benign operation, but it has a mortality rate of 19.1 deaths per 100,000 procedures, which is high considering a reported mortality of 3:100,000 elective hernia repairs. The most common cause of death is pulmonary thromboembolism, which is responsible for 23% of deaths following liposuction. Anesthesia-related deaths make up 10% of the total mortality and cardiorespiratory failure occurs in 5.4% of patients who die during or following liposuction procedures. Technically, lipoplasty requires training and skill to perform, as abdominal and viscus perforation is reported 15% of the time as a cause of mortality. Certainly, "large-volume" aspirations are best performed by those surgeons who routinely perform them, with a team of professionals (including an anesthesiologist) who have experience in managing these patients perioperatively.

The prophylactic use of pneumatic compression stockings applied to the lower extremities is advised, particularly under general anesthesia. Some groups have explored the use of additional measures to reduce the incidence of thromboembolism, including intravenous ethanol, steroids, or both, with limited success.

Intraoperative hypothermia is of major concern, especially with the removal of large aspirates. Thus "wetting" solutions are warmed prior to infiltration and patients are subjected to heat conserving measures by being given warm intravenous fluids and by allowing the operating room's ambient temperature to rise.

Clinical Caveat: Liposuction Morbidity/Mortality

Liposuction is best performed by an experienced team of professionals who are clearly capable of differentiating the "science" from the "art" of providing perioperative care to patients undergoing liposuction. A mortality of 19.1 deaths per 100,000 procedures is ominous. Liposuction has been compared to an extensive "burn" that occurs subcutaneously – unrecognized third-space losses contribute to hypovolemia, which increases the risk of thromboembolism. Lidocaine toxicity from "tumescent" wetting solutions is manifested as cardiorespiratory collapse following central nervous system depression.

RHYTIDECTOMY AND FACIAL LASER RESURFACING

Most surgical face-lifts (rhytidectomy), endoscopically performed forehead and brow lifts, and facial laser resurfacing procedures are performed in free-standing outpatient surgery facilities and in surgeons' offices under monitored anesthesia care with the administration of local anesthetics to the area of surgical incision. Anxiolysis is maintained under conscious or deep sedation by employing the pharmacologic and predictable advantages of an ultra-short-acting sedative hypnotic such as propofol or the ultra-short-acting opioid analgesic remifentanil. Anxiolysis is attained with midazolam; its short half-life and quick onset are suitable for office-based surgical anxiolysis.

During the infiltration of local anesthesia on the face and neck, excellent analgesia may be attained with the intravenous infusion of remifentanil (not exceeding 0.25 μg/kg/min). The injection of local anesthesia into the subcutaneous tissues of the face and neck (often referred to as "compact infiltration," "artificial infiltration," or "hard infiltration") is exceedingly painful; intense analgesia is achieved with the administration of propofol (25–100 μg/kg/min) and/or remifentanil (0.05–0.25 μg/kg/min). Both may be administered by a bolus technique (propofol 0.5–1.5 mg/kg, remifentanil 0.2–1.0 μg/kg) and then a continuous infusion of both or each alone may be initiated to maintain analgesia as multiple local anesthetic injections are performed throughout the face and neck.

Often, a local anesthetic (lidocaine 0.5%) containing epinephrine 1:400,000 is employed to selectively block facial nerves such as the supraorbital, supratrochlear, and mental nerves, followed by multiple "field blocks" around the surface of the face. During these blocks the patient's vital signs and respiratory status are judiciously observed.

The patient may require an intermittent jaw thrust to avoid upper airway obstruction and the patient's facial expressions are observed for painful grimaces suggestive of the need for additional analgesia.

About 60–90 minutes prior to surgery the patient is given 5–10 mg of oral diazepam to achieve anxiolysis and 1.5 μg/kg of clonidine, a centrally acting alpha-2-adrenergic partial agonist that significantly contributes to the patient's anxiolysis and central anesthesia while reducing the central sympathetic outflow of catecholamines, which are capable of increasing the patient's heart rate and blood pressure. During the operative procedure blood pressure is maintained in the low normal range, with systolic pressures between 90 and 130 mmHg. Heart rate is maintained between 55 and 90 beats/min, and oxygen is administered if the oxygen saturation falls below 90–92%. Clearly, a major surgical postoperative concern is hematoma formation requiring surgical evacuation. Often labetalol, in 5 mg increments, atenolol in 2.5 mg increments, or propanolol in 0.25 mg increments is given intravenously to maintain both the heart rate and systolic blood pressure within the ideal range in order to reduce the incidence of hematoma formation.

More than 50% of hematoma formation occurs within the first 15 hours following surgery, although clearly hematomas may occur 48 hours following surgery when head dressings and drains are removed. The increased incidence of hematoma formation on the first postoperative day is probably related to the increased level of activity that occurs following a night's peaceful sleep. During anesthesia, whether general anesthesia or conscious sedation, it is important to maintain blood pressure, at the lowest normotensive level for the patient. Doing so allows the surgeon to identify intraoperatively bleeding vessels that may possibly contribute to hematoma formation postoperatively. Systolic pressures above 150 mmHg are treated intraoperatively to prevent postoperative bruising and hematoma formation.

Patients are allowed to emerge smoothly by eliminating the incidence of coughing and "straining" on the endotracheal tube following general anesthesia by intravenous lidocaine, 1.0–1.5 mg/kg upon emergence; coughing or "bucking" on the endotracheal tube will increase venous pressure and thus possibly contribute to postoperative bleeding, particularly if the superficial temporal vessels have been compromised intraoperatively. Nausea, and in particular vomiting, increases venous pressure and contributes to postoperative hematoma formation. Ondansetron, metoclopramide, anzemet, and dexamethasone have been employed to decrease the incidence of postoperative nausea and vomiting following rhytidectomy.

A total intravenous anesthetic technique for outpatient facial laser resurfacing may be employed with the use of intravenous ketamine and propofol. Ketamine is an arylcyclohexylamine, very similar structurally to phencyclidine, and thus a "dissociative" anesthetic that provides profound analgesia. When employed as a continuous infusion (35 µg/kg/min) with propofol (100 µg/kg/min), the total dose of opioid employed to attain analgesia is reduced; therefore the patient is at reduced risk of developing respiratory depression. This is significant in that during rhytidectomy the patient's airway is not readily available to the anesthesiologist, particularly when administering monitored anesthesia care under deep sedation. A small percentage of patients will experienced "vivid but pleasant dreams" despite the concomitant administration of midazolam and propofol.

Clinical Caveat: Anesthetic Management for Face-lift

Preoperative evaluation focused on a history of hypertension and its medical management

Ideal candidate without history of bleeding disorders

Maintain normotension intraoperatively, provide a smooth emergence, reduce those physical actions of the patient that increase venous pressure in the head and neck, and closely monitor respirations while under conscious sedation

Patients who undergo facelifts under monitored anesthesia care while receiving oxygen via a nasal cannula at 2 L/min are at risk of flash fires during facial surgery when electrocautery is employed at low settings. Thus patients without any underlying cardiorespiratory disease may undergo conscious sedation without supplemental oxygen as long as their oxygen saturations are at or above 90–92%. Under such circumstances, oxygen may be administered when clinically necessary, or when the patient has a mild underlying cardiorespiratory disease that is medically stable, since the incidence of such flash fires is extremely rare. Patients undergoing face lifts during general anesthesia should have lower extremity intermittent compression devices to reduce the incidence of deep vein thrombosis and pulmonary embolus.

BREAST RECONSTRUCTION

Anesthesia for breast reconstruction typically occurs in an outpatient surgical facility and is often for breast augmentation. Breast reduction mammoplasty is often performed in an inpatient hospital setting because the risk of bleeding intraoperatively and postoperatively is so much greater although clearly reduction mammoplasty may be performed in an outpatient facility when the risk of hemorrhage is minimal.

All surgery on the breast may be performed with general endotracheal anesthesia, under conscious and deep sedation with the infiltration of "tumescent" local anesthetic, under thoracic paravertebral (T1–T7) block, or with continuous thoracic epidural anesthesia (catheter placement high at T3–T4 or low at T6–T7). Procedures using transverse rectus abdominis myocutaneous (TRAM) and latissimus dorsi flaps are performed under general endotracheal anesthesia in an inpatient hospital location without the use of vasoconstrictors, to maintain a stable blood pressure. These "flaps" require a quiet surgical field during arterial anastomosis.

Breast augmentations performed in an outpatient surgical facility are often carried out using an inframammary partial retropectoral approach. The goal of both surgery and anesthesia is to return the patient to normal daily activity as soon as possible. This includes allowing the patient to raise her arms above her head within 24 hours of surgery and certainly to drive a vehicle within 48 hours. The type of anesthesia employed is patient- and surgeon-specific. Breast augmentation is truly a fine surgical procedure; the goals of which are to minimize bleeding (which contributes to the inflammatory response around the saline-filled implant) and excessive tissue trauma. By minimizing both bleeding and excessive trauma, the inflammatory response around the implant is minimized and the patient suffers less pain and is in need of less (opioid) analgesia, so she may recover quickly without added morbidity that eventually delays recovery and adds additional expense to the procedure.

Axillary and inframammary approaches are performed surgically such that all dissections are completed under direct or endoscopic vision to preserve the neurovascular bundles. All pocket dissections are completed with a monopolar, hand-switching, needle-tip electrocautery forceps. A strict no-touch technique regarding the periosteum and perichondrium is followed in subpectoral pocket dissections to eliminate bleeding from small surface vessels on rib periosteum or costal cartilage perichondrium, and all retraction instrumentation and techniques are designed to minimize retraction forces, bleeding, and trauma to tissue caused by the retractors.

Some surgeons believe that the use of short-acting muscle relaxants (mivacurium and rocuronium) under general anesthesia is required to minimize retractor forces on the tissues directly engaged with the retractor. These surgeons have zero tolerance of bleeding and tissue trauma. Retractor placement is exquisitely precise in order to visualize the location of vessels to prevent unwanted bleeding.

Breast augmentation is a fine surgical technique requiring the surgeon and anesthesiologist to work closely together in order to minimize the time and expense of the procedure. The anesthesiologist, by knowing the length of time the surgeon takes to create the implant pocket, will not necessarily need to reverse the muscle relaxant with an anticholinergic that might contribute to postoperative nausea and vomiting and thus delay the patient's discharge home. By minimizing bleeding and tissue trauma there is less of an inflammatory response and therefore less pain postoperatively; many patients are discharged home on nonsteroidal anti-inflammatory drugs such as ibuprofen. Postoperative hemorrhage requiring hematoma evacuation is rare and most patients do not even have signs of ecchymoses on the breast surfaces following augmentation.

Some surgeons are capable of performing breast augmentation under local anesthesia and intravenous sedation while infiltrating "tumescent" local anesthetic cocktails that reduce the amount of blood loss (with the use of dilute epinephrine) and provide analgesia with large doses of very dilute local anesthetics. Regardless of the anesthetic technique, the goal is always the same – to assist the surgeon in creating a bloodless field and to meet the patients expectations by reducing pain and providing intense analgesia in a safe and comfortable environment.

ABDOMINOPLASTY

An abdominoplasty is a surgical procedure of the skin; it may be performed under conscious sedation with a tumescent local anesthetic technique of lidocaine and epinephrine. Although many surgeons prefer the administration of general endotracheal anesthesia, clearly the skin can be anesthetized like any other organ. When the rectus fascia is plicated and the skin flap is created, tumescent infiltration is achieved along with additional concentrated local anesthetic injection into the skin and the perforating nerves before dividing them. In order to be successful with this anesthetic technique for abdominoplasty, the surgeon and anesthesiologist need to possess a clear understanding of the important role each contributes to in order to be successful in achieving an esthetically pleasing result.

SUMMARY

With the priority of cost containment measures in the administration of acute care services and the greater expense of care being provided directly by the consumer, our anesthetic approaches to a multitude of plastic surgery procedures have evolved and will continue to do so for many years to come. Our plastic surgery patients are price-conscious and value-oriented; it is our goal to provide anesthesia for our surgeons that is conducive to their surgical technique and skills and to meet our patient's expectations while providing a safe anesthetic. During plastic surgery we practice our profession under circumstances where the "art" of anesthesia is just as important as the "science" of surgical technique.

Case Study

A 29-year-old healthy woman underwent suction lipectomy of the abdomen, hips, and trochanteric area under uneventful general endotracheal anesthesia. A total of 600 mL of adipose tissue was removed with very little blood loss, a total of 1,600 mL of crystalloid was administered intraoperatively, and her urine output perioperatively was 500 mL. One hour following surgery the patient, while breathing room air, became anxious and dyspneic (25 breaths/minute), and her oxygen saturation decreased from 93% to 82%. A pulmonary embolism was ruled out by pulmonary angiography. There were no petechiae, and computed tomography of the chest revealed patchy bilateral ground-glass densities, macronodular opacities, and alveolar consolidation without pleural effusion.
- Is this patient at risk of developing acute respiratory distress syndrome (ARDS)?
- If yes, would you possibly expect to see global neurologic dysfunction?
- How would pulmonary lipases contribute to this patient's ARDS?

SUGGESTED READING

American Society of Anesthesiologists Task Force on Sedation and Analgesia by Non-Anesthesiologists. Practice guidelines for sedation and analgesia by non-anesthesiologists. *Anesthesiology* 2002;96:1004-1017.

De Jong R, Grazer M. Perioperative management of cosmetic liposuction. *Plast Reconstr Surg* 2001;107:1039-1044.

Fourme T, Vieillard-Baron A, Loubieres Y, et al. Early fat embolism after liposuction. *Anesthesiology* 1998;89:782-784.

Grazer F, de Jong R. Fatal outcomes from liposuction: census survey of cosmetic surgeons. *Plast Reconstr Surg* 2000;105:436-446.

Iverson R. Sedation and analgesia in ambulatory settings. *Plast Reconstr Surg* 1999;104:1559-1564.

Karmo F, Milan M, Silbergleit A. Blood loss in major liposuction procedures: a comparison study using suction-assisted versus ultrasonically assisted lipoplasty. *Plast Reconstr Surg* 2001;108:241-247.

Klein JA. The tumescent technique for liposuction surgery. *Am J Cosmetic Surg.* 1987;4:263.

Klein JA. Tumescent technique for local anesthesia improves safety in large volume liposuction. *Plast Reconstr Surg* 1993;92:1085-1098.

Klein SM, Bergh A, Steele SM, et al. Thoracic paravertebral block for breast surgery. *Anesth Analg* 2000;90:1402-1405.

McDevitt N. Deep vein thrombosis prophylaxis. *Plast Reconstr Surg* 1999;104:1923-1928.

Marcus J, Tyrone J, Few J, et al. Optimization of conscious sedation in plastic surgery. *Plast Reconstr Surg* 1999;104:1338-1345.

Pechter EA. The clinical outcome of abdominoplasty performed under conscious sedation: increased use of fentanyl correlated with longer stay in outpatient unit. *Plast Reconstr Surg* 2000;105:1577–1579.

Rees TD, Barone CM, Valauri FA, *et al*. Hematomas requiring surgical evacuation following face lift surgery. *Plast Reconstr Surg* 1994;93:1185–1190.

Tebbetts J. Achieving a predictable 24-hour return to normal activities after breast augmentation: part II. Patient preparation, refined surgical techniques, and instrumentation. *Plast Reconstr Surg* 2002;109:293–305.

Teimourian B, Adham MN. A national survey of complications associated with suction lipectomy: what we did then and what we do now. *Plast Reconstr Surg* 2000;105: 1881–1884.

Trott SA, Beran SJ, Rohrich RJ, *et al*. Safety considerations and fluid resuscitation in liposuction: an analysis of 53 consecutive patients. *Plast Reconstr Surg* 1998;102:2220– 2229.

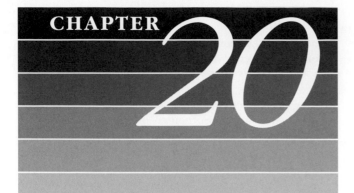

CHAPTER 20

Anesthesia in Remote Locations

AISLING M. CONRAN

YULIA DEMIDOVICH

Anesthesiologists can optimize completion of diagnostic studies and therapeutic interventions, and at the same time alleviate patient discomfort and maximize patient safety, by administering anesthetics in remote areas of the hospital.

ANESTHESIA FOR GASTROENTEROLOGY PROCEDURES

Gastroenterology procedures that may require consultation with an anesthesiologist include endoscopic retrograde cholangiopancreatography (ERCP), endoscopic gastric duodenum examination with ultrasound-guided biopsy (EUS), or colonoscopy. A diagnostic ERCP may be performed to evaluate choledocholithiasis, as well as biliary strictures. A therapeutic ERCP may include biliary stent placement, stone removal, and sphincter of Oddi manometry. In addition to the usual off-site anesthetic concerns, most of the above cases involve sharing the airway with the endoscopist.

The patient population undergoing these procedures consists of patients with known or suspected cancer (pancreatic, hepatic, gallbladder, gastric), patients at risk of developing Barrett's esophagus or colonic polyps, and patients with gastroesophageal reflux. In addition, these patients may have other comorbidities (diabetes, coronary artery disease, stroke, renal disease, hepatitis, pregnancy) that need to be considered in the anesthetic preoperative evaluation. Another segment of the adult gastrointestinal patient population consists of liver transplant patients. They may come to the gastrointestinal laboratory for follow-up exams to evaluate biliary strictures.

Fentanyl and midazolam are a common combination used in gastrointestinal procedure areas; droperidol, meperidine, and others are used as well. Guidelines for the administration of droperidol in gastrointestinal procedures are included in the *Guidelines for the Use of Deep Sedation and Analgesia for GI Endoscopy*

Procedures published by the American Society for Gastrointestinal Endoscopy. Droperidol has been reported to cause *torsade de pointes* in patients and its use by anesthesia care providers has diminished.

A failed sedation case occurs when a sedation protocol is followed without successfully completing the examination. The combination of medications used may not have resulted in the desired level of sedation, or may have caused side effects such as respiratory depression/ hypoxia or hypotension, and/or created an uncooperative patient who is disinhibited. Prolonged therapeutic procedures such as ERCP have the highest rate of these problems.

Anesthesiologists are usually consulted (Box 20-1) when any of the following pertinent items in the history are obtained:

- An obvious/known difficult airway
- Previous failed sedation by the gastroenterology team
- Problems associated with prior anesthetic exposure
- Morbid obesity
- Stridor, snoring, or sleep apnea
- Gastroesophageal reflux/aspiration risk

and for procedures performed in the prone position.

Patients may be tolerant to sedative medications if they are chronic users of benzodiazepines, narcotics, alcohol or other drugs. Patients with neurologic diseases may be more susceptible to sedative medications and may hypoventilate. Patients with psychiatric disorders or extremely anxious patients may not cooperate during the procedure. Patients who have had a previous unsatisfactory experience with sedation for this procedure may request general anesthesia. Patients who have a known difficult airway or who have features suggestive of a difficult airway/difficult mask (small mouth opening; head and neck cancer patients, particularly after radiation therapy; patients with cervical fusions and limited airway/extension of the neck) are frequently scheduled with an anesthesiologist from the beginning.

Propofol and inhalation agents, including nitrous oxide, have been used for endoscopic procedures. Propofol has been used in combination with other drugs for upper endoscopies and colonoscopies but without any distinct advantages over other drug regimens. However, its use during ERCP and EUS has resulted in shorter recovery times, allowed patients to transfer independently, and allowed a faster return to baseline oral intake and activity level. Propofol has been administered for these procedures by other physicians and nurses with advanced airway skills and even by patient-controlled sedation. Typically, these patients are American Society of Anesthesiologists (ASA) I or II, without coexisting significant morbidities. For an ASA III or IV patient, emergency procedures, or in the circumstances discussed earlier, anesthesia care providers are typically consulted.

The choice of general anesthesia does have some limitations for ERCP as well as some advantages. Increased time scheduled for the procedure allows for a thorough preoperative evaluation, as well as induction and positioning of the intubated patient in the prone position. The procedure room must incorporate enough space for the addition of anesthesia personnel and equipment. The cost per procedure is increased. However, in a small study of 65 patients, the use of general anesthesia resulted in fewer complications, such as a decreased incidence of acute pancreatitis post-ERCP. In addition, patients who have had an unsuccessful sedation for ERCP in the past may successfully complete the procedure with propofol sedation or with a general anesthetic.

An ERCP may be performed in the lateral or prone position. The prone position is preferred by many endoscopists, giving easier scope manipulations. At our institution, we have worked with our gastroenterologists and generally agree that the choice of monitored anesthesia care versus general anesthesia is decided upon by the anesthesiology team based upon the patient's preoperative evaluation. This choice determines the patient's position.

If the patient is thin, has a good airway, and, in the anesthesiologist's opinion, is a good candidate for sedation with spontaneous respirations then the procedure is performed in the prone position. The patient positions him/herself prone, the monitors are applied, the patient's head is turned toward the endoscopist and both arms are placed alongside the torso. Oxygen is applied via nasal cannula and the oropharynx is anesthetized topically with a local anesthetic spray. Intravenous sedation is then administered. A common choice of intravenous sedation at our institution includes a midazolam premedication with a propofol infusion, and perhaps fentanyl.

Box 20-1   Guidelines for Anesthesiology Assistance During Gastrointestinal Endoscopy

Anesthesiologist assistance may be considered in the following situations:

- Prolonged or therapeutic endoscopic procedure requiring deep sedation
- Anticipated intolerance to standard sedatives
- Increased risk for complication because of severe co-morbidity (American Society of Anesthesiologists [ASA] class III or higher)
- Increased risk for airway obstruction because of anatomic variant (see text)

With permission from Guidelines for the use of deep sedation and anesthesia for GI endoscopy. *Gastrointest Endosc* 2002;56:6161

If the patient is morbidly obese, has a difficult airway, and/or has gastroesophageal reflux, then general anesthesia with orotracheal intubation is the anesthetic plan. After anesthesia is induced and the trachea is intubated, the patient is positioned in the lateral position. One of the advantages of the lateral position is a lower likelihood of injury to hospital/gastrointestinal personnel and the patient, while positioning. Positioning a patient in the lateral position is easier than positioning an intubated patient prone. Our gastroenterology colleagues are used to having patients position themselves and, as a consequence, are not well versed in properly positioning an unconscious patient, both with regards to the patient's positioning and padding and their own position during this process. This means that the anesthesiologist must be even more vigilant regarding positioning injuries and in supervising positioning by others. A disadvantage of this approach is that the examination is more difficult for the endoscopist to perform and may take longer as a result.

ANESTHESIA FOR ELECTROCONVULSIVE THERAPY

Electroconvulsive therapy (ECT) was first introduced in 1938 and now assumes a significant role in the treatment of major depression, bipolar disorder, schizophrenia, and many other psychiatric disorders. For almost 30 years, ECT was performed without anesthesia. General anesthesia is now commonly employed not only for its amnestic qualities but more importantly for muscle relaxation and attenuation of the physiological responses commonly seen during ECT treatments.

Electroconvulsive Therapy and Physiologic Responses

The mechanism of action of ECT is not fully understood, although theories abound, including increased levels of circulating neurotransmitters and direct stimulation of various systems of the brain. A generalized seizure is induced during ECT by application of an electric current to one or both sides of the brain via transcutaneous electrodes. A motor seizure of 20–30 seconds has long been thought necessary to achieve clinical efficacy with this therapy, although there is some recent evidence that seizure length does not correlate with the antidepressant effect of ECT.

The resultant tonic–clonic responses are accompanied by marked cardiovascular responses. The sympathetic response results in transient tachycardia and hypertension and lasts 5 minutes or longer. Sympathetic stimulation is preceded by parasympathetically induced bradycardia or even asystole. This reaction can precipitate acute myocardial ischemia, infarction, and cardiac arrhythmias if induced in a susceptible patient, as well as depressing left ventricular systolic and diastolic functions for 20 minutes to 6 hours after ECT, even in patients without cardiac disease. Other complications that may result include intracerebral hemorrhages, cortical blindness, neurologic ischemic deficits, short-term memory loss, fractures, dislocation, muscle aches, nausea, headaches, and even sudden death.

Anesthetic Management

The main goal of anesthesia for ECT patients is to combine adequate amnesia, sedation, muscle relaxation, and attenuation of the sympathetic system response. These anesthetic goals require a rapid return to spontaneous ventilation and consciousness without interfering with the quality and duration of the seizure. These goals favor the use of short-acting medications. Methohexital is by far the most widely used general anesthetic for ECT. The current recommended induction dose is 0.75–1.0 mg/kg; however, patients who chronically use alcohol and centrally active drugs may manifest increased anesthetic requirements and elderly patients may require a dose reduction. Compared to methohexital, thiopental (induction dose of 1.5–2.5 mg/kg) shortens ECT seizure duration. Propofol (0.75–2.4 mg/kg) has been compared to methohexital in numerous studies, and it decreases the seizure duration. However, in two small studies, the use of propofol correlated with an improved therapeutic outcome, as compared to methohexital. Etomidate (0.15–0.3 mg/kg) is generally associated with a prolonged seizure effect, which may be helpful in those patients with a short seizure time. However nevertheless, etomidate has provides cardiovascular stability and the acute hemodynamic response to ECT could be unfavorably accentuated. In addition, the intermediate recovery from etomidate (between methohexital and thiopental), and its increased rate of emesis, as compared to thiopental make etomidate a less optimal choice for ECT.

Ketamine is an unfavorable drug in this setting because its sympathomimetic activity increases hemodynamic responses as well as intracranial pressure following administration of the electrical stimulus. Benzodiazepines should be avoided prior to ECT because of their anticonvulsant properties; however, their effect can be readily reversed when flumazenil is given prior to ECT treatment.

Inhalation anesthesia is rarely used in ECT treatment since current intravenous therapy is a more convenient form of general anesthetic in a remote location. While inhalational anesthetics are not employed often in routine ECT treatments, they are used with patients in late stages of pregnancy to minimize the uterine contractions triggered by ECT.

In order to minimize myalgias and to prevent severe musculoskeletal injuries as a result of a vigorous seizure, a muscle relaxant is commonly used during ECT. Succinylcholine (0.5–1.5 mg/kg) remains one of the most popular choices because of its rapid onset of action and short duration. However, when significant contraindications exist (malignant hyperthermia, neuroleptic malignant syndrome, hyperkalemia), mivacurium (0.08–0.2 mg/kg) is a good alternative. One must remember that both of these medications are metabolized by plasma cholinesterase and an alternative muscle relaxant should be chosen if the patient is plasma-cholinesterase-deficient.

As mentioned above, parasympathetic and sympathetic outbursts are seen following an induced seizure. Several drugs are used to abolish or diminish the undesired effects. Glycopyrrolate (0.2 mg intravenously) is the preferred anticholinergic agent; it attenuates the post-ECT hypersalivation, bradycardia, or asystole that results from the initial parasympathetic surge. In contrast, atropine has central nervous system activity with pronounced side effects and may produce excessive postprocedural delirium when given in combination with tricyclic antidepressants.

Beta-blockade is commonly used to reduce the acute sympathetic discharge. Esmolol (1–1.3 mg/kg) and labetalol (0.1–0.2 mg/kg) are frequently administered prior to induction with successful diminution in the cardiovascular response to ECT. However, both have been found to reduce the electroencephalogram (EEG) seizure duration. Interestingly, in older patients with known hypertension, combining labetalol with nifedipine or nicardipine has been shown to be an effective treatment for post-ECT hemodynamic excitement without altering seizure duration, as opposed to diltiazem, which shortens seizure length. Verapamil 0.1 mg/kg prior to ECT treatment reduces the peak heart rate and mean arterial blood pressure after ECT but does not affect seizure duration.

Pretreatment of patients with dexmedetomidine, an alpha-2-adrenergic agonist, prior to the therapy (0.5–1.0 µg/kg intravenously) produced dose-related sedation but failed to decrease peak mean arterial blood pressure and heart rate responses after ECT stimulus and resulted

Table 20-1   Implications of Psychotropic Drug Use for Electroconvulsive Therapy Anesthesia

Drug (Medication) Class	Mechanism of Action	Side Effects	Anesthetic Concerns
Phenothiazines (chlorpromazine)	Antagonizes dopamine in the basal ganglia and forebrain	Extrapyramidal; neuroleptic malignant syndrome (NMS); lowers seizure threshold	Malignant hyperthermia has a similar presentation to NMS; *cardiovascular* – peripheral alpha-blockade, direct smooth relaxation, direct cardiac depression
Butyrophenones (droperidol and haloperidol)	Decreases dopamine actions postsynaptically	Extrapyramidal; cerebral vasoconstrictor *cardiovascular* – peripheral alpha-blockade	Antiemetic; *torsade de pointes* with droperidol
Lithium	Substitutes for Na⁺ intracellularly → decreased cAMP	Polyuria, polydipsia	Narrow therapeutic range; toxicity leads to sedation, muscle weakness, nausea and ECG changes
Tricyclic antidepressants (amitriptyline, doxepin, etc.)	Potentiates norepinephrine and serotonin in the central nervous system by blocking reuptake	Anticholinergic; *cardiovascular* – orthostatic hypotension; slight ↑ heart rate; sedation	Indirect-acting sympathomimetics (ephedrine) produce ↑ response – use direct-acting medications (phenylephrine)
Monoamine oxidase inhibitors (pargyline, selegiline, phenelzine, etc.)	Inhibit monoamine oxidase, increasing levels of neurotransmitters	Sedation, blurred vision, orthostatic hypotension	Indirect-acting sympathomimetics (ephedrine) and direct-acting drugs produce ↑ response; meperidine may produce hyperthermia upon interaction with MAOIs
Serotonin reuptake inhibitors (fluoxetine, trazodone)	Inhibit uptake of serotonin	Slight slowing of cardiac conduction; slight anticholinergic effect	

cAMP, cyclic adenosine monophosphate; ECG, electrocardiographic; MAOI, monoamine oxidase inhibitor.

in a prolonged recovery time. Clonidine (0.05–0.3 mg), an alpha-2-adrenergic agonist, produces a dose-related decrease in mean arterial blood pressure prior to electrical stimulation but no significant effect on post-ECT heart rate.

Opioid medications such as alfentanil (10 µg/kg), when used in combination with methohexital and propofol, reduce the induction doses and prolong the ECT-induced seizure duration. Remifentanil (1 µg/kg) and methohexital 0.5 mg/kg in combination show an increase in duration of the seizure. Both alfentanil and remifentanil allow for a decreased induction dose without significant changes in hemodynamic values or recovery times in elderly patients. On the other hand, fentanyl (1.5 µg/kg) in combination with methohexital reduces seizure duration and fails to address the ensuing hemodynamic changes post-ECT. Thus, it appears that the increased seizure duration seen with short-acting opioids is most probably related to a decreased anesthetic dose required for induction.

Patients may arrive with current drug therapy for their psychiatric illness. Medications may include phenothiazines, butyrophenones, lithium, tricyclic antidepressants, serotonin reuptake inhibitors and monoamine oxidase inhibitors. Each class of medication has its own side effects and potential anesthetic interactions (Table 20-1).

Anesthetic Technique

As stated above, the role of the anesthesiologist during ECT is to provide a safe therapeutic environment for a patient undergoing the procedure. Amnesia, analgesia, and attenuation of hemodynamic responses, while minimizing interference with the seizure activity, are achieved with the drugs described above. Rapid onset of unconsciousness and prompt recovery are achieved using fast-onset, short-acting medications (succinylcholine, methohexital, propofol, esmolol), which should be drawn and readily available to the provider.

Patients presenting for ECT should follow ASA nil-by-mouth guidelines; however, those with cardiovascular diseases should be encouraged to take their antihypertensive medications, except diuretics, as per routine, with small amounts of clear fluids. To prevent or ease post-ECT myalgias, patients may be premedicated with acetaminophen or nonsteroidal anti-inflammatory drugs.

Patients may be poor historians because of their current disease process. The history may be obtained from the chart, psychiatric staff and family members. Nil-by-mouth status may be verified by staff. Because of the short and noninvasive nature of the procedure, the MAC approach or a brief general anesthetic is appropriate. Kadar *et al.* evaluated more than 650 general anesthetics, without intubation, administered to obese patients undergoing ECT with no evidence of regurgitation or aspiration. If the patient is pregnant or has significant risks of aspiration, tracheal intubation with a rapid sequence induction is the recommended approach.

Appropriate resuscitative equipment, including laryngoscope, endotracheal tube, laryngeal mask airway (LMA), oral and/or nasal airways, face mask with a standard circuit or a bag-valve system, and a functional suction system must be available. Standard monitors such as electrocardiogram (ECG), pulse oximeter, and noninvasive blood pressure monitor should be applied to the patient prior to induction together with electroencephalogram (EEG) and electromyographic monitor. During the induction, ventilation is assisted with a standard circuit or an Ambu/Jackson–Reese system. A bite block must be placed prior to the application of stimuli in order to protect the teeth and prevent lacerations of the tongue. A tourniquet may be used to isolate the circulation in an extremity before the muscle relaxant is administered. The tourniquet system is used by the psychiatrist to quantify the durations of the motor seizure, which correlates with the EEG seizure.

The recovery period can be complicated by agitation, and amnesia. Central nervous system side effects after ECT include headaches, confusion, and cognitive impairment. Nausea, vomiting, and dizziness are infrequent. Acute cardiovascular or neurological events are rare. Patients should be monitored for 15–30 min following recovery from ECT.

Complicated Patients for Electroconvulsive Therapy

Cerebral Aneurysm
Patients with cerebral aneurysms are at risk of having an aneurysm rupture or enlarge because of the increase in cerebral blood flow that takes place during ECT. The increase in cerebral blood flow velocity is less with propofol than with thiopental.

Subdural Hemorrhage and Intracranial Mass Lesion
In patients with cerebral mass lesions, premedication with steroids and diuretics, followed by hyperventilation, are recommended prior to unilateral stimulus application. However, raised intracranial pressure is a relative contraindication for ECT, since cerebral blood flow increases during ECT as a result of the seizure. Consultation with neurosurgical colleagues, as well as close follow up with computed tomography (CT) scans is advised.

Cardiovascular Disease
As discussed above, patients with history of coronary artery disease should be pretreated with beta-blockers or a combination of beta-blockade and calcium channel blockade in order to attenuate a post-ECT sympathetic response and decrease the incidence of ischemia, arrhythmias, and hypertension. One of the absolute contraindications to ECT is the patient with an untreated pheochromocytoma.

Therefore, anyone with symptoms of hypertension, flushing, and headaches should be deferred from ECT until the diagnostic workup is completed.

In patients with chronic atrial fibrillation, full anticoagulation is recommended since they are at higher risk of embolism. Those with a history of bradyarrhythmias (sick sinus syndrome) may need to be pretreated with atropine, as well as patients with myasthenia gravis who are receiving pyridostigmine.

Permanent pacemakers should temporarily be converted to fixed-rate pacing before the treatment in order to minimize the risk of interference with pacemaker function. Automatic internal defibrillators should be deactivated before the initiation of therapy. Consultation with the patient's cardiologist is advised on the proper method of deactivation.

Pregnancy

Rapid sequence endotracheal intubation must be used for airway protection in the second- and third-trimester parturient for general anesthesia. Maintenance of general anesthesia with inhalation agents may reduce the risk of uterine contractions following ECT. Nevertheless, tocolytic prophylaxis should be considered to prevent spontaneous abortion in patients with a history of premature labor or uterine contractions. Fetal monitoring should be considered with gestational ages more than 20 weeks.

Conclusion – Electroconvulsive Therapy

Electroconvulsive therapy is a commonly performed procedure in many inpatient and outpatient centers and, when administered appropriately, can be a beneficial and safe procedure. However, the current patient population continues to grow older and presents with a variety of coexisting diseases that should be considered thoroughly. Thus, no matter how easy the procedure appears, anesthetics should be chosen with careful consideration and tailored to the patient's physiology.

ANESTHESIA IN THE CARDIAC CATHETERIZATION LABORATORY

Cardioversions

Cardioversions can restore sinus rhythm and are performed more frequently now in patients than in the past. The direct current necessary to convert atrial fibrillation or atrial flutter to sinus rhythm is painful for the patient. This is typically a very brief procedure. Even if more than one attempt is required, these can be done in quick succession. In summary, a brief general anesthetic is required for this uncomfortable procedure.

The patient population requiring a cardioversion often has associated diseases that place them in a higher risk

category. Hypertension, diabetes mellitus, coronary artery disease, congestive heart failure, renal insufficiency or end-stage renal disease, strokes (via paradoxical emboli), and chronic obstructive pulmonary disease are likely to be found in the patient's medical history. A reasonable number of patients older than 70 years is to be expected.

Airway issues, including airway patency, dentures/bridges/caps/dentition, and range of motion of the cervical spine need to be addressed. Wall oxygen and suction, the ability to perform bag-mask ventilation, and intubation equipment must be readily available during the performance of the procedure. Monitoring of the electrocardiogram, pulse oximetry, and blood pressure is necessary. Most practitioners rely on portable end-tidal carbon dioxide (ET-CO$_2$) monitors for confirmation of tracheal intubation in the rare instances in which intubation is required. A short period of postprocedure monitoring is generally required to assure wakefulness, stable vital signs, and oxygen saturation.

American Society of Anesthesiologists nil-by-mouth guidelines should be followed. For healthy patients without aspiration risk, nil-by-mouth for 6 hours or more is sufficient. Patients with gastroesophageal reflux may benefit from longer fasting times, premedication with a nonparticulate antacid, metoclopramide, and an H$_2$ antagonist, and consideration of rapid sequence induction with endotracheal intubation.

Short-acting induction agents such as propofol and methohexital are tailor-made for a brief general anesthetic in which spontaneous respirations are not only acceptable but desirable. A successful technique may include preoxygenation, propofol or methohexital for induction, brief direct current shock for cardioversion, and rapid recovery of the patient. In cases where more than one shock is required, a repeated dose of propofol or methohexital after reassessment of the patient's degree of wakefulness will still allow for a fast recovery with little to no "hang-over" drug effect from the sedative medication.

Both of these medications produce hypnosis. Propofol 1 mg/kg will in most cases provide an unconscious, spontaneously breathing patient who recovers from the anesthetic quickly. Methohexital 0.5–0.6 mg/kg has been given by non-anesthesiologists with additional airway/sedation training, with good results. Complications of direct-current cardioversion include unplanned admission, awareness, respiratory complications (includes intubation), bradyarrhythmias, ventricular fibrillation, and embolic stroke.

Electrophysiology Studies

Patients may be evaluated for re-entry pathways, tachycardias, or other arrhythmias. Ascertaining the reason for the anesthesia consultation is clearly necessary here, since, for the most part, anesthesiologists are infrequently involved in adult electrophysiology studies. Common reasons are found in Box 20-2.

Monitored anesthesia care is often acceptable, with oxygen via nasal cannula and general anesthesia as a backup plan. Discuss sedative medications and inhalation agents with the electrophysiologist (Table 20-2). Certain anesthetics/sedative medications can suppress the dysrhythmia or re-entry pathways that the cardiologist is trying to map. Perhaps an easier question to ask is whether there is a particular medication that the electrophysiologist would like one to avoid in the current patient.

Monitoring for electrophysiology studies includes electrocardiogram, automated noninvasive blood pressure, oxygen saturation, placement of a preinduction arterial line versus monitoring the arterial line placed by cardiologist. R2 pads need to be placed so that dysrhythmias can be rapidly controlled electrically if necessary.

Discussion and ongoing communication with the cardiologist needs to take place regarding treatment of arrhythmias. As the electrophysiology mapping occurs, the dysrhythmia being evaluated will be produced. Treating it with antiarrhythmic agents may result in completely abolishing the arrhythmia for a time and delay-

ing its successful mapping. Certainly, any hemodynamic instability should be communicated directly to the cardiologist, who may cease the electrical stimulation. If the dysrhythmia persists, the R2 pads on the patient are available to electrically cardiovert or defibrillate the patient as necessary. In addition, one may be asked by the cardiologist to initiate an infusion such as isoproterenol, which may stimulate the patient's heart and produce the tachyarrhythmia that is being sought.

Cardiac Catheterization

Adult cardiac catheterizations for coronary angiography are generally performed with conscious sedation and local anesthetics administered by the cardiologist. These procedures are well tolerated by the patient. On occasion, if significant ischemia, an allergic reaction to the intravenous contrast, or significant respiratory or hemodynamic instability occurs, the patient may require emergent intubation and/or transport to the operating room for emergency cardiac surgery. In this urgent scenario, an anesthesiologist will be consulted quickly to help with controlling the airway, resuscitation, and transport to the operating room.

Atrial Septal Defect and Ventricular Septal Defect Device Closures

Device closures of septal defects (mostly atrial) or the occasional patent ductus arteriosus are performed in adult patients. At our institution, these procedures are performed by the pediatric interventional cardiologists in the pediatric catheterization laboratory. Often, patients receive very light conscious sedation from the sedation nurse, supervised by the cardiologist. Local anesthetic is used by the cardiologist for the femoral arterial and venous access necessary for the procedure. On occasion,

Table 20-2 Medications for Anesthesia in Remote Locations

	Induction Agents	Muscle Relaxants	Reflux Precautions	Antiemetics	Resuscitation	Sedation/ Anxiolysis
General	Thiopental Propofol Etomidate	Succinylcholine Nondepolarizer	Sodium bicarbonate Metoclopramide Pepcid	Metoclopramide Ondansetron	Epinephrine Ephedrine Phenylephrine Sodium bicarbonate Calcium Lidocaine	Propofol Midazolam
	Anticoagulation and Reversal	**HR Control**	**Antibiotics**	**Diuretics**	**Pretreatment for Dye Allergies**	**BP Control**
Catheterization Laboratory	Heparin Protamine	Adenosine Esmolol Isoproterenol	Antibiotics	Furosemide	Steroids Diphenhydramine	Sodium nitroprusside Nitroglycerin
Neuroradiology	Heparin Protamine	Esmolol Labetalol		Furosemide Mannitol	Steroids Diphenhydramine	Sodium nitroprusside

an anesthesiologist will be consulted if the patient has a difficult airway, is critically ill, or has failed to achieve adequate analgesia/anesthesia with the catheterization laboratory's sedation protocol.

Critically ill patients include those who develop a post-infarct ventricular septal defect. These patients have a significant mortality if undergoing an operative repair with cardiac bypass. Instead, these patients now come to the catheterization laboratory for a device closure of the ventricular septal defect. They are often intubated and are typically on a ventricular assist device for support of the acute volume overload on the right heart.

Rarely, a device can embolize. The cardiologist can often re-secure the device for removal via a specialty catheter with a wire enclosure. If this is not successful, the patient may go to the operating room for removal of the device and possible operative repair of the defect.

INTERVENTIONAL RADIOLOGY

A recent study surveyed interventional radiologists' use of sedation/analgesia in Europe and compared this data to a similar survey in the United States. Sedation was used much more frequently in the United States. Many European procedures are performed with the patient in the awake, alert state. The procedures likely to require a general anesthetic were the same but a higher percentage required general anesthesia in the United States. In this type of setting, anesthesia providers are most often consulted when the patient has failed the radiologist's sedation protocol.

Biliary Tubes/Stents

Biliary tube placements or exchanges require a higher analgesic dose to achieve sufficient analgesia for the procedure (Box 20-3). These biliary procedures resulted in the highest incidence of respiratory complications in a study of conscious sedation by radiologists for these procedures. Respiratory complications included placement of an oral airway, use of an Ambu bag, or use of the jaw-thrust maneuver.

Transjugular Intrahepatic Portosystemic Shunt

Transjugular intrahepatic portosystemic shunt (TIPS) is performed commonly at our institution and increasingly in interventional radiology suites across the country (Box 20-4). A TIPS procedure is performed in a patient with portal hypertension, as evidenced by esophageal/gastric varices or severe ascites, that has failed medical therapy. This procedure connects the portal and systemic venous systems, thus decompressing the portal circulation.

Catheterization of the hepatic veins is performed via the right internal jugular vein. A long, curved needle is passed from the hepatic vein through liver parenchyma into an intrahepatic branch of the portal vein. Pressures are measured in the systemic and portal veins. In order to dilate the connection between the hepatic and portal veins, a stent is placed and dilated until adequate decompression of the portal system is obtained.

A TIPS procedure is often used as definitive therapy, as well as a bridge to transplantation. Anesthesiologists are consulted because of the patient's severe systemic disease (typically ASA PS III or IV) or Child–Pugh classification, the potential for significant blood loss, and the need for suspension of respirations.

Suspension of respiration at certain points facilitates the right internal jugular access and the transhepatic connection necessary for this procedure; therefore general anesthesia with endotracheal intubation is a reasonable anesthetic plan. Patients with the associated sequelae of severe liver disease, such as esophageal varices or significant ascites with increased abdominal pressure, or patients with other medical disorders, such as gastroesophageal reflux and diabetic gastroparesis, may benefit from a rapid sequence induction. Preoxygenation is very important in this group of critically ill patients, who may desaturate quickly because of decreased functional residual capacity (due to the ascites and increased abdominal girth).

Complications occur during approximately 10–15% of procedures. Mortality is typically a result of hemorrhage (<2%). Major complications (3%) can include hemoperitoneum (3%), gall bladder puncture (0.5%), stent malposition (1%), free stent migration within the vascular tree and

---

Box 20-3   Common Procedures in Interventional Radiology

Biliary drainage tube placement and exchange
Tunneled catheters
Diagnostic arteriography; vascular angiography
Therapeutic vascular procedures (angioplasty + embolization); thrombolysis
Other catheter insertions

Box 20-4   Other Interventional Radiology Procedures

TIPS
Fistulography
Liver biopsy (via IJ)
Nephrolithotomy

perforation, hemobilia (2%), hepatic artery injury, and death (11%). Minor complications include transient contrast reaction controlled by medical therapy (15–25%), fever (2%), transient pulmonary edema (1%), and entry site hematoma (2%). Other complications include tamponade, intra-abdominal hemorrhage, and decreased hepatic function.

A successful TIPS may be determined by technical success (a connection made between hepatic veins and a branch of the intrahepatic portal vein), hemodynamic success (post-TIPS decrease in the gradient between the portal-to-systemic venous systems), or clinical success (decrease in variceal bleeding and in refractory ascites). Long-term patency of TIPS is an issue.

Blood products should be available. Fresh frozen plasma may be necessary if the patient has an elevated prothrombin time, reflecting a systemic coagulopathy due to decreased coagulation factor production by the failing liver. Packed red blood cells should also be available, since substantial blood loss can occur. If this complication happens, volume resuscitation must begin immediately, with blood products, colloid, and crystalloid.

INTERVENTIONAL NEURORADIOLOGY

Interventional neuroradiology procedures include:

- Embolization of arteriovenous malformations, carotid cavernous fistulas, cerebral aneurysms, and tumors of the head and neck
- Sclerotherapy of venous malformations
- Angioplasty of carotid stenosis or vasospasm from subarachnoid hemorrhage
- Test occlusions of cerebral aneurysms and brain tumors
- Super-selective angiography of arteriovenous malformations and aneurysms.

Many of these procedures are dangerous, and complications can occur. While the anesthetic considerations are similar to those of neurosurgical repairs in the operating room, significant differences exist between the two areas.

Interventional neuroradiology involves arteriography of the head and neck, with access usually achieved via the femoral vessels. A femoral introducer is placed, then a catheter through the introducer. The tip of the catheter is placed in the carotid or vertebral artery in question, and then a smaller catheter is placed distally that will allow more selective angiograms to take place and clearly define the anatomy of the abnormal vessels.

High-resolution fluoroscopy and high-speed digital subtraction angiography allow a map of the patient's vascular anatomy to be made. A scout film is made before each run to remove bone and other nonvascular structures from subsequent angiograms in the run (only specified vessels are visible). The selective catheters are placed and a map is made of the patient's vascular anatomy. The computer superimposes this image on the live image so that the radiologist can see the progress of the tip of the radio-opaque catheter. Any movement during this time results in a much poorer quality image. Frequently, conscious sedation is employed, except for specific procedures or in uncooperative adults.

Aneurysm Coiling

Cerebral aneurysms may be obliterated by coil closure in the interventional radiology suite. Percutaneous access for the necessary angiograms is obtained via the femoral vessels. One may be able to monitor the arterial line via the femoral access. While the aneurysm is being evaluated, the patient may need to be able to cooperate with frequent assessments. After a consultation between the neuroradiologist and a neurosurgeon, the aneurysm may be determined to be amenable to coiling. Patient immobility is desired so that the coils do not dislodge/embolize because of patient movement at an inopportune time.

General anesthesia is often chosen to provide an immobile patient. In addition, this procedure can be quite time-consuming, with numerous coils needed. An advantage of this plan is that it allows one to hyperventilate the patient, if necessary, for added brain protection. In addition, allowing the patient to cool to about 35.5° C provides for further brain protection. Clearly, tight blood pressure control is important in the patient with a known cerebral artery aneurysm. Just as in an operative repair of cerebral aneurysms, a quick "wake-up" is desired so that the patient may undergo neurologic evaluation.

Deliberate hypotension may be needed for arteriovenous malformations or if ischemia occurs during the procedure. Pharmacologic agents should be available during the procedure in order to manipulate blood pressure as needed. If bleeding occurs because of aneurysm rupture, deliberate hypotension may be required until the bleeding is under control.

The device or coils can embolize but may be retrieved by the radiologist and further angiograms obtained. If the coils cannot be retrieved, the patient is transported to the OR for removal of the coils and possible operative clipping of the aneurysm.

For the preanesthetic evaluation, one must obtain the specific history set out in Box 20-5, in addition to the usual anesthetic considerations. During the physical examination, evaluate the airway carefully. If the procedure is tumor embolization in the airway, consider the impact of postprocedural edema and discuss this issue with the interventional neuroradiology

Box 20-5   Preprocedure Evaluation for Interventional Neuroradiology

Neurosurgical considerations
Anticoagulation or coagulation disorders
Protamine allergy (insulin use, previous vasectomy, fish allergy)
Recent steroid use
Contrast reactions (iodine, shellfish allergies, atopy)
Neck, back or joint problems → patient may not be able to lie still for several hours → general anesthetic
Control of preoperative hypertension → essential for perioperative control
Baseline electrocardiogram
Pregnancy test for women of childbearing age

From Young WL, Pile-Spellman J. Anesthetic considerations for interventional neuroradiology. *Anesthesiology* 1994;80:427–456.

team. In addition to any laboratory tests suggested by the preoperative evaluation, consider obtaining coagulation studies.

Premedication may include an anxiolytic, glycopyrrolate (antisialagogue), and/or medication for blood pressure control and deliberate hypotension. At least one large intravenous line, 18-gauge, should be placed for an interventional neuroradiology procedure, with a couple of extensions. Other cases may require two large-bore intravenous lines. An arterial line may be required for various medical reasons, or if deliberate hypotension or hypertension are going to be used for posterior fossa cases. One can usually follow the femoral arterial line accessed by the radiologist.

Positioning issues include padding and placing a pillow under the patient's knees after femoral access is achieved, to increase patient comfort for a potentially lengthy procedure. Protect against inadvertent movements of the head if the patient startles by placing paper tape as a "reminder" restraint over the forehead. Careful attention must be paid that the tape is not too tight for the patient to turn the head if necessary. This might lead to aspiration if vomiting occurs during the procedure.

If an endotracheal tube is in place, or will be placed, take advantage of the fluoroscopy to confirm its position, as well as the position of any central venous catheters. Other monitors include ECG with ST trending, pulse oximetry, ET-CO$_2$, temperature and a Foley catheter. Medications should include agents to control blood pressure, diuretics, protamine, sedatives, induction agents, and muscle relaxants (see Table 20-2). Extensions should be placed on all intravenous lines and on the circuit to avoid disconnections during movement of the table.

Embolization of Intracranial Arteriovenous Malformations

Patients often have large arteriovenous malformations with several feeder arteries. The goal is to embolize as many of the feeders as possible in preparation for surgery. This may facilitate surgery by decreasing bleeding and allowing the brain adequate time to accommodate to the changing hemodynamics of an arteriovenous malformation with decreased flow.

Anesthetic goals include a comfortable patient, and this goal may be met by allowing sedation to fluctuate as necessary to allow for neurologic assessments. The neuroradiologist may use glue, coils, alcohol particles, or silk thread to embolize the arteriovenous malformation in preparation for surgery. Hypotension may be utilized to decrease flow in the arteriovenous malformation so that the glue will be distributed only in the arteriovenous malformation and not distally.

Deliberate Hypotension

This technique is used to slow the flow into the arterial side of an arteriovenous malformation before the injection of glue and to test the cerebrovascular reserve in patients undergoing carotid occlusion. Sedation is decreased and the patient is allowed to become more alert to allow for neurologic evaluation. Nausea and vomiting are a significant problem in the awake patient. The use of neurolept anesthesia employing droperidol may allow benefit from the antiemetic effect of droperidol in this instance, although another dose may now be required (see Table 20-2).

In the awake patient, hypotension may be more challenging to achieve than in patients undergoing a general anesthetic. Esmolol (1 mg/kg) bolus followed by an infusion of 0.5 mg/kg/min titrated to systemic blood pressure is one option. Supplemental boluses of labetalol, 50–100 mg, may be needed (see Table 20-2).

Adrenergic blockers have the advantage of not affecting cerebral blood flow directly. Sodium nitroprusside can be used but may result in significant hypotension. Treating severe systemic hypotension in the awake period is difficult because of the nausea and vomiting that develops. The motion from emesis can result in dislodged catheters, vessel damage, and vessel perforation.

Deliberate Hypertension

A situation may arise in which cerebral ischemia occurs. Raising the systemic blood pressure will improve flow to the ischemic area via collateral blood vessels. The collateral pathways include the circle of Willis, and absence of parts of the circle is a normal variant. Therefore, deliberate hypertension may not be successful.

Phenylephrine (1 μg/kg) bolus followed by an infusion titrated to effect on the systemic blood pressure is a logical choice of pharmacological agent (see Table 20-2).

Raising the systemic blood pressure to levels that reverse the deficit and keeping the blood pressure at this level is the main goal at this point. Observe the ECG for signs of myocardial ischemia.

Deliberate Hypercapnia

The addition of inspired CO_2 produces excess cerebral venous outflow. This creates a pressure gradient that promotes flow of the sclerosing agent or chemotherapy away from vital intracranial structures. If inspired CO_2 is not available, hypoventilation may be employed. An inspired oxygen concentration of 100% and positive end-expiratory pressure may help with oxygenation.

Anticoagulation

Patients are anticoagulated to decrease the risk of thromboembolic complications and thrombosis that may result from damage to vessels by catheters. Some institutions obtain a baseline activated coagulation time (ACT) and follow the ACT hourly, redosing heparin as necessary. Others dose the heparin initially at 5,000 units/70 kg and follow-up dosing is based on time. If the patient will remain heparinized overnight, the large femoral introducer will remain in place until the heparin effect has worn off. If the procedure ends prematurely, or the lesion is not amenable to repair by interventional radiology techniques, then the heparin is reversed with protamine, the femoral introducer is removed, and pressure is held.

Contrast Reactions

Low osmolality non-ionic contrast is commonly used today in radiology and the catheterization laboratories. This contrast medium has one-third of the osmolality of the older agents. Fatal reactions can still occur (1:100,000 exposures) but there is a much lower rate of mild-to-moderate reactions with the lower-osmolality non-ionic contrast agents. Euvolemia is important to maintain in these patients to avoid renal side effects of the contrast.

Patients may have a history of a previous reaction to contrast. Pretreatment with steroids and antihistamines should take place prior to the procedure. Prednisone 50 mg the night before and prednisone 50 mg and diphenhydramine 50 mg intravenously are given prior to the procedure.

Neurologic Catastrophes

Communication between the neuroradiologist and anesthetist must be quick and effective. Airway control is a priority. In addition, the anesthesiologist must ascertain if the problem is bleeding or thrombosis. If bleeding or hemorrhage is occurring, the heparin must be quickly reversed with protamine. An emergency reversal dose of protamine 1 mg to 100 units of heparin may be given. While the bleeding is ongoing, the blood pressure must be kept lower while maintaining cerebral perfusion pressure. Thiopental will decrease the chance of seizures, which may occur from subarachnoid hemorrhage. Once the bleeding is under control, systemic blood pressure should be brought up. Consult with the neuroradiologist on current blood pressure goals at this point.

If cerebral ischemia is occurring as a result of vascular occlusion, then systemic blood pressure must be raised significantly. This increase in systemic blood pressure will improve perfusion to the ischemia area via collaterals. A rapid induction with thiopental and succinylcholine will not only allow for rapid control of the airway, but the use of thiopental will provide brain protection.

Sclerotherapy of Venous Angiomas

Sclerotherapy can result in significant postprocedure edema. If the angioma is in the airway, the patient may be unable to maintain a patent airway. Ethanol is used in sclerotherapy and side effects include hypoglycemia and alcohol intoxication.

Anesthetic Techniques (Plans)

Conscious Sedation

Goals include adequate analgesia, anxiolysis, patient immobility, and the ability to produce rapid changes in level of alertness/sedation as necessary for neurologic evaluation.

Analgesia

Procedures are not very painful except for chemotherapy and sclerotherapy. Patient discomfort may arise from lying still for long periods of time. Padding and placing a blanket under the knees, after femoral access is achieved, may relieve back discomfort. The femoral access and the urinary catheter are two specific points that bother the patient during the procedure.

Anxiolysis

These procedures are very stressful for the patient. Many patients have already had a previous episode of intracranial bleeding or cerebrovascular accident.

Anesthetic agents

Droperidol and fentanyl (2–4 μg/kg) as a combination for neurolept anesthesia has been used with success to obtain immobility with adequate spontaneous ventilation. Propofol infusion, beginning at 10–20 μg/kg/min and then titrated slowly upwards, gives an unconscious patient who is usually able to maintain his/her airway. There is still a risk of airway obstruction, leading to further airway interventions. Supplemental oxygen via nasal cannula should be provided during sedation techniques.

General Anesthesia

Uncooperative patients may require general anesthesia. Certain procedures such as aneurysm coiling, sclerotherapy, and some chemotherapy cases require general anesthesia to produce immobility and improve radiographic image quality. Occasionally, brief periods of apnea are required. The use of controlled ventilation allows some cerebral protection, and its use has already been reviewed earlier. The associated use of nitrous oxide during general anesthesia carries the risk of expanding air emboli that may be introduced during the procedure.

COMPUTED TOMOGRAPHY

Computed-tomography-guided biopsies may be performed in conjunction with general anesthesia. Radiofrequency ablation and percutaneous administration of 95% ethanol are methods of pain palliation for metastatic neoplasms that use CT imaging. The decision to use general anesthesia or conscious sedation with local anesthetics may depend on the number of electrode placements for radiofrequency ablation or their location (one or two sites, proceed with conscious sedation; more than two sites, proceed with general anesthesia). Image-guided percutaneous biopsies of the lung have a far greater complication rate (5% pneumothorax requiring chest tube) than all other biopsies (0.5%). Other complications include infection and bleeding.

RADIATION THERAPY

Radiation therapy involves truly remote anesthesia. It does require that patients stay completely still, and frequently hold their breath, but the treatment is administered in seconds to minutes in a large room. Most adults are able to cooperate with radiation therapy and so this discussion will focus on intraoperative radiation therapy.

Some institutions are able to deliver radiation therapy in the same room the operation takes place in but in others the patient must be transported from the operating room to the radiation therapy suite and back. Transportation of an intubated patient under general anesthesia has obvious risks but an added one in this case is infection, since the wound is only superficially closed, although covered with a sterile dressing. Intravenous anesthetics are used for ease of transportation. Ventilation with 100% oxygen allows for a greater safety margin and may make the cancer cells more sensitive to the radiation therapy.

Patient immobility, provided by general anesthesia with endotracheal intubation and muscle relaxation, helps to avoid inappropriate patient movement and decreased movement of the area where the radiation is to be directed. Intraoperative radiation therapy allows lower doses of radiation to be directed at a very specific area, decreasing the potential damage to nearby structures.

Remote monitoring must be performed via cameras and electronic monitoring. The simplest technique is to have two cameras in place. One is directed at the patient,

although it can be difficult to appreciate chest wall movement. The second camera is directed at the anesthesia machine and monitors. Blood pressure, electrocardiogram, oxygen saturation, respiratory rate and ET-CO_2 are easily viewed on the display when the camera is appropriately focused and the monitor is directed towards the camera. A back-up monitor in the control room may be connected to the monitor attached to the patient and display the same information.

Again, radiation therapy is often administered in seconds to minutes. The room may be entered at any time if one is concerned. The radiation technician will turn off the radiation and the room can be entered within 20 seconds.

MAGNETIC RESONANCE IMAGING

Magnetic resonance imaging is based on the fact that all atomic nuclei have a charge (from protons) and mass (from protons and neutrons), and that the rotation of the protons and neutrons around the nucleus produces a local magnetic field. These nuclei line up with the static but powerful magnetic field of the magnet after a radiofrequency pulse. The excess of parallel versus antiparallel atoms provides the basis for magnetic resonance imaging (MRI). Different nuclei produce differing magnetic fields and so different areas can be distinguished from each other.

Magnetic resonance imaging is advantageous for many reasons. No intervention takes place. It is repeatable. Most notably, and in contrast to other modalities, any plane may be obtained (sagittal, coronal, transverse, or oblique). The brain, spinal cord, soft tissues, and blood vessels are well defined by MRI.

The patient lies within the magnet bore. The part to be examined, for example the brain, may be set within a smaller coil. This coil limits patient movement and can limit access to the airway. The pertinent body part that will be examined is placed at the center of the magnet.

Radiofrequency filters and screens built into the MRI suite prevent the other equipment (monitors, ventilators) from causing interference with the study. MRI-compatible monitors and anesthesia machines within the magnet room are composed of nonferrous metal and use fiberoptic technology (or radiofrequencies that are not close to the one used in the study). Electrical connections to the patient from monitors can distort the MRI image by acting as antennas for radiofrequency signals.

Ferromagnetic objects are attracted to the center of the magnet, often with great force. Therefore, caution must be exercised at all times in the MRI suite. Stethoscopes, scissors, pagers, batteries in the laryngoscope, and oxygen tanks contain ferromagnetic metals. Identification badges and credit cards contain a magnetic strip that may be wiped clean by exposure to the magnetic field. Watches will slow down as the metal hand is pulled by the magnetic field and the watch may become a flying object. All these objects must be left outside the scanning room. They can cause injury to the patient if brought into the magnet room, since the patient being examined is in the core of the magnet, the area of greatest attraction. Reports of severe, even fatal injuries can be found related to such items being brought into the magnetic room by an unsuspecting individual who has not been well educated in MRI safety. Since the magnetic field takes 72–96 hours to reactivate, at great expense, it is only shut down during emergencies.

Magnetic objects can heat up in magnetic fields and cause burn injuries to the patient. Awake patients can report if an object becomes warm but the unconscious or anesthetized patient cannot. Coiled ECG leads and pulse oximeters have produced burn injuries. Prevention of burn injuries includes avoidance of coiled monitor wires, ensuring intact insulation, separating cables from the skin by padding, and keeping monitors away from the site of examination (away from the core), for example placing the pulse oximeter on the toe during a brain MRI.

Implants may or may not be a problem in the MRI scanner. Pacemakers, automatic implantable defibrillators, nerve stimulators, cochlear implants, and infusion pumps may not function appropriately in the MRI field. It is important to determine in advance if an implant or foreign material in the body contains ferrous metal. Many implants, cardiac valves, prosthetic joints, and clips are made of nonferrous metal. Even ones that contain ferrous metal may be able to be scanned if they have been in place a long time (scarred in), e.g., a cardiac valve. In addition, the force exerted by the magnet on the valve may be less than the mechanical force of the heart. However, patients with vascular clips for intracranial aneurysms, foreign objects in the eye, and pacemakers should not be subjected to MRI. The possible consequences, such as intracranial bleeding, loss of sight, and pacemaker malfunction, disconnection, or even microshock, are too severe (Figure 20-1).

The magnetic strength is measured at the core of the magnet but a magnetic field does exist beyond the magnet itself. This peripheral field decreases in intensity with decreasing distance from the core, sometimes quite rapidly. It is important to be aware of the extent of this field and to avoid bringing noncompatible equipment, e.g., ferromagnetic oxygen tanks, too close to the magnetic field.

Patients should be examined for metallic objects both on their person (ECG leads, metallic snaps on gowns, hair pins) and for scars that may indicate the presence of metallic objects (implants) within their body. Metallic objects near the scanned body part will cause interference and distortion of the image or cause injury to the patient. Even tattoos or eye makeup with metallic components can cause local irritation or interfere with the MR scan, as can the metallic spring in the cuff of an LMA.

The loud noises generated by magnetic resonance imaging can be combated by MRI-compatible ear plugs. The noise level may necessitate a deeper level of anesthesia.

Pregnant patients may undergo an MRI, if a MRI level 2 personnel-designated radiologist and the referring doctor discuss the risk/benefit ratio as per Kanal's White Paper on MR safety.

Indications for anesthesia care in adults include claustrophobia (up to 70% of awake patients), severe muscle spasm and inability to maintain adequate oxygenation. Obesity may add to claustrophobic feelings in the patient and make it difficult to position the patient, monitors, airway and intravenous line. Confused or uncooperative patients may also need sedation/general anesthesia in order to obtain the MRI. Occasionally, the administration of oxygen, particularly 100% oxygen, can affect the imaging of cerebrospinal fluid. The radiologist should be aware of this phenomenon and be aware that the study was performed under general anesthesia with supplemental oxygen.

Monitors and Equipment

Some monitors produce radiofrequency emissions which overlap those of the MRI scanner and cause image degradation. Monitors need to be evaluated in the specific MRI scanner in which they will be used (even similar monitors). Monitors which function well in one MRI environment may not in another, and vice-versa.

Electrocardiography

Electrocardiography monitoring is the monitor that shows the most frequent problems. ECG monitoring is fraught with difficulty and is often suboptimal for ST segment monitoring throughout. During radiofrequency pulsing, it is difficult monitoring the QRS complex. Newer monitors have gated signals that subtract the MRI field and radiofrequency signals to leave the patient's ECG intact. Follow the manufacturer's directions with regard to lead placement – typically three leads in a horizontal row. The wire leads can act as antennae and therefore can produce radiofrequency interference with the MR image. In addition, the leads provide a potential source of electrical shock. It is necessary to ensure that the leads are well insulated, that coiling is avoided, and that there are no cracks in the insulation.

Noninvasive blood pressure monitors with long tubing and plastic connectors are also placed as far from the magnet as possible. Arterial and central venous pressure lines may be left in place. Some transducers,

Medical History Questionnaire

Patient Name:_____ MR #:_____ Date:_____

If someone will be going with the patient to the exam room, please print your name here and state your relationship to the patient.

_____   _____

(YOUR NAME)   *(RELATIONSHIP)*

Please answer these important safety questions and give this form to the MRI staff when you arrive. *If you circle "YES" to ANY of these questions, please notify the MRI facility immediately!*

1. Do you have a heart pacemaker, electrodes, any type of muscle or nerve stimulator, or an implanted chemotherapy pump?	YES UNSURE NO
2. Have you had a clip placed on a large blood vessel in your brain?	YES UNSURE NO
3. Do you have an artificial heart valve?	YES UNSURE NO
4. Have you had a blood clot filter, a "plug," or any other metal device placed inside a blood vessel?	YES UNSURE NO
5. Have you had a cataract removed from your eye? Have you had an intraocular lens implanted?	YES UNSURE NO
6. Have you ever had surgery on your eyes or ears? Have you ever had a metal object implanted in an eye or ear?	YES UNSURE NO
7. Have you ever had a piece of metal stuck in your eyes from grinding, drilling, or welding? Do you have permanent eye-liner?	YES UNSURE NO
8. **Are you claustrophobic (fear of tight places)?**	YES UNSURE NO
9. Is there a bullet, shrapnel, or any other type of metallic projectile within your body?	YES UNSURE NO
10. Are you pregnant or breast-feeding?	YES UNSURE NO
11. Do you have sickle cell disease, thalassemia, or any other disease of the red blood cells?	YES UNSURE NO
12. Do you have abnormal kidney or liver function?	YES UNSURE NO
13. Do you weigh 300 lb or more? What is your current weight? _____	YES UNSURE NO
14. Are you bringing a sedative with you to your appointment?	YES UNSURE NO
15. Have you ever had an operation or surgical procedure? If yes, please list below.	YES UNSURE NO

Type of procedure	Date	Hospital/Surgeon	Metallic implants

16. Do you have any known drug allergies?	YES UNSURE NO

_____   _____   _____   _____
Patient or Parent Signature   Date   MRI Staff Signature   Date

Figure 20-1   Medical history questionnaire. This is a standardized form used in the Radiology Department at the University of Chicago Hospitals.

however, are not MRI-compatible and will have to be disconnected.

Various anesthesia machines are available on the market for use inside the MRI magnet room. These MRI–compatible anesthesia machines are composed of nonferrous metal, powered by oxygen, and volume controlled. The backup oxygen cylinders are made of aluminum. Long extension tubing, in addition to the regular circuit, make the breathing circuit feasible even when the patient's head is deep inside the center of the magnet.

Capnography is available. The tubing is quite long, but the monitor provides an accurate respiratory rate and will alarm with circuit disconnections. Respirations may also be monitored in the spontaneously breathing patient under general anesthesia by placing the bag on the ventilator in view of the camera. Inhalation agent monitoring is also available.

Intravenous infusion pumps may not function as programmed in a MRI field. One may place them outside the scanner and use long extension tubing to connect the infusion to the patient's intravenous line. MRI-compatible pumps are also available.

Anesthesiology Checklist for Magnetic Resonance Imaging

It is important to thoroughly check out one's anesthesia equipment and the general area to ensure that the appropriate MRI-compatible equipment is available (Boxes 20-6 and 20-7). An induction area outside the scan room is very helpful (Box 20-8).

Occupational Exposure

Magnetic resonance imaging does not require ionizing radiation. Studies in mice have not revealed any complications from long-term exposure. Healthcare practitioners may be involved in patient care within the scan room but are advised to stay out of the magnet core and to stay out of the magnet room while scans are being performed.

Patient Accessibility

The main difficulty is access to the patient. The patient is in the magnet core and the anesthetist is monitoring

---

Box 20-6   Anesthetic Checklist for Magnetic Resonance (MR) Procedures

Remove metallic objects (including paging devices), nondigital watches and credit cards. Check your pockets for dangerous metallic objects (scissors, artery forceps, pens, needles, paperclips, etc.). Do not take credit cards, computer floppy discs, or other magnetic data storage devices near the magnet.

1. Ensure that:
   a. Anesthetic/monitoring equipment is working ☐
   b. There is a suitable area for induction recovery ☐
   c. The breathing system in the magnet area is long enough to allow transfer from the oxygen cylinder outside the 50 Gauss line ☐
2. Consent form signed ☐
3. Day case criteria satisfied if needed ☐
4. MR safety checklist completed; contraindications excluded ☐
5. Magnetic and metallic objects removed from patient, including eye makeup and prosthetic devices if appropriate ☐
6. Placement of MR-compatible monitoring leads – if patient already has monitoring on, these leads may need to be removed ☐
7. Interposition of appropriate lengths of extension line to intravenous access site (and infusion pumps, if appropriate) ☐
8. Induction of anesthesia on an MR-compatible trolley ☐
9. Move patient to magnet area and position for examination. **Check that the ferrous oxygen cylinder is removed and that infusion pumps are at a safe distance from the magnet** ☐
10. Connect monitoring devices and anesthetic breathing system and check function ☐
11. Ensure that intravenous access will still be available when the patient goes into the magnet bore ☐
12. Patient moved into magnet bore – monitoring and receiver coil leads are separate, and there are no nonessential cables or potentially dangerous inductive loops. ☐
13. MR procedure complete – remove patient to induction/recovery area with transfer to cylinder gases outside 50 Gauss line ☐
14. Reversal of anesthesia and recovery – check monitoring sites for burns and record their presence or absence in the notes ☐

From Menon DK, Peden CJ, Hall AS, *et al*. Magnetic resonance for the anaesthetist. *Anaesthesia* 1992;47:240–255, with permission of Blackwell Publishing Ltd.

Box 20-7 Appropriate Anesthesia Equipment for Magnetic Resonance Imaging (MRI)

Plastic stethoscope
Nonferrous MRI-compatible anesthesia machine
Nonferrous oxygen tanks on anesthesia machine
MRI-compatible monitors
Suction
Wall-based oxygen source

Box 20-8 Equipment for Induction Area Outside Magnetic Resonance Imaging Scanner

Suction
Anesthesia machine
Monitors
Wall oxygen
Backup oxygen tank for transportation
Laryngoscope and airway equipment

---

from the control room. While the patient is in the magnet core, the airway, intravenous access, and monitor placement may be inaccessible, particularly during a brain or spine MR scan. Extensions should be added to the intravenous tubing to ensure that a port is accessible when the patient is being scanned. In addition, it can be difficult to visualize the patient on camera at all times.

If there is a problem with the patient or the airway, the magnet room is easily entered at any time. The patient may be pulled out of the scanner by using the MRI cart controls and the quick undocking mechanism. Taking the patient back outside the magnet room to the induction room allows one to focus on the patient and the urgent problem without having to remember all the rules regarding MRI suites. This induction/emergence area has suction and an anesthesia machine with operating-room-type monitoring. All airway equipment can be used with ease here.

Temperature/Monitors/Anesthesia Machines

The scan room is kept cool for the magnet, but the scan itself warms tissue locally. Core temperatures should be monitored as needed.

Many MRI-compatible monitors and anesthesia machines are now available. The most important component of MRI-compatible anesthesia machines is the aluminum or nonferrous metal used in their construction.

Anesthetic Techniques in Magnetic Resonance Imaging

Monitored Anesthesia Care

American Society of Anesthesiologists standards for basic intraoperative monitoring should be followed. Supplemental oxygen via nasal cannula should be provided during sedation techniques. Many sedation techniques are available.

General Anesthesia

An induction area outside the scan room allows one to operate in a familiar environment and focus on the patient and the airway. Endotracheal intubation or an LMA may be used. The cuff on the LMA must be taped to the circuit, since it contains a metal spring. This spring can cause a signal dropout or interference with a head/brain MR image.

All anesthesia staff, including anesthesiologists, nurse anesthetists, residents, and technicians, should receive education in MRI safety prior to participating in patient care in this unique environment. These individuals need to be screened to ensure their own safety in the MRI magnet room. A good beginning is taking the MRI screening questionnaire. All objects taken into the scan room need to be clearly labeled as MRI-compatible and nonferromagnetic if they are metallic, recognizing that specific magnet strengths – 1.5 tesla, for example – are usually specified. The MR technician or MR radiologist supervises all others within the control room and magnet room regarding issues of MR safety.

ANESTHESIA CONSULTATIONS IN REMOTE LOCATION

As reviewed above, there are many reasons for anesthesia consultation in a remote location of the hospital. These consultations are occurring more frequently as the complexity and duration of such cases increases. Some of the reasons are noted in Box 20-9.

Radiation Exposure

In off-site locations, outside the operating rooms, anesthesiologists may participate in prolonged cases in close proximity to a source of radiation. Therefore, one needs to limit one's own exposure while at the same time providing a safe anesthetic to the patient. Interventional radiology and the cardiac catheterization laboratory are the areas that provide the greatest radiation exposure.

One's overall radiation exposure should be limited to 50 mSv per year, unless one is pregnant. Pregnant women should limit exposure to 0.5 mSv/month. A cumulative lifetime dose should not exceed 10 mSv × age in years. If one is frequently the anesthesiologist for remote

Box 20-9 Reasons for Anesthesia Services in Remote Locations

Failed sedation
Immobility required
Difficult airway
Critically ill patient
Airway protection
Claustrophobia and anxiety
Loud noises
Obese patients
Poor access to airway

locations, particularly interventional radiology, a radiation badge that is monitored each month for overall exposure should be obtained through the radiology department.

Methods to decrease one's radiation exposure at each encounter include such basics as wearing a lead apron and thyroid shield. These should be provided by the radiology/cardiac/gastrointestinal department where the procedure is being performed. Movable protective screens are also available when the anesthesia provider remains in close proximity to the patient. Distancing oneself from the fluoroscopy equipment (more than 5 feet) will also decrease exposure. In certain situations such as MRI or radiation therapy, observing the patient via remote monitors and cameras will decrease exposure. Also, in CT, viewing the patient through the leaded window will decrease exposure. Alternatively, remaining in the CT scanner with the patient but wearing a lead apron and a thyroid shield is another viable option (Box 20-10).

Monitored Anesthesia Care Versus General Anesthesia

The decision to proceed with monitored anesthesia care versus general anesthesia is always based on a combination of patient factors and procedural requirements. A common requirement is for patient immobility for limited or extensive periods of time. Adult patients are generally cooperative but in certain cases a mentally impaired or developmentally delayed adult patient may not be able

Box 20-10 Radiation Protection

Lead aprons
Thyroid shields
Movable screens (leaded glass)
Closed-circuit TV
Leaded windows
Exposure badges

to cooperate fully with the examination/procedure. In remote locations, one also needs to consider limited access to the patient, as found in radiation therapy or MRI.

The ability to fully monitor a patient needs to be insured. A plan of general anesthesia necessitates monitoring of $ET\text{-}CO_2$, as noted in the ASA guidelines. Continuous monitoring of $ET\text{-}CO_2$ is available via a separate monitor but is most easily come by in an anesthesia machine. This allows one to have a ventilator, as well as convenient and familiar monitors, including $ET\text{-}CO_2$. These machines, however, are not easily transportable. One can move them from location to location but this takes up valuable time and can be backbreaking. If the anesthesia department provides services frequently in one area, radiology for example, investing in a machine for this location would allow for ease of anesthesia planning with fewer limitations on providing care.

Logistics

A variety of paramedical personnel may be part of the patient care team at each location. Certainly, in interventional radiology, the gastrointestinal lab or the cardiac catheterization lab, a physician will be performing the procedure and working closely with the anesthesia team. However, in MRI, CT, and radiation therapy, a radiology technician will be performing the scan/treatment under the guidance of a radiologist/radiation therapist, who will be in the area but perhaps not the immediate vicinity. Even in the interventional radiology suite during induction and emergence, the radiologist is available but not in the room. A radiology technician will be with the patient. During electrophysiology studies and device closures in the cardiac catheterization laboratory, a nurse is generally present while the patient is in the laboratory.

All these paramedical personnel may be, and often are, very well trained but they may not be aware of common anesthesia needs or concerns. For example, in the operating rooms, the circulating nurse remains present during induction and emergence to provide any assistance that might be required. This same understanding may not be found in remote locations. Groundwork needs to be laid and, at each procedure, if something specific is required, e.g., cricoid pressure for a rapid sequence induction, there must be communication with the personnel and physician responsible for the procedure at hand. The goal is to maintain the same standards that one has in the operating rooms. Ascertaining the medical training of paramedical personnel is important. For instance, MRI technicians are CPR-certified. One needs to be aware of the personnel who can be helpful in an emergency. They may know how to call the code team and the location of the code cart, along with other more common procedural details such as where the lead aprons and the patient holding areas are located.

Consents

Certainly, consent for anesthesia must always be obtained from patients, discussing with them the options, risks, and benefits, and answering their questions. How that consent is documented varies among institutions. In the operating rooms, separate consents for surgery and anesthesia may be obtained, or a combined consent may be signed by the patient. When practicing anesthesia in remote locations, one needs to ascertain whether or not the procedural consent includes a consent for anesthesia. If it does not, a separate consent for anesthesia must be obtained. In certain areas, most commonly MRI and CT, no consent may be obtained for the examination itself. Particularly in these cases, do not overlook documenting the verbal consent obtained for providing anesthesia services to the patient.

Transportation

Transportation of the patient from a remote location to the recovery room or an intensive care unit may involve covering a significant distance and an elevator ride. A portable monitor should be available that is capable of monitoring oxygen saturation, ECG, and blood pressure. An oxygen tank and a means to ventilate the patient (Ambu bag and mask) should be present on the trip. For a MAC case, the patient may only need oxygen by nasal cannula, while for a general anesthetic the patient may require 100% oxygen by face mask. Medications should be available for sedation, analgesia, induction and intubation, and resuscitation, as well as medication for continued blood pressure control if this has been an issue (Box 20-11).

Total Intravenous Anesthesia

Total intravenous anesthesia (TIVA) is a valuable anesthetic plan in remote locations. Medical gases (oxygen and nitrous oxide) may not be available, at least not from a wall source. It is always advisable to have an oxygen tank available as a backup source for oxygen, just as one would have it at hand in the operating room. Nitrous oxide may only be available from a tank on the anesthesia machine. Certainly, TIVA is a very portable anesthesia plan and allows for ease of patient transportation.

When using either nitrous oxide or halogenated anesthetic gases, the ability to scavenge these vapors must be considered. Typically, the remote sections of the hospital to which anesthesiologists now travel to provide sedation/anesthesia do not have either the passive or active scavenging systems that are present in the operating rooms. Activated charcoal canisters are available that easily attach to the anesthesia machine. These activated charcoal canisters will scavenge halogenated agents (not nitrous oxide) and last for approximately 8 hours. A more exacting/efficient use of these canisters may be obtained by routinely weighing them. A certain increase in weight, noted on the canister, indicates when the charcoal has been exhausted as an effective scavenging agent.

SUMMARY

Increasingly, anesthesia care providers are consulted in remote areas of the hospital. Complex or uncomfortable diagnostic and therapeutic procedures often require the close monitoring, vigilance and skills of an anesthesiologist to complete successfully. Remote areas entail specific considerations for the individual location and procedure (radiation protection), as well as general considerations for remote anesthesia (transport, consents, recovery). The pros and cons of monitored anesthesia care versus general anesthesia must be considered for each individual case. Anesthesia care providers and technicians must be educated in the risks and special considerations of each site. Awareness of the problems, the types of case, and the patient population one may encounter at these remote locations allows the anesthesia care provider to anticipate and prepare effectively for these cases.

Box 20-11 Equipment Required for Transportation

Oxygen tank
Portable monitor
Ambu bag plus mask
Medications:
- Sedation
- Analgesia
- Induction
- Muscle relaxant
- Resuscitation
- Blood pressure control

Case Study

A 56-year-old man is scheduled for a transjugular intrahepatic portosystemic shunt. His past medical history is significant for alcohol abuse, esophageal varices, cirrhosis, and hypertension. Medications include octreotide, famotidine, multivitamins, folate and vitamin B_{12}. Heart rate is 90. Blood pressure is 140/90. On physical examination, the cachetic patient is awake and has significant ascites. The lungs are clear. Hemoglobin is 8.5 g/dL.
- Is any further preoperative testing necessary?
- What blood products would you like to be available?
- What anesthetic technique will you recommend?
- What type of intravenous access would you like?
- Is any special monitoring needed?

SUGGESTED READING

American College of Radiology. *White paper on MR safety*. AJR 2002;178.

American Society of Anesthesiologists. *Guidelines for non-operating room anesthetizing locations*. Park Ridge, IL: ASA, 1994.

American Society of Anesthesiologists. *Standards for basic anesthesia monitoring*. Park Ridge, IL: ASA, 1998.

American Society of Anesthesiologists. *Standards for post-anesthesia care*. Park Ridge, IL: ASA, 1994.

American Society of Anesthesiologists. *Updated practice guidelines for sedation and analgesia by non-anesthesiologists*. Park Ridge, IL: ASA, Aug. 2001.

Arepally A, Oechsle D, Kirkwood S, Savader SJ. Safety of conscious sedation in interventional radiology. *Cardiovasc Intervent Radiol* 2001;24:185–190.

Bashein G, Russell AH, Momii ST. Anesthesia and remote monitoring for intraoperative radiation therapy. *Anesthesiology* 1986;64:804–807.

Conran AM. GI endoscopy/EGD non-operating room anesthesia. In: Roizen MF, Fleisher LA, eds *Essence of anesthesia*. New York: WB Saunders, 2002, 405.

Etzkorn KP, Diab F, Brown RD, *et al*. Endoscopic retrograde cholangiopancreatography under general anesthesia: indications and results. *Gastrointest Endosc* 1998;47:363–367.

Fu W, White PF. Dexmedetomidine failed to block the acute hyperdynamic response to electroconvulsive therapy. *Anesthesiology* 1999;90:422–424.

Haslam PJ, Yap B, Mueller PR, Lee MJ. Anesthesia practice and clinical trends in interventional radiology: a European survey. *Cardiovasc Intervent Radiol* 2000;23: 256–261.

Jorgensen NH, Messick JM, Gray J, *et al*. ASA monitoring standards and magnetic resonance imaging. *Anesth Analg* 1994; 79:1141–1147.

Kadar AG, Ing CH, White PF, *et al*. Anesthesia for electroconvulsive therapy in obese patients. *Anesth Analg* 2002; 94:360–361.

Menon DK, Peden CJ, Hall AS, *et al*. Magnetic resonance for the anaesthetist. *Anaesthesia* 1992;47:240–255.

Patteson SK, Chesney JT. Anesthetic management for magnetic resonance imaging: problems and solutions. *Anesth Analg* 1992; 74:121–128.

Standards of Practice Committee, American Society for Gastrointestinal Endoscopy. Guidelines for the use of deep sedation and anesthesia for GI endoscopy. *Gastrointest Endosc* 2002;56:613–617.

Walder B, Seeck M, Tramèr MR. Propofol versus methohexital for electroconvulsive therapy: a meta-analysis. *J Neurosurg Anesthesiol* 2001;13:93–98.

Young WL, Pile-Spellman J. Anesthetic considerations for interventional neuroradiology. *Anesthesiology* 1994;80: 427–456.

SPECIAL CONSIDERATIONS

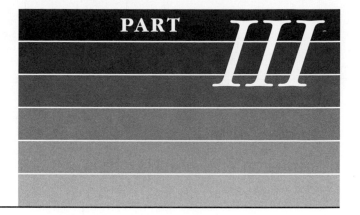

CHAPTER 21

Malignant Hyperthermia

LINDA J. MASON

DESCRIPTION

Malignant hyperthermia is a clinical syndrome, classically observed during general anesthesia, whose hallmark is rapidly increasing temperature (1° C/5 min) and a high mortality rate. This syndrome results from acute uncontrolled increases in skeletal muscle metabolism resulting in increased oxygen consumption, lactate accumulation, heat production, and rhabdomyolysis. Therapy with dantrolene has reduced the mortality from 70% to 10%.

BACKGROUND

The overall incidence of malignant hyperthermia during general anesthesia has been reported as 1:50,000–100,000 for adults as compared to 1:3,000–15,000 children. A Danish survey indicates an incidence of fulminant malignant hyperthermia as 1:250,000 total anesthetics, 1:80,000 anesthetics with inhalational agents alone, and 1:60,000 anesthetics with inhalational agents and succinylcholine. The incidence of suspected malignant hyperthermia is 1:16,000 total anesthetics, 1:6,000 with inhalational agents alone and 1:4,000 with inhalation agents and succinylcholine. Of interest, the majority of patients who were referred to the malignant hyperthermia hotline during 1990–1994 were children 0–10 years of age.

The most common presenting symptoms include skeletal rigidity, temperature elevation, increased end-tidal CO_2 (ET-CO_2) and arrhythmias. Laboratory abnormalities include an increased creatinine kinase level, respiratory acidosis, myoglobinuria, metabolic acidosis, and hyperkalemia. About 66% of symptoms occur during induction, 13% during the procedure, and the rest postoperatively. Halothane was used in 69% and succinylcholine in 75% of cases.

ETIOLOGY AND GENETICS

Malignant hyperthermia is an inherited metabolic defect transmitted as an autosomal dominant genetic disorder with reduced penetrance and variable expression. Reduced penetrance means that fewer offspring are affected than would be predicted by a perfectly dominant pattern. Variable expression is a difference of susceptibility between families with little variation within the same family. The genetic abnormality of malignant hyperthermia can be transmitted by more than one gene and allele.

In pigs, the porcine stress syndrome, or pale soft exudative pork syndrome, is an animal model for malignant hyperthermia. Certain breeds of pig show a classic presentation of malignant hyperthermia on induction of anesthesia with potent inhalation agents and succinylcholine. These breeds (Poland, China, Landrace, Pietrain) have deliberately been inbred for desirable traits and have had a single point mutation that occurs at the *RYR1* gene locus. It is then transmitted as an autosomal recessive genetic disorder. This syndrome can be triggered by stressors other than anesthesia (e.g., shipping, preparation for slaughter).

413

In humans the most common genetic abnormality of malignant hyperthermia relates to the ryanodine receptor (RYR1) on chromosome 19 (Figure 21-1). This receptor is the major component of the ionized calcium release pathway between the sarcoplasmic reticulum and the sarcolemma. Although 50% of malignant hyperthermia patients have a genetic mutation of the *RYR1* gene, these mutations do not always relate to a positive *in vitro* contracture test to halothane. No clinical correlation exists between the clinical presentation and the genetic mutation observed. Malignant hyperthermia in humans is not a single disease as in the pig but a syndrome with multiple sites of causation and multiple mutations at these sites.

Even the presentation of malignant hyperthermia is not the same in all patients. Some 30% of malignant hyperthermia patients have had up to three uneventful anesthetics. A spectrum can occur from minor reactions to rapid temperature rise, muscle rigidity acidosis, arrhythmias, and death. Some reactions have greater latency to onset and may not manifest for up to 24 hours postoperatively. Malignant hyperthermia may not occur always in response to triggering agents. Also, malignant hyperthermia may occur without any signs of temperature elevation or rigidity. Thus, there may be different genes causing malignant hyperthermia in different families or other predisposing factors being expressed differently in patients or families. Malignant hyperthermia may be described as a heterogeneous genetic disorder with a highly variable clinical presentation. This makes the possibility of a specific DNA test for the condition unlikely.

PATHOPHYSIOLOGY

Malignant hyperthermia demonstrates the signs of hypercarbia, oxygen desaturation, tachycardia, tachypnea, cyanosis, mottling, cardiac arrhythmias, rigidity of muscles, fever, rhabdomyolysis, and shock. The pathogenesis involves defects in the release and reuptake of calcium from the sarcoplasmic reticulum (Figure 21-2). With normal muscle contraction, ionized calcium is released into the sarcolemma after discharge from the sarcoplasmic reticulum. The rapid increase in intracellular ionized calcium initiates muscle contraction, while the reuptake causes relaxation and requires adenosine triphosphate (ATP). It appears that during malignant hyperthermia excess calcium is released, with a concomitant defect in calcium reuptake. The muscles respond with a marked increase in energy production in an attempt to return the calcium to the sarcoplasmic reticulum. Hypermetabolism and muscle contractures (rigidity) are a result.

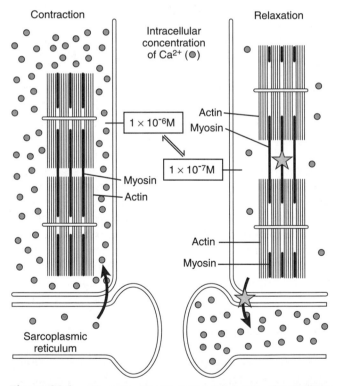

Figure 21-2   The actin–myosin movement during calcium-stimulated muscle contraction is illustrated. Biochemically, the relaxation phase is the energy-using process, and contraction is a more passive event. It is the failure of lowering myoplasmic calcium, which occurs normally during the relaxation phase, that leads to the development of malignant hyperthermia in a patient. The stars indicate the sites of action of dantrolene. (Redrawn from Bissonnette B, Ryan JF: Temperature regulation: normal and abnormal (malignant hyperthermia). In: Coté CJ, Rodrea ID, Goudsouzian NG, Ryan JF, eds. *A practice of anesthesia for infants and children*, 3rd ed. Philadelphia: WB Saunders, 2001:621.)

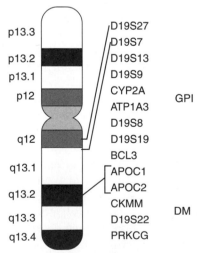

Figure 21-1   The location of malignant hyperthermia susceptibility to DNA markers from the 19q12–13.2 region of human chromosome 19, as reported by McCarthy *et al.*, has a maximum likelihood of 450,000:1, favoring linkage of susceptibility to the cytochrome P450 (CYP2A) locus. (Redrawn from McCarthy TV, Healy JM, Heffron JJ, *et al.* Localization of the malignant hyperthermia susceptibility locus to human chromosome 19q12–13.2. *Nature* 1990;343:562–564.)

The high myoplasmic ionized calcium level combines with troponin and causes muscle contracture. Continuous muscle contracture requires a constant energy supply by ATP. Acceleration of glycogenolysis and phosphorylase kinase produces ATP and heat. The muscle enters into a hypermetabolic state that exhausts aerobic metabolism, and anaerobic metabolism begins with lactate accumulation. The metabolic rate causes a high rate of oxygen consumption, CO_2 production, and generation of heat. Dantrolene blocks the release of calcium from the sarcoplasmic reticulum, attenuating the hypermetabolic state.

At the beginning of an episode of malignant hyperthermia, normal circulatory responses may allow for heat dissipation but, in an effort to supply the increased demand for oxygen to the muscles, blood is shunted from the skin and consequently body temperature rises. Oxygen demand exceeds oxygen delivery. A peripheral venous sample draining skeletal muscle will show a combined metabolic and respiratory acidosis with venous desaturation. $ET\text{-}CO_2$ is the most sensitive and useful monitor for early diagnosis of a hypermetabolic state, and is elevated before any clinically evident change in pulse or respirations. Pulse oximetry may show a pattern of desaturation as a result of marked oxygen extraction.

Skeletal muscles may exhibit rhabdomyolysis, with massive swelling and leakage of intracellular potassium, calcium, myoglobin, sodium and creatinine phosphokinase. Hyperkalemia is the major cause of mortality in an early malignant hyperthermia episode. It is usually reversible with the onset of treatment with dantrolene. Exogenous calcium must be administered with caution for treatment of hyperkalemia-induced arrhythmias. Other causes of cardiac arrhythmias are hyperpyrexia, acidosis, hypoxemia, and autonomic hyperactivity. Calcium channel blockers have a profound interaction with dantrolene and can cause hyperkalemia and direct myocardial depression; they are contraindicated during an episode of malignant hyperthermia. Other complications are hemolysis, myoglobinemia, and renal failure. Disseminated intravascular coagulation can be prevented with early dantrolene treatment.

Death in the initial few hours is usually due to hyperkalemia-induced ventricular fibrillation. Several hours after the initial episode, death may be due to pulmonary edema, coagulopathy, or acid–base or electrolyte imbalance. Before dantrolene therapy was introduced, a sharp decrease in plasma potassium was typically observed several hours after treatment, due to the return of intracellular potassium. Deaths that occur days after the malignant hyperthermia episode are due to multiple organ failure, brain damage, or renal decompensation. The magnitude of the fever has no predictive value on outcome.

TRIGGERING AGENTS

Drugs that trigger malignant hyperthermia include the potent inhalational agents and succinylcholine (Table 21-1). The onset may be explosive if succinylcholine is used during the induction of anesthesia, and acceleration of symptoms may be seen in 5–10 minutes. However, there may be a normal response to succinylcholine and an inhalational agent may be the trigger. The use of nitrous oxide is safe in these patients.

All local anesthetics, whether amides or esters, are safe in patients susceptible to malignant hyperthermia. Vasopressors and other catecholamines are not involved in triggering malignant hyperthermia. Nondepolarizing muscle relaxants and their reversal agents are not a problem in malignant-hyperthermia-susceptible patients. Neither ketamine or propofol are triggers for the condition. Although caffeine induces contracture responses *in vitro*, it seems that these related effects do not apply to related compounds such as theophylline and aminophylline. The incidence of awake triggering of malignant hyperthermia in humans is very low. The anxiety reaction may apparently precipitate a malignant hyperthermia response. There are four case reports of unusual events

Table 21-1   Safe Anesthetic Agents and Triggering Agents for Malignant Hyperthermia

Triggering Agents	Safe Drugs
All volatile agents	Althesin
Succinylcholine	Antibiotics
	Antihistamines
	Antipyretics
	Atracurium
	Barbiturates
	Benzodiazepines
	Cisatracurium
	Droperidol
	Etomidate
	Ketamine
	Local anesthetics
	Opioids
	Nitrous oxide
	Pancuronium
	Propofol
	Propranolol
	Rocuronium
	Vasoactive drugs
	Epinephrine/ norepinephrine
	Vecuronium

Modified from Rosenberg H, Fletcher JE, Seitman D. Pharmacogenetics. In: Barash PG, Cullen BF, Stoelting RK, eds. *Clinical anesthesia*, 3rd ed. Philadelphia: Lippincott Williams & Wilkins, 1997:492.

relating to heat stroke, sudden and unexpected death, unusual stress, fatigue, or myalgias representing possible awake episodes of malignant hyperthermia.

DIAGNOSIS OF THE CLINICAL SYNDROME

Malignant hyperthermia is a disorder of increased metabolism with increased oxygen consumption and CO_2 production. The cardiovascular and respiratory systems respond to this by increasing cardiac output and respiratory rate. In a spontaneously breathing patient, the first clinically evident signs of malignant hyperthermia are an increase in ET-CO_2, tachycardia, and tachypnea (Table 21-2). The CO_2 absorber in a semiclosed system may become hot and the canister absorber will be exhausted. Without hypercapnia the diagnosis of malignant hyperthermia is questionable.

Tachycardia may be attributed to "light" anesthesia and cause a delay in the diagnosis. It is reasonable to deepen the anesthesia while assessing other possible causes of tachycardia. Keep in mind that rapid increases in desflurane and sevoflurane concentrations can cause tachycardia and also delay diagnosis.

It is important to draw a simultaneous venous and arterial blood gas to determine if a hypermetabolic state is present. A mixed venous sample will reflect the muscle effluence and will give an earlier indication of the metabolic abnormality. The ET-CO_2 should return quickly to normal with hyperventilation if airway obstruction is the

Table 21-3 Common Laboratory Findings in Malignant Hyperthermia

Arterial blood gases	Acidosis – both respiratory and metabolic
	Hypercapnia
	Hypoxemia
	Base deficit
Electrolytes	Hyperkalemia
	Hypermagnesemia
	Hypercalcemia (early)
	Profound hypocalcemia (late)
	Hypernatremia
Enzymes	Increased creatinine kinase – 20,000 IU/L is diagnostic
Blood profile	Decreased hemoglobin
	Thrombocytopenia
Coagulation profile	Prolonged prothrombin and partial thromboplastin time
	Decreased fibrinogen
	Increased fibrin split products

Modified from Bell C, Kain ZN, eds. *The pediatric anesthesia handbook*, 2nd ed. St Louis: Mosby/Year Book, 1997:492.

problem but not with a hypermetabolic state. Arrhythmias are caused by sympathetic stimulation and hypercarbia. Premature ventricular contractions and ventricular tachycardia are common and as hyperkalemia progresses the electrocardiogram will show peaked T-waves and widening of the QRS complex.

Initially there is an increase in blood pressure from sympathetic stimulation but, as malignant hyperthermia progresses, hypotension may develop secondary to cardiac depression from severe acidosis and hyperkalemia.

Measurements of myoglobin and creatinine kinase must be done. A creatinine kinase level of more than 20,000 IU/L is thought to be diagnostic (Table 21-3), but it may be elevated with a major surgical procedure *per se*.

Differential Diagnosis

A moderate increase in temperature may be due to simple explanations such as excessive draping of the patient, air/mattress warming devices, or occlusive plastic wrap. Conversely, the onset of high fever may be due to sepsis, neurologic injury, thyroid storm, metastatic carcinoid syndrome, or pheochromocytoma. Usually acid–base abnormalities and muscle rigidity are not observed with these syndromes.

Malignant hyperthermia rarely begins as an abrupt cardiac arrest after the use of succinylcholine during induction of anesthesia. If cardiac arrest on induction occurs,

Table 21-2 Signs and Symptoms of Malignant Hyperthermia

Specific for Malignant Hyperthermia	Less Specific for Malignant Hyperthermia
Generalized muscle rigidity (early sign)	Tachycardia
Rapidly increasing ET-CO_2 (early sign)	Tachypnea
	Arrhythmia
Rapidly developing fever (late sign)	Hypotension
	Hypertension
Cola-colored urine (myoglobinemia, late sign)	Cyanosis
	Metabolic acidosis
Increased serum creatinine kinase (late sign)	Hyperkalemia
	Coagulopathy

Modified from Bissonnette B, Ryan JF: Temperature regulation: normal and abnormal (malignant hyperthermia). In: Coté CJ, Rodrea ID, Goudsouzian NG, Ryan JF, eds. *A practice of anesthesia for infants and children*, 3rd ed. Philadelphia: WB Saunders, 2001:621.

generally this is a response to an occult myopathy that responds to succinylcholine with abrupt rhabdomyolysis, and acute, massive hyperkalemia. Many of these patients are found to have a myopathy, usually Duchenne muscular dystrophy. These patients are very difficult to resuscitate and will require extensive therapy with calcium chloride, hyperventilation, sodium bicarbonate, glucose and insulin, and vasopressors. Several hours of resuscitation may be necessary and cardiopulmonary bypass may be required. Glucose must be administered carefully because of the potential for cerebral ischemia and worse neurologic outcomes with hyperglycemia. Thus the current recommendation is that succinylcholine should not be used routinely in children, particularly males, below the age of 8 except for treatment of laryngospasm, emergency airway management, or as an intramuscular adjuvant when intravenous access is not available.

Symptoms of the neuroleptic malignant syndrome include fever, rhabdomyolysis, tachycardia, hypertension, muscle rigidity, and acidosis. The mortality rate is high – 20%. The differences between the neuroleptic malignant syndrome and malignant hyperthermia include that malignant hyperthermia is acute and the neuroleptic malignant syndrome occurs after a long exposure to phenothiazines and haloperidol alone, or in combination. The neuroleptic malignant syndrome is thought to be due to dopamine depletion in the central nervous system by psychoactive agents. Bromocriptine, a dopamine agonist, has been used to treat this syndrome, as well as discontinuance of psychotropic drugs, control of acid–base and intravenous fluid balance, and dantrolene.

Association with Other Disorders

Linkage of malignant hyperthermia with other diseases has been problematic: only central core disease appears to be truly linked and now even this link is not consistent. There is also less certainty concerning patients with exertional heat stroke or exercise-induced rhabdomyolysis. These patients may have abnormalities similar to malignant hyperthermia and may need testing.

Masseter Muscle Spasm/Rigidity/Tetany

Masseter spasm following succinylcholine administration has been recognized as a marker for possible occurrence of malignant hyperthermia; however, succinylcholine increases jaw muscle tone in all patients but this generally relaxes over a matter of seconds (Figure 21-3). It appears now there is an extreme variant of masseter spasm that can be called masseter tetany. Inability to open the mouth despite loss of train of four is highly suggestive of masseter tetany. Further administration of succinylcholine will not relieve the problem. If there is rigidity of other muscles in addition to the jaw, then the diagnosis of malignant hyperthermia must be considered, the anesthetic halted, and treatment begun immediately.

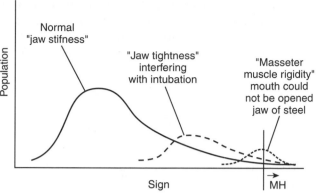

Figure 21-3   The spectrum of masseter muscle responses to succinylcholine varies from a slight jaw stiffness that does not interfere with endotracheal intubation to the extreme "jaws of steel," which is masseter muscle tetany, not allowing the mouth to be opened. It is likely that the latter response is more highly associated with malignant hyperthermia. It should be noted that, even with the inability to open the mouth, the patient should still be able to be ventilated by bag and mask, since all other muscles are relaxed. (Redrawn from Kaplan RF. *Malignant hyperthermia. Annual Refresher Course Lectures.* Washington, DC: American Society of Anesthesiologists, 1993.)

However, what about patients who have masseter spasm and no other muscle rigidity? The differential diagnosis must include:

- Underdosing of succinylcholine or insufficient time for onset
- Myotonic syndrome
- Temporomandibular joint dysfunction
- Malignant hyperthermia.

The incidence of masseter muscle spasm may be as high as 1/12,000 anesthetics when succinylcholine is used (in children and adults).

Even though these patients have masseter spasm they can still be ventilated with a face mask, which sustains oxygenation until the masseter muscles relax, which can take several minutes to half an hour. Between 31% and 50% of patients who experience masseter spasm test positive by muscle biopsy for malignant hyperthermia.

The decision to cancel or proceed with nontriggering agents after masseter muscle spasm depends on the anesthesiologist, surgeon, and family. If the procedure is elective, cancellation may be the safest choice. If the decision is made to continue, all triggering agents should be discontinued and the patient should be observed for 15–20 minutes to be sure that no signs of malignant hyperthermia occur. Dantrolene must be available but it is not necessary to administer it unless other signs of malignant hyperthermia are present (tachycardia, hypercapnia, acidosis). Temperature and ET-CO$_2$ must be closely monitored. The patient should be admitted for 24 hours with creatinine kinase levels assessed at 12 and 24 hours, as well as myoglobin tested in the urine. If the creatinine kinase is greater than 20,000 IU/L without a concomitant myopathy, the diagnosis of malignant hyperthermia is very probable, with an 80% chance that the patient will be malignant-hyperthermia-positive by the caffeine/halothane contracture test.

The presence of neuromuscular disease must be evaluated with a formal neurologic consultation and a possible electromyography. These patients should be considered for muscle biopsy testing. With the decreased use of succinylcholine, masseter muscle spasm has decreased in incidence. Also, induction with a thiobarbiturate instead of an inhalational agent decreases the incidence of masseter muscle spasm and myoglobinemia.

Muscle Biopsy Testing

Muscle biopsies have been used to determine whether there is a consistent marker of muscle function associated with malignant hyperthermia. The most widely accepted test is the quantitation of forces of muscle contraction after exposure of the muscle biopsy to halothane, caffeine, or both. Indications for referral for this test are:

- Clinical history suspicious for malignant hyperthermia
- The patient is a first-degree relative of a patient with documented malignant hyperthermia
- Masseter muscle rigidity.

Traditionally, the standard is to perform the actual biopsy within 1 hour of the testing center. However, recent data shows that, with cold preservation of the tissue, the test is still effective for up to 24 hours. A list of malignant hyperthermia muscle biopsy testing centers can be obtained from the Malignant Hyperthermia Association of the United States.

Skeletal muscle 1–3 g is biopsied from the vastus lateralis muscle. It is important that the patient has not taken dantrolene, as this drug can normalize a positive response. The excised muscle is placed in a physiologic bath at 37° C to verify viability. After a 15–60 minute equilibration period, in which the preparation is oxygenated with O_2/CO_2 (95/5%) mixture, halothane is added to the gas, either as a bolus dose or in an incrementally increasing concentration. A second set of muscle strips is equilibrated and exposed to incrementally increasing concentrations of caffeine. Caffeine strips should be tested early because they tend to be more unstable over time.

There are differences in the North American Malignant Hyperthermia Group (NAMHG) and European Malignant Hyperthermia Group (EMHG) protocols. Both protocols and interpretations are prone to a small number of false positives: EMHG 7% and NAMHG 22%. Both have 97–99% sensitivity (frequency of positive results in patients with clinically established malignant hyperthermia) and acceptable 78–94% specificity (frequency of negative results in low risk controls). The false-negative result is less than 1% for the European and less than 3% for the North American protocol.

The ryanodine contracture test appears to add further sensitivity to the testing, since the muscle of an individual susceptible to malignant hyperthermia is more sensitive to caffeine and develops larger contractures to halothane and ryanodine than that of a normal individual. The Ca^{2+} responses to caffeine or 4-chloro-*m*-cresol in B lymphocytes has shown significant differences between malignant-hyperthermia-susceptible and malignant-hyperthermia-negative individuals. These results suggest that enhanced Ca^{2+} responses are associated with mutations in the *RYR1* gene in some malignant-hyperthermia-susceptible individuals. This may have promise in heralding "noninvasive" testing for susceptibility to malignant hyperthermia. A number of new tests are being investigated, including histologic examination of muscle, electromyography, platelet ATP depletion, and Ca^{2+} uptake from muscle strips. The validity of these tests has not been confirmed.

MANAGEMENT OF A MALIGNANT HYPERTHERMIA CRISIS

A full blown episode of malignant hyperthermia demands immediate aggressive therapy. The main approach includes immediate cessation of triggering agents, delivery of 100% oxygen, hyperventilation, and treatment with sodium dantrolene. A call for extra personnel is necessary because assistance may be needed in mixing the dantrolene. Dantrolene is a poorly soluble solution combined with sodium hydroxide, pH 9–10 (otherwise it won't dissolve), and mannitol (150 mg/mg dantrolene – 3 g per vial) for isotonicity. It must be mixed as 20 mg dantrolene in 50 mL of sterile distilled water (not saline or D5W). If it does not dissolve immediately, producing a clear orange color, it should be heated under tap water. The first dose of dantrolene should be 2.5 mg/kg intravenously, and repeated as needed to a dose of 10 mg/kg. This initial dose can be repeated every 5–30 minutes using heart rate, body temperature and P_aCO_2 as the best guideline to clinical therapy. Following intravenous dantrolene it typically takes 6–20 minutes to see a response, the first being a decrease in the ET-CO_2 with an improvement in blood gas analysis in 20 minutes. The half life of dantrolene in children and adults is 10–12 hours.

Other supportive measures are also essential – active cooling, correcting acidosis (2–4 meq/kg bicarbonate) and correcting the electrolyte imbalance. The most effective way to treat hyperkalemia is reversal of malignant hyperthermia by effective doses of dantrolene. Persistent hyperkalemia can be treated with hyperventilation, bicarbonate, intravenous glucose, and insulin (10 units regular insulin in 50 mL 50% glucose or 0.15 units/kg regular insulin in 1 mL/kg 50% glucose) titrated to effect. Calcium is indicated only for life-threatening arrhythmias and poor cardiac function at a dose of 2–5 mg/kg of calcium chloride. Arrhythmias may be treated with procainamide 1.5 mg/kg every 5 minutes to a total dose of 15 mg/kg or lidocaine 1 mg/kg. Beta-blockers such as esmolol may also be used for tachyarrhythmias. Calcium channel blockers are contraindicated with the use of dantrolene as they cause hyperkalemia and myocardial depression.

While treatment is ongoing, monitoring lines for arterial pressure and central venous pressure, or pulmonary artery pressure, should be inserted. A urinary catheter should be inserted and urine output maintained. Volume expansion should include 10–15 mL/kg of intravenous cold saline every 10 minutes, not lactated Ringer's. Body temperature should be managed by surrounding the patient with ice packs and instituting gastric, wound, and rectal lavage. Gastric lavage is the quickest most practical means for rapid temperature control. Peritoneal dialysis or cardiopulmonary bypass may be needed. Cooling should be stopped when the body temperature reaches 38° C to avoid hypothermia.

Changing of the CO_2-absorbent and anesthesia circuit may remove trace triggering agents. Although arterial blood gases are useful for determining the level of acidosis, central mixed venous blood gas determinations serve as a better guideline for therapy. Further blood studies should be sent (electrolytes, creatinine kinase, liver profile, blood urea nitrogen, lactate, glucose), coagulation studies (prothrombin time, activated fibrinogen, partial thromboplastin time, fibrinolytic split products, platelet count, serum hemoglobin and myoglobin, and urine hemoglobin and myoglobin.

The important fact is that within 45 minutes the patient should be completely normal; if not, intensive therapy should be pursued. Recrudescence may occur in 25% of patients, usually within 4–8 hours after the initial episode but recrudescence as late as 36 hours has been reported. Patients may smolder, with symptoms such as continued hyperkalemia, residual muscle rigidity, massive fluid requirements, and oliguria progressing to anuria. Dantrolene should probably be repeated even if the initial episode is under control – 1–2 mg/kg intravenously every 6 hours over a 24-hour period. If there are no signs of recurrence, dantrolene can be discontinued after 24 hours; however some recommend continuing oral dantrolene 1 mg/kg every 4–8 hours for 48 hours.

Disseminated intravascular coagulation may occur, probably resulting from release of thromboplastins secondary to shock and/or release of cellular contents or membrane destruction. The usual regimen for treating disseminated intravascular coagulation should be followed.

Myoglobinuric renal failure may occur, due to intense myoglobinuria, within 4–8 hours after the episode. Continuing the dantrolene preparation may be helpful (3 g of mannitol per vial). Furosemide 0.5–1.0 mg/kg intravenously can also be given. Creatinine kinase elevations (which may not manifest for 6–12 h) may be followed as a rough guide for therapy and how long to continue the dantrolene.

Dantrolene

In 1979 intravenous dantrolene was approved by the Food and Drug Administration for treatment of malignant hyperthermia. Prior to 1979 dantrolene was used primarily for the treatment of muscle spasticity. Dantrolene acts within the muscle cell itself, reducing intracellular calcium. It prevents the release of calcium from the sarcoplasmic reticulum and antagonizes calcium at the actin–myosin or troponin–tropomyosin level, or both (see Figure 21-2).

A recent study did not identify the ryanodine receptor as the site of dantrolene's action so it may have an intermediary role at this receptor site. Dantrolene's action is specific for skeletal muscle. In clinical doses it has little effect on myocardial contractibility. Dantrolene does not effect neuromuscular transmission but can produce muscle weakness which may potentiate nondepolarizing muscle relaxants. It must be used cautiously in patients with neuromuscular disease.

At doses of 5–15 mg/kg, intravenous dantrolene produces significant muscle relaxation and even oral dantrolene may produce feelings of weakness (Box 21-1). Intravenous doses of dantrolene up to 15 mg/kg have no effect on the cardiovascular system and there is no respiratory depression if the dose is less than 30 mg/kg. One of dantrolene's most important effects is that cellular metabolism returns to an aerobic process, respiration normalizes and acidosis is reversed. This rapidly reduces potassium levels because with correction of acidosis, potassium returns to the cells and produces cardiac stability.

Box 21-1 Dantrolene

DRUG INTERACTION

Verapamil; myocardial depressant

SIDE EFFECTS

Dizziness, lightheadedness, drowsiness, hepatic
 dysfunction

Modified from Bissonnette B, Ryan JF: Temperature regulation: normal and abnormal (malignant hyperthermia). In: Coté CJ, Rodrea ID, Goudsouzian NG, Ryan JF, eds. *A practice of anesthesia for infants and children*, 3rd ed. Philadelphia: WB Saunders, 2001:626.

ANESTHESIA FOR THE MALIGNANT-HYPERTHERMIA-SUSCEPTIBLE PATIENT

Anesthesia for these patients should consist of agents such as nitrous oxide, barbiturates, etomidate, propofol, opiates, tranquilizers, and/or nondepolarizing muscle relaxants. All volatile anesthetic agents and succinylcholine must be avoided.

The current consensus is that pretreatment with dantrolene is not needed if nontriggering agents are used. This avoids dantrolene's side effects of muscle weakness and nausea. If, however, a surgical procedure is planned in a known malignant-hyperthermia-susceptible patient and pretreatment with dantrolene sodium is desired because of the patient's or anesthesiologist's concern arising from the severity of a previous episode of malignant hyperthermia, dantrolene can be administered orally or intravenously. The oral dosage is 4.8 mg/kg/day in three or four divided doses for 48 hours prior to anesthesia, or a single intravenous dose of 2.5 mg/kg can be given before induction. Since oral absorption of dantrolene is erratic and patient side effects are so prominent, the intravenous route is preferred.

To prepare a "clean" anesthesia machine, all vaporizers should be removed and the CO_2 absorbers should be changed as well as the fresh gas outlet hose, the circuit, and the mask. The machine should be purged with a flow of 100% oxygen at 10 L/min for 10 minutes.

Other modalities used to avoid triggering malignant hyperthermia are:

- Moderate to heavy premedication with tranquilizers, barbiturates, benzodiazepines, or opiates
- Balanced anesthesia technique (nitrous oxide/oxygen, barbiturate, opioid, and any nondepolarizing muscle relaxant).

The use of ketamine and propofol is acceptable. In addition, careful monitoring is the most important aspect of management, especially heart rate, ET-CO_2, pulse oximetry, and central core temperature. It is important to have dantrolene immediately available.

Regional or local anesthesia with ester or amide local anesthetics is acceptable. In obstetrical anesthesia, regional conduction anesthesia is the best choice for labor and cesarean section but if a general anesthetic must be administered succinylcholine should be avoided. Dantrolene pretreatment is not needed but if deemed necessary should be given after the cord is clamped to avoid a floppy infant.

It is acceptable to perform surgery in ambulatory centers on patients susceptible to malignant hyperthermia as long as they are monitored for at least 1 hour after the procedure, and dantrolene and appropriate monitoring devices are available.

FAMILY COUNSELING AND PATIENT SUPPORT SERVICES

In the event of a malignant hyperthermia crisis, it is important that a formal letter describing the event, laboratory documentation, treatment, and future recommendations be given to the family and mailed to the primary physician. The patient should be encouraged to wear a medical alert bracelet. This may need to be extended to other family members, depending on the results of further testing.

Following the episode the malignant hyperthermia patient and family must be referred to an agency or center who can give information, counseling, and possible future testing for the patient and all first- or second-degree relatives. The Malignant Hyperthermia Association of the United States is such an agency. They publish a quarterly newsletter, *The Communicator*, with information and updates for patients from the medical literature. The address is:

11 East State Street
Box 1069
Sherbourne, NY 13460.

For nonemergency and patient referrals the number is 1 800-98MHAUS or 607-674-7901. Their FAX number is 1-800-440-9990. The website is: http//www.mhaus.org. There is also a hotline for physicians to call during emergency situations, through which you will be put in touch, 24 hours a day, with a knowledgeable specialist who can answer questions. The number is 1-800-MHHYPER (1-800-6449737) or 00113154647079 outside the US.

SUMMARY

Malignant hyperthermia can occur not only in young infants and children but also in adults and the elderly. A high index of suspicion and knowledge of current treatment is the key to successful management of these patients.

SUGGESTED READING

Beebe JJ, Sessler DI. Preparation of anesthesia machines for patients susceptible to malignant hyperthermia. *Anesthesiology* 1988;69:395.

Bissonnette B, Ryan JF. Temperature regulation: normal and abnormal (malignant hyperthermia). In: Coté CJ, Rodrea ID, Goudsouzian NG, Ryan JF, eds. *A practice of anesthesia for infants and children*, 3rd ed. Philadelphia: WB Saunders, 2001:621.

Denborough M. Malignant hyperthermia. *Lancet* 1998;352: 1131-1136.

Fruen BR, Mickelson JR, Louis CF. Dantrolene inhibition of sacroplasmic reticulum Ca^{2+} release by direct and specific action at skeletal muscle ryanodine receptors. *J Biol Chem* 1997;272:26965-26971.

Islander G, Twetman ER. Comparison between the European and North American protocols for diagnosis of malignant hyperthermia susceptibility in humans. *Anesth Analg* 1999;88:1155-1160.

Islander G, Henriksson KG, Ranklev-Twetman E. Malignant hyperthermia susceptibility without central core disease (CCD) in a family where CCD is diagnosed. *Neuromusc Disord* 1995;5:125-127.

Kaplan RF, Rushing E. Isolated masseter muscle spasm and increased creatine kinase without malignant hyperthermia susceptibility or other myopathies. *Anesthesiology* 1992;77:820.

Larach MG, Allen GC, Kunselman AR, *et al*. Do patients who experience masseter muscle rigidity as part of a malignant hyperthermia episode differ from patients with isolated masseter muscle rigidity? *Anesthesiology* 1996;85:A1057.

Larach MG, Rosenberg H, Gronert GA, *et al*. Hyperkalemic cardiac arrest during anesthesia in infants and children with occult myopathies. *Clin Pediatr (Phila)* 1997;36:9-16.

Lazzell VA, Carr AS, Lerman J, *et al*. The incidence of masseter muscle rigidity after succinylcholine in infants and children. *Can J Anaesth* 1994;41:475.

Malignant hyperthermia. In: Bell C, Kain ZN, eds. *The pediatric anesthesia handbook*, 2nd ed. St Louis: Mosby, 1997;492.

Ording H. Investigation of malignant hyperthermia susceptibility in Denmark. *Dan Med Bull* 1996;43:111.

Ryan JF, Tedeschi LG. Sudden unexplained death in a patient with a family history of malignant hyperthermia. *J Clin Anesth* 1997;9:66.

Sei Y, Brandom BW, Bina S, *et al*. Patients with malignant hyperthermia demonstrate an altered calcium control mechanism in B lymphocytes. *Anesthesiology* 2002;97:1052-1058.

Wedel DJ, Quinlan JG, Iaizzo PA. Clinical effects of intravenously administered dantrolene. *Mayo Clin Proc* 1995;70:241-246.

CHAPTER 22

Allergic Reactions

LINDA J. MASON

INTRODUCTION

The anesthesiologist is in a unique position when it comes to recognition and treatment of allergic reactions. First, patients are exposed to multiple foreign substances in the perioperative period. This exposure includes anesthetic drugs, antibiotics, protamine, blood products, and latex, all which have the potential to produce adverse or allergic reactions. Secondly, anesthesiologists are one of the few groups of physicians who personally administer these agents and can immediately see the effects and must respond with appropriate management. In a 5-year review of 83,844 anesthetics, anaphylaxis was listed fifth as one of the common serious problems that can occur during anesthesia – the top four were problems with intubation, difficult emergence, arrhythmias, and hypotension. This puts into perspective the importance of early recognition and management of allergic reactions in relationship to successful anesthetic outcomes.

DEFINITIONS

Adverse Drug Reaction

The risk of an adverse drug reaction is an inevitable consequence of drug administration, with up to 30% of patients developing some form of adverse drug reaction during hospitalization.

Predictable adverse drug reactions are often dose-dependent, occur in normal patients, are related to the known pharmacologic actions of the drug, and account for 80% of adverse drug effects. The most serious of these are either overdose or inadvertent wrong route of administration. However, side effects are the most common adverse drug reactions – the undesirable, but unavoidable pharmacologic action of drugs prescribed at usual dosages (e.g., opioid-induced respiratory depression). Secondary effects are indirect but not inevitable consequences of the drug's pharmacologic actions (e.g., drug-mediated histamine release from mast cells). Drug interactions also are a problem for anesthesiologists (e.g., combining sedative/hypnotics with opioids can produce synergistic respiratory depression and hypotension as compared to either drug administered alone).

Unpredictable adverse drug reactions are dose-independent, not related to the drug's pharmacologic actions, and, in the case of an allergic reaction, involve the immunologic response of the patient with an untoward physiologic response not related to the pharmacologic action of the drug.

Anaphylaxis

Anaphylaxis is an immune-mediated hypersensitivity response that involves the production of IgE antibodies. Subsequent exposure to the same or chemically similar antigens results in antigen–antibody interactions with degranulation of mast cells and basophils. This is a life-threatening reaction. The liberated mediators produce a symptom complex of bronchospasm, upper airway edema, vasodilatation, increased capillary permeability, and urticaria. Initial manifestations usually occur within 10 minutes of exposure to antigens but in the case of latex allergy may have a delayed onset (typically longer than 30 minutes). An allergic reaction must be considered when there are abrupt decreases in systemic blood pressure and increases in heart rate that exceed 30% of the control value. In 10% of patients hypotension may be the only presenting symptom during anesthesia. The unusual problem with anaphylaxis is the unpredictability of occurrence, the severity of the attack, and the fact that there may be no prior allergic history.

During anaphylaxis plasma IgE initially decreases, initially because of complexing with the new antigens; after which there is an overshoot of IgE (Figure 22-1). Further

evidence of anaphylaxis is an increase in plasma tryptase levels. Tryptase is liberated into the systemic circulation during anaphylactic but not anaphylactoid reactions, showing that mast cell activation with mediator release has occurred. Another marker, histamine, is elevated in the plasma for about 30–60 minutes but is elevated in the urine for much longer.

Identification of offending antigens is often difficult. Skin testing must be carried out with preservative-free solutions with antigen concentrations of 10–20 μl. A positive intradermal test (wheal and flare more than 4 mm in diameter) confirms the presence of IgE antibodies. The radioallergosorbent test (RAST) and enzyme-linked immunosorbent assay (ELISA) are antigen preparations that combine with antibodies in the patient's plasma that are specific for test antigens.

Anaphylactoid Reaction

An anaphylactoid reaction reflects massive release of histamine from basophils or mast cells in response to administration of certain drugs (muscle relaxants, opioids, and protamine), independent of IgE. One cannot distinguish between an anaphylactic and an anaphylactoid reaction on the basis of clinical observation.

Nonimmunologic release of histamine can occur in response to different agents in a dose-dependent fashion. Intravenous administration of morphine, atracurium, or vancomycin can produce urticaria and vasodilatation along the vein of administration. Pretreatment with H_1- and H_2- receptor antagonists is more effective in controlling symptoms with local drug-induced histamine release than systemic anaphylactoid reactions. Systemic reactions can be treated with intravascular volume administration and/or catecholamines. The newer neuromuscular blocking agents such as rocuronium that are devoid of histamine releasing effects still may cause anaphylaxis.

Another non IgE mechanism for allergic reactions may be polymorphonuclear leukocyte (neutrophil) activation. Complement fragments of C3 and C5, called anaphylatoxins, release histamine from mast cells and basophils, contract smooth muscles, and increase vascular permeability. This can occur following complement activation of immunologic antibody-mediated IgM and IgG activator or nonimmunologic (heparin–protamine) pathways. These aggregated leukocytes can cause microvascular occlusion and also liberate inflammatory products such as prostaglandins and leukotrienes. This polymorphonuclear activation may be responsible for clinical manifestations of transfusion reactions and pulmonary vasoconstriction following protamine reactions.

Thus, although more than one mechanism may be involved in the production of allergic drug reactions in the same patient, the manifestations and treatment are identical. A comparison is detailed in Table 22-1.

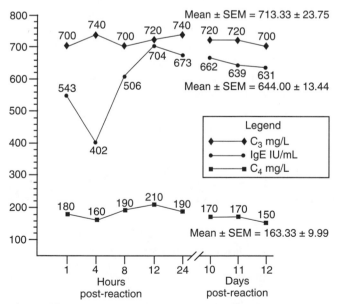

Figure 22-1   A patient experiencing an anaphylactic reaction to thiopental manifested a decrease followed by an overshoot in the plasma concentration of immunoglobulin E (IgE). Concentrations of complement proteins C3 and C4 were unchanged. (From Lilly JK, Hoy RH. Thiopental anaphylaxis and regain involvement. *Anesthesiology* 1980;53:335–337, with permission.)

Table 22-1   Types of Allergic Drug Reaction

Type of reaction	Cause	Example
Anaphylaxis	IgE-mediated	Penicillin, latex, muscle relaxants
Anaphylactoid	Nonimmunologic	Opioids, muscle relaxants, protamine
	Release of histamine from mast cells and basophils	
Polymorphonuclear leukocyte activation	Complement activation	Transfusion reactions, protamine
	IgG or IgM or nonimmunologic	

DIAGNOSIS

Recognition of allergic reactions under general anesthesia may be difficult. The onset and severity of the reaction relate to the mediator's end-organ effects. A spectrum of reactions can occur and anesthetic drugs may confound the scenario by altering vasoactive mediator release, possibly delaying early recognition. Thus, hypotension and cardiovascular collapse may be the first manifestation during anesthesia of an allergic reaction. Signs and symptoms of an allergic reaction are listed in Table 22-2, and mediators of an allergic reaction in Table 22-3.

TREATMENT

Treatment for anaphylaxis or anaphylactoid reactions must include reversal of hypoxemia, optimizing intravascular volume, preventing further release of vasoactive mediators, and airway maintenance. Oxygen (100%) administration, intravascular volume expansion, and epinephrine are the first line treatment. Box 22-1 lists the necessary items to have available.

When the reaction is life threatening, epinephrine 5–100 μg in incremental intravenous doses may be needed, depending on the severity and response to the initial dose. Epinephrine increases cyclic adenosine monophosphate, restores membrane permeability and decreases the release of vasoactive mediators. It relaxes bronchial smooth muscle due to its beta-2 effects. If anaphylaxis is not life-threatening a standard adult dose of epinephrine is 0.3–0.5 mg in a 1:1,000 dilution can be administered subcutaneously.

Antihistamines may decrease the side effects of histamine (hypotension, pruritus, and bronchospasm) by competing with receptor sites occupied by histamine. However, once vasoactive mediators have been released antihistamines may not be effective. In addition, bronchospasm and the negative cardiac inotropic effects of histamine are due to subsequent leukotriene release, not histamine *per se*. The role of H_2 antagonists once anaphylaxis has occurred remains unclear.

Corticosteroids may enhance the beta-2-agonist effects of other drugs and inhibit release of arachidonic acid, which is responsible for leukotriene and prostaglandin release. They also may be helpful if the underlying cause activates the complement system.

Aminophylline is a weak bronchodilator that increases right and left ventricular contractility and decreases pulmonary vascular resistance. It may be useful with persistent bronchospasm and hemodynamic stability however the inhaled beta-2 agonists seem to be superior and should be used as the initial treatment. An intravenous

Table 22-2   Signs and Symptoms of an Allergic Reaction

Systems	Symptoms	Signs
Respiratory	Dyspnea, chest pain	Cough, wheezing, laryngeal edema, pulmonary edema, decreased pulmonary compliance
Cardiovascular	Dizziness, retrosternal pain	Diaphoresis, loss of consciousness, hypotension, tachycardia, cardiac arrest, dysrhythmias, pulmonary hypertension, decreased systemic vascular resistance
Cutaneous	Itching, burning	Urticaria, flushing, oral and periorbital edema

Modified from Levy JH. *Anaphylactic reactions in anesthesia and intensive care*. Stoneham: Butterworth-Heinemann, 1992

Table 22-3   Causative Mediators of an Allergic Reaction

Vasoactive Mediator	Physiologic Effect
Histamine	Peripheral vasodilatation
	Bronchospasm
	Increased capillary permeability
Leukotrienes	Increased capillary permeability
	Bronchospasm
	Negative inotropy
	Possible coronary artery vasoconstriction
Prostaglandins	Bronchospasm

Modified from Stoelting RK, Dierdorf SF. Diseases related to immune system dysfunction. In: *Anesthesia and co-existing disease*, 4th ed. Philadelphia: Churchill Livingstone, 2002:613.

Box 22-1   Requirements for Treatment of Anaphylaxis or Anaphylactoid Reactions

Oxygen
Balanced salt solutions
Colloids
Epinephrine
Diphenhydramine
Inhaled beta-2 agents
Corticosteroids
Sodium bicarbonate

Modified from Stoelting RK, Dierdorf SF Diseases related to immune system dysfunction. In: *Anesthesia and co-existing disease*, 4th ed. Philadelphia: Churchill Livingstone, 2002:614.

Box 22-2   Treatment of Anaphylaxis

PRIMARY THERAPY

1. Think of it!
2. Withdraw the antigen
3. Maintain airway with 100% oxygen
4. Discontinue all anesthetic agents, blood, and antibiotic and muscle relaxant infusions
5. Intravascular volume expansion – crystalloid up to 4 L in adults, 10–20 mL/kg in children
6. Epinephrine 5–10 μg intravenously adults, children 0.5–5 μg/kg intravenously – double dose every 3 minutes until satisfactory blood pressure is obtained – if no intravenous access present can be given intratracheally

SECONDARY TREATMENT

Antihistamine: Diphenhydramine 0.5–1 mg/kg adults and children
Bronchodilators: Albuterol or terbutaline inhaler
Corticosteroids: 0.25–1 g hydrocortisone or 1–2 g methylprednisolone (adults), 0.5 mg/kg hydrocortisone or 1 mg/kg methylprednisolone (children)
Sodium bicarbonate: 0.5–1 mEq/kg for persistent hypotension and acidosis
Catecholamine infusion: Epinephrine 5–10 μg/min (adult), 0.05–4 μg/kg/min (children); norepinephrine 5–10 μg/min (adults), 0.05–0.1 μg/kg/min (children); isoproterenol is contraindicated because of its vasodilatory properties, unless refractory bronchospasm is present
Airway evaluation before extubation

loading dose of 5–6 mg/kg over 20 minutes is followed by an infusion of 0.5–0.9 mg/kg/hr. Milrinone may have a role in the treatment of right ventricular dysfunction and pulmonary hypertension but may cause systemic vasodilatation and hypotension. Box 22-2 summarizes the treatment of anaphylaxis.

ROLE OF PRETREATMENT FOR ALLERGIC REACTIONS

Patients with a history of allergy, atopy, or asthma are more likely to develop life-threatening hypersensitivity reactions during anesthesia. There is no data in the literature to show that pretreatment with antihistamines and/or corticosteroid is effective for true anaphylaxis. Most of the literature on pretreatment efficacy is from patients with previous radiocontrast media reactions (nonimmunologic mechanisms). Otherwise, pretreatment

has not been shown to be beneficial and may give physicians a false sense of security.

DRUG ALLERGIES IN THE PERIOPERATIVE PERIOD

Almost all drugs administered during anesthesia have been reported to have caused allergic drug reactions except for the benzodiazepines and ketamine. Latex sensitization is thought to be present in as many as 15% of patients undergoing anesthesia and many allergic reactions attributed to drugs may be actually due to latex.

Muscle Relaxants

Muscle relaxants may present with allergic reactions by both anaphylactic and anaphylactoid mechanisms. They may be responsible for up to 60% of drug-induced allergies during anesthesia. In a recent report of anaphylaxis during anesthesia from a 2-year survey in France, neuromuscular blocking agents were responsible for 69.2% of reactions, as opposed to latex, which was present in 12.1%. It is also known that up to 50% of patients who experience allergic reactions to one muscle relaxant are also allergic to other muscle relaxants. The structural similarities between muscle relaxants may in part explain this cross-sensitivity (e.g., quaternary ammonium groups).

In the French study the most common cause of severe anaphylaxis was succinylcholine. The next most severe reaction was due to rocuronium, with vecuronium and pancuronium being the least often implicated. Although atracurium and mivacurium reactions were reported, most were mild immune-mediated adverse reactions, possibly due to mast cell histamine release rather than IgE antibodies, which were present in a high number of rocuronium, succinylcholine, and vecuronium patients.

If the reaction is due to drug-induced histamine release from mast cells and basophils, decreasing the rate of administration of intravenously administered drugs may decrease this reaction.

Induction Agents

Allergic reactions to barbiturates are rare (1:30,000 anesthetics) and usually present in patients with a history of food allergies, rhinitis, or asthma. Methohexital may be less likely to induce histamine release than other intravenous barbiturates.

Allergic reactions to propofol can occur during the first or subsequent exposure. Patients with a history of allergies to other drugs seem to be more vulnerable to propofol allergic reaction, which can be life-threatening. Bronchospasm is more common with this drug than with other anesthetic agents, particularly with the preparation containing preservative.

Local Anesthetics

Only 1% of reactions to local anesthetics are true allergic reactions. Most reactions are due to inadvertent intravascular injection with resultant toxicity or systemic absorption of epinephrine in the local anesthetic solution resulting in tachycardia and hypertension.

Ester-based local anesthetics are more likely to produce true allergic reactions than amide-based drugs because of their metabolism to paraamino benzoic acid (PABA), which is highly antigenic. However, preservatives used in these local anesthetic solutions may be the true culprit because of their structural similarity to PABA, which may make them antigenic. Cross-reactivity does not seem to exist between amide and ester local anesthetics.

Opioids

True anaphylaxis is rare following opioid administration. However, anaphylactoid reactions are more common with morphine and its derivatives than with fentanyl. Allergic reactions have been seen with fentanyl following systemic or neuraxial administration.

Volatile Anesthetics

Halothane hepatitis has clinical manifestations that suggest drug-induced allergic reaction. These include eosinophilia, fever, or rash with prior exposure. The patient's plasma may contain antibodies that react with halothane-induced liver antigens. Subsequent antigen–antibody reactions are responsible for the liver injury. There may be cross-reactivity with other volatile agents, which is possibly related to the magnitude of metabolism of the agent. The most predictable agent to cause anesthetic-induced hepatitis, because of the degree of hepatic metabolism, would be enflurane, with the risk being minimal with isoflurane and rare with desflurane. Sevoflurane has not shown production of oxidative metabolites like the other agents, so the risk is considered small with this agent.

Protamine

Anaphylactic reactions to protamine are more likely in patients with seafood allergies (protamine is derived from salmon sperm), or those patients who take a protamine-containing insulin preparation, although the risk is very small (0.6–2%). In vasectomized men, although circulating antibodies to sperm may be seen, an increase in allergies to protamine is not seen.

Protamine also may directly evoke histamine release by activating the complement system, leading to pulmonary hypertension and bronchospasm. The rate of administration may decrease the severity of this reaction.

Antibiotics

Penicillin and cephalosporins have structural similarity, both having beta-lactam rings. Cephalosporin allergic reactions are low (0.02%) and are only minimally increased in patients with penicillin allergy. Vancomycin may produce life-threatening allergic reactions even if the rate of intravenous administration is slow.

Blood and Plasma Volume Expanders

Cross-matched blood has an incidence of allergic reactions of 3%, with pruritus, urticaria, pulmonary edema, and fever being the common symptoms. Synthetic plasma solutions that include dextran and hydroxyethyl starch have both been reported to cause anaphylactic and anaphylactoid reactions. Low molecular-weight dextran does not induce antibodies but may react with antibodies already present, and may also activate the complement system.

Intravascular Contrast

The iodine in these agents evokes allergic reactions in 5% of patients. The risk of allergies to these agents is increased in patients with other food and drug allergies. Many of these reactions are actually anaphylactoid and can be modified by pretreatment with corticosteroids or diphenhydramine, and limiting the iodine dose.

LATEX ALLERGY

The patient with latex allergy who comes for surgery presents a specific list of problems for the anesthesiologist. Latex allergy is a type I anaphylactic reaction. It is IgE-mediated, antigen-stimulated, and has mast cell activation. Clinical signs are listed in Box 22-3.

In addition, a type IV hypersensitivity reaction or cell-mediated immunity has been seen with latex contact dermatitis due to exposure to latex gloves. This reaction is a T-cell-mediated reaction and presents 6–48 hours after contact.

Groups at risk for latex allergy include:
- *Patients* (particularly children) *with neural tube defects* (meningomyelocele, spina bifida, congenital urologic anomalies) *and cerebral palsy*: The incidence is 18–56%. Patients with prolonged exposure to latex – constant or repeat urinary catheterizations and multiple surgery – are also at increased risk. Spina bifida patients with more than six surgeries and/or atopy history have increased risk. Patients on home mechanical ventilation may also be at increased risk because of their constant latex exposure.
- *Patients with a history of atopy*: 35–83% of latex allergy patients. Children with a banana, chestnut, or avocado allergy suggest a protein cross-reactivity with latex.

- *Healthcare workers*: Up to 8% of physicians, 5.6% of nurses, and 13.7% of dental personnel. The IgE-antibody-positive rate is as high as 12.5% in anesthesiologists.
- *Patients with a history of multiple exposures*: This may be from multiple surgical procedures or repeated examinations involving mucous membrane contact with latex products. Risk factors for latex sensitization in this group are atopy, a history of allergy to selected fruits, and a history of skin symptoms with latex glove use.
- *Workers in the rubber industry*: Chronic exposure to latex antigens leads to a 10% incidence in this population.

Routes of Exposure and Clinical Manifestations

- *Direct skin contact*: Contact dermatitis with occupational latex glove exposure, a localized or generalized skin response in the form of urticaria.
- *Absorption from mucous membranes* (nose, bowel, mouth, vagina, or rectum): Can present as conjunctivitis, rhinitis, stomatitis, or asthma with angioedema. May result in cardiovascular collapse intraoperatively.
- *Inhalation of latex protein*: Starch aeroallergens may cause desaturation, wheezing, bronchospasm, and hypoxemia – worse with powdered gloves.
- *Direct intravascular absorption of antigen*: Prolonged exposure to surgical gloves results in tachycardia, hypotension, and cardiorespiratory collapse.

Diagnosis of Latex Allergy

Preoperative diagnosis is usually made by a history of balloon or glove intolerance or allergies to medical products e.g., urinary catheters. Tests to determine latex sensitivity are listed in Box 22-4.

Box 22-3   Clinical Signs of Latex Allergy

Increased vascular permeability (urticaria and laryngeal edema)
Contraction of smooth muscle (bronchospasm)
Vasodilatation (flushing and hypotension)
Stimulation of sensory nerve endings (pruritus)
Cardiac histamine receptor stimulation (tachycardia and arrhythmias)

Box 22-4   Tests to Determine Latex Sensitivity

***IN VIVO* TESTS**

Skin prick test (SPT) – most reliable, nonammoniated latex reagent (NAL) diagnosed latex allergy with no adverse effect
Patch test – scratch covered by latex glove piece
Use test – if the product produces allergic symptoms

***IN VITRO* TESTS**

Radioallergosorbent test (RAST; radioactivity to detect antibodies to IgE)
Enzyme-linked immunosorbent assay (ELISA)
Alstat – latex-specific IgE antibodies – takes $3\frac{1}{2}$ hours, sensitivity (94%), specificity (81%)

Patients who are positive for latex allergy should wear a Medic-alert bracelet.

Preoperative Preparation

There is still controversy about pretreating patients with H_1- and H_2-blockers and steroids. This is currently not recommended, since avoidance of latex exposure is the most important aspect of preparation. If pretreatment is deemed useful the protocols listed in Box 22-5 are suggested.

Management

Treating patients at high risk for latex allergy (e.g., spina bifida and myelodysplasia patients) in a latex-free environment from their first surgical procedure may decrease the incidence of latex sensitization and intraoperative allergic reactions.

The patient's chart should be labeled "allergic to latex." Scheduling is important, since latex is an aeroallergen and is present in the operating room for at least an hour after the use of latex gloves. When possible, the patient should be scheduled as first case of the day. Two and a half hours of nonuse of the operating room and anesthesia machine reduces levels of latex aeroallergens by 96%. Many hospitals now have a latex-free environment in place. Necessary latex precautions are listed in Box 22-6.

Box 22-6 Latex Precautions in the Operating Room

Use of nonlatex gloves – most important!

If latex-free intravenous tubing is unavailable, use stopcocks and tape over latex ports

Avoid multidose vials – it does appear to be safe to puncture a multidose vial one time but repeated punctures are unacceptable

Wrap blood pressure connecting tube with Webril or use latex-free cuffs

Use Velcro tourniquets

Avoid histamine-releasing drugs

Use neoprene bellows for the Ohmeda ventilator – if not available use gas flows lower than 10 L/min and consider washing the ventilator bellows bag

A circuit filter such as a Pall TM BB25, which will prevent inhalation of latex particles, should be placed between the breathing circuit and the endotracheal tube.

Place a sign on operating room door indicating that the patient is allergic to latex

A latex allergy cart can be very helpful – it should include:
- Latex-free syringes, glass syringes
- Drugs in glass ampules
- Intravenous tubing without latex injection ports
- Neoprene reservoir bags
- Webril
- Neoprene gloves
- Ambu bags with silicone valves
- Neoprene bellows for ventilator

Box 22-5 Pretreatment for Latex Allergy

ADULTS

Methylprednisolone 1 mg/kg intravenously every 6 hours – maximum dose 60 mg

Diphenhydramine 1 mg/kg intravenously every 6 hours – maximum dose 50 mg

Ranitidine 0.5 mg/kg intravenously every 6 hours – maximum dose 150 mg

CHILDREN

<1 year old
None

1–12 years old
Prednisone 1 mg/kg by mouth every 6 hours – maximum dose 40 mg

Hydroxyzine 0.7 mg/kg by mouth every 6 hours – maximum dose 50 mg

12 years–Adult
Prednisone 1 mg/kg by mouth every 6 hours – maximum dose 40 mg

Loratadine 10 mg by mouth the night before

Diagnosis of Latex Anaphylaxis

The onset of anaphylaxis due to latex is generally 20–60 minutes after exposure to the antigen (range 5–290 min). It usually presents as a clinical triad
- Hypotension – most common
- Rash – urticaria
- Bronchospasm

Treatment of Intraoperative Latex Anaphylaxis

Treatment for anaphylaxis is the same as described earlier in this chapter. If the patient has been pretreated with an H_2-blocker such as ranitidine or takes this medication for another medical problem (e.g., gastroesophageal reflux) and a latex allergic reaction occurs during anesthesia the presenting symptom may be a 3:1 heart block. H_2-receptor stimulation mediates coronary vasodilatation and increases heart rate and myocardial contractility. The use of H_2-receptor antagonists prior to anaphylaxis may predispose a patient to development of heart block by preventing the H_2-receptors from counteracting the cardiorespiratory depressant actions of anaphylactic mediators, and also predispose to myocardial ischemia in patients with coronary artery disease.

Remember that antibiotic or muscle relaxant allergies can be present in the latex-allergic patient, and may be the cause of the allergic reaction – not latex.

SUGGESTED READING

Anne S, Reisman RE. Risk of administering cephalosporin antibiotics to patients with histories of penicillin allergy. *Ann Allergy Asthma Immunol* 1995;74:167–170.

Birmingham PK, Dsida RM, Grayhack JJ, *et al*. Do latex precautions in children with myelodysplasia reduce intraoperative allergic reactions? *J Pediatr Orthoped* 1996;16:799–802.

Brown RH, Schauble JF, Hamilton RG. Prevalence of latex allergy among anesthesiologists. Identification of sensitized but asymptomatic individuals. *Anesthesiology* 1998;89:292–299.

Delfico AJ, Dormans JP, Craythorne CB, Templeton JJ. Intraoperative anaphylaxis due to allergy to latex in children who have cerebral palsy: a report of six cases. *Dev Med Child Neurol* 1996;39:194–197.

Fasting S, Gisvold SE. Serious intraoperative problems – a five-year review of 83,844 anesthetics. *Can J Anesth* 2002;49: 545–553.

Fisher MM, Baldo BA, Silbert BS. Anaphylaxis during anesthesia: use of radioimmunoassays to determine etiology and drugs responsible in fatal cases. *Anesthesiology* 1991;75:1112–1115.

Holzman RS. Clinical management of latex allergic children. *Anesthesiology* 1997;85:529–533.

Laxenaire MC, Mertes PM, Groupe d'Etudes des Reactions Anaphylactoides Peranesthesiques. Anaphylaxis during anaesthesia. Results of a two-year survey in France. *Br J Anaesth* 2001;87:549–558.

Levy JH. *Anaphylactic reactions in anesthesia and intensive care*. 2nd ed. Stoneham: Butterworth-Heinemann, 1992.

Levy JH, Adelson DM, Walker BF. Wheal and flare responses to muscle relaxants in humans. *Agents Actions* 1991;34:302–308.

Levy JH, Schieger IM, Zaidan JR, *et al*. Evaluation of patients at risk for protamine reactions. *J Thorac Cardiovasc Surg* 1989;98:200–204.

Patterson LJ, Milne B. Latex anaphylaxis causing heart block: role of ranitidine. *Can J Anesth* 1999;46:776–778.

Porri F, Pradal M, Lemiere C, *et al*. Association between latex sensitization and repeated latex exposure in children. *Anesthesiology* 1997;86:599–602.

Stoelting RK, Dierdorf SF. Diseases related to immune system dysfunction. In: *Anesthesia and co-existing disease*, 4th ed. Philadelphia: Churchill Livingstone, 2002:611–620.

Weiss ME, Nyhan D, Peng Z, *et al*. Association of protamine IgE and IgG antibodies with life-threatening reactions to intravenous protamine. *N Engl J Med* 1989;320:886–892.

CHAPTER 23

Obesity

KENNETH KUCHTA

INTRODUCTION

While obesity is increasingly being recognized as a disease with significant public health implications, anesthesiologists have long respected the challenges and perioperative risk associated with the obese patient. The common anesthetic issues range from potential airway nightmares to cardiac and pulmonary compromise. Moreover, the list of diseases associated with the overweight patient is so lengthy as to make the approach to these patients a sobering process. These reservations notwithstanding, overweight and obese patients will continue to present to surgery for a variety of disease processes, whether comorbid with, or unrelated to, their overweight status. For the foreseeable future the incidence of surgery for the treatment of obesity will likely increase as diet, behavior modification, and drug therapy continue to fail in a significant number of patients. As we enter the first decade of the new millennium, despite nearly a quarter century of emphasis on the identification and treatment of the overweight adult, the prevalence of this problem is increasing. From the late 1970s to 1999 the percentage of adults in the United States who met the National Institutes of Health (NIH) definition of overweight or obesity rose from 47% to 61%. This combined with growing evidence of the tremendous health costs (both human and monetary) led the Surgeon General to announce a "call to action" in 2001 to stem what is now being labeled an epidemic.

DEFINITION AND EPIDEMIOLOGY

While various measures have been used to define overweight and obesity, the most generally recognized definitions are based on the body mass index (BMI). The BMI is calculated by dividing the weight in kilograms by the square of the height in meters. Substituting pounds and the square of height in inches requires that the result be multiplied by a conversion factor of 703. Although there are a variety of specific definitions of overweight and obesity, the one most widely recognized was provided by the NIH in 1998. The NIH defines "overweight" as a BMI of 25 or more, while obesity is defined as a BMI of 30 or greater. The commonly used term "morbid obesity" is not found in the text of the NIH report, although obesity is further divided into class I (30–34.9 BMI), class II (35–39.9 BMI) and class III, also called "extreme obesity" (40 or greater BMI).

While the BMI provides a single easily obtainable estimate of total body fat that can be used irrespective of gender, it may overestimate body fat in the case of very muscular individuals and underestimate body fat in those who have lost body mass (as is commonly seen in the elderly). There is evidence that the distribution of fat is important, with abdominal distribution (android obesity) representing a greater oxygen consumption and greater health risk than fat distributed to the thighs and buttock (gynecoid obesity).

Despite these limitations, it is important to not lose sight of the general utility of the index and obesity classification. The NIH BMI classes were chosen because they correlated with increased risk for the complications of obesity: risk increased if the BMI was more than 25 and increased at a greater rate when the BMI was above 30. The comorbidities of obesity are important health risks that point to potential coexisting diseases that have anesthetic implications. Being overweight or obese increases the chance of hypertension, dyslipidemia, type II diabetes, coronary artery disease, congestive heart failure, stroke, gallstones, osteoarthritis, and obstructive sleep apnea. Rates for cancer of the colon, breast, endometrium, and gallbladder are also increased for obese patients. Obesity is associated with menstrual dysfunction and increases the morbidity of both the parturient and child in pregnancy. Social stigmatization and emotional problems can further complicate the lives of the obese.

CARDIOVASCULAR CHANGES

To meet the increased oxygen demand imposed by extra tissue, absolute blood volume is increased while volume per weight actually decreases (from 75 mL/kg to 50 mL/kg; Table 23-1). This is not surprising as much of the added weight is poorly perfused adipose tissue. While blood flow to the splanchnic circulation increases, renal and cerebral blood flow remain unchanged. For the cardiovascular system the net result is an increased peripheral oxygen consumption requiring an increased cardiac output. Since heart rate is usually unchanged, this augmentation in cardiac output is accomplished by an increase in stroke volume. The response of the heart to the increased stroke volume and perhaps to the larger preload often seen in obesity is chamber dilation and eccentric hypertrophy. Meanwhile systemic vascular resistance (SVR) is usually decreased. If the patient also develops systemic hypertension (a common comorbidity

of obesity) the patient will probably develop a concentric hypertrophy and a normal to elevated SVR.

The long-term impact of these physiologic derangements is profound. Even without left ventricular hypertrophy, the obese have diastolic dysfunction as seen on echocardiography. Left ventricular hypertrophy adds systolic dysfunction, limits coronary reserve, and increases the incidence and complexity of ventricular arrhythmias. The pulmonary pathophysiological consequences of obesity with its propensity for hypoxia and hypercarbia can result in pulmonary hypertension, tricuspid regurgitation, right ventricular hypertrophy, and/or failure.

As previously noted, other long-term cardiovascular consequences of obesity include an increased risk of coronary artery disease, hypertension, congestive heart failure, and stroke.

"Fen-phen"

In the mid 1990s drug therapy for obesity changed dramatically with a switch from short- to long-term therapy. The use of dexfenfluramine and fenfluramine increased rapidly. Phentermine was often combined with fenfluramine ("fen-phen") to minimize the side effects of each drug. In 1995-96 an estimated 14 million prescriptions were written for either dexfenfluramine or fenfluramine, with between 1.2 and 4.7 million patients exposed to these drugs. Reports of regurgitant valvular heart lesions (mostly left-sided) led to the Food and Drug Administration requesting a voluntary recall of these two drugs from the market. Additional concerns over reports of pulmonary hypertension have also surfaced. While these drugs are now off the market, the sheer volume of patients exposed to these products indicates that we should continue to consider their potential long-term side effects when interviewing any obese patient.

Table 23-1	Summary of the Cardiovascular Changes Associated with Obesity	
		Change
Absolute blood volume		↑
Relative blood volume (ml/kg)		↓
Splanchnic blood flow		↑
Renal and cerebral blood flow		↔
Cardiac output		↑
Stroke volume		↑
Heart rate		↔
Systemic vascular resistance without hypertension		↓
Systemic vascular resistance with hypertension		↔ or ↑

Drug Interactions: Possible Adverse Effects of Weight-loss Pharmacotherapy

Valvular heart disease, pulmonary hypertension, and neurotoxicity with dexfenfluramine and fenfluramine (both withdrawn from the market)

Increased heart rate and blood pressure with sibutramine

Decreased absorption of fat-soluble vitamins with orlistat

Patients should be questioned specifically about the use of over-the-counter and herbal weight-loss medications

RESPIRATORY CHANGES

While the evolution of cardiac pathophysiological changes of obesity present significant comorbidities for the patient, which can impact anesthesia care, the pulmonary pathophysiology of obesity presents immediate concerns for the anesthesiologist (Table 23-2). While these problems are linked to the even more pressing concerns presented by the airway, we will attempt to discuss these issues separately but in succession for clarity. Obese patients tend to have decreased functional residual capacity (FRC) with an even more marked decrease when recumbent. Expiratory reserve volume is decreased, as is total lung capacity. Unless reactive airway disease intervenes, the lung pathology is restrictive in nature. With the increased oxygen demand mentioned in the prior section, the decreased FRC results in a markedly reduced reserve, translating to a picture all too familiar to anesthesiologists, one of early desaturation on induction and emergence and increased risk throughout the perioperative period. The decreased FRC places the patient at a suboptimal portion of the lung compliance curve, and, accordingly, the obese have a tendency to take shallow and rapid breaths. The result can be hypercarbia and, with the development of ventilation perfusion mismatch, hypoxia. Further progression can result in the pickwickian syndrome – massive obesity resulting in alveolar hypoventilation and severe hypoxia and hypercarbia, daytime somnolence, periodic respirations, secondary polycythemia, right-heart hypertrophy, and failure.

Airway

While cardiac changes found in obesity can contribute to significant cardiovascular pathology and the respiratory pathophysiology can provide challenges in maintaining ventilation and oxygenation, the overriding concern for anesthesiologists rests in the profound changes that can occur with respect to airway management for these patients. A careful airway examination of an obese patient conducted by even a junior anesthesiology resident often contains more than one feature

---

Box 23-1 Summary of Anatomic Changes That Can Affect Airway Management

Short neck with limited range of motion
Large breasts
Enlarged tongue
Thickened cheeks
Thickened palatal, pharyngeal, or supralaryngeal tissue

---

for concern. The list of possible findings may include a short, thick neck with limitation of motion, suprasternal fat or large, pendulous breasts, an enlarged tongue, thickened cheeks, and redundant or thickened palatal, pharyngeal, or supralaryngeal tissue (Box 23-1). Some authors have gone so far as to consider obesity itself to be a risk factor for difficult intubation. Others have not found obesity, in and of itself, to be a sole predictor of problems with intubation.

A prudent approach would dictate a very careful airway examination and a relatively conservative approach (i.e., fiberoptic intubation when there is any reasonable doubt) based upon the judgment and experience of the anesthesiologist. An interesting consideration in airway evaluation and management is appearing more prominently in the literature, the issue of obstructive sleep apnea (OSA).

Current Controversies: Airway Management

Some have found that the obese are more difficult to intubate, while others have claimed that it is not an independent variable
Awake fiberoptic intubation is proposed as the preferred method of airway management by some, while others note that many obese patients can be intubated via direct laryngoscopy following anesthetic induction
All would agree that caution and a very careful airway examination (possibly with additional attention to obstructive sleep apnea) is essential

---

Obstructive Sleep Apnea and Obesity

While OSA is defined by the number of apneic spells (more than five per hour, each lasting longer than 10 seconds), its relevance during the perioperative period lies in its pathophysiology.

In the normal state, phasic contraction of the tensor palatini, genioglossus, and hyoid muscle maintain a patent airway, despite the negative intra-airway pressure

---

Table 23-2 Summary of the Respiratory Changes Associated with Obesity

	Change
Functional residual capacity upright	↓
Functional residual capacity supine	↓ ↓
Expiratory reserve volume	↓
Total lung capacity	↓

of inspiration, by pulling the palate, tongue, and hyoid anteriorly. Fat deposited in the walls of pharyngeal structures in the obese decrease the pharyngeal area and may make it harder for the phasic contraction of the pharyngeal muscles to maintain airway patency as described above (Figure 23-1). One author has even suggested that a change in the orientation of the airway in some patients with OSA may significantly influence the ease in which it can be opened. A change from a normally horizontal ellipse to a vertical orientation (as seen with OSA) can result in less of an increase in area as the anterior wall of the airway is pulled forward by the phasic contraction outlined above (Figure 23-2).

With the onset of normal sleep, a generalized decrease in muscle tone progresses to a generalized loss of muscle tone during the very deep rapid eye movement (REM) stage of sleep. For those with OSA this normal decrease in muscle tone can instigate apneic periods (with hypercapnia and hypoxia) that are punctuated with arousal. The fact that this occurs in or prior to the restorative REM sleep can result in daytime sleepiness, as well as cognitive and behavioral changes. Patients can also develop arrhythmias (bradycardia and ventricular ectopy) during the apneic episodes. In the long term, pulmonary and systemic hypertension can result from the hypoxia associated with OSA. Most anesthetics decrease the tone of the pharyngeal muscles and thus make the patient with OSA more susceptible to airway closure in the perioperative period. Furthermore, narcotics will decrease the arousal response to these apneic episodes in the first 3 days after surgery. Meanwhile REM sleep is initially depressed only to rebound in postoperative days 4–6, thus enhancing the risk for these patients.

Although recognition of OSA is increasing, most patients with this disorder are not yet diagnosed. It is not uncommon for the anesthesiologist to be the first to raise the possibility of OSA when interviewing a patient. Since obesity is so closely related to OSA in adults, the anesthesiologist dealing frequently with the obese should search for symptoms of OSA during the interview. A definitive diagnosis, however, requires a sleep study.

There are many implications of OSA in the perioperative period. For those not formally diagnosed, yet presenting a suspicious history and physical examination, surgery may be delayed for appropriate referral to diagnose and manage this disorder. An acceptable alternative may be to proceed with surgery and assume that the suspected diagnosis is correct. Regional anesthesia may be considered, not only to avoid tracheal intubation, but also to obviate the need for large amounts of sedatives and narcotics. This must be weighed against the possibility of the patient not tolerating the procedure without the need for heavy sedation or an urgent and potentially more difficult intraoperative induction of general anesthesia and airway management.

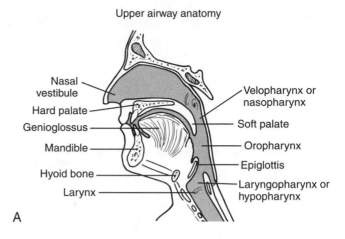

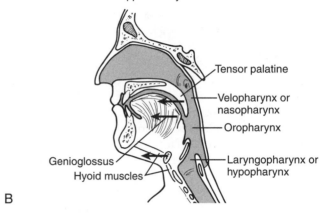

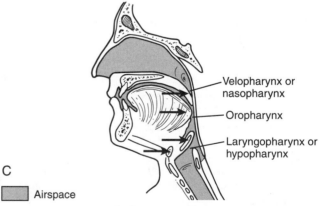

Figure 23-1   A, Important upper airway anatomy. The nasopharynx ends at the tip of the uvula; the oropharynx extends from the tip of the uvula to the epiglottis; the laryngopharynx extends from the tip of the epiglottis to the posterior cricoid cartilage. **B,** Action of the most important dilator muscles of the upper airway. The tensor palatine, genioglossus, and hyoid muscles enlarge the nasopharynx, oropharynx, and laryngopharynx, respectively. **C,** Collapse of the nasopharynx at the palatal level, the oropharynx at the glottic level and the laryngopharynx at the epiglottic level. (Redrawn with permission from Benumof J Obstructive sleep apnea in the adult obese patient: Implications for airway management. *J. Clinic Anesthesia* 2001; 13: 144–156. © 2001 with permission from Elsevier.)

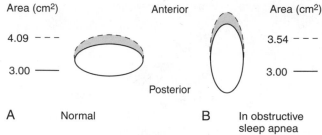

Figure 23-2   The effect of a 5 mm change in the anteroposterior (AP) diameter of the airway on airway cross-sectional area is shown for two equally elliptical airways with different lateral/AP ratios. **A**, Lateral/AP ratio = 2. **B**, Lateral/AP ratio = 0.5. The lateral dimension of each ellipse was held constant. The solid line represents the starting area (3 cm² in both ellipses), and the dotted line represents the area after a 5 mm increase in AP diameter. The area change is greater in the ellipse with a more lateral orientation (**A**). (Redrawn with permission from Leiter JC Upper airway shape. Is it important in the pathogenesis of obstructive sleep apnea? *Am J Respir Crit Care Med* 1996; 153: 894–898. © American Lung Association.)

The pathology of OSA clearly contributes in some degree to difficulties in intubating obese patients and additional caution may be warranted. The decision about extubation in the operating room versus in the recovery room or even the intensive care unit is also widely debated and needs to be individualized based upon good judgment and experience. The need to monitor the patient with OSA more closely in the perioperative period and the most prudent postoperative pain management strategy are also controversial. The above-mentioned controversies regarding the perioperative management of the obese patient with presumed or documented OSA only points to the risk that this disorder may add to the already complicated management of obesity.

Clinical Caveats: Obstructive Sleep Apnea

Most obstructive sleep apnea is not recognized
Diagnosis can only be made with a formal sleep study
As the anesthesiologist may be the first to suggest the diagnosis, knowledge of the signs and symptoms is essential – findings suggesting obstructive sleep apnea:
- Snoring*
- Snorting or apnea during sleep*
- Daytime sleepiness or fatigue
- Nocturnal diaphoresis and enuresis
- Frequent nocturia
- Morning headaches
- Cognitive or behavioral abnormalities
- Obesity
- Systemic and/or pulmonary hypertension
- Enlarged neck circumference (>40–42 cm)

* May be reported only by relatives or others in a position to observe the patient's sleep pattern.

ENDOCRINE

While obesity may be due to a number of endocrine disorders such as Cushing's syndrome, hypothyroidism, hypothalamic disorders, hypogonadism, and insulinomas, the predominant endocrine disorder that coexists in obese patients is type II diabetes mellitus. The chances of being a diabetic increase as weight increases, and with weight loss glucose intolerance in nondiabetic patients improves. Glucose regulation also improves with weight loss in some diabetics.

GASTROINTESTINAL

Conventionally, it is taught that increased intra-abdominal pressure, along with low gastric pH and increased residual gastric volume, are reported in obese patients, putting them at increased risk of aspiration. However, recent data has actually claimed a higher incidence of low pH and high gastric volume in lean versus obese patients. As many other factors (intra-abdominal pressure, hiatal hernia, difficult airways and their management, etc.) may also influence the risk of aspiration, it is difficult to interpret these new data and what their clinical implications are with regard to aspiration risk for obese patients.

OBESITY AND ANESTHETICS

Much of the literature regarding the effect of obesity on anesthetic agents attempts to address the issue of pharmacokinetics with little conclusive information available. Opioid distribution in some cases seems to be related to total body weight, while elimination may be more related to lean body weight. This has a rationale in that there is a greater volume of distribution for obese patients, while much of the metabolism occurs in lean tissues.

Prolonged duration of action is reported for a number of neuromuscular agents including metocurine, doxacurium, vecuronium, and rocuronium. Atracurium is sometimes advocated as the ideal agent for the obese patient because of a reported similar duration of action when compared to lean patients. Since pancuronium's duration of action has also been reported to be unaffected by weight, this argument is perhaps somewhat simplistic. Perhaps a more appropriate course of action may be to choose relaxants on the basis of all their characteristics as they relate to a particular patient and procedure and then dose cautiously (some have suggested 20% more than lean body mass) while carefully monitoring to avoid the complications of overdosing, which may be more difficult to manage in the obese.

For inhalation agents there are similar concerns stated in the literature that are either not relevant, because of the properties of newer agents, or simply overstated. For example, fluoride levels are increased in the obese after methoxyflurane, halothane, and enflurane anesthesia, yet these agents are rarely used in contemporary anesthetic practice. Similarly there is much written about fat-soluble volatile anesthetic agents overly prolonging anesthesia recovery in obese patients. That studies have failed to confirm this is perhaps not surprising when one calculates that the contribution of halothane from fat stores to venous blood after a 3-hour anesthetic is less than 1% of the minimum alveolar anesthetic concentration (MAC). Other factors related to the individual patient, or familiarity with a particular drug and skill in its administration, may be more important in choosing which inhalation agent to use.

OBESITY AND SURGERY

Anesthesiologists have at least three opportunities to encounter obese patients in the operating room. Patients may present for surgery totally unrelated to their obesity. Secondly, since obesity is related to a wide variety of conditions that may require surgery, obese patients may present for cholecystectomy, various carcinomas, coronary artery bypass, procedures for obstructive sleep apnea, or orthopedic operations related to osteoarthritis, etc. Finally those who have failed weight loss via diet, exercise, drug treatment, or behavioral therapy may seek surgical treatment (bariatric surgery) of their obesity.

By NIH guidelines surgery is considered an option for those patients with a BMI greater than 40, or with comorbidities and a BMI greater than 35. Candidates for bariatric surgery should be well informed, motivated, and have acceptable perioperative risk (without other significant risk factors). Earlier procedures emphasized malabsorption as their goal and were complicated by significant long-term side effects. By contrast, modern procedures are designed to reduce food intake. Various gastric banding or partitioning operations may be used, often combined with gastric bypasses (usually Roux-en-Y) to achieve this goal. Results of 50–100 kg weight loss over 6–12 months can be achieved. Although failure to maintain this reduction in weight can occur, surgery has produced the best results of all therapies. In addition to the significant perioperative risks in this population, there are several potential significant long-term complications (malabsorption, "dumping syndrome", gallstones) and a need for lifelong medical follow-up.

PERIOPERATIVE ANESTHETIC MANAGEMENT – BRINGING IT ALL TOGETHER

Perioperative management of the obese patient begins with a careful preoperative history. One should attempt to elicit signs and symptoms of coexisting disease, including cardiac, pulmonary, and endocrine disorders. This may not be easy, as these patients may have chest pain, dyspnea on exertion, and decreased exercise tolerance due to their obesity alone. Attempts to further clarify their symptoms may also be hampered. Breath and heart sounds may sound distant and peripheral edema may be hard to characterize in light of the patient's obesity. Echocardiography may be limited because of an inability to obtain adequate images. Moreover, we have seen patients whose cardiac workup was halted because they exceeded the weight limit of the available angiography table.

Perhaps the most important part of the preoperative visit is a mandatory and thorough airway examination. While some feel that obesity and OSA are both strong predictors of a difficult airway and advocate awake intubation as the airway management of choice in these patients, many anesthesiologists have been surprised by the ease of routine intubation. They have also been relieved, since any error with regard to predicted ease of intubation could easily lead to a rapid airway catastrophe.

Nonetheless, an awake intubation is not always the easy fallback for the obese patient. Sedation may be desired for patient acceptance as well as concern prompted by comorbid conditions (e.g., cardiac disease); however, many obese patients tolerate sedation poorly with complete loss of the airway a result. Regional anesthesia is another consideration, in order to avoid intubation and minimize sedation and opiate analgesia. This needs to be balanced against the relative difficulty in successfully performing these techniques, as well as the probability of conversion to a general anesthetic during the case (when time may be limited and airway access more difficult).

A variety of airway management options should be readily available and one should consider informing backup personnel of a possible difficult airway. Some have gone so far as recommending that two anesthesiologists are present at induction. A short-handled laryngoscope is often useful. Optimal positioning is crucial and may take extra time because of the size of the patient. A head-up position is useful for keeping the airway open as well as allowing better ventilation. (It should be noted that an extreme head-up position often requires elevating steps for the intubating anesthesiologist and may lessen the chance of aspiration.) It is also vital that at least one other person in the room knows exactly how to lower the head of the table in case this is needed for better airway access.

Depending upon the distribution of fat, intravenous access and invasive monitoring placement may be difficult. In this case Doppler probes and two-dimensional ultrasound may be helpful. Blood pressure cuffs must be the proper size and, while difficulty in obtaining a reliable reading is to be expected, it seems prudent to assume that failure to obtain a reading is hypotension until proven otherwise. Invasive arterial monitoring should be considered early as an alternative when obesity-related equipment failure occurs. Patient positioning is also problematic and the operating room may have to acquire special equipment to accommodate obese patients. Some positions (e.g. prone) may simply be physiologically impossible for the patient to tolerate and compromises regarding the surgical approach may be mandatory.

A rapid emergence with minimal time in the second stage of anesthesia is crucial for the obese patient if extubation in the operating room is desired. As other authors have correctly noted, it is important that extubation occurs with the patient truly awake and not merely thrashing about. It is also important to minimize the second stage of anesthesia as it can be physiologically dangerous to the patient and physically dangerous for all in the room. With this in mind (barring other overriding considerations), it seems prudent to use rapid recovery agents such as desflurane while carefully avoiding an overdose of intravenous agents. Postoperative pain management can be efficiently titrated in the recovery room while closely monitoring the patient's level of sedation. Postoperative regional analgesia, if selected, may contribute to successful emergence and extubation.

Finally, we have found that, while obstructive sleep apnea is to be respected as a possible confounding problem, extubation and management of sleep apnea on a regular surgical ward is possible in selected patients. Our aggressive continuation of preoperative continuous positive airway pressure into the postoperative period, as well as the availability of nursing staff very familiar with the care of obese patients, probably contributes to the success of this approach.

SUMMARY

The obese patient presents many challenges to the anesthesiologist. The epidemiology of obesity and the frequent failure of nonoperative treatment of this disease indicate that anesthesiologists will be caring for larger numbers of these patients in the foreseeable future. A wide range of associated comorbidities can affect many of these patients, the cardiac and respiratory derangements being especially prominent. Changes in the airway can make decisions about management difficult and challenging. Awareness of both the pathophysiology of obesity and the mechanism of obstructive sleep apnea will allow the anesthesiologist to optimally care for the obese patient.

Case Study

A 35-year-old female is scheduled for a Roux-en-Y gastric bypass. She has a long-standing history of obesity that is not responsive to diet and exercise and used "fen-phen" for 18 months several years ago. She was evaluated for atypical chest pain with a stress test that showed a normal ejection fraction and a questionable area of ischemia versus artifact. Her husband notes that she frequently snores at night. Other problems include osteoarthritis, chronic low back pain, depression, and borderline hypertension. Her BMI is 41 and vital signs reveal a blood pressure of 140/95, pulse of 85 and respiratory rate of 22. On physical examination she has a thick neck with a Mallampati score of II–III, and very distant breath and heart sounds. A follow-up note from her cardiologist has just arrived via fax noting that an angiogram was scheduled but that she exceeded the weight limit for their table and that she is cleared for surgery.

- Does her history of "fen-phen" use concern you? Would you want any further evaluation?
- Is the issue of her chest pain resolved? If not, what would you do now?
- Does the snoring history concern you? Given this finding, what else would you like to know?

SUGGESTED READING

Benumof J. Obstructive sleep apnea in the adult obese patient: implications for airway management. *J Clin Anesth* 2001;13:144–156.

Messerli F. Cardiovascular effects of obesity and hypertension. *Lancet* 1982;1:1165–1168.

National Institutes of Health/National Heart, Lung and Blood Institute. Clinical guidelines on the identification, evaluation, and treatment of overweight and obesity in adults. HHS, Public Health Service, 1998. Available online at: http://www.nhlbi.nih.gov/guidelines/obesity/ob_home.htm.

Laparoscopic Surgery

PARWANE S. PARSA

INTRODUCTION

Because minimally invasive techniques have diagnostic and therapeutic applications in many surgical specialties, laparoscopic surgery is being performed with increasing frequency on inpatients and outpatients. However, although laparoscopic procedures provide significant advantages for patients, they also generate challenges for anesthesiologists. This chapter will discuss the anesthetic management of uncomplicated laparoscopic procedures, as well as the diagnosis and treatment of complications during or after such procedures.

PHYSIOLOGIC RESPONSES DURING LAPAROSCOPIC SURGERY

Hemodynamic and ventilatory stresses are observed in patients undergoing laparoscopic procedures (Table 24-1). Insufflation of carbon dioxide, which creates and maintains the pneumoperitoneum to allow visualization during the procedure, is a primary cause of physiologic changes. Insufflation of CO_2 to establish the pneumoperitoneum causes an increase in intra-abdominal pressure that is dependent on the gas insufflation pressure limit. Consequences include an initial increase then a decrease in preload as the intra-abdominal pressure increases, and an increase in systemic vascular resistance. The cardiac output decreases while the blood pressure increases. The patient's position can alter these responses. In the Trendelenburg position, the decrease in preload and increase in afterload is less striking than in the reverse Trendelenburg position.

Respiratory effects play a major role during laparoscopic procedures. CO_2, the insufflating gas to establish pneumoperitoneum, is nonflammable and blood soluble. After CO_2 insufflation is started, hypercapnia occurs within several minutes but stabilizes within the first hour of surgery, usually presenting an increased CO_2 load of up to 30%. Consequences include sympathetic stimulation, the potential for dysrhythmias, and respiratory acidosis; these problems can usually be corrected by increasing the minute ventilation. An additional impact of pneumoperitoneum is the mechanical effect of increased intra-abdominal pressure. Pulmonary compliance and functional residual capacity are reduced, and dead space is increased.

ADVANTAGES OF LAPAROSCOPIC PROCEDURES

Compared to similar open surgeries, laparoscopic procedures result in smaller incisions and decreased postoperative pain. Postoperative pulmonary function is preserved and atelectasis less after laparoscopic procedures. Postoperatively, patients also regain bowel function faster, have shorter hospital stays, and return to

437

Table 24-1 Hemodynamic and Ventilatory Changes with Insufflation

Parameter	Change	Therapy/Comments
End-tidal CO_2	↑ initially then stable	Increase minute ventilation
P_aCO_2	↑ initially then stable	Consider checking arterial blood gas; potential for increased P_aCO_2–ET- CO_2 gradient in certain patients
Compliance	↓	
Systemic vascular resistance	↑ initially then return toward baseline	Vasopressin release; Modify with vasoactive agents, volume loading
Pulmonary vascular resistance	↑	
Venous return	Initial ↑ then ↓	Additional volume before insufflation
Cardiac output	↓	Additional volume before insufflation

ET-CO_2, end-tidal carbon dioxide.

their regular activities sooner. The magnitude of these benefits varies with the patient group and the type of procedure.

COMPLICATIONS DURING LAPAROSCOPIC PROCEDURES

Most complications relate directly or indirectly to the need to insufflate CO_2 to create an operating space. If CO_2 enters a vessel rapidly, it will remain as insoluble gas and embolism can result. Insoluble gas can accumulate within the right heart, causing hypotension and possible cardiac arrest. A massive CO_2 embolus may be detected with a precordial stethoscope (murmur), transesophageal echocardiography, and end-tidal CO_2 monitoring (CO_2 transiently increases, followed by a decrease). Treatment includes stopping CO_2 insufflation, basic support measures (hyperventilation with 100% oxygen, fluid resuscitation), changing the patient's position to right side up, and placing a central venous catheter for aspiration of gas.

If gas intended for pneumoperitoneum escapes outside that space or if the laparoscopic procedure involves extraperitoneal insufflation (as for adrenalectomy or hernia repair), subcutaneous emphysema can occur. The end-tidal CO_2 increases to high levels and crepitus is noted, which usually resolves without intervention. Another serious concern is pneumothorax if gas enters the thorax through a tear created during surgery or from cervical subcutaneous tissue. Intervention is not always necessary because pneumothorax often resolves after insufflation is discontinued. Surgical mishaps can also complicate laparoscopic procedures. Conversion to an open procedure is necessary in cases of uncontrolled bleeding or visceral perforation (e.g. uterus, bowel, stomach).

ANESTHETIC TECHNIQUE

Preoperative Evaluation

As should be the custom before all anesthetics, an airway examination and a complete medical history are necessary. Because of the hemodynamic and respiratory stresses imposed on a patient during a laparoscopic procedure, preoperative evaluation should specifically focus on the identification of patients with severe lung disease and impaired cardiac function.

Intraoperative Management

Frequently, patients undergo laparoscopic procedures under general anesthesia with standard monitoring. Noninvasive blood pressure measurement and capnography are especially important to follow the hemodynamic and respiratory effects of pneumoperitoneum and positioning changes. In selected circumstances, invasive arterial blood pressure monitoring should be considered (Box 24-1). If the gradient between arterial and end-tidal CO_2 is large, sampling blood gases to measure the level of hypercapnia at intervals can guide ventilator adjustments during the procedure. Similarly, central venous pressure

Box 24-1 Indications for Arterial Line During Laparoscopic Procedures

Poor cuff fit over the upper extremity
Severe pulmonary disease
Higher than expected arterial to end-tidal CO_2 gradient
Reduced ventricular function

monitoring, pulmonary artery catheter placement, or transesophageal echocardiography may be useful in patients with impaired cardiac function or pulmonary hypertension.

Adequate intravenous access is important during laparoscopic surgeries. Although it is tempting to proceed with any available intravenous line because modest blood loss is expected, adequate intravenous access is key if fluid resuscitation is necessary for uncontrolled hemorrhage or gas embolus. Central venous access should be considered in patients with poor peripheral veins.

To prevent pulmonary aspiration, and to maintain the airway, an endotracheal tube should be placed. Placement of an orogastric or nasogastric tube after the airway is secured decompresses the stomach, decreasing the chance of gastric injury and improving the view during the procedure. As the intra-abdominal pressure increases with the pneumoperitoneum, the endotracheal tube allows positive-pressure ventilation at adequate pressures to avoid hypoxemia and to excrete the excess CO_2 absorbed. Pneumoperitoneum can cause unintended endobronchial intubation in patients with short tracheas when the carina moves cephalad. Placing the tube in the midtrachea in these patients and rechecking its position is suggested.

Anesthesia is typically maintained with a volatile agent, intravenous opioids, and muscle relaxants. Nitrous oxide is usually avoided during laparoscopic procedures because it increases bowel distension and the risk of postoperative nausea.

Clinical Caveats: Nitrous Oxide

Causes bowel distention during laparoscopic procedures
Increases postoperative nausea

During laparoscopic procedures the patient is often placed in the Trendelenburg or reverse Trendelenburg position. Nerve injuries to the patient should be avoided by securing and padding all extremities. In addition, airway pressures can increase with changes in positioning and ventilation often needs adjustment.

Two main goals during maintenance of patients for laparoscopic surgery under general anesthesia are preservation of normocapnia and treatment of hemodynamic derangements. Hypercapnia usually begins several minutes after insufflation of CO_2. To normalize the CO_2, the tidal volume and/or respiratory rate is increased, while peak airway pressures are kept at an acceptable level and end-tidal CO_2 is monitored. If hypercapnia

continues to worsen, in difficult cases the procedure may be converted to an open one. Stable hypercapnia is acceptable if end-tidal levels correlate with arterial CO_2.

Hemodynamic changes must be anticipated and managed during laparoscopic procedures. To ensure stability, augmenting the intravascular volume before insufflation avoids large decreases in preload. If the blood pressure increases, treatment options include deepening inhalational anesthesia and administering agents such as nitroprusside, esmolol, or calcium channel blockers. Treatment with alpha agonists such as clonidine or dexmedetomidine is another strategy. To minimize hemodynamic problems, the intra-abdominal pressure should be kept as low as feasible. Although healthy patients tolerate hemodynamic variations, patients with poor cardiac function can be adversely affected and may benefit from invasive monitoring (arterial line, central line, transesophageal echocardiography) during the procedure.

Drug Interactions

ALPHA AGONISTS
Reduction in minimum alveolar concentration (MAC) for inhaled anesthetics
Potential for bradycardia

NITROPRUSSIDE
Reflex tachycardia
Potential for cyanide toxicity

Postoperative Management

In the postanesthesia care unit, hypercapnia can persist for up to 45 minutes after the procedure is completed, imposing an extra ventilatory load on patients. Postoperative nausea and vomiting after laparoscopic procedures is affected by the type of procedure, residual pneumoperitoneum, and patient characteristics. Several agents alone or in combination to prevent or treat this complication include metoclopramide, ondansetron, and dexamethasone. To decrease the incidence of postoperative nausea and vomiting, minimize opioid doses and consider a propofol-based anesthetic. Because many laparoscopic procedures are planned on an outpatient basis, evaluation for discharge that day may also be needed.

The Laryngeal Mask Airway

Ventilation with the laryngeal mask airway for anesthesia during laparoscopic cases is controversial. Placement of a laryngeal mask airway is uncomplicated and atraumatic and provides an adequate airway in most patients. The concern is the potential for gastric distention, regurgitation, and pulmonary aspiration during positive-pressure ventilation in the presence of increased intra-abdominal pressure. However, in a study of patients who had laparoscopic cholecystectomy, gastric distention graded at the beginning and end of the procedure was not significantly different between patients managed with a laryngeal mask airway and those with endotracheal intubation.

Current Controversies: Laryngeal Mask Airway

The laryngeal mask airway can provide adequate ventilation without excess gastric distention but its use is not widespread during laparoscopic procedures.

Regional Anesthesia

Regional anesthesia is not used routinely for laparoscopic procedures because irritation to the diaphragm from CO_2 insufflation may cause shoulder pain. In addition, recovery times for complete return of function may be unacceptably prolonged for the ambulatory setting. With a low-dose lidocaine and opioid spinal technique, one study found that postoperative pain after gynecologic laparoscopy was less than with a comparable desflurane-based general anesthetic.

Pain Management

The analgesic requirement after laparoscopic procedures is generally less than after comparable open surgery. The modalities used for analgesia must treat pain that may be incisional, visceral, or a result of residual gas from pneumoperitoneum. Pain management begins before or during the surgical procedure. Administering intravenous opioids (fentanyl, morphine) in combination with intravenous nonsteroidal anti-inflammatory compounds helps to insure patient comfort at the end of the procedure. Infiltration of a local anesthetic such as bupivacaine at the port sites in the skin and peritoneum blocks somatic and visceral pain.

Postoperative analgesia is continued with intermittent intravenous opioids or oral pain medications. Certain patients may benefit from placement of an epidural catheter for postoperative pain management. Similarly, intrathecal opioids as a component of a spinal anesthetic technique can provide several hours of analgesia.

SPECIAL PATIENT POPULATIONS

Laparoscopic procedures are performed for pediatric patients, pregnant women, and the morbidly obese—patient populations that may present specific anesthetic challenges.

Morbidly Obese Patients

The morbidly obese may benefit from the laparoscopic approach for certain procedures. After a laparoscopic procedure, postoperative pulmonary function may be better, there is less risk of a wound infection with a smaller incision, and hospital stay may be shorter than after open surgery. Several studies have compared laparoscopic and open procedures in obese and nonobese individuals. Obese patients did just as well after laparoscopic colectomy as did their normal weight counterparts. In other studies, laparoscopic and open Roux-en-Y gastric bypass were found to be equally safe. Patients who had the laparoscopic procedure had less pain and returned to preoperative levels of pulmonary function more quickly than patients undergoing the analogous open procedure.

On the other hand, laparoscopic procedures pose specific risks in the morbidly obese. Ventilation of these patients is already difficult and oxygenation may be worsened with creation of pneumoperitoneum. Hypercapnia with an enlarged arterial to end-tidal CO_2 gradient during the procedure is also an issue.

Pregnant Patients

In the pregnant patient scheduled for laparoscopic surgery, the principal concerns are the impact on the fetus and the effect of pneumoperitoneum. Any pregnant patient who needs surgery is at risk of preterm labor; the incidence of this complication is greater in gravid patients who have undergone surgery than in those who have not. However, it is reassuring that in several series no difference in the rate of preterm labor or other significant fetal complications was found when patients who had laparoscopic procedures were compared with patients who had conventional open surgeries. Monitoring the fetal heart rate and uterine activity pre- and postoperatively is recommended.

Ventilation in the presence of pneumoperitoneum can be more difficult in the gravid patient, possibly leading to hypoxemia and hypercapnia, with the potential for fetal acidosis, distress, and death. Maintenance of the maternal end-tidal CO_2 within a normal range during the laparoscopic procedure should be sufficient to avoid fetal acidosis, because the correlation between end-tidal and arterial CO_2 is close. Placement of an arterial catheter and measuring maternal blood gases can be considered in selected cases. Finally, the gravid patient should be positioned carefully with uterine displacement to avoid hypotension from compression of the inferior vena cava, which can be compounded by the increased intra-abdominal pressures with pneumoperitoneum.

Pediatric Patients

Common laparoscopic procedures for pediatric patients include Nissen fundoplication, pyloromyotomy, appendectomy, and hernia repair. Advantages of the laparoscopic method in children have been demonstrated for laparoscopic appendectomy and hernia repair.

The impact of pneumoperitoneum in children is generally similar to that in adults. Vagal responses are greater during insufflation because of higher resting vagal tone. To lessen the impact, atropine premedication can be considered. Hypercapnia caused by CO_2 absorption is accentuated, requiring changes in minute ventilation to correct it. If the surgical site is amenable, caudal blockade can be successful for postoperative pain relief.

SUMMARY

Minimizing the intraoperative stresses imposed by pneumoperitoneum and reducing postoperative pain and nausea are major goals of anesthetic management for laparoscopic procedures. Patients benefit from these minimally invasive surgeries with reduced pulmonary complications, shorter hospital stays or same day discharge, and rapid return to their preoperative level of function.

Case Study

A 44-year-old woman is scheduled for laparoscopic Roux-en-Y gastric bypass. Her medical history is significant for sleep apnea managed with continuous positive airway pressure at night, hiatal hernia, and hypertension. She reports dyspnea after walking a short distance. On examination, the blood pressure and heart rate are 173/86 and 85 respectively; height is 5 ft 3 in and weight is 180 kg. Airway examination indicates a potentially difficult airway: Mallampati class 4; small oral

Case Study—cont'd

aperture; short, thick neck. Results of the cardio-pulmonary examination are normal. Preoperative medications include omeprazole, enalapril, and hydrochlorothiazide. Preoperative electrocardiogram reveals normal sinus rhythm with evidence of left ventricular hypertrophy.
- Discuss airway management plans for this patient.
- Are any further tests recommended before proceeding with surgery?
- What types of monitoring would be appropriate during the procedure?
- Discuss postoperative pain management options.

SUGGESTED READINGS

Bogdonoff DL, Schirmer B. Laparoscopic surgery. In: Stone DJ, Bogdonoff DL, Leisure GS, *et al.*, eds. Perioperative care: anesthesia, medicine, and surgery. St Louis: Mosby, 1998:547-558.

Huang JC, Shieh JP, Tang CS, *et al.* Low-dose dexamethasone effectively prevents postoperative nausea and vomiting after ambulatory laparoscopic surgery. *Can J Anesth* 2001;48:973-977.

Jones SB, Jones DB. Surgical aspects and future developments of laparoscopy. *Anesthesiol Clin North Am* 2001;19:107-124.

Joris JL. Anesthesia for laparoscopic surgery. In: Miller RD, ed. *Anesthesia*, 5th ed. Philadelphia: Churchill Livingstone, 2000:2003-2023.

Joris JL, Chiche JD, Canivet JL, *et al.* Hemodynamic changes induced by laparoscopy and their endocrine correlates: effects of clonidine. *J Am Coll Cardiol* 1998;32:1389-1396.

Joshi GP. Complications of laparoscopy. *Anesthesiol Clin North Am* 2001;19:89-105.

Lennox PH, Vaghadia H, Henderson C, *et al.* Small dose selective spinal anesthesia for short-duration laparoscopy: recovery characteristics compared with desflurane anesthesia. *Anesth Analg* 2002;94:346-350.

Maltby JR, Beriault MT, Watson NC, Fick GH. Gastric distension and ventilation during laparoscopic cholecystectomy: LMA-Classic vs. tracheal intubation. *Can J Anesth* 2000;47:622-626.

Pennant, JH. Anesthesia for laparoscopy in the pediatric patient. *Anesthesiol Clin North Am* 2001;19:69-88.

Smith, I. Anesthesia for laparoscopy with emphasis on outpatient laparoscopy. In: Anesthesia for minimally invasive surgery. *Anesthesiol Clin North Am* 2001:19:21-40.

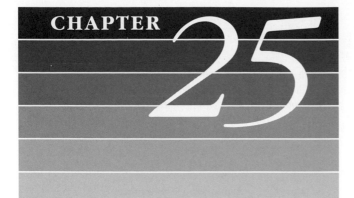

CHAPTER 25

Laser Surgery

KIANUSCH KIAI

INTRODUCTION

The development of the argon laser in 1959 opened the door to the many applications of laser medicine. Today there are many different types of laser used in all branches of medicine. In order to be able to give an effective and safe anesthetic, it is important for the anesthesiologist to understand what a laser is, how it functions, and how it affects the body. This chapter will review basic laser theory, discuss the different types of laser and their use in medicine, and consider the implications of anesthetizing a patient for a laser procedure.

BASIC LASER PHYSICS

The laser beam is an intense source of electromagnetic radiation that can be focused on a small area of interest, resulting in precisely controlled coagulation, an incision, or vaporization of tissue. In order to produce this high-intensity energy beam, a laser medium is necessary. The laser medium can be a solid, liquid or gas. The basic principle is that the atoms or molecules of the medium are excited to a higher energy level by absorption of energy. This absorption of energy causes electrons to move to a higher state of excitation and an unstable configuration. The excitation energy may be produced by the collision of the electrons of radiation energy, such as visible light, or produced by electrical excitation. Since the electrons of the atoms in the medium are now in a more unstable position, they will collapse to a lower, more stable energy position spontaneously; this process is called spontaneous emission. The energy released and the wavelength produced are determined by the specific characteristic of the atoms and thus the medium used.

The adjacent molecules and atoms may absorb this released energy. Those atoms that are already in a higher energy phase will be stimulated to release their energy. This process is called stimulated emission. The energy released is in phase with the incident energy and the two packets of energy combine to give amplification. This is *l*ight *a*mplification by *s*imulated *e*mission of *r*adiation, otherwise known as laser. The laser beam is then focused and directed to a specific site of interest (Figures 25-1 to 25-3).

Types of Laser

The type of laser is dependent on the medium used; this can be solid, liquid, or gas. The resulting beam will have different wavelengths and thus different energy on application. Although there are many different varieties of lasers in production, a limited number are used in medicine. Some commonly used laser types are listed in Table 25-1.

MEDICAL USES OF LASERS

Laser technology is used in many different areas of medical specialties, including:
- Cardiology
- Cardiothoracic surgery
- Dentistry
- Dermatology

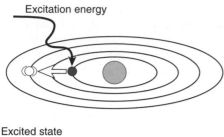

Figure 25-1   Excitation to a more unstable configuration.

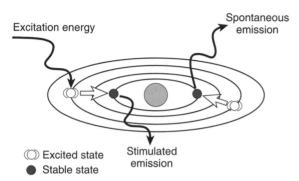

Figure 25-2   Spontaneous and stimulated emission of energy.

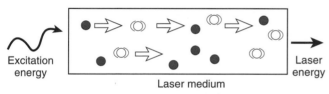

Figure 25-3   Production of laser beam.

- Gastroenterology
- Gynecology
- Neurosurgery
- Oncology
- Ophthalmology
- Orthopedics
- Otolaryngology and head and neck surgery
- Pulmonary Medicine
- Urology.

We will look at the specific uses of laser in these specialties and the anesthetic considerations for each. Many of the uses are quite straightforward from an anesthesiologist's perspective; however, there are a few that present significant challenges to the practice of anesthesiology.

Cardiology and Cardiothoracic Surgery

A substantial number of patients with coronary artery disease respond well to medical therapy. However, some patients need more invasive procedures such as angioplasty, stent placement, or a surgical procedure such as

Table 25-1	**Types of Laser, Their Wavelengths and Their Medical Uses**	
Wavelength	**Laser**	**Medical use**
Ultraviolet to blue		
125–350 nm	Eximer	Ophthalmology
	ArF, XeCl	Dermatology
488–514 nm	Argon	Ophthalmology
		Dermatology
		Cardiothoracic
		General surgery
Green to yellow		
510 nm	Copper vapor	Photodynamic therapy
514 nm	Argon	Ophthalmology
		Photodynamic therapy
532 nm	KTP-YAG	Gynecology
		General surgery
578 nm	Copper vapor	Dermatology
Red		
627.8 nm	Gold vapor	Photodynamic therapy
630 nm	Copper vapor	Photodynamic therapy
632.8 nm	Helium neon	Acupuncture
647 nm	Krypton	Ophthalmology
Infrared		
800–904 nm	Semiconductor	Physiotherapy
	GaAs	Sports injury
1,060 nm	Nd:YAG	Gynecology
		Ophthalmology
		Cardiothoracic surgery
		General surgery
		Gastroenterology
2,100 nm	Holmium YAG	Orthopedic
		Gynecology
		General surgery
10,600 nm	Carbon dioxide	Head and neck surgery
		Dermatology
		General surgery
		Gynecology

coronary artery bypass grafting. A few patients do not respond satisfactorily to either medical or surgical treatment. Typically, these patients have diffuse disease within their coronary circulation, which affects the distal part of the vessels. In these cases, there is an experimental procedure that is being attempted. The theory behind this procedure is direct perfusion of the myocardium through transmural perfusion. In other words, in areas of severe, reversible ischemia, the surgeon will make multiple small holes, using a laser, that allow blood from the heart to reach the ischemic area.

The patients are studied thoroughly by angiography as well as by nuclear perfusion study to determine the areas of ischemia. The procedure is usually carried out in the operating room under general anesthesia using a left anterolateral thoracotomy. Recent advances have made it possible to carry out this procedure using thoracoscopic techniques. The laser probe is placed on the predetermined area, over the surface of the left ventricle, and is activated when the ventricle is maximally distended with blood. The density of the laser channels within each of the ischemic zones is about one every 1.0 cm². Subsequent histological evaluation of these hearts show that the channels close postprocedure and thus direct perfusion is not likely. The current theory is that angiogenesis is the mechanism for symptomatic improvement. Other theories revolve around denervation as well as the placebo effect.

Anesthetic considerations for these cases are similar to most thoracotomy cases. A thoracic epidural may be of benefit for postoperative pain control. The procedure requires general anesthesia with a double lumen tube to isolate the left lung. This is necessary for the surgeon to have access to the left ventricle. An arterial line is a requirement. It is important to review the patient's pulmonary function preoperatively to determine if they can tolerate one lung ventilation. Good intravenous access and a central venous catheter are indicated, as there is a serious risk of rupture of the left ventricle. A pulmonary artery catheter may be indicated, dependent on myocardial function. Some practitioners use transesophageal echocardiography to evaluate the heart and the effectiveness of the laser treatment.

Ophthalmology

Ophthalmology was one of the first medical specialties to use laser technology, and currently ophthalmologists use the laser for treatment of almost all aspects of ocular pathology. This section will list the most common uses of laser in ophthalmology and its anesthetic implications.

Use of the laser in the treatment of cataracts is a recent development that is becoming more popular. Although the ultrasound phacoemulsification technique is still the most widely used, some ophthalmologists use the laser surgical technique, as they believe it is a safer surgical modality. Ultrasound phacoemulsification cataract surgery is an effective, safe procedure but it requires considerable skill and can result in injury to the cornea, iris, and posterior capsule. Laser-based surgery produces less heat and vibration and thus decreases the risk of injury to nearby structures. The discomfort is less and recovery is much quicker with the laser technique. There is also less chance of wound complication and astigmatism with this technique. The discomfort with this procedure is relatively small and the procedure can easily be completed with a topical anesthetic, thus decreasing anesthetic risks.

Recent developments have allowed the laser to be used to treat corneal disease. Laser technology can be used to remove opacities, scarring, and epithelial abnormalities in the cornea, or for reshaping the cornea to treat astigma-tism. The most common use for laser in corneal surgery is the LASIK (laser-assisted *in situ* keratomileusis) procedure for vision correction. This involves creating a hinged flap of the anterior corneal tissue, lifting the flap, performing a laser ablation upon the stromal bed, and repositioning the flap without sutures. The anesthetic considerations of LASIK are few. These cases can easily be performed under topical anesthesia or a retrobulbar block.

Proliferative retinopathies are caused by a variety of retinal vascular diseases. These diseases are usually due to retinal ischemia and neovascularization of the posterior segment. Neovascularization can cause blindness, hemorrhage, and macular and retinal detachment. There was no meaningful treatment for proliferative retinopathy until the advent of the laser. Laser surgery remains the safest and most effective treatment for these types of disorders. Laser has also been used for treatment of diabetic retinopathy, thus decreasing the vision loss previously so common with this disorder. Other retinal diseases treated with laser include retinal venous occlusions, choroidal neovascularization and other macular disease. In general these cases require general anesthesia, although some less involved cases can be performed with a retrobulbar block. The considerations for the anesthesiologist are those for general anesthesia and are patient-specific.

The laser is being used experimentally to treat intraocular tumors. As sole mode of treatment, the laser does not treat the tumor completely and complications are numerous and disabling. Presently this modality is of some help in conjunction with other treatments. From an anesthetic perspective these procedures require general anesthesia.

The anesthetic needs for ophthalmic laser surgery are identical to those of general ophthalmologic cases. There are no specific anesthetic concerns other that those of regional or general anesthesia.

Current Controversies

The use of laser for treatment of intraocular tumors, especially pigmented tumors, are at best controversial. There is increased risk of complication and vision loss and the cure rate is less than other treatments.

Dermatology and Plastic Surgery

Cutaneous laser techniques have become quite popular for skin disorders. This technology is quite versatile and has applications in both adult and pediatric patients in the operating room as well as office-based procedure rooms. The laser can be used to treat both congenital and acquired vascular lesions, and pigmented lesions or tattoos (Box 25-1).

Box 25-1   Common Skin Lesions Treatable by Laser

VASCULAR LESIONS

Congenital	**Acquired**
Hemangiomas	Telangiectasias
Port-wine stains	Cherry angiomas
Venous malformations	Pyogenic granulomas
Lymphangioma	Venous lakes
	Poikiloderma
	Kaposi's sarcoma

PIGMENTED LESIONS AND TATTOOS

Epidermal	**Dermal**	**Mixed**	**Tattoos**
Lentigines	Nevi of Ota or Ito	Postinflammatory pigment	Professional – organometallic dye
Ephelides	Melanocytic nevi	Melasma	Amateur – India ink
Café-au-lait macule	Blue nevi	Nevus spilus	Cosmetic – iron or titanium oxide
Becker's nevus			Traumatic – carbon, metals, dirt
			Medicinal – India ink

The laser has made revision of scars and striae much easier and more effective. The various categories of scars include:

- *Erythematous*: Pink to red in color, shiny, few skin markings, and flat
- *Pigmented*: Tan to brown in color, shiny, few markings, and flat
- *Hypertrophic*: White, pink or red in color, shiny, minimal skin markings, raised, and firm
- *Keloid*: Deep red or purple in color, shiny, minimal to no skin markings, raised, firm
- *Atrophic*: White to pink in color, shiny, wrinkled with few skin markings, indented, or pitted in morphology.

The most commonly performed cutaneous laser surgery is laser-assisted hair removal. This therapy offers a safe, effective, painless, and permanent way to eliminate unwanted hair.

Facial resurfacing with lasers has become a very common procedure, both as an office-based procedure and in an operating room. This procedure encompasses a wide spectrum of treatment needs. Some patients require only a small area treated, such as the eyelids or around the mouth; others require treatment throughout the face. Cutaneous laser surgery has also been very effective in treating disfiguring lesions in children.

All the above cutaneous laser treatments can vary from mildly unpleasant to significantly painful and uncomfortable, depending on the depth of treatment. Children in general do not tolerate laser treatments without anesthesia. Since the magnitude of discomfort is variable, the method of intraoperative analgesia and anesthesia is quite varied. For many adults and older children, the discomfort associated with the treatment is tolerable. Most treatments however do require some pain management. Topical cutaneous anesthesia can be provided using EMLA® cream, a mixture of lidocaine 2.5% and prilocaine 2.5%. The EMLA® cream needs to be applied to the area for at least 1 hour prior to surgery to be effective. This treatment is contraindicated in small infants, as prilocaine can lead to methemoglobinemia. The effectiveness of analgesia provided by the EMLA® cream is non-uniform for laser surgeries.

Local infiltration of the lesion and the area of treatment is also possible, depending on the size and the location of the lesion. Any of the short-acting local anesthetics such as lidocaine or procaine are good choices, since the duration of the treatment is short. As the treatment area becomes large, systemic toxicity of the local anesthetics can become important. Also, injection of large areas with local anesthetic can cause significant discomfort and thus is not well tolerated by the patient.

Intravenous sedation and analgesia may be necessary in patients with a high level of anxiety and discomfort. Short-acting medications such as fentanyl and midazolam are a good choice for most patients. Another excellent adjunct is a propofol infusion. This medication is short-acting and creates significant amnesia, which can be important during the procedure. With procedures on the face, one must be careful with deep levels of sedation that may require oxygen. Having oxygen near the laser increases the risk of fire.

Drug Interaction

In a high oxygen environment the laser can cause fire and thus injury to the patient

Most pediatric patients, adults with large areas to be treated, or areas that are very sensitive, require general anesthesia. If the area involved is on the face, general anesthesia with facemask is not recommended, again because of the risk of fire. General anesthesia using either a laryngeal mask airway or an endotracheal tube are the best options. The risks of anesthesia for these procedures are those of general anesthesia and thus are dependent on the patient's medical needs.

Head and Neck Surgery

Head and neck surgeons use the laser for minor cutaneous application to major procedures in the tracheobronchial tree. Application of the laser technology in head and neck surgery include:

- Cutaneous procedures
- Ossicular surgery
- Paranasal sinus surgery
- Surgery in the oral cavity
- Surgery in the pharynx
- Laryngeal surgery
- Surgery in the tracheobronchial tree
- Inner ear surgery.

Cutaneous applications of the laser by the head and neck surgeons are very similar to its use by dermatologists. These have been discussed above.

Lasers have been used in otology since the late 1970s. The applications in otology are varied and include:

- *Laser stapedectomy*: The laser is used to create a small fenestra in the stapes footplate
- *Malleus fixation*: There is usually a bony connection between the malleus and the attic; the laser is used to vaporize this connection
- *Middle ear scar and cholesteatoma*: Laser is used to vaporize any scarring or the cholesteatoma
- *Middle ear tumors*: Small tumors can be treated with the laser
- *Drum adherence to the malleus*
- *Ossicle and cartilage sculpting*.

Use of the laser in these procedures has been shown to decrease bleeding and injury to nearby structures. Laser procedures also decrease postoperative vertigo and the hospital stay. General anesthesia is needed for these procedures, as the surgeries can be very stimulating and uncomfortable. Other than intense stimulation for a relatively short period of time, there is no special anesthetic need for these procedures.

Laser technology, especially the different YAG lasers, is frequently used for endoscopic sinus surgery. The laser allows the surgeon to burn the lesion with good coagulation, and thus minimizes the risk of bleeding. Endoscopic sinus surgery requires a very straightforward general anesthetic, with intense stimulation for a relatively short period of time.

Laser surgery is also extensively used for surgeries involving the airway. The laser is used for both benign and malignant lesions of the mouth, nose, oral pharynx, nasal pharynx, larynx, and tracheobronchial tree. In the area of the nose and the mouth, the laser allows for quick excision of the lesion with excellent hemostasis. The use of the laser in the pharynx has allowed many of these surgeries to be office-based, with less pain and discomfort for the patient. This technology allows quick and easy treatment of benign masses in the oral cavity with good hemostasis and much less discomfort and scarring.

Uvulopalatopharyngoplasty is a treatment for obstructive sleep apnea and snoring. The laser can be used to resect and ablate the soft tissue of the uvula and the soft palate. Laser-assisted tonsillectomy is being performed more frequently. This procedure ablates the tonsillar crypts and grossly reduces the tonsillar tissue. This removes the reservoirs and foci of infection and thus reduces chronic inflammation of the area. The use of laser for these procedures decreases bleeding, edema, and postoperative discomfort.

Laser technology has proved to be very valuable in microlaryngeal surgery. Its applications are numerous both in adult and pediatric populations. The laser can be used for excision of nodules, polyps, and cysts. The superiority of laser over other microsurgical techniques is especially noted for vascular lesions. The hemostasis achieved by the use of the laser allows for a faster and more precise procedure. The laser can be used to treat laryngeal stenosis and is also beneficial for the excision of granulation tissue from the larynx and cervical trachea, and excision of benign neoplasia such as recurrent respiratory papillomatosis.

For laser cases involving the pharynx and larynx a small endotracheal tube that is out of the way of the surgeon is used. The anesthesiologist must use the smallest-diameter endotracheal tube that can safely be used for that patient. The MLT-tube (microlaryngeal tube) is beneficial in these cases. These endotracheal tubes have a small external diameter with a large cuff to protect the airway.

The biggest challenge of surgery involving the airway arises when the surgeon uses laser in the field. Regardless of the type of laser used, there is risk of fire in the airway. For laser procedures in the airway, especially when the surgical field is in close proximity to the endotracheal tube, a laser tube is essential. All endotracheal tubes are made from a silicon-based material and thus can ignite and burn. A laser tube is a regular endotracheal tube wrapped with a nonflammable, metal covering which protects it from the heat of the laser. The balloon cuff of the endotracheal tube is the only exposed part of the tube that is flammable. Laser endotracheal tubes have been designed with two balloon cuffs. It is recommended that the balloons are inflated with a known quantity of saline or water. This is a safeguard against the laser igniting the cuff. If a fire does occur the liquid inside the cuff should put out the fire and the second cuff is still intact to protect the airway.

Laser treatment of lesions of the tracheobronchial tree is common. Surgeons treat neoplasms, tracheal stenosis, and vascular lesions. Planning of anesthesia for laser procedures in the airway is more involved and more concerning. Many of the procedures can be performed under sedation and injection of local anesthetic. The main concern when this technique is used is to provide enough sedation to allow the surgeon to operate and the patient to remain comfortable without compromising the safety of the patient and loss of the airway. Most cases, however, require general anesthesia. For cases involving the oral cavity, it is best to intubate through the nares or to find a small tube that can be positioned away from the surgical field. Since the anesthesiologist is sharing the airway with the surgeon, and for most of the procedure the airway is away from the anesthesiologist, it is important to safely secure the endotracheal tube. This may involve having the surgeon suture the tube to the gums.

Drug Interaction

In a high oxygen environment the laser can cause fire and thus injury to the patient

Nitrous oxide can support a fire just like oxygen and thus is contraindicated when using the laser

---

When surgery involves a laser in the proximity of the airway, the anesthesiologist must use the lowest inspired concentration of oxygen that is safe for the patient and as close to room air as possible. Nitrous oxide should be avoided. Both oxygen and nitrous oxide can support a fire. In case of an airway fire, the anesthesiologist must act quickly, stop ventilation and remove the oxygen source. Extubate the trachea – this is to remove the burning endotracheal tube and to avoid inhalational injury. Flood the mouth with normal saline and suction all the liquid and the debris from the airway. Ventilate the patient by mask and reintubate the trachea. Ventilate with air until all the fire is out, then ventilate with 100% oxygen. Examine the airway for injury with a fiberoptic scope.

Some laser procedures require free surgical access to the trachea and thus intubation is not possible. The anesthesiologist has few options in these cases. All have the potential risk of fire and the practitioner must be ready for such an event.

- The first option is to have the patient under deep anesthesia with spontaneous ventilation. Intravenous anesthetics can be used or anesthetic gases can be connected to the surgical bronchoscope and thus delivered to the patient.

- The second option is intermittent ventilation and apnea, where the surgeon operates and then stops, and allows the anesthesiologist to ventilate the patient before commencing with surgery. A risk with this technique is that it requires high F_iO_2 in order to allow the surgeon enough time to operate in between ventilations. The high oxygen environment increases the risk of airway fire substantially.

- The third option, the one most commonly used by thoracic surgeons, is jet ventilation. This allows continuous ventilation while the surgeon is operating. The jet ventilator connects to the side of the bronchoscope and provides high frequency bursts of gas that travel to the alveoli and provide gas exchange. Obese patients or patients with chronic obstructive pulmonary disease may not tolerate jet ventilation. Also, patients with chronic obstructive pulmonary disease may be at risk of developing a pneumothorax.

As a final reminder, the use of a laser in the airway with high oxygen and/or nitrous oxide concentration is dangerous and airway fires are a real threat. The anesthesiologist must be diligent and prepared to deal with the fire in case it occurs.

Clinical Caveats: Airway Fire

Turn off the ventilator

Extubate the trachea

Flood the mouth with normal saline

Suction all liquid and debris from airway

When the fire is out, ventilate the patient with 100% oxygen

Reintubate the trachea

Examine the airway for injury

Examine pharynx, larynx and the tracheobronchial tree using a fiberoptic scope

---

Other Areas of Medicine

Laser technology is used by many other surgical subspecialties and new roles are found every day for this versatile instrument.

- Orthopedic surgeons use the laser extensively in joint surgery, especially arthroscopy.

- General surgery uses the laser in laparoscopic surgery. The laser can easily be directed to a focal area through remote control, without the need for a large incision.

- Urology and gynecology depend on the laser to perform their less invasive surgery. Gynecologists frequently use the laser for excision of hyperplasia and excisional biopsies. Urologists use the laser for bladder and urethral lesions such as hyperplasia, small tumors, or stone disease. The use of the laser for transurethral resection of the prostate is also becoming more popular.

- The laser is also used by gastroenterologists for ablation of small lesions at the time of endoscopy.

The anesthetic needs for the above procedures are similar to those for similar procedures without the use of a laser. For less invasive and less sensitive procedures, such as excisional biopsies, local anesthesia can be used. More invasive procedures require general anesthesia. There are no special considerations for use of the laser in these applications.

SUMMARY

In medicine today, laser technology is used widely. In many surgical specialties, lasers are a basic technology and frequently used. Other fields of surgery and medicine find new uses for this technology every day. Lasers are versatile and safe in trained hands and allow for concise treatment of the medical problem.

Anesthesiologists must also understand this technology. They must understand the needs and the potential problems of lasers in order to make sure that the patient is safe. This chapter reviewed the common uses of laser in medicine as well as the new areas of medicine into which it is being introduced. We have also shown the potential anesthetic issues and what may be important for the anesthesiologist to consider. Physicians involved, including anesthesiologists, must keep up with the advances in order to continue a safe practice.

SUGGESTED READING

Aaberge L, Aakhus S, Nordstrand K, *et al*. Myocardial performance after transmyocardial revascularization with CO_2 laser: a dobutamine stress echocardiographic study. *Eur J Echocardiogr* 2001;2:187-196.

Blomquist S, Algotsson L, Karlsson S. Anaesthesia for resection of tumours in the trachea and central bronchi using the Nd-YAG-laser technique. *Acta Anaesthesiol Scand* 1990;34:506-510.

Clarke S, Schofield P. Laser revascularisation. *Br Med Bull* 2001; 59:249-259.

Cohen M, Steiner M. Local anesthesia techniques. *World J Urol* 2000;18(Suppl. 1):S18-S21.

Diethrich E. Classical and endovascular surgery: indications and outcomes. *Surg Today - Jpn J Surg* 1994;24:949-956.

Epstein R, Halmi B, Lask G. Anesthesia for cutaneous laser therapy. *Clin Dermatol* 1995;13:21-24.

Friedberg B. Facial laser resurfacing with the propofol-ketamine technique: room air, spontaneous ventilation (RASV) anesthesia. *Dermatolic Surg* 1999;25:569-572.

Hermens J, Bennett M, Hirshman C. Anesthesia for laser surgery. *Anesth Analg* 1983;62:218-229.

Kattner M, Clark G. Recurrent respiratory papillomatosis. *Nurse Anesth* 1993;4:28-35.

Keon T. Anesthetic considerations for laser surgery. *Int Anesthesiol Clin* 1988;26:50-53.

Keon T. Anesthetic management during laser surgery. *Int Anesthesiol Clin* 1992;30:99-107.

Ossoff R. Laser safety in otolaryngology - head and neck surgery: anesthetic and educational considerations for laryngeal surgery. *Laryngoscope* 1989;99:1-26.

Ossoff R, Reinisch L, eds. Laser applications in otolaryngology. *Otolaryngol Clin North Am* 1996;29.

Padfield A, Stamp J. Anaesthesia for laser surgery. *Eur J Anaesthesiol* 1992;9:353-366.

Paes M. General anaesthesia for carbon dioxide laser surgery within the airway. *Br J Anaesth* 1987;59:1610-1620.

Parsons D, Lockett J, Martin T. Pediatric endoscopy: anesthesia and surgical techniques. *Am J Otolaryngol* 1992;13:271-283.

Rabinowitz L, Esterly N. Anesthesia and/or sedation for pulsed laser therapy. *Pediatr Dermatol* 1992;9:132-153.

Shikowitz M, Abramson A, Liberatore L. Endolaryngeal jet ventilation: a 10-year review. *Laryngoscope* 1991;101:455-461.

Sosis M. Anesthesia for laser surgery. *Int Anesthesiol Clin* 1990;28:119-131.

CHAPTER 26

Drug Interactions in Anesthetic Practice

DAVID M. SIBELL

JEFFREY R. KIRSCH

INTRODUCTION

Anesthesiologists require a comprehensive knowledge of pharmacology. In order to care appropriately for a wide variety of patients in the critical perioperative period, the intensive care unit, and the acute and chronic pain settings, anesthesiologists must be especially sensitive to pharmacological interactions. These interactions may take several forms, principally physicochemical, pharmacokinetic, synergistic, and additive.

It would be impractical to attempt to list all possible interactions in one short practice-oriented chapter, as entire textbooks have been written on this subject. However, by understanding principles behind the most relevant interactions, an anesthesiologist can anticipate and avoid the problematic interactions, and take advantage of the most beneficial interactions.

PHYSICOCHEMICAL INTERACTIONS

In physicochemical interactions, the physical properties (e.g., acid–base compatibility, contact between drugs, and anesthesia machine components) of medication combinations predispose them to precipitation or other chemical reactions. Although these are not the most common interactions, they are particularly relevant to anesthesiologists, because several of the drugs used by anesthesiologists are prone to such interactions.

Sodium thiopental is an alkaline solution (pH 10–11). It will precipitate with several acidic anesthetic medications, including lidocaine (pH 3.3–5.5) and acidic solutions of steroid nucleus muscle relaxants, such as pancuronium or rocuronium (pH 3.8–4.2). Therefore, any instances of coadministration of these medications must account for this: if they share a port or injection tubing, the areas must be flushed between injections to avoid combination of the drugs. Failure to observe this precaution can result in precipitation in the intravenous tubing. This can at least cause loss of the intravenous site (particularly problematic during induction of anesthesia in small children) and, in theory, crystal embolism.

An additional set of physicochemical interactions includes two important chemical reactions between volatile anesthetic agents and carbon dioxide absorption material in the anesthetic circuit. Traditional CO_2 absorbing material is strongly basic in nature and acts to remove a proton from anesthetic molecules, which then hastens chemical breakdown of these agents. Under low-flow conditions, sevoflurane interacts with CO_2 absorbers (e.g., soda lime, Baralyme®), to form compound A. The production of this potentially toxic substance was initially reported in the early 1990s but has been reviewed recently. Compound A is nephrotoxic in animal models but humans may be less susceptible to this toxicity under most clinical conditions. The majority of reports of nephrotoxicity due to compound A in humans have demonstrated only transient increases in laboratory indicators of kidney dysfunction.

Desflurane may also interact with CO_2 absorbers, causing elevated concentrations of carbon monoxide in the inspiratory limb of the anesthesia circuit. This is most likely to result in clinically significant concentrations of CO when the CO_2 absorber is desiccated, as may be the case on a Monday morning after high flows of oxygen have been maintained through an unused circuit over a weekend. Baralyme® is also more likely to cause CO accumulation than are other absorbers. Enflurane, no longer used in the United States, also produces CO under similar conditions, but CO levels are highest with desflurane. Rehydrating the desiccated absorbent prior to use can prevent this chemical reaction.

PHARMACOKINETIC INTERACTIONS

The more common interactions are pharmacokinetic in nature, in which metabolic effects of one drug alter the biotransformation of another. These interactions principally entail one of two categories: enzymatic induction and inhibition.

Enzymatic induction refers to the process of one compound causing increased *de novo* synthesis of a catabolic enzyme, causing enhanced biotransformation of another compound. This increase in catabolism causes a reduction in pharmacodynamic activity of the affected compound.

Inhibition may be caused by one of four potential mechanisms:

- Competition between multiple parent compounds for biotransformation
- Formation of a metabolite intermediate compound that, although catalytically inactive, reduces the availability of the enzyme to the parent compound
- Mechanism-based, or "suicide" inhibition, in which the metabolite of a parent compound diminishes activity of the enzyme catabolizing it
- Depletion of cofactors.

Several common medications cause induction of cytochrome P450 enzymes. Others compete for biotransformation at these sites. In the last three decades, this class of enzymes has been further divided into subtypes. Many current antidepressant medications interact at this enzyme, as does tramadol (an oral analgesic). Patients who mix these medications may experience serious adverse effects, including seizures, ventricular tachyarrhythmias, and the serotonin syndrome (characterized by the sudden onset of mental status changes, autonomic instability, and neuromuscular changes such as myoclonus, hyperreflexia, rigidity, and trismus). Since these medications are common in patients being treated for pain and chronic diseases, anesthesiologists must be aware of this potential hazard.

Additionally, protein binding can cause pharmacokinetic interactions. For instance, chronic phenytoin induces an increase in plasma levels of alpha-1-acid glycoprotein. The increased alpha-1-acid glycoprotein binds with several medications, including nondepolarizing muscle relaxants, decreasing their free levels in the bloodstream. This is just one of the several mechanisms that contribute to a reduced duration of action for nondepolarizing muscle relaxants in patients who receive anticonvulsants on a chronic basis.

ADDITIVE AND SYNERGISTIC INTERACTIONS

The most classic additive drug interactions relevant to anesthesiology result from MAC (minimum alveolar anesthetic concentration) reduction studies. In these studies, administration of analgesic and/or sedative medications results in reduced requirement for volatile anesthetic agents. Opioids have an additive interaction with volatile agents, as evidenced by these experiments. Although volatile anesthetic medications have additive interactions with each other, this is largely irrelevant to modern clinical practice: current anesthesia machines are designed to prevent mixing of volatile anesthetics

Of note, while they do not reduce MAC, monoamine oxidase inhibitors (MAOIs) may interact with vasoactive agents such as ephedrine to cause hypertensive crisis. The mechanism for this interaction relates to the ability of MAOIs to increase presynaptic accumulation of catecholamines and the fact that ephedrine increases blood pressure indirectly by release of presynaptic vesicles. These combinations interact further with volatile agents, especially halothane, to increase susceptibility to ventricular tachyarrhythmias. Additionally, meperidine, still in moderate use despite numerous interactions and adverse metabolic and central nervous system effects, interacts with MAOIs and catecholamines, which can cause a potentially lethal hypertensive crisis.

Nondepolarizing muscle relaxants have synergistic interactions with each other. The greatest synergy is seen with combinations between benzylisoquinolone and steroid nucleus drugs, with less synergistic or additive effects within these classes. Although both groups of muscle relaxants affect the nicotinic receptor, their slightly different site of action on the receptor accounts for the synergist response to coadministration. Historically, these interactions have been exploited to reduce cost by combining two older, generic drugs instead of using a single, more expensive drug. These combinations are not used frequently in contemporary practice, as there are safety considerations due to their prolonged duration of action compared with modern, short-acting agents.

There are important safety concerns regarding the interaction between opioids and other medications with sedative properties. Generally speaking, these reactions are synergistic, and although these interactions can be beneficial, they can also result in unacceptable sedation and respiratory depression.

Opioids interact with one another at the receptor level, with both additive and synergistic results. For instance, the L enantiomer of methadone is synergistic with morphine and morphine metabolites but is additive with fentanyl and oxycodone. Midazolam and fentanyl, a common mixture used in sedation, react synergistically, and can be a common cause of potentially serious respiratory depression.

Two more short-acting medications share a rather different interaction. In the presence of clinically significant propofol blood levels, remifentanil's volume of distribution and distribution clearance is reduced by 41%, and its elimination clearance is reduced by 15%. However, given the rapid metabolism of both substances, the clinically significant aspect of the interaction is only relevant during the bolus dosing. There is a clinically insignificant concentration difference during maintenance phase and only a negligible difference on recovery profiles.

Certain antiemetic medications have synergy for respiratory depression with opioids. For example, promethazine has independent effects on respiratory mechanics and when it is coadministered with opioids these effects are enhanced synergistically. Droperidol has been implicated in respiratory depression, especially in association with neuraxial opioids. This risk of synergy for respiratory depression is enhanced in patients with respiratory disease, sleep apnea, or at extremes of age.

SPECIAL CONSIDERATIONS IN ACUTE AND CHRONIC PAIN TREATMENT

In the setting of acute postoperative pain, many interactions are possible; but not all are problematic. In fact, most acute pain management specialists advocate multimodal analgesia for optimization of pain control while minimizing adverse effects from larger doses of single medications. Although not studied during all perioperative conditions, both acetaminophen and non steroidal anti-inflammatory drugs (NSAIDs) have been found to have opioid-sparing effects (approximately 20–30%). While no studies have defined the exact mechanism for the dose reduction caused by coadministration of NSAIDs and acetaminophen with opioids, there remains a rationale for opioid dose reduction in this manner. Neuraxial medications represent a special case. The nature of neuraxial opioid interactions is similar to those with systemic opioids. However, since neuraxial administration of opioids, especially more hydrophilic opioids, can cause significant elevations in cerebrospinal fluid levels, these patients are more predisposed to both acute and delayed respiratory depression.

The most common epidurally administered synergistic combination is an opioid and a local anesthetic. Combining these two classes allows the use of lower doses of each individual drug than would be appropriate if it were used as a single agent. This improves analgesia, and spares adverse effects.

Additionally, neuraxially administered local anesthetic and clonidine can each cause hypotension, especially in the presence of other causes of hypotension, such as hypovolemia. However, clonidine has additive analgesic and antihyperalgesic effects that make it attractive to use, via the neuraxial route, in combination with opioids and/or local anesthetics in the management of pain.

For patients taking medications to treat chronic pain, the situation can be more complicated. These patients may be taking high doses of opioids, antidepressant combinations, and anticonvulsants. While documentation of specific interactions in these cases is rare, the risks certainly increase with polypharmacy. Furthermore, patients with high preoperative pain ratings are predisposed to higher postoperative pain ratings, as are patients with preoperative emotional distress. Therefore, patients with chronic pain generally require more involved pain treatment in the acute setting, and higher doses of medication.

Fortunately, patients taking chronic opioids have a relatively high tolerance for the dose-related adverse effects of opioids, predominantly sedation and respiratory depression. While these patients generally tolerate higher doses of opioids than opioid naïve patients, they still require adequate monitoring for these adverse events. This is especially true for coadministration of sedating medications with opioids.

COMPLEMENTARY AND ALTERNATIVE MEDICINE

Approximately half of adults surveyed in the United States, Western Europe, and Australia have used at least one type of complementary or alternative medicine. Therefore, in contemporary anesthetic practice, vigilance includes awareness of interactions between frequently used herbal remedies and dietary supplements with conventional anesthetic agents and operative conditions. A complete review of all possible interactions goes beyond the scope of this chapter. However, there are several commonly used herbal agents and dietary supplements that can affect anesthetic outcome and medication choices significantly.

The most commonly used herbal agents and dietary supplements in the United States are, in order, ginkgo, St John's wort, ginseng, garlic, echinacea, saw palmetto, and kava. Several of these have significant drug–drug interactions, or associated coagulation or hemodynamic effects. The vigilant anesthesiologist must remember that patients will often not think of these dietary supplements as medications, and will therefore not include them on medication lists. It is therefore incumbent on the anesthesiologist to inquire the patient directly regarding the use of herbal agents.

Table 26-1 Common Drug Interactions Relative to Anesthetic Practice

	Cisatracurium	Cyclosporine	Droperidol	Fentanyl	Isoflurane	Lidocaine	Meperidine	Midazolam	Mivacurium	Morphine	Pancuronium	Quinidine	Rocuronium	SSRI	St Johns wort	TCA	Thiopental	Tramadol
Cisatracurium					A/S				A		S	S	S					
Cyclosporine				I			I	I		I		S			E			
Droperidol				S			S	S		S						A		
Fentanyl		I	S		A		A	S		A								A
Isoflurane	A/S			A		A	A	A	A/S	A	A/S		A/S					A
Lidocaine					A													
Meperidine		I	S	A	A					A				I		A	A	A
Midazolam		I	S	S	A									I				A
Mivacurium	A				A/S						S	S	S		I			
Morphine		I	S	A	A		A											A
Pancuronium	S				A/S				S				A				P	
Quinidine	S	S							S							I		
Rocuronium	S				A/S				S		A						P	
SSRI							I	I								I		I
St John's wort		E							I									
TCA			A				A					I		I				I
Thiopental							A				P		P					I
Tramadol				A	A		A	A		A				I		I	I	

A, additive; E, enzymatic induction; I, inhibited catabolism; P, physiochemical; S, synergistic; SSRI, selective seratonin reuptake inhibitors; TCA, tricyclic antidepressants.

Several herbal agents are used as anticoagulants, and have pharmacological activity on either the coagulation cascade (e.g., garlic) or platelet activity (e.g., ginkgo). These can cause spontaneous hemorrhages, and can also interact with other anticoagulants to exacerbate anticoagulated states. There are also concerns involving regional anesthetic techniques in these patients. At this time, however, the American Society of Regional Anesthesia and Pain Medicine's consensus guidelines do not recommend altering regional anesthetic plans based on herbal therapy.

St John's wort is taken for a variety of mood symptoms, most commonly depression. This is significant, as the compound has an effect similar to MAOIs. In addition, St John's wort may cause the serotonin syndrome in patients also taking selective serotonin reuptake inhibitors (SSRIs), and can also cause hypertension in the perioperative period, similar to an MAOI. St John's wort also has many interactions based on its induction of P-glycoprotein. This reduces blood levels of warfarin, cyclosporin, and digoxin, among other drugs. This has been associated with acute rejection in the perioperative period for organ transplant patients.

However, while there are numerous case reports and retrospective articles addressing concerns about these interactions, to date, there has been no systemic, prospective study of the incidence of serious adverse effects in the perioperative period attributed to this compound. This has not prevented some authors from advising a 2-week period of abstinence prior to experiencing general anesthesia, as has been advised regarding MAOIs. More current opinions have retreated from this position, as the pharmacological activity appears to be insignificant compared with that of MAOIs.

The last area of major concern to anesthesiologists in regards to complementary and alternative medicine is the vasoactive nature of several of these agents. Aside from the effect that enzymatic induction has on certain vasoactive agents the patient may be taking ginkgo as a peripheral vasodilator. Despite this, there are case reports of paradoxical hypertension related to ginkgo use.

With any of these agents, the perioperative physician must understand that there is no meaningful Food and Drug Administration study of the pharmacological properties of the agents. With the passage of the Dietary Supplement Health and Education Act of 1994, these agents are listed as dietary supplements, not medications. Neither the dosage of the active ingredients nor the presence of additives and/or contaminants is documented rigorously.

CONCLUSION

Even the most adept and studious clinician can find it impossible to list or memorize all the potential drug–drug interactions that may be seen in anesthetic practice. Rather, as some of the older medications, with their concurrent interactions (e.g., halothane and epinephrine) phase out, entire new sets of interactions emerge. Some of the more common or important interactions are listed in Table 26-1, but this is merely a sample of what could possibly occur in the complicated perioperative pharmacological milieu. Therefore, in the name of patient safety, it is insufficient for the practicing anesthesiologist to understand only the common interactions. It is incumbent on the anesthesiologist to understand the basic principles of such interactions and to keep a vigilant eye out for new possibilities.

SUGGESTED READING

Ang-Lee MK, Moss J, Yuan CS. Herbal medicines and perioperative care. JAMA 2001;286:208–216.

Bailey PL, Pace NL, Ashburn MA, et al. Frequent hypoxemia and apnea after sedation with midazolam and fentanyl. Anesthesiology 1990;73:826–830.

Bolan EA, Tallarida RJ, Pasternak GW. Synergy between μ opioid ligands: evidence for functional interactions among μ opioid receptor subtypes. J Pharmacol Exp Ther 2002;303:557–562.

Bouillon T, Bruhn J, Radu-Radulescu L, et al. Non-steady state analysis of the pharmacokinetic interaction between propofol and remifentanil. Anesthesiology 2002;97:1350–1362.

Cohen SE, Rothblatt AJ, Albright GA. Early respiratory depression with epidural narcotic and intravenous droperidol. Anesthesiology 1983;59:559–560.

De Leon-Casasola OA, Myers DP, Donaparthi S, et al. A comparison of postoperative epidural analgesia between patients with chronic cancer taking high doses of oral opioids versus opioid-naive patients. Anesth Analg 1993;76:302–307.

Fang ZX, Eger EI, Laster MJ, et al. Carbon monoxide production from degradation of desflurane, enflurane, isoflurane, halothane, and sevoflurane by soda lime and Baralyme®. Anesth Analg 1995;801:1187–1193.

Freund PR, Bowdle TA, Posner KL, et al. Cost-effective reduction of neuromuscular-blocking drug expenditures. Anesthesiology 1997;87:1044–1049.

Gentz BA, Malan TP. Renal toxicity with sevoflurane: a storm in a teacup? Drugs 2001;61:2155–2162.

Jamison RN, Taft K, O'Hara JP, Ferrante FM. Psychosocial and pharmacologic predictors of satisfaction with intravenous patient-controlled analgesia. Anesth Analg 1993;77:121–125.

Kim KS, Chun YS, Con SU, Suh JK. Neuromuscular interaction between cisatracurium and mivacurium, atracurium, vecuronium, or rocuronium administered in combination. Anaesthesia 1998;53:872–878.

Liu SS, Carpenter RL, Mackey DC, et al. Effects of perioperative analgesic technique on rate of recovery after colon surgery. Anesthesiology 1995;83:757–765.

Nemeroff CB, DeVane CL, Pollock BG. Newer antidepressants and the cytochrome P450 system. Am J Psychiatry 1996;153:311–320.

Sedation

SARA ARNOLD

DANIEL J. COLE

JEFFREY R. KIRSCH

Monitored anesthesia care (MAC) usually refers to the use of intravenous agents for sedation and/or analgesia by an anesthetist (an anesthesiologist or certified registered nurse anesthetist), concurrently with local anesthetics by the surgeon to allow comfort and safety for a variety of surgical, diagnostic and endoscopic procedures. When a nurse, without specific anesthesia training, provides this care it is usually referred to as "sedation and analgesia". Occasionally, MAC refers to the provision of the expertise of an anesthetist to monitor the patient who has a particularly complex medical condition and no intravenous medications are given. The relatively loose use of the term MAC creates a great deal of confusion for the surgeons, nurses without anesthesia training, and third-party payers.

INTRODUCTION

The term "conscious sedation" was coined by Bennett to describe the use of intravenous drugs to produce a minimally depressed level of consciousness with maintenance of the patient's protective airway reflexes.

It is now recognized that sedation exists along a continuum with subtle differences between lighter and deeper levels. The principle objectives of sedation are to relieve anxiety, promote cooperation, produce a degree of amnesia, and maintain consciousness and patency of the airway. Painful procedures require the concomitant use of sedation and analgesia. When providing sedation, the potential for general anesthesia always exists. Vigilant monitoring of the patient's vital signs by appropriately trained personnel, appropriate facilities, and equipment for resuscitation are therefore necessary for the safe provision of sedation (Table 27-1 and Box 27-1).

PATIENT SELECTION

Preoperative evaluation includes both the physical and emotional needs of the patient. Risks of complications arising from sedation and the procedure must be individually evaluated. Extreme anxiety, a history of failed sedation, confusion, mental illness, and extremes of age may warrant modification of plans for sedation or even cause the anesthetist to choose to use general anesthesia in an otherwise acceptable situation. A thorough history and physical examination should be performed and documented. Sleep apnea, morbid obesity, pregnancy, gastroesophageal reflux; severely compromising respiratory disease, known difficult endotracheal intubation, or airway examination suggestive of a difficult intubation may indicate that sedation without airway protection would place the patient at an unacceptable risk for aspiration or loss of airway.

Nil-by-mouth guidelines are the same for sedation as general anesthesia: 2 hours for clear liquids, 6 hours

Table 27-1   Continuum of Depth of Sedation

	Minimal Sedation (Anxiolysis)	Moderate Sedation/Analgesia (Conscious Sedation)	Deep Sedation/Analgesia	General Anesthesia
Responsiveness	Normal response to verbal stimulation	Purposeful response to verbal or tactile stimulation	Purposeful response after repeated or painful stimulation	Unarousable, even with painful stimulus
Airway	Unaffected	No intervention required	Intervention may be required	Intervention often required
Spontaneous ventilation	Unaffected	Adequate	May be inadequate	Frequently inadequate
Cardiovascular function	Unaffected	Usually maintained	Usually maintained	May be impaired

Box 27-1   Definitions

LIGHT SEDATION (ANXIOLYSIS)

A drug-induced state with a minimally depressed level of consciousness that retains the patient's ability to maintain a patent airway independently and continuously and to respond appropriately to physical stimulation or verbal command.

MODERATE SEDATION/ANALGESIA (CONSCIOUS SEDATION)

A drug-induced depression of consciousness in which patients respond purposefully to verbal commands, either alone or accompanied by light tactile stimulation. No interventions are required to maintain a patent airway, and spontaneous ventilation is adequate. Cardiovascular function is usually maintained.

DEEP SEDATION/ANALGESIA

A controlled drug-induced state of depressed consciousness or unconsciousness from which the patient is not easily aroused, and which may be accompanied by a partial or complete loss of protective reflexes, including the ability to maintain a patent airway independently and to respond purposefully to physical stimulation or verbal command. Cardiovascular function is usually maintained.

GENERAL ANESTHESIA

Composed of three components: hypnosis, analgesia, and muscle relaxation. Awareness is obliterated, movement does not occur with incision, and sympathoadrenal responses to surgical stimulation are blunted or eliminated

NEUROLEPSIS

A state characterized by quiescence, reduced motor activity, reduced anxiety, and indifference to surroundings.

DISSOCIATIVE STATE

Characterized by sedation, catalepsy (maintenance of muscle tone), amnesia, and analgesia.

for solids and nonclear liquids. Adequacy of intravenous access should be insured. Renal and hepatic function should be reviewed to assist with drug selection and dosing. Concurrent medications and current pain level should be reviewed. Known medical allergies should be reviewed. History and evidence for cardiovascular disease may suggest the need for more invasive monitoring. The type of surgery, its expected duration and positioning, idiosyncrasies, and the speed of the surgeon may have great impact on the success and safety of sedation. A thorough PARQ (procedure, alternatives, risks, questions) conference is mandatory and discussion should include the possibility of general anesthesia and airway control. Good communication prior to and during the sedation can go a long way towards the goal – anxiolysis, sedation, and cooperation with the procedure.

DRUGS

DPT Cocktail

The DPT (Demerol, Phenergan, Thorazine) cocktail is an older form of intramuscular sedation that is primarily indicated for children. Although most children would rather not receive a needlestick, this technique can be useful in children over 1 year of age. This cocktail typically consists of meperidine (Demerol, 2 mg/kg), promethazine (Phenergan, 1 mg/kg), and chlorpromazine (Thorazine, 1 mg/kg). With many contemporary alternatives available, this cocktail is not recommended by the American Academy of Pediatrics because of its narrow therapeutic index. Promethazine and chlorpromazine are very long-acting drugs and produce profound sedation and analgesia at the time of the procedure and sedation and respiratory depression for several hours afterwards. Chlorpromazine can induce seizures in those with an underlying seizure focus.

Clinical Caveat: Narrow Therapeutic Index

DPT is rarely used because it has a narrow therapeutic index and may cause apnea at sedative doses, may cause prolonged sedation, and there are no specific reversal agents available.

Barbiturates

By enhancing the inhibitory tone of gamma-amino butyric acid (GABA), barbiturates depress impulse transmission within the central nervous system (CNS). They may produce various levels of mood alteration from excitation to mild sedation, hypnosis, or coma. They do not provide analgesia. They are widely distributed to all tissues and body fluids and are metabolized within the liver. These drugs are potent inducers of hepatic microsomal enzymes.

Clinical Caveat: Narrow Therapeutic Index

Barbiturates have a narrow therapeutic index and may cause apnea at sedative doses. The anesthetist should be prepared to manage the patient's airway and support respiratory function with mechanical ventilation. In general, other sedatives are preferred for procedure-related sedation.

Potential adverse reactions include: hypotension, CNS alterations (prolonged sedation, paradoxical restlessness and agitation), enhanced depressant effects when combined with other CNS depressants, acute intermittent porphyria, and nausea/vomiting. Drug interactions include increased metabolism of warfarin, phenytoin, phenylbutazone, prednisone, hydrocortisone, and digoxin. Barbiturate metabolism is inhibited by concomitant use of valproic acid or chloramphenicol. Contraindications to the use of barbiturates include: hypersensitivity to barbiturates, porphyria, severe hepatic dysfunction, and severe pulmonary disease.

Phenobarbital

Phenobarbital is a long-acting barbiturate that may be dosed orally (1–2 mg/kg) but has an hour-long onset and duration of 6–12 hours. Intramuscular doses (1–2 mg/kg) have onset in minutes and last 4–10 hours. Intravenous dosing is the same as intramuscular.

Pentobarbital

Pentobarbital is a medium-duration barbiturate (0.5–4 hr). Oral and rectal doses (<4 years 3–6 mg/kg; >4 years 1.5–3 mg/kg to max 100 mg) have onset in 15–60 minutes and last 1–4 hours. Intravenous doses have onset in 1 minute and last more than 30 minutes.

Thiopental

Thiopental is dosed intravenously only, has a 1-minute onset, and has a short duration of action (2–10 min).

Methohexital

Methohexital may be dosed per rectum with a 10–30-minute onset of action, lasting 1–3 hours; or by the intravenous route with a 1-minute onset and 5–6-minute duration of action.

Benzodiazepines

Classed as sedative hypnotics, benzodiazepines bind to specific receptors to facilitate neurotransmission at GABA synapses – the inhibitory system in the brain – depressing excitable neurons. Depending on the dose and drug employed, administration gives rise to CNS depression, which leads to sedation in larger doses, respiratory depression and induction of general anesthesia. Benzodiazepines have anticonvulsant properties and cause amnesia. In sedative doses a small reduction in tidal volume occurs, which is compensated by an increased respiratory rate; in larger doses effects vary from a small decrease in minute volume to apnea. Effects on the cardiovascular system include a small decrease is systemic blood pressure secondary to a decrease in systemic vascular resistance.

Benzodiazepines are mainly metabolized by the liver. Their use in patients with hepatic failure may lead to prolonged sedation and coma. An enhanced and prolonged sedative effect may also occur in patients treated with antidepressants, antipsychotics, antihistamines, alpha-blockers, and opioid analgesics. Dosing for the elderly should be selected with caution because of their increased sensitivity to these drugs and their altered ability to metabolize them to nonactive products.

Diazepam

Diazepam was the first benzodiazepine to be used for sedation. It has a duration of action of 3–4 hours, but it has active metabolites with a duration of action of 21–37 hours. It has a high incidence of venous irritation and resultant phlebitis and thrombosis. Attempts to reduce the irritation by formulating diazepam in a lipid emulsion have had limited success in decreasing the pain of injection. Its use for sedation has been limited since the advent of midazolam.

Midazolam

Midazolam has a half-life of 2–4 hours but without active metabolites. It is water-soluble and does not cause venous irritation. The usual adult dose is 0.5–2.5 mg – up to 5 mg – titrated over several minutes to the desired effect: somnolence and anxiolysis. The pediatric dose is 0.25–1.0 mg/kg to a maximum of 20 mg orally (or per rectum), or 0.1–0.15 mg/kg intramuscularly. Intravenous pediatric dosing is: initial dose 0.025–0.05 mg/kg then titrated to a maximum of 0.4 mg/kg.

Paradoxical excitement may occur, more frequently in adolescent children and the elderly. Midazolam is also known to occasionally precipitate hostility and violence instead of tranquility. In a review of patients receiving midazolam for intraoperative sedation and control of restlessness, the incidence of paradoxical events is approximately 10%. The paradoxical event usually occurs within minutes and is fully reversed by flumazenil, within 30 seconds of administration.

Midazolam has been found to be somewhat unreliable for sedation in young children. In one study intravenous doses as high as 0.6 mg/kg were found to be unreliable in achieving sleep in children before general anesthesia. In another study only 50% of children treated with rectally administered midazolam for computed tomography were sedate enough to complete the study.

Midazolam may be administered by a variety of different routes. The intravenous route is reliable and effective. However, this route may not be practical for use in children preoperatively, since sedation is frequently required prior to placement of an intravenous catheter. The intramuscular route is somewhat less predictable than the intravenous route and is associated with pain at the site of injection. However, in an emergency, an intramuscular injection may provide a necessary means to the initiation of sedation. In addition, use of a Bioject® air-injector, appears to be associated with less injection pain when used to administer small volumes of drug (1 mL or less). Oral administration of midazolam, although requiring an increased dosage and 15–30 minutes for onset of action, is effective for the cooperative patient. However, the bitter taste of midazolam is difficult to mask with reasonable volumes of different-favored solutions. It is common for anesthesiologists to mix midazolam with flavored liquid acetaminophen in order to take advantage of both the analgesic and flavor properties of this secondary agent. Nasal administration is possible but usually causes a burning sensation in the nasal mucosa and is, therefore, less commonly used as a route for midazolam administration.

Opioids

Opioids provide analgesic and sedative effects via agonist activity at specific opioid receptors within the nervous system. They all also have direct inhibitor effects on cardiovascular and respiratory control centers in the brain, causing bradycardia and a decrease in respiratory rate. Individual opioids may also cause hypotension and reflex tachycardia related to their tendency to cause histamine release. Analgesia is associated with binding at mu receptors and sedation with binding at kappa receptors.

Morphine

Morphine acts on the brain by interfering with the transmission and interpretation of pain impulses. It also causes CNS depression, which leads to drowsiness and sedation. It has a depressant action on the medullary respiratory center, causing a reduced sensitivity to a rise in partial pressure of carbon dioxide in blood. Patients who become apneic secondary to this mechanism will often breathe on command but not spontaneously. Mild hypotension secondary to decreased systemic vascular resistance may occur related to histamine release. Morphine affects the gastrointestinal system via delayed gastric emptying and prolonged transit time through the colon. It also causes increased pressure in the biliary ducts, resulting in decreased flow and production of bile. Therefore, morphine should not be used in patients undergoing biliary procedures or in those with biliary colic. When used for sedation, the usual adult dose of morphine is 2–5 mg intravenously over 5 minutes which may be repeated at 5-minute intervals to a maximum of about 20 mg. It has an onset of 2–5 minutes, a peak analgesic activity and respiratory depression in 20 minutes, and a duration of 4–5 hours. The delay in onset of analgesia and respiratory depression, relatively long half-life, and histamine release limit its use for routine sedation.

Fentanyl

Fentanyl is a synthetic opioid 80–100 times as potent as morphine. It has an onset time of 1–2 minutes and duration of action of 30–60 minutes. It has high lipid solubility, so it readily crosses the blood–brain barrier, allowing its rapid time of onset. The usual adult dose for sedation is 25–50 μg intravenous. over 2 minutes, which may be repeated at 3–5-minute intervals. Fentanyl can also be administered via the transmucosal route (e.g., fentanyl lollipop). Chest-wall rigidity has been reported with rapid administration of fentanyl.

Sufentanil

Sufentanil is a highly selective mu receptor agonist that is 10–15 times more potent than fentanyl. Its effects resemble those of fentanyl, but because of its mu receptor selectivity its respiratory depression may be more profound. Clearance is rapid via hepatic metabolism. Obesity may increase the volume of distribution and prolong the half-life of sufentanil.

Alfentanil

Alfentanil is a mu receptor agonist one-tenth as potent as fentanyl. Because it crosses to the brain very rapidly (about 1 min compared with about 6 min for fentanyl) it has a rapid onset of action. Redistribution is also rapid and extensive, leading to a short duration of action after a single bolus. A single dose of 500–1000 μg can allow the placement of a retrobulbar block for eye surgery. It may be administered as a continuous infusion.

Remifentanil

Remifentanil is a mu receptor agonist that is ultra-short-acting because of its hydrolysis by blood and tissue esterases. It appears to have decreased clearance and increased potency in the elderly. Because of the short duration of action, patients may experience significant pain once the infusion is stopped. The dose used for sedation and analgesia is 0.01–0.5 μg/kg/min intravenously. When combined with propofol or a benzodiazepine the dose requirement is decreased by approximately 50%. A single dose of up to 1 μg/kg may be given 90 seconds before retrobulbar block.

Meperidine

Meperidine has an onset time of 1–5 minutes and a duration of action of 2–3 hours. An active metabolite, normeperidine (renal excretion), has a long half-life and, with accumulation, has caused seizure. Therefore, administration of meperidine is contraindicated in patients with a history of seizures or renal failure. Meperidine administration is also associated with tachycardia (histamine and direct effect) and should therefore be used with caution in patients with ischemic heart disease. The usual adult dose is 25–50 mg intravenously over 1–2 minutes. Common routes of administration are intravenous, intramuscular injection, transmucosal (lollipop), and intranasal.

Clinical Caveat: Benzodiazepine + Opioid – Synergy of Action

When administered together, a significantly decreased dose of both drugs is required for sedation and analgesia

Incidence of side effects such as hypotension and respiratory depression is increased

---

Other Agents

Propofol

Propofol, 2,6-diisopropylphenol, is insoluble in water, so is prepared in an egg–lecithin emulsion. It is associated with pain on injection that may be minimized by a prior dose of 1% lidocaine or using larger veins for injection. It is rapidly cleared by hepatic and possibly lung metabolism. The recommended infusion rate for hypnosis is 100–200 μg/kg/min and for sedation is 25–75 μg/kg/min. Propofol may produce a subjective feeling of euphoria. There is a dose-dependent depression of ventilation. Cardiovascular effects include decreased vascular resistance (arterial and venous dilation) and direct myocardial depressant effects, which appear to be more pronounced in the elderly. Beneficial side effects include antiemetic properties and antipruritic properties.

An area of controversy is the use of propofol infusion for prolonged periods, for instance for patients in the intensive care unit. There have been many case reports documenting the development of metabolic acidosis, rhabdomyolysis, and cardiovascular collapse in pediatric patients sedated in the intensive care unit. Sometimes called the "propofol infusion syndrome," this set of clinical features, which may include hyperkalemia, hepatomegaly, lipemia, with metabolic acidosis, myocardial failure, and rhabdomyolysis, has also been reported in critically ill adults. Current recommendations include avoidance of propofol for sedation in pediatric intensive care unit patients and limiting the total dose and duration of infusion in critically ill adults.

Ketamine

Ketamine, D1-2-(O-chlorophenyl)-2-(methyl–amino)-cyclohexanone is classed as a dissociative anesthetic. It produces analgesia and amnesia via binding sites on the N-methyl-D-aspartate (NMDA) receptor. Analgesic effects may be obtained with injection of 0.1–0.5 mg/kg intravenously or an intravenous infusion of 4 μg/kg/min. Ketamine is extensively metabolized in the liver to norketamine, which may accumulate. It is associated with psychomimetic reactions, which may be minimized by pretreatment with a benzodiazepine. Ketamine can activate epileptogenic foci. It stimulates the sympathetic nervous system and may increase heart rate, blood pressure and pulmonary artery pressure.

Ketamine has a direct inhibitory effect on the myocardium that is minimized in patients with normal sympathetic tone because of its effect on the sympathetic nervous system. However, profound hypotension may occur following ketamine administration in patients who have endured prolonged stress (e.g., critically ill patients) where there is inadequate concurrent sympathetic reserve. Ketamine does not usually depress ventilation and has bronchodilating properties, but tends to increase oral secretions and may be associated with laryngospasm.

Ketamine is a popular sedative for children, especially for procedures such as laceration repair and fracture reduction in the emergency department. Delivered by intravenous or intramuscular injection it is generally considered highly effective, with a wide margin of safety.

Its use in this setting is sometimes associated with airway complications, emesis, and recovery agitation. A review of children given intramuscular ketamine for emergency room procedures found the incidence of transient airway complications to be 1.4% (airway malalignment 7/1022, laryngospasm 4/1022, apnea 2/1022, and respiratory depression 1/1022). Emesis occurred in 6.7% without evidence of aspiration. Mild recovery agitation occurred in 17.6%, while moderate to severe agitation occurred in 1.6%. In this study acceptable sedation was achieved in 98%.

In addition, a large review of children sedated with ketamine at a major university emergency department sought predictors for adverse outcomes. It found no univariate associations with airway complications. Emesis was associated with younger age (3.5% in children less than 5 years, 1% in children older than 5 years). Recovery agitation was associated with the presence of underlying medical condition (17.9% in ASA class 1 and 33.3% in ASA class 2 or greater) and inversely correlated with increasing age (22.5% for children less than 5 years, 12.1% for children 5 years or older).

Etomidate

Etomidate, (R)-(+)-ethyl-1-(1-phenylethyl)-1H-imidazole-5-carboxylate, is a nonbarbiturate hypnotic. It is thought to work at the GABA receptor to produce hypnosis without analgesia. It is frequently used as an agent for induction of general anesthesia. It is sometimes used in smaller doses (0.10–0.20 mg/kg) as a sedative for brief procedures (e.g., emergency room procedures, cardioversion). It can provide effective, deep sedation with little hemodynamic compromise. There is risk of respiratory depression, especially in older individuals and with higher cumulative doses.

The use of etomidate infusion for prolonged sedation has been associated with adrenal suppression, low levels of cortisol, and increased mortality. Even small doses, such as those given for induction of anesthesia, have resulted in inhibition of adrenal steroidogenesis. Therefore, it is recommended that physicians should not use etomidate for prolonged sedation and should consider treating selected patients with corticosteroids if etomidate is used.

Nitrous Oxide

Isolated in 1772, this gas was introduced for use for dental extractions in 1844. Since this time it has enjoyed varying degrees of favor as an adjunct anesthetic (it lacks the potency necessary for a full anesthetic) and sedative agent. Currently it is used in a 50:50 mixture with oxygen as an inhaled sedative for painful procedures such as venous cannulation, lumbar puncture, bone marrow aspirations and dressing changes. Used in these circumstances there are minimal side effects and a short recovery time.

Sevoflurane

An anesthetic gas first used in 1971, sevoflurane can be used for inhalational sedation in a manner similar to nitrous oxide because it is less noxious than the other flurane anesthetic gasses. When used as a 1% concentration in patients undergoing dental extraction, investigators have shown an equivalent acceptance with nitrous oxide.

Dexmetomidine

Dexmetomidine is a potent, selective alpha-2 agonist with sedative, anxiolytic, and analgesic properties. It was recently approved for sedation of critically ill patients. Activation of alpha-2 adrenoreceptors in the CNS, present in large concentrations in key arousal centers such as the locus ceruleus, decreases centrally mediated sympathetic activity and induces sedation. Sedation with dexmetomidine infusion can offer hemodynamic stability with minimal effects on respiratory and cognitive function. A suggested dosing regimen for the intubated intensive care unit patient is: loading dose of 1.0 μg/kg over 10 minutes then a maintenance infusion of 0.2–0.7 μg/kg/hr, intravenously. Decreased cardiac output and heart rate occur with larger doses of dexmetomidine and decreases in both regional and global cerebral blood flow have been described.

Chloral Hydrate

Chloral hydrate is a sedative hypnotic agent used widely for pediatric sedation. Studies have shown it to be a more reliable sedative than midazolam for young children. It may be administered by a variety of routes including oral, rectal, and intravenous, although dosing becomes unreliable via the rectal route after age 3 years. Cardiac rhythm abnormalities have been noted during chloral hydrate sedation but a study of the efficacy and safety of chloral hydrate sedation in children undergoing echocardiography observed no clinically significant hemodynamic changes and a 6% incidence of vomiting. Repetitive dosing and the use of chloral hydrate for long-term sedation has been questioned because of possible accumulation of trichloroethanol, which is a metabolite with a half life between 9 and 40 hours.

Toxicity from chloral hydrate overdose, primarily documented in adults, includes liver disease and gastric irritation as well as cardiac irritability and central nervous depression. The CNS toxicities of chloral hydrate are worsened by coadministration of benzodiazepines, barbiturates and ethanol. Deaths due to chloral hydrate overdose have been documented in adults, usually after more than 10 g has been ingested; the cause of death is usually resistant cardiac arrhythmia. There is also potential carcinogenicity associated with chloral hydrate use. The evidence for carcinogenicity of chloral hydrate is from large doses given to rodents and the clinical relevance is questionable.

Clinical Caveat: Prepare for Escalation of Care

The possibility of respiratory depression, loss of protective airway reflexes, and hemodynamic instability mandates the availability of counteractive drugs and equipment in any area where sedation and analgesia are provided
Drugs: Flumazenil, naloxone, oxygen, resuscitation drugs
Equipment: Suction, airway equipment, intravenous therapy supplies, Trendelenburg capability, external defibrillator, telephone
A plan for increased intensity of care

Reversal Agents

Flumazenil

Flumazenil is the specific reversal agent for benzodiazepines, released for use by the Food and Drug Administration in 1991. It competitively inhibits the binding of benzodiazepines, resulting in a rapid and effective reversal of the sedation with a partial reversal of the respiratory depression. The initial adult dose is 0.2 mg intravenously over 15 seconds and may be repeated at 1 minute intervals to a maximum of 1 mg. It should not be used in patients with elevated intracranial pressure or people with epilepsy on benzodiazepine therapy. Adverse effects include: dizziness, agitation, hypertension, arrhythmias, and seizures. The duration of action of flumazenil, 45–90 minutes, may be shorter than the duration of action of the benzodiazepine. Therefore the patient must be monitored for re-sedation and potentially re-dosed with flumazenil.

Naloxone

Naloxone is the specific reversal agent for the opioids via opioid receptor antagonism. It causes partial to complete reversal of the respiratory depression, sedation, and hypotension caused by opioids. The dose must be titrated carefully to avoid the sudden return of severe pain. Adverse effects include tachyarrhythmias, hypertension and noncardiogenic pulmonary edema. The usual adult dose is 40 μg intravenous repeated every 2–3 minutes until the desired effects are achieved. The duration of action of naloxone, 30–90 minutes, may be shorter than the duration of action of the opioid. Therefore, the patient must be monitored and potentially re-dosed. A continuous intravenous infusion of 0.05–0.10 μg/kg/min can be titrated in patients to maintain the desired level of consciousness.

Physostigmine

Physostigmine is a tertiary amine anticholinesterase that crosses the blood–brain barrier and acts to increase levels of acetylcholine. It can be used to treat postoperative delirium and agitation associated with anticholinergic administration (atropine or scopolamine toxicity). It may also reverse prolonged postoperative somnolence associated with diazepam and droperidol or any of a number of drugs that cross the blood–brain barrier and have antimuscarinic activity (antihistamines, tricyclic antidepressants, tranquilizers). The central anticholinergic syndrome presents as dry mouth, blurred vision and mydriasis, hot dry skin, and fever. Mental symptoms range from sedation to coma or anxiety, restlessness, and delirium. If lethal poisoning has occurred, convulsions and ventilatory arrest may ensue. Physostigmine should be given slowly in 1 mg doses, not exceeding 3 mg in a 70 kg adult to avoid producing peripheral cholinergic activity.

MONITORING

Most adverse effects can be detected early if appropriate monitoring is employed, and prompt action can be taken. Several working groups have presented recommendations for the use of sedation in various environments such as endoscopy and radiology. Most agree on the basic necessary monitoring.

The emergency equipment required for sedation and analgesia is listed in Box 27-2.

Level of Sedation

There are risks to both over-sedation and inadequate sedation. The over-sedated patient is at risk of respiratory and cardiovascular depression, loss of airway, and aspiration. The inadequately sedated patient is at risk of agitation, sympathetic activation, and failure to comply with the procedure. A variety of methods have been employed to evaluate and measure the level of sedation, basically of two types: observation and mechanical. The Wilson Sedation Scale (Table 27-2) is an example of observation-based evaluation of level of sedation.

Advantages of this type of evaluation include sensitivity during lower levels of sedation and an absence of a mechanical device. Disadvantages include the need to disturb the patient during the procedure and observer subjectivity.

The alternative methods for level of sedation evaluation include mechanical devices such as the BIS (bispectral index) monitor, auditory evoked potentials, and power spectral measure. These devices have the potential advantage of objectivity but currently lack sensitivity during lower levels of sedation.

Box 27-2 Emergency Equipment for Sedation and Analgesia

INTRAVENOUS ACCESS EQUIPMENT

Gloves, tourniquets, alcohol wipes, sterile gauze pads, intravenous catheters, intravenous tubing, intravenous fluid, assorted needles, syringes, and tape

BASIC AIRWAY MANAGEMENT EQUIPMENT

Source of compressed oxygen (tank with regulator or pipeline supply with flow meter), source of suction, suction catheters, Yankauer-type suction, face masks, self-inflating breathing bag-valve set, oral and nasal airways, lubricant

ADVANCED AIRWAY MANAGEMENT EQUIPMENT

Laryngeal mask airways, laryngoscope handles and blades, endotracheal tubes, stylet

PHARMACOLOGIC ANTAGONISTS

Naloxone and flumazenil

EMERGENCY MEDICATIONS

Epinephrine, ephedrine, vasopressin, atropine, nitroglycerine, amiodarone, lidocaine, glucose (50%), diphenhydramine, hydrocortisone, methylprednisolone or dexamethasone, diazepam or midazolam
From ASA Task Force. Practice guidelines for sedation and analgesia by non-anesthesiologists. *Anesthesiology* 2002;96:1004-1017.

Ventilation

Monitoring of pulmonary function by observation or auscultation can help detect drug-induced ventilatory depression and airway obstruction. When the patient must be physically separated from the observer, exhaled carbon dioxide monitoring can be employed.

Table 27-2 Wilson Sedation Scale

Score	Description
1	Fully awake and oriented
2	Drowsy
3	Eyes closed but rousable to command
4	Eyes closed but rousable to mild physical stimulation (earlobe tug)
5	Eyes closed but unarousable to mild physical stimulation

From Wilson E, David A, Mackenzie N, Grant IS. Sedation during spinal anesthesia: comparison of propofol and midazolam. *Br J Anaesth* 1990;64:48-52.

Oxygenation

Blood oxygen saturation may be monitored using pulse oximetry with appropriate alarms.

Hemodynamic

Early detection of changes in the patient's heart rate and blood pressure may enable the practitioner to detect problems and intervene in a timely fashion. Noninvasive blood pressure measurements at 3-5-minute intervals and continuous electrocardiographic monitoring are usually appropriate.

RECOVERY

Pulse, blood pressure, respirations, level of consciousness, and oxygen saturation should be monitored and recorded every 15 minutes until recovery is complete. Recovery is complete when the patient is awake and oriented. There should be discharge criteria protocols in place. These usually include the following

- The patient is alert and oriented
- Observations have been stable for at least 30 minutes
- The patient is able to walk without dizziness
- The patient can take oral fluids
- Nausea is absent
- A responsible adult will escort the patient home
- Verbal and written instructions have been given to the patient and escort (because of the amnestic effects of sedation).

There should be a mechanism in place for the need for extended monitoring or medical care, including airway support/ventilation.

SUMMARY

Sedation is the art of providing anxiolysis and pain relief when necessary, and promoting patient comfort and cooperation with medical interventions. When providing sedation it is important to realize that sedation exists along a continuum that can end with loss of the protective airway reflexes. Sedation providers should be trained to manage the airway and all aspects of resuscitation. Appropriate monitors should be used to detect problems early and plans should be in place for escalation of care. It is important to know the pharmacology of the available sedation and reversal medications and their interactions when combined (Table 27-3). The sedation plan should be tailored to the individual patient and procedure and include the flexibility to adapt to the changing level of stimulation during the intervention.

Table 27-3 Summary of Drug Dosing Guidelines for Procedure-Related Sedation and Analgesia

Medication	Adult Dose	Pediatric Dose	Onset (min)	Duration (hr)	Adverse Reactions	Warnings*
Sedatives						
Phenobarbital	1–2 mg/kg	1–2 mg/kg	IV: 5–10; IM: minutes; PO:hours	IV: 4–10; IM: 4–10; PO: 6–12	RD, hypotension, drug interactions	Avoid in patients with porphyria
Pentobarbital (Nembutal)	IV: 2–3 mg/kg IM: 2–6 mg/kg	IV: 1–3 mg/kg, max 100 mg PO/PR: 2–6 mg/kg, max 100 mg	IV: 1–2; IM:10–15; PO/PR: 15–60	IV: 30+ min; IM: 1–4; PO/PR: 1–4	RD, hypotension, drug interactions	Avoid in patients with porphyria
Thiopental (Pentothal)	IV: 0.5–2 mg/kg	IV: 0.5–2 mg/kg	IV: 1	2–10 min	RD, hypotension, drug interactions	Avoid in patients with porphyria
Methohexital (Brevital)	IV: 1–2 mg/kg	IV: 1–2 mg/kg PR: 15–30 mg/kg	IV: 1; PR: 10–30	IV: 5–6 min; PR: 1–3	RD, hypotension, drug interactions	Avoid in patients with porphyria
Chloral hydrate	PO: 500–1000 mg	PO/PR: 50–100 mg/kg (max 2 g)	30–60	4–8	RD	
Midazolam (Versed)	IV: 0.05–0.1 mg/kg IM: 0.05–0.1 mg/kg	IV: <6 months 0.01–0.02 mg/kg; 6 months–5 yr 0.05–0.1 mg/kg 6–12 yr 0.025–0.05 mg/kg IM: 0.1–0.15 mg/kg Nasal: 0.3–0.7 mg/kg PO/PR: 0.2–0.5 mg/kg	IV: 1–2; IM:5–15; Nasal: 8–12;PO/PR:15–20	IV: 1–2; IM:1–6; Nasal/ PO/PR: 30–45 min	RD	
Lorazepam (Ativan)	IV/IM: 0.02–0.05 mg/kg PO: 0.02–0.05 mg/kg	IV/IM: 0.02–0.05 mg/kg PO: 0.02–0.05 mg/kg	IV: 1–2; IM: 5–15; PO: 15–20	IV: 6–8; IM:10–20; PO: 10–20	RD	
Diazepam (Valium)	IV: 0.1–0.2 mg/kg PO: 0.2–0.3 mg/kg	IV: 0.1–0.2 mg/kg PO: 0.2–0.3 mg/kg	IV: 1–4; PO: 20–60	IV: 2–4; PO: 1–2	RD	
Nonopiate Analgesics						
Ketorolac (Toradol)	IV/IM: 30–60 mg load, 1/2 load q 6 hr PO: 10 mg	Not recommended	IV: 5; IM: 5–10; PO: 20–40	IV: 4–6; IM: 4–6; PO: 4–6	Abnormal hemostasis, gastrointestinal discomfort	Avoid in hypovolemic patients

Agent	Dose	Dose	Onset (min)	Duration (hr)	Side Effects	Comments
Opiate Analgesics						
Morphine	IV: 0.1–0.2 mg/kg IM/SQ: 0.1–0.2 mg/kg	IV: 0.1–0.2 mg/kg IM/SQ:0.1–0.2 mg/kg	IV: 5–10; IM/SQ: 15–40	IV: 2–4; IM/SQ: 2–4	RD	Enhanced effect with sedatives
Fentanyl (Sublimaze)	IV/IM: 50–100 µg	IV: 1 µg/kg,then 0.5 µg/kg q 5 min PO: 5–15 µg/kg	IV: 1–2; IM:7–15; PO: 5–15	IV: 30–90 min; IM: 1–2; PO: 60–90 min	RD, chest rigidity	Enhanced effect with sedatives
Alfentanil (Alfenta)	IV: 10–15 µg/kg	IV: 5–25 µg/kg	IV: 1–2	IV: 15–30 min	RD, chest rigidity	Enhanced effect with sedatives
Meperidine (Demerol)	IV: 1–1.5 mg/kg SQ: 1–2 mg/kg IM:0.5–2 mg/kg	IV: 0.5 mg/kg SQ: 0.5 mg/kg IM: 0.5 mg/kg	IV: 5–10; SQ: 40–60; IM: 20–40	IV: 2–3; SQ: 2–4; IM: 2–3	RD, elliptogenic metabolite	Enhanced effect with sedatives, do not give to patients on MAOIs
Methadone (Dolophine)	IV: 0.1–0.2 mg/kg PO: 0.1–0.2 mg/kg	IV: 0.1 mg/kg PO: 0.1 mg/kg	IV: 1–2 PO: 30–60	IV: 6–8 PO: 6–8	RD	Enhanced effect with sedatives
Other						
Ketamine (Ketalar)	Not recommended	IV: 1.0–1.5 mg/kg IM: 2–5 mg/kg	IV: 1; IM: 5	IV: 1–2; IM: 1–2	Emergence delirium, tachycardia, salivation	
Nitrous oxide	20–50%	20–50%	Immediate	3–5 min	Inhibits methionine synthase	Avoid in patients with closed air spaces
Propofol (Diprivan)	IV: 100–150 µg/kg/min load, followed by 25–75 µg/kg/min	IV: 100–150 µg/kg/min load, followed by 25–75 µg/kg/min	IV: 1	IV: 2–10 min	Pain at injection site	Intralipid allergy
Diphenhydramine (Benadryl)	IV: 25–100 mg PO: 25–100 mg	IV: 1 mg/kg; PO: 1 mg/kg	IV: 3–5; PO: 1–2 hr	IV: 4–8 hr; PO: 4–8 hr	Dry mouth, urinary retention	
Reversal Agents						
Naloxone (Narcan)	IV/IM/SQ/trach: 0.01 mg/kg, q 2 min (max 2 mg)	IV/IM/SQ/tracheal: 0.01 mg/kg, q 2 min (max 2 mg)	IV: 1–2; IM/SQ/ trach:2–5	IV: 20–60 min; IM/SQ/ trach: 20–60 min	Pulmonary edema, opioid withdrawal	
Flumazenil (Romazicon)	IV: 0.2 mg q 1 min (max 1 mg)	IV: 0.1 mg/kg (max 0.2 mg) q 1 min (max 1 mg)	IV:1–5	IV: 20–60 min	Benzodiazepine withdrawal	Avoid in patients on benzodiazepines

*Alterations in dosing may be indicated based on the clinical situation and the practitioner's clinical experience with these agents. Individual agent dosages may vary when used in combination with other agents, especially when benzodiazepines are combined with narcotics. RD, respiratory depression; IV, intravenous; IM, intramuscular; PO, by mouth; PR, per rectum; min, minutes; hr, hours.

SUGGESTED READING

American Society of Anesthesiologists. Practice guidelines for sedation and analgesia by non-anesthesiologists. *Anesthesiology* 2002;96:1004–1017.

Hashimoto T, Gupta DK, Young WL. Interventional neuroradiology-anesthetic considerations. *Anesthesiol Clin North Am* 2002;20:347–359.

Ibrahim EH, Kollef MH. Using protocols to improve the outcomes of mechanically ventilated patients. Focus on weaning and sedation. *Crit Care Clin* 2001;17:989–1001.

Izurieta R, Rabatin JT. Sedation during mechanical ventilation: a systematic review. *Crit Care Med* 2002;30:2644–2648.

Jackson DL, Johnson BS. Inhalational and enteral conscious sedation for the adult dental patient. *Dent Clin North Am* 2002;46:781–802.

Kaplan RF, Yang CI. Sedation and analgesia in pediatric patients for procedures outside of the operating room. *Anesthesiol Clin North Am* 2002;20:181–194.

Maze M, Scarfini C, Cavaliere F. New agents for sedation in the intensive care unit. *Crit Care Clin* 2001;17: 881–897.

Webb MD, Moore PA. Sedation for pediatric dental patients. *Dent Clin North Am* 2002;46:781–802.

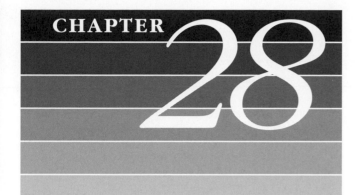

Geriatrics

RONALD W. PAULDINE

INTRODUCTION

The life expectancy of the population in Western countries is increasing. This fact, in combination with advances in surgical and anesthetic techniques, is resulting in an increasing number of geriatric patients presenting for elective and emergency surgery. Currently 14% of those living in Western nations are over the age of 65. This number is growing, such that by 2030 it has been estimated that 20% of the population of the United States will be over 65. Considering that currently one-third of all surgical procedures are performed on older adults, it is no surprise that there is an increasing emphasis on the care of the geriatric surgical patient. This chapter will briefly review age-related alterations in physiology most frequently affecting anesthetic care, the impact of age-related disease, pharmacological considerations in aging, and current controversies in perioperative management.

THEORIES OF AGING

The progressive decline in an organism's internal condition leads to an increased risk of death. This process represents changes that occur in increasing magnitude with advancing age and are present in all individuals. These changes are referred to as aging and are differentiated from the concept of age-related disease. Age-related disease is the term describing an increased incidence of chronic illness such as hypertension and diabetes in an aging population. It is important to note that the changes specifically associated with aging are in general well compensated but do result in a number of implications for anesthetic management. These will be addressed below.

The biochemical processes involved in aging are poorly understood. The process seems to be multifactorial as it is unlikely that one specific mechanism can account for all observed phenomena. While a comprehensive discussion of the biology of aging is beyond the scope of this chapter, several aspects have received attention recently. Evolutionary theory accounts for changes in the genetic profile associated with aging. This theory postulates a series of events affecting genes responsible for controlling functions such as DNA repair and protection from oxidative damage. The net result is a life-long accumulation of random damage to cells due to a progressive limitation in the processes responsible for cell maintenance. Significant evidence is mounting regarding the role of reactive oxygen species in promoting aging. The interactions and influence of oxidative stress on numerous cellular pathways have been described. However,

465

the exact role and interaction in human aging is not known. Other evidence suggests that telomeres, terminal DNA sequences involved in maintaining chromosomal stability and consistent replication, may play an important role in initiating senescence. Telomeres shorten with each cell division and cell division ceases when telomeres reach a critical length. Through such a mechanism it has been suggested that telomeres may function to limit the number of times a cell may divide.

PHYSIOLOGICAL CONSIDERATIONS IN AGING

Central Nervous System

Central nervous system dysfunction in aging is often subtle and highly variable. The etiology is unclear. Continued controversy exists as to whether memory decline is a result of normal aging or represents a separate clinical entity. However, recent findings suggest that memory decline is not inevitable. Morphologically, atrophy is frequently evident but does not necessarily correlate to cognitive decline. The decrease in number of neurons is matched by a reduction in the cerebral metabolic rate and cerebral blood flow. Cerebral metabolic rate and cerebral blood flow remain coupled. Reduced levels of neurotransmitters and specific receptors have been demonstrated in different regions of the brain. Serotonin receptors are decreased in the cortex. Dopamine and dopamine receptors are reduced in regions of the basal ganglia. Acetylcholine and cholinergic receptors are also decreased. The overall effect of these changes on anesthetic management is a significant increase in the sensitivity to a number of anesthetic agents.

Cardiovascular System

Age-related changes in cardiovascular physiology in the absence of superimposed cardiovascular disease have the net result of preserving cardiac output but do so in a manner that limits cardiac reserve capacity. Changes occur in both the heart and vasculature (Box 28-1), and a number of adaptive responses ensue. Understanding these changes has important implications for perioperative care and pharmacological intervention. Numerous alterations at the cellular level affect calcium homeostasis, excitation–contraction coupling, cell growth, and matrix composition. These changes in turn lead to altered cardiac and vascular morphology and ultimately affect cardiovascular function. In the heart, mechanical and contractile efficiency is decreased, cardiac relaxation is prolonged (diastolic dysfunction), and beta-adrenergic responses are attenuated.

In youth, the vascular system is compliant and is mechanically coupled to the heart such that there is very

Box 28-1 Age-related Cardiovascular Changes

VASCULAR SYSTEM

Increased vascular impedance
- Increased pulse wave velocity
- Early wave reflection
- Increased afterload

HEART

Changes largely secondary to primary alterations in vascular system
- Left ventricular hypertrophy
- Decreased diastolic compliance
- Shortened diastolic filling time
Increased end-diastolic volume
- Preserved cardiac output

AUTONOMIC NERVOUS SYSTEM

Decreased resting parasympathetic tone
Increased resting sympathetic tone
- Underlying decrease in beta-adrenergic receptor responsiveness
- Decreased response to exercise and metabolic stress
- Decreased baroreceptor responsiveness
- Impaired protective reflexes in response to hypotension

little cost in terms of the energy required to pump blood through the peripheral circulation. With aging there is an increase in vascular stiffness, resulting in increased pulse wave velocity and early reflection of pulse waves from the periphery. Reflected waves increase load on the heart during late systole, decreasing efficiency and promoting cardiac hypertrophy. These effects have been demonstrated in studies of vascular impedance and represent a progressive "detuning" of the heart from the vasculature. In response to this increase in impedance, systolic time is increased thereby preserving stroke volume but at the expense of diastolic time in the setting of impaired early diastolic filling. Under these conditions late diastolic filling and atrial "kick" increase in importance and help to explain why dysrhythmias are often poorly tolerated in the elderly.

End diastolic volume is elevated in older men but not in women. This results in increased stroke volume and preserves cardiac output in the setting of a reduced heart rate observed with aging in men. Women, however have a slightly reduced cardiac output. With exercise peak heart rate, ejection fraction and cardiac output are decreased, chiefly as a result of decreased beta-adrenergic response. Autonomic control of cardiovascular function becomes less effective. Resting parasympathetic tone is decreased and sympathetic nervous system activity increases, albeit in the setting of decreased beta-adrenergic receptor responsiveness. The overall effect is a decrease in baroreceptor responsiveness to changes in blood pressure with a reduced protective reflex in response to hypotension.

Further, increased resting sympathetic nervous system activity may contribute to increases in systemic vascular resistance along with mechanical stiffening of the peripheral vasculature. This in turn may make the elderly patient more sensitive to interventions that affect the sympathetic nervous system.

Clinically these changes lead to a greater likelihood of intraoperative hemodynamic lability and decreased ability to meet the metabolic demand of exercise or surgical stress.

Respiratory System

A number of clinically relevant changes occur in the respiratory system with aging (Box 28-2). Alterations in control of respiration, lung structure, mechanics, and pulmonary blood flow place the elderly at increased risk for perioperative pulmonary complications. Reduced central

---

Box 28-2   Age-related Respiratory Changes

CONTROL OF RESPIRATION

Impaired response to hypoxia
Impaired response to hypercarbia

PULMONARY BLOOD FLOW

Decreased cross sectional area of pulmonary capillaries
• Increased pulmonary vascular resistance
• Increased pulmonary artery pressure
• Decreased hypoxic pulmonary vasoconstriction

LUNG AND CHEST WALL STRUCTURE

Decreased alveolar surface area
• Increased anatomical dead space
• Decreased diffusing capacity
Decreased elastic recoil of lung
Increased chest wall stiffness
• Increased intrapleural pressure
• Diaphragmatic flattening

PULMONARY MECHANICS

Decreased forced expiratory time in 1 second
Increased residual volume
Decreased vital capacity
No change or slightly increased functional residual capacity
Increased closing capacity
• Increased ventilation/perfusion mismatch
• Decreased resting arterial oxygen tension

---

nervous system activity leads to impaired ventilatory responses to hypoxia, hypercapnia, and mechanical stress. The well-known effects of benzodiazepines, opioids, and volatile anesthetics on ventilatory response are further exaggerated. It follows that the usual mechanisms to protect against hypoxemia are profoundly impaired after anesthesia and surgery in the elderly.

Structural changes result from the additive effects of oxidative damage. These effects lead to a progressive loss of alveolar surface area, resulting in increased anatomical dead space and decreased diffusing capacity. Reorganization of collagen and elastin in lung parenchyma combined with altered surfactant production lead to a loss of elastic recoil and greater lung compliance. Loss of the cross-sectional area of the pulmonary capillary bed results in increased pulmonary vascular resistance and elevated pulmonary artery pressures. The chest wall becomes stiffer and less compliant with age. The net effect of decreased elastic recoil and increased chest wall stiffness is to elevate intrapleural pressure by 2–4 cmH$_2$O, leading to the typical barrel chest appearance with diaphragmatic flattening. The flattened diaphragm is mechanically less efficient and is further affected by a significant loss of muscle mass associated with aging.

Forced expiratory volume in 1 second (FEV$_1$) is decreased by 6–8% per decade. Residual volume (RV) is increased by 5–10% per decade while total lung capacity (TLC) is unchanged. Vital capacity (VC) is therefore decreased. Functional residual capacity (FRC) is unchanged or slightly increased with aging. Closing capacity (CC), the volume at which small dependent airways start to close, is increased in aging. Closing capacity is unaffected by body position. Functional residual capacity changes with a number of factors including body position, obesity and anesthesia. In the young, CC is below FRC. Closing capacity equals FRC in the supine position at 44 years of age and at 66 years of age in the upright position. When CC encroaches on tidal breathing, ventilation/perfusion mismatch will occur. Likewise, when FRC is below closing capacity, shunt will increase and arterial oxygenation will fall. These changes result in increased ventilation/perfusion mismatch with aging and represent the most important mechanism for the increase in the alveolar–arterial gradient for oxygen observed in aging. Clinically these alterations contribute to decreased effectiveness of preoxygenation. Additionally, hypoxic pulmonary vasoconstriction is blunted in the elderly and may result in difficulty with one lung ventilation.

Hepatic System

With aging there is an overall reduction in hepatic mass, accounting for a 40% decrease by age 80. This is matched by a reduction in hepatic and splanchnic blood flow. Hepatic microsomal enzymes participating in phase

I oxidation reactions exhibit decreased activity. These changes may influence drug metabolism.

Renal System

The kidney loses nephrons at a rate of 0.5–1% per year, mostly from the cortex. Renal blood flow decreases. Glomerular filtration rate is decreased by about 35% over a person's lifetime. Urine concentrating ability and sodium absorption are decreased. Thirst perception is blunted. Total body water is decreased by 10–15%. Loss of muscle mass in the elderly makes serum creatinine an unreliable predictor of renal function. Creatinine clearance in men can be estimated from the formula:

$$\text{Creatinine clearance (ml/min)} = \frac{(140 - \text{age}) \times \text{body weight (kg)}}{72 \times \text{serum creatinine (mg/dL)}}.$$

Creatinine clearance for women = 0.85 × above value.

Age-related alterations in renal physiology account for an impaired ability for the geriatric patient to protect against significant dehydration and tend to decrease the clearance of drugs with renal routes of elimination.

Thermoregulation

Numerous adverse effects of hypothermia have been demonstrated, including increased myocardial oxygen demand with shivering, increased systemic vascular resistance, increased incidence of postoperative myocardial infarction, cardiac dysrhythmias, coagulopathy, increased incidence of postoperative infection, and prolonged effect of neuromuscular blocking agents. The basal metabolic rate is reduced about 1% per year in the elderly, causing decreased heat production and increasing susceptibility to hypothermia. Elderly patients are likely to become more hypothermic during surgery, shiver less postoperatively, and take longer to rewarm.

AGE-RELATED DISEASE CONSIDERATIONS

There is a higher incidence of chronic illness in the elderly. Pathophysiology associated with a particular process or processes will be superimposed on those alterations in physiology that are already present as part of the normal aging process. The reduction in the functional reserve of nearly every major organ system translates to impaired compensation in the face of disease (Box 28-3). Diseases such as Alzheimer's-type dementia, Parkinson's disease, stroke, hypertension, coronary artery disease, congestive heart failure, chronic obstructive pulmonary disease, diabetes, renal insufficiency, osteoarthritis, and malignancy are all more prevalent in the elderly. Generally, the man-

Box 28-3 Clinical Correlates of Effects of Aging

Effects of aging on major organ systems generally result in decreased reserve capacity with specific implications for anesthetic management

Central nervous system changes lead to increased sensitivity to many anesthetic agents and increased risk of postoperative delirium and prolonged cognitive decline

Cardiovascular changes lead to a greater likelihood of hemodynamic lability and decreased ability to meet the increased metabolic demand of exercise or surgical stress

Pulmonary changes contribute to decreased ventilatory responses to hypoxia and hypercarbia and decreased effectiveness of preoxygenation

Hepatic and renal effects may influence drug clearance

Renal effects promote likelihood of dehydration

Alterations in thermoregulation put the elderly patient at risk for hypothermia

agement issues regarding specific diseases in the elderly will involve many of the same considerations as in younger patients. However, there are a number of issues that are more important or unique to the aged population. Several of these will be addressed below.

With the increasing frequency of disease comes an increased use of prescription medication. Elderly patients often present for surgery with a long list of medications. The use of multiple medications, often termed polypharmacy, increases the possibility of drug interactions and risk of adverse medication related events.

Drug Interactions

Polypharmacy is commonly seen in elderly patients

Polypharmacy increases the likelihood of adverse drug reactions

Polypharmacy has been associated with postoperative delirium

Newer medications prescribed for the treatment of Alzheimer's disease act via inhibition of cholinesterase and may prolong the effect of succinylcholine or alternatively decrease the effectiveness of nondepolarizing neuromuscular blockers – monitor neuromuscular function with a peripheral nerve stimulator

Central nervous system diseases such as dementia place the elderly patient at greater risk of postoperative delirium. The risk for postoperative delirium is also increased in patients receiving multiple medications.

Medications with significant anticholinergic effects may be particularly problematic. Newer medications used in the management of Alzheimer's disease act via inhibition of cholinesterase. These drugs may prolong the effect of succinylcholine or antagonize the effect of nondepolarizing neuromuscular blockers. This is rarely a significant problem clinically, and it is not necessary to stop these medications perioperatively, but monitoring of neuromuscular function with a peripheral nerve stimulator allows assessment to ensure recovery from succinylcholine and guides dosing of nondepolarizing relaxants.

Patients with a prior history of stroke often experience temporary exacerbation of pre-existing deficits following anesthesia. Older patients also have a higher incidence of impaired vision and hearing. Difficulties with hearing often interfere with accurate and effective communication between the operating team and patient. Visual impairment has important implications for a patient's ability to function independently and also places patients at greater risk of delirium.

The elderly patient with hypertension may have exaggerated responses to medications used to control blood pressure. The older patient is also more likely to experience orthostatic hypotension. Therefore, additional care should be taken when encouraging ambulation after surgery.

Patients with coronary artery disease may not exhibit classic symptoms. The elderly are more likely to have silent ischemia and infarction and also more frequently experience nonspecific complaints or vague patterns of chest pain related to myocardial ischemia.

As mentioned above, diastolic relaxation is impaired in the aging heart. In addition to this age-related change, severe diastolic heart failure can result. Cardiac relaxation is an energy-requiring process and diastolic dysfunction has been observed in conditions, including hypertension with left ventricular hypertrophy, ischemic heart disease, hypertrophic cardiomyopathies, and valvular heart disease. The primary problem is lack of left ventricular compliance during diastole, resulting in greatly increased left ventricular diastolic pressure. This pressure can be conducted retrograde to the pulmonary circulation, resulting in pulmonary venous congestion and pulmonary edema. This is often a pressure-related event and does not necessarily imply volume overload. The diagnosis can be difficult to make since the clinical picture can mimic left ventricular systolic failure. Making the correct diagnosis is important as interventions commonly employed in systolic failure such as diuretics and inotropes may exacerbate diastolic dysfunction. Echocardiography is the diagnostic modality of choice. Classically, echocardiography will demonstrate preserved or hyperdynamic left ventricular systolic function and characteristic changes of early (E) and atrial (A) contraction-related flow velocities at the mitral valve.

Clinical Caveats: Diastolic Dysfunction

Clinically may resemble left ventricular systolic dysfunction, obscuring diagnosis
Echocardiography is diagnostic test of choice
Diuretics and inotropes may exacerbate symptoms
Beta-blockers and calcium channel blockers may be beneficial

Non-flow-limiting calcification around the aortic and mitral valves is a common echocardiographic finding in the elderly. It has recently been demonstrated that there is a high incidence of aortic valve sclerosis in the elderly, which is correlated to a 50% increase in the risk of death from cardiovascular causes and the risk of myocardial infarction. It has been suggested that this may represent a marker for coronary artery disease. A similar association has been postulated for mitral annular calcification.

Diabetes is frequently underdiagnosed in the elderly. The older patient is also at higher risk for significant hypoglycemia due to decreased counterregulatory responses and reduced glycogen stores related to poor nutrition. Some patients may be unable to report symptoms due to cognitive impairment. This has obvious consequences for management in the perioperative period.

The presence of arthritis and increased fragility of the skin require that great care be taken in positioning of the patient. Use of adequate padding during surgery is a must.

PHARMACOLOGICAL CONSIDERATIONS IN AGING

Clinically, it is apparent that the elderly are more sensitive to anesthetic agents. Lower anesthetic doses are required to achieve a desired clinical effect, untoward effects of anesthetics such as hemodynamic perturbations occur in greater magnitude, and the pharmacologic effects of anesthetics are often prolonged. These responses are the result of alterations in distribution and clearance of drugs (pharmacokinetics) as well as increased sensitivity of the target organs to a drug (pharmacodynamics). Expected compensatory or reflex responses may be blunted or absent. The relative influence of pharmacokinetic changes and pharmacodynamic alterations will depend on the specific agent's physical properties and mechanisms for metabolism and elimination.

Pharmacokinetic Changes

Body composition is altered in aging such that there is a decrease in lean body mass, an increase in body fat, and a decrease in total body water. These changes indicate a smaller central compartment, leading to increased serum concentrations after bolus administration of a drug. Moreover, there should be a greater volume of distribution, potentially prolonging the clinical effect of a drug. Alterations in hepatic clearance occur as a result of decreased hepatic blood flow, especially important for drugs that undergo first-pass metabolism, and decreased activity of enzymes participating in phase I biotransformation reactions. Renal clearance is dramatically decreased, as mentioned previously. Protein binding is altered as a result of increases in alpha-1-acid glycoprotein and decreases in albumin. The net effect will depend on the extent to which a drug is protein bound and to which serum protein it predominantly binds.

Pharmacodynamic Changes

For a number of anesthetic agents, increased cerebral sensitivity results in decreased dose requirements. This is true for opioids, benzodiazepines, and propofol. Thiopental and muscle relaxants demonstrate no increased target organ sensitivity. Hemodynamic responses to intravenous anesthetics may be exaggerated because of interactions with the aging heart and vasculature.

CONSIDERATIONS FOR SPECIFIC AGENTS

Hypnotics

Pharmacological considerations for the use of hypnotics in elderly people are summarized in Table 28-1.

Thiopental

Thiopental has been extensively studied. The recommended induction dose for the elderly is decreased by about 15%. There is no apparent increase in cerebral sensitivity to thiopental. The reduction in dose is the result of a decrease in the central volume of distribution leading to higher serum levels from a given dose of drug. Recovery from thiopental infusion is not prolonged. Thiopental administration may lead to significant hypotension in

the elderly through effects on sympathetic nervous system tone.

Propofol

With aging the brain becomes more sensitive to the effects of propofol. Clearance is decreased in the elderly as well. Pharmacokinetic compartment modeling demonstrates a decreased rapid equilibration compartment, with delayed intercompartmental clearance. The net result is a 30–50% decrease in the required propofol dose. Recovery from a propofol infusion is markedly delayed in the elderly.

Midazolam

Brain sensitivity to midazolam is significantly increased in aging. Protein binding is slightly reduced. Clearance is decreased by as much as 30% by 80 years of age. Recovery from infusion is dramatically prolonged. The net effect is a nearly 75% reduction in the dose of midazolam needed for elderly patients.

Etomidate

There is no evidence for increased brain sensitivity to etomidate. However, the dose required for induction is reduced by about 20%. This is due to a decreased central compartment accounted for by decreased protein binding. Clearance is reduced as a result of there being a larger volume of distribution. Etomidate causes less cardiovascular depression than barbiturate induction agents and may be especially useful in the elderly.

Opioids

Pharmacological considerations for the use of opioids in elderly people are summarized in Table 28-2.

Fentanyl

There is increased central sensitivity to fentanyl. Only minimal changes in pharmacokinetics have been demonstrated. The increased pharmacodynamic effects account for a 50% reduction in induction dose by age 85.

Alfentanil

Changes are similar to those for fentanyl.

Sufentanil

Sensitivity is increased by about 50%. A small decrease in central compartment volume has been demonstrated.

Table 28-1 Pharmacologic Considerations in Aging: Hypnotics

Drug	Altered Pharmacokinetics	Altered Pharmacodynamics	Recommend Adjustment in Dose
Thiopental	Yes	No	Decreased 15%
Propofol	Yes	Yes	Decreased 30–50%
Midazolam	Yes	Yes	Decreased 75%
Etomidate	Yes	No	Decreased 20%

Table 28-2 Pharmacologic Considerations in Aging: Opioids

Drug	Altered Pharmacokinetics	Altered Pharmacodynamics	Recommend Adjustment in Dose
Fentanyl	Minimal	Yes	Decreased 50%
Alfentanil	Minimal	Yes	Decreased 50%
Sufentanil	Yes	Yes	Decreased 50%
Remifentanil	Yes	Yes	Induction dose decreased 50%, maintenance dose decreased 33%

Remifentanil

Brain sensitivity is increased. Pharmacokinetic changes include decreased central compartment volume and decreased clearance. Induction dose is reduced by about half as with fentanyl, alfentanil, and sufentanil. Maintenance infusion is only one-third of that required in younger patients.

Neuromuscular Blockers

There is no evidence for increased receptor sensitivity to neuromuscular blocking agents. Alterations in dose requirements are due to changes in pharmacokinetic parameters. Pharmacological considerations for the use of neuromuscular blocking agents in elderly people are summarized in Table 28-3.

Pancuronium

The clearance of pancuronium depends on renal function and decreases with advancing age. The clinical effect is prolonged.

Vecuronium

Clearance is decreased by approximately 30%. Data is conflicting in regard to changes in the volume of distribution. Clinically the loading dose is similar to that used in younger patients but with continuous administration lower infusion rates are required.

Rocuronium

Clearance and volume of distribution are decreased and the duration of action is significantly prolonged.

Cisatracurium

Cisatracurium undergoes Hofmann degradation. This process is nonenzymatic and occurs spontaneously. Because of this organ-independent elimination, dose adjustment for aging is not necessary and clinical effect is not prolonged.

Mivacurium

Mivacurium is metabolized by plasma cholinesterase. Plasma cholinesterase levels are decreased with aging, leading to decreased clearance and increased duration of action. Lower rates for maintenance infusion are needed.

Volatile anesthetics

Brain sensitivity to volatile agents is increased and is expressed in terms of lower values for minimum alveolar concentration (MAC) and MAC-awake. Induction may be slowed by decreased rate of rise in alveolar concentration caused by ventilation/perfusion inequalities in the aging lung. Emergence may be delayed as the volume of distribution is increased.

Table 28-3 Pharmacologic Considerations in Aging: Neuromuscular Blockers

Drug	Altered Pharmacokinetics	Altered Pharmacodynamics	Recommend Adjustment in Dose
Pancuronium	Yes	No	Dose dependent on renal function
Vecuronium	Yes	No	Similar loading dose, decreased clearance, lower infusion rates
Rocuronium	Yes	No	Decreased clearance
Cisatracurium	No	No	No adjustment necessary
Mivacurium	Yes	No	Decreased clearance, lower maintenance infusion rate

Clinical Caveats: Pharmacology

Changes in clinical response to agents administered to elderly patients may be the result of alterations in pharmacokinetics, pharmacodynamics, or both
Regardless of the cause, the predominant effect is an exaggerated response that usually mandates the administration of lower doses

PERIOPERATIVE CONSIDERATIONS IN AGING

Preoperative Considerations

It is readily evident that the geriatric population is quite heterogeneous. Age alone does not imply a given level of function. Age alone also does not necessarily imply increased perioperative risk. Age has been included as a minor predictor in some risk assessment indices. However, increased perioperative risk has been more closely correlated with other factors, including the need for emergency surgery and, most importantly, coexisting disease. Therefore, the preoperative approach to the geriatric patient is similar to that for other patients. Identifying comorbid conditions and ensuring optimal preoperative management are central to successful management.

Placing this information in context with age-related changes in physiology allows for an evaluation directed at determining the functional reserve of organ systems. Functional reserve can be thought of as the difference between the basal level of functioning of an organ system and the maximum level of function sustainable to meet a given challenge. Assessing functional capacity can be quite challenging in some elderly patients. Some patients are sedentary and may limit activity enough to not provoke cardiopulmonary symptoms. These patients often will deny the presence of symptoms. It is also important to clarify the level of activity and a pattern of decreasing activity or increasing frequency of symptoms in assessing stability of disease over time. This is further complicated by the greater likelihood of atypical cardiopulmonary symptoms in the elderly. Assessing a baseline level of function also provides a reference for postoperative outcome. The goal of any procedure should be to return the patient to at least their baseline abilities after surgery.

The American College of Cardiology and the American Heart Association published guidelines for preoperative cardiovascular evaluation in 1996. An update to the guidelines was published in 2002 and provides an excellent approach to cardiovascular evaluation and risk assessment. These guidelines offer recommendations for the evaluation and testing of patients with and without known coronary artery disease and with and without prior coronary intervention. While a complete overview is beyond the scope of this chapter, the guidelines are an important resource. The recommended stepwise approach considers major, intermediate, and minor clinical predictors, patient functional capacity, and the nature of the proposed surgical procedure to direct preoperative testing and intervention. The guidelines stress that preoperative intervention is rarely necessary as a means to lower surgical risk unless the intervention would have been indicated regardless of the proposed surgery. Importantly, there have been several studies demonstrating benefit of perioperative beta-blocker administration in patients with known coronary artery disease and with significant risk factors for coronary artery disease. These studies as well as the guidelines are useful, but are not specific to the geriatric population.

Current controversy exists as to the nature and extent of preoperative testing that is necessary to provide safe, cost-effective perioperative care. Greater evidence is evolving that standard laboratory testing based only on patient age may not be necessary, especially for low-risk procedures. A recent study demonstrated no difference in perioperative morbidity and mortality for cataract surgery when standard laboratory tests, including electrocardiogram, complete blood count, serum electrolytes, urea nitrogen, creatinine, and glucose, were not performed preoperatively. This is a low-risk procedure performed under local anesthesia and extrapolation of these results beyond cataract surgery may not be appropriate. Another study investigated the prevalence and predictive value of abnormal laboratory tests in a prospective cohort study of 544 consecutive patients undergoing noncardiac surgery. A low prevalence of electrolyte abnormalities and thrombocytopenia (0.5–5%) was observed. There was a higher prevalence of low hemoglobin, elevated creatinine, and elevated glucose but no abnormal test was associated with adverse outcome. When adjusted for elderly ASA physical class I and II patients, the prevalence of abnormal values was that of the general population. These studies suggest that standard preoperative laboratory screening for hemoglobin, glucose, creatinine, platelets, and electrolytes may not be necessary. It is important to note that these studies do not advocate that no testing be performed but rather that preoperative testing be based on a particular patient's underlying condition as determined by history and physical, the proposed surgical procedure (low, intermediate, or high risk, likelihood of blood loss), and the likelihood that a test result will result in a change of care.

Intraoperative Considerations

Anesthetic Technique: Regional Versus General Anesthesia

Considerable controversy remains regarding whether regional anesthesia is associated with improved outcomes when compared to general anesthesia for patients undergoing major surgery. Early studies suggested survival benefit for neuraxial regional techniques. Many potential benefits of neuraxial blockade have been proposed, including attenuation of the neurohumoral stress response associated with surgery and trauma, initiation of pre-emptive analgesia, decreased intraoperative blood loss, decreased incidence of deep venous thrombosis, decreased incidence of postoperative peripheral vascular graft thrombosis, and improved pulmonary function.

In spite of these potentially beneficial effects few recent studies have been able to demonstrate differences in major morbidity and mortality between regional and general anesthesia. A recent meta-analysis of 141 clinical trials, where patients were randomized to receive either neuraxial regional anesthesia or general anesthesia, observed a 33% decrease in mortality at 30 days related to a decreased incidence of pulmonary emboli, cardiac events, stroke, and pulmonary complications for patients who received neuraxial regional anesthesia. The results are difficult to generalize since the study did not specifically examine outcomes in elderly patients and the analysis included a wide variety of studies with different surgeries and anesthetic techniques conducted over a number of years. The study could not distinguish whether the observed improvement was the result of direct beneficial effects of regional technique or avoidance of deleterious effects of general anesthesia. Further, it is unclear if the effect was related to intraoperative management, continuation of postoperative regional analgesia, or both. Other recent studies have not corroborated these results.

Clinical Considerations

Considerations in the intraoperative management of the aged patient will be the result of the cumulative effects of aging and age-related disease leading to a decrease in organ reserve capacity as mentioned above. Decisions regarding invasive monitoring and intravenous access will be based on underlying patient functional status and the nature of the anticipated surgery. Careful attention should be paid to assessment of intravascular volume as the elderly often present with hypovolemia due to impaired conservation of free water, decreased thirst, and treatment with diuretics. Increased ventricular stiffness and diastolic dysfunction will make the elderly patient more sensitive to both relative hypovolemia as well as volume overload.

Premedication in the elderly should be considered carefully. Use of midazolam has been associated with delayed discharge from postanesthesia recovery and a greater incidence of postoperative arterial desaturation.

Preoxygenation may be impaired because of increased closing capacity. Hemodynamic responses to volatile and intravenous agents may be exaggerated by their effects on vascular preload, direct myocardial depression, and chemical sympatholysis. Protective reflex mechanisms may be ablated because of decreased baroreceptor gain and altered vagal tone. Decreased venous return associated with positive-pressure ventilation may be poorly tolerated.

Dosage adjustments for the majority of medications administered during anesthesia must be considered as outlined above. Gradual titration of intravenous agents to effect is preferred over large-bolus administration. Consideration of increased circulation time and delayed onset of clinical effect may be important, especially in patients with impaired left ventricular systolic function. Every effort should be made to defend the patient's temperature by maintaining acceptable ambient operating room temperature, use of forced air warmers, humidity moisture exchangers, and warming intravenous fluids as appropriate.

Elderly patients may be more sensitive to the sympatholytic effects of neuraxial regional anesthesia, responding with a greater degree of hypotension due to impaired compensatory mechanisms and a higher resting sympathetic tone. Epidural test doses containing epinephrine may not elicit the expected heart rate response to an intravascular injection. It appears that the blood pressure response is not impaired. With neuraxial regional anesthesia, a decrease in the dose required to achieve a similar extent of both intrathecal and epidural block has been demonstrated in elderly patients as compared to their younger counterparts.

Clinical Caveats: Intraoperative Management

At risk for significant volume depletion preoperatively
Preoxygenation less effective
More sensitive to hypotensive effect of intravenous induction agents and neuraxial local anesthetics
Dosage adjustments frequently required for nearly all anesthetic agents
Intravenous medications may have a longer circulation time and delayed onset of effect
Carefully titrate medications to effect
At risk for greater hemodynamic lability with positive pressure ventilation
At increased risk for hypothermia – defend patient temperature
Heart rate response to epidural test dose may be absent – blood pressure response preserved

---

Postoperative Considerations

Older patients are more likely to experience a variety of postoperative complications. Concerns more specific to the geriatric population include pulmonary and central nervous system complications.

Pulmonary complications including pneumonia and the adult respiratory distress syndrome are the most common problem in the elderly following surgery. Physiologic changes as outlined previously place the geriatric patient at risk for hypoxemia, decreased pulmonary toilet, and aspiration. The presence of pre-existing chronic lung disease, smoking, and obesity are significant risk factors.

Postoperative neurologic dysfunction is a very important problem in the geriatric surgical population. Delirium has been reported as a frequent postoperative event, occurring in as many as one-third of patients after repair of hip fracture. Delirium may actually be underdiagnosed in the surgical patient. It is easy to identify patients who are obviously confused and agitated. However a number of patients appear calm but, when rigorously assessed, are

Box 28-4   Risk Factors for Postoperative Delirium

Prior history of dementia or organic brain disease
Use of physical restraints
Indwelling urinary catheters
Polypharmacy

clearly confused. The patient with delirium may be at higher risk of injury from falls, be unable to cooperate with therapy, and interfere with necessary interventions such as intravenous catheters and wound dressings. Postoperative delirium has been associated with increased morbidity, mortality, and utilization of healthcare resources.

Factors associated with postoperative delirium include a preoperative history of dementia, use of physical restraints, indwelling urinary catheters, and polypharmacy (Box 28-4). The use of multidisciplinary care teams, including daily follow-up from a geriatrician, appears to be beneficial. The contribution of intraoperative management in preventing postoperative delirium is unclear. It seems prudent to avoid anticholinergic medications whenever possible. Studies have failed to demonstrate a lower incidence of delirium with regional versus general anesthesia.

Postoperative cognitive dysfunction is not limited to the immediate postoperative period. The International Study of Post Operative Cognitive Decline (ISPOCD1) included 1,218 patients and demonstrated cognitive dysfunction in 25.8% and 9.9% of patients at 1 week and 3 months after surgery respectively. These values compared to controls of 3.4% and 2.8%. Risk factors for early cognitive dysfunction included age, duration of anesthesia, lower level of education, repeat surgery, postoperative infection, and respiratory complications. Late cognitive dysfunction was associated only with advancing age. Cerebral hypoperfusion has been previously suggested a possible mechanism contributing to postoperative cognitive decline. However, hypoxemia and hypotension were not associated with postoperative cognitive decline in this study. These results have important implications for the ability of patients to return to their baseline level of function.

SUMMARY

An increasing number of elderly patients are presenting for surgery and the number is expected to increase. Understanding age-related changes in physiology and the importance of age-related disease, as well as adverse perioperative events associated with an older patient population, has important consequences for the anesthesiologist. In general, the presence of coexisting disease and a given patient's functional status are more important than age alone in assessing anesthetic risk and planning for appropriate perioperative care. There is a clear need for increased understanding into the mechanisms and nature of postoperative delirium and long-term cognitive decline. The debate over the impact of regional versus general anesthesia continues. The role of peripheral nerve blocks in the elderly is an area that needs to be defined, as does the contribution of postoperative analgesia. Education and awareness of problems specific to the geriatric population is necessary for all healthcare professionals involved in their care.

Case Study

An 80-year-old woman is scheduled to undergo placement of a bipolar hip prosthesis for treatment of a femoral neck fracture. Past medical history is significant for long-standing hypertension, hypercholesterolemia, and mild dementia. The family reports that she comfortably performs activities around the house but has become increasingly forgetful. Medications include lisinopril, pravastatin, and donepezil. Heart rate is 76. Blood pressure is 172/90. On examination the heart rate is regular, without murmurs. The lungs are clear. Hemoglobin is 11.4 g/dL.

- Is any further preoperative testing necessary?
- What anesthetic technique will you recommend?
- Are you concerned about any specific drug interactions?
- How will you counsel the patient's family regarding perioperative risk?

SUGGESTED READING

Dzankic S, Pastor D, Gonzalez C, Leung J. The prevalence and predictive value of abnormal laboratory tests in elderly surgical patients. *Anesth Analg* 2001;93:301-308.

Eagle KA, Berger PB, Calkins H, *et al*. ACC/AHA guideline update for perioperative cardiovascular evaluation for noncardiac surgery—executive summary. A report of the American College of Cardiology/American Heart Association Task Force on Practice Guidelines (Committee to Update the 1996 Guidelines on Perioperative Cardiovascular Evaluation for Noncardiac Surgery). *Anesth Analg* 2002;94:1052-1064.

Katz PR, Grossberg GT, Potter JF, *et al*. *Geriatrics syllabus for specialists*. New York: American Geriatrics Society, 2002.

Liu L, Leung J. Predicting adverse postoperative outcomes in patients aged 80 years or older. *J Am Geriatr Soc* 2000; 48:405-412.

Moller JT, Cluitmans P, Rasmussen LS, *et al*. Long-term postoperative cognitive dysfunction in the elderly: ISPOCD1 study. *Lancet* 1998;351:857-861.

Priebe HJ. The aged cardiovascular risk patient. *Br J Anaesth* 2000;85:763-778.

Rodgers A, Walker N, McKee A, *et al*. Reduction of postoperative mortality and morbidity with epidural or spinal anesthesia: results from an overview of randomized trials. *Br Med J* 2000;321:1-12.

Schein OD, Katz J, Bass EB, *et al*. The value of routine preoperative medical testing before cataract surgery. *N Engl J Med* 2000;342:168-175.

Shafer SL. The pharmacology of anesthetic drugs in elderly patients. *Anesthesiol Clin North Am* 2000;18:1-29.

Von Zglinicki T, Bürkle A, Kirkwood TBL. Stress, DNA damage and ageing – an integrative approach. *Exp Gerontol* 2001; 36:1049-1062.

INTRODUCTION

Resuscitation, according to Webster's definition, is "to revive, particularly to recover from apparent death or unconsciousness". We think of resuscitation as being necessary following sudden traumatic or unforeseen circumstances that lead to cardiac arrest or severe injury but, as anesthesiologists, recognize that it occurs in a controlled setting daily for the anesthesia care provider. Recovery from unconsciousness following general anesthesia is expected by patients, families, surgeons, and the anesthesia team. Our understanding of the depths or degrees of unconsciousness during anesthesia is a question of importance for the anesthesia community and research is ongoing to develop monitoring that will accurately measure levels of unconsciousness and may impact how we "resuscitate" people on a daily basis.

Anesthesia providers are often asked to participate in patient care for individuals who are in danger of impending or apparent death from trauma, infections, or complications of major disease processes. This may be a frequent occurrence for practitioners in a busy level 1 trauma center where patients often present with life-threatening injuries. These events require resuscitative skills that incorporate many of the algorithms taught by Advanced Cardiac Life Support (ACLS) courses throughout the country.

While the mechanics and elements of resuscitation are not as foreign to the anesthesia provider as they may be to other health-care providers, the need for continual medical education is necessary to enable all practitioners to perform well in these often extremely stressful circumstances where individuals require resuscitation. These algorithms are meant for first responders both in the field and within the hospital. In the last 20 years they have been continually upgraded and their last update was done by an international group, utilizing an evidence based approach for development of guidelines.

This reference will review the history of resuscitation and the current treatment algorithms for resuscitation in adults, emphasizing the most recent changes, and explore areas of current research that may impact future guidelines and our management of resuscitation. We will only briefly touch on basic life support and techniques for airway management, as anesthesia care providers are already highly trained in this area. Additionally, pediatric and neonatal resuscitation have been left entirely out of this chapter. The reader is referred to the ILCOR guidelines for further discussion in these areas.

HISTORY

Resuscitative algorithms have changed many times since the concept of modern cardiopulmonary resuscitation began over 40 years ago. The most recent consensus statement was published in 2000 by a new group, the International Liaison Committee on Resuscitation (ILCOR). This group brought together experts from many countries practicing in several different disciplines, who critically examined the available research in the area of resuscitation to develop the first international guidelines.

These efforts had been carried out many times previously by distinct groups, including the American Heart Association (AHA) and the European Resuscitation Council. These groups and several others came together in an effort to produce an international consensus and guidelines for the lay responder as well as the experienced practitioner. This global, uniform thinking reflects the core philosophy that these guidelines need to be easier to teach and practice to enhance the ultimate goal: improved patient care and survival. The reader will find many structural similarities between the current guidelines and those previously published. There are still a large number of algorithms that require rhythm recognition but several areas have been simplified, ultimately to improve patient care through more appropriate and rapid intervention.

Previous recommendations by AHA were published in 1974, 1980, 1986, and 1992 prior to merging with ILCOR for development of the current recommendations. Undoubtedly, future guidelines will emerge as research is vigorous in all aspects of resuscitation. New guidelines may include entirely new specific areas such as therapeutic hypothermia. Two recent studies have led to the publication of recommendations by the Advanced Life Support (ALS) Task Force of ILCOR in April 2003, which are discussed below.

It was not until the 1960s that resuscitation evolved to include emergency care for cardiovascular collapse. A series of fortuitous, related observations would lead to the development of cardiopulmonary resuscitation (CPR) as we have understood it for several years – combining the elements of respiratory resuscitation via mouth-to-mouth ventilation and closed chest compressions. The development of the defibrillator, which was first described in the 1950s, would add to the armamentarium of the lay responder with the development and deployment of automatic external defibrillators (AEDs) in the 1990s.

Kouwenhoven first demonstrated the ability to produce arterial pulsations with forceful chest compressions in the early 1960s. This gave new hope to simplifying the technique of open cardiac massage, which had been used successfully previously but required highly trained personnel and specialized equipment. Interestingly, the technique of open cardiac massage is enjoying a resurgence of research interest and will be discussed later in this reference. While Kouwenhoven was studying closed cardiac compressions, Safer and Elam had been revitalizing and extrapolating a technique for adults that had been used successfully by midwives on infants. This technique was ultimately validated as a means of providing ventilatory support for the apneic patient. Together, Kouwenhoven and Safer appreciated the rationale for combining their techniques and the foundation of basic CPR was established.

BACKGROUND

Implicit in the publications of previous AHA and current ILCOR guidelines are classifications of the various interventions presented. Every intervention is classified according to evidence available and the review and interpretation of this evidence by the expert panels in each technical area. Changes throughout the years recognize new information, which may either upgrade or downgrade the relative class an intervention is placed within. Interventions are classified in five groups (Table 29-1).

Interventions rated as acceptable, safe, and useful would be rated as class I. An example of this would be early defibrillation by first responders. Several commonly used drugs, such as epinephrine and lidocaine, have had their classification changed since the 1992 guidelines were published. These are both now class Indeterminate (available evidence insufficient) for the ventricular tachycardia algorithm based on the evaluation by ILCOR's panel of experts of the available literature on these two drugs. These new changes are spelled out in detail in the complete ILCOR document and the advanced reader may wish to read only the section that describes the changes between the 2000 consensus statement and previous versions. The complete document covers all areas of basic life support (BLS) and ACLS as well as specialized areas such as hypothermia and stroke.

BASIC LIFE SUPPORT

A good illustration of how critical appraisal of the data has led to a change in guidelines is within the BLS guidelines for the carotid pulse check. Table 29-2 details the accuracy of lay responders in identifying a pulse accurately. Because of the high overall error rate, the potential for a significant delay while the assessment is made and the potential for inappropriate interventions (no chest compressions when a pulse is absent or chest compressions when a pulse is present), the carotid pulse check is no longer part of BLS training for the lay provider. Health-care providers, however, will continue to be instructed to assess the pulse.

Another important change is within the guidelines for confirmation of endotracheal tube placement. Anesthesia personnel are well aware of the inherent dangers of misplaced or dislodged endotracheal tubes. Both these complications can lead to catastrophic consequences for any patient within a short period of time. ILCOR recognized that both these possibilities could occur during resuscitation attempts and have changed their recommendations accordingly. Guidelines now mandate confirming endotracheal tube placement by using non-physical-examination

Table 29-1 Classes of Recommendations 2000: Classification of Therapeutic Interventions in CRP and ECC

1. Search for Evidence: Locates the Following	2. Consensus Review by Experts: Intervention is Placed in Following Class	3. Interpretation of This Class of Recommendation when Used Clinically
Minimum evidence required for a Class I recommendation: • Level of evidence: 1 or more RCTs • Critical assessment: *excellent* • Results: homogenous, consistently positive, and robust	**Class I: Excellent** *Definitely recommended* Supported by excellent evidence Proven efficacy and effectiveness	**Class I** interventions are always acceptable, proven safe, and definitely useful
Minimum evidence required for a Class IIa recommendation: • Level of evidence: higher • Number of studies: multiple • Critical assessment: *good to very good* • Weight of evidence/expert opinion: more strongly in favor of intervention than Class IIb • More long-term outcomes measured than Class IIb • Results: positive in majority of studies • Observed magnitude of benefit: higher than Class IIb	**Class IIa: Good to very good** *Acceptable and useful* **Good/very good** evidence provides support Note: "Contextual" factors: In addition to level of evidence, these additional factors are considered in making final class of recommendation. Contextual factors include small magnitude of benefit, high cost, education and training challenges, large difficulties in implementation, and impractical, unfavorable cost-benefit ratios.	**Class IIa** interventions are acceptable, safe, and useful. • Considered standard of care: reasonably prudent physicians can choose • Considered **intervention of choice** by majority of experts • Often receive AHA support in training programs, teaching materials, etc. *"Contextual" or "mismatch" factors may render an intervention Class IIa in one context and Class IIb in another (see Note)*
Minimum evidence required for a Class IIb recommendation: • Level of evidence: lower/intermediate • Number of studies: few • Critical assessment: *fair or poor* • Weight of evidence/expert opinion: less in favor of usefulness/efficacy • Outcomes measured: immediate, intermediate, or surrogate • Results: generally, but not always, positive	**Class IIb: Fair to good** *Acceptable and useful* **Fair to good** evidence provides support Note: Contextual/mismatch factors should not be used to avoid the trouble and expense of adopting new but clinically beneficial interventions	**Class IIb** interventions are acceptable, safe, and useful. • Considered within "standard of care": reasonably prudent physicians can choose • Considered **optional or alternative interventions** by majority of experts
Evidence found but available studies have one or more shortcomings • Promising but low-level • Fail to address relevant clinical outcomes • Are consistent, noncompelling, or report contradictory results • May be high-level but report conflicting results	**Class Indeterminate** *Preliminary research stage* Available evidence insufficient to support a final class decision Results promising but need additional confirmation Evidence: no harm but no benefit No recommendation until further evidence is available	Note: Interventions classed **Indeterminate** can still be recommended for use, but reviewers must acknowledge that research quantity/quality falls short of supporting a final class decision. Do not use *Indeterminate* to resolve debates among experts, especially when evidence is available but experts disagree on interpretation. *Indeterminate* is limited to promising interventions.
Positive evidence completely absent or evidence strongly suggests or confirms harm	**Class III: Unacceptable, no documented benefit, may be harmful** *Not acceptable, not useful, may be harmful*	Interventions are designated as **Class III** when evidence of benefit is completely lacking or studies suggest or confirm harm.

RCT, randomized controlled trial.

From American Heart Association/International Liaison Committee on Resuscitation (ILCOR) Guidelines 2000 for cardiopulmonary resuscitation and emergency cardiovascular care. An international consensus on science. *Circulation* 2000;suppl:1–357:1-5.

Table 29-2   Sensitivity, Specificity, and Reliability of Pulse Check: Performance of Pulse Check as a Diagnostic Test

	Pulse is Present	Pulse is Absent	Totals
Rescuer thinks pulse is present	81 (Sensitivity: correct positive result of pulse check ÷ all times a pulse was actually present) _a_	6 _b_	87 (No. of times rescuer thought pulse present = a + b)
Rescuer thinks pulse is absent	66 _c_	53 (Specificity: correct negative result of pulsecheck ÷ all times there actually was no pulse) _d_	119 (No. of times rescuer thought pulse absent = c + d)
Totals	147 (Total number of study opportunities where a pulse was actually present = a + c)	59 (Total number of study opportunities where a pulse was actually absent = b + d)	206 (Total study opportunities = a + b + c + d)

Calculations derived from above:

_a_ **Positive predictive value**: Of the total times the rescuer thinks a pulse is present (total 87 times), a pulse _is_ present = 81/87 times = 93%

_b_ **Negative predictive value**: Of the total times the rescuer thinks a pulse is absent (total 119 times), a pulse _is_ absent = 53/119 times = 45%

_c_ **Sensitivity**: Rescuer's ability to detect a pulse when one actually is present = 81/147 = 55%

_d_ **Specificity**: Rescuer's ability to recognize that a pulse is absent when a pulse actually is absent = 53/59 = 90%

Accuracy = "Rescuer correct"/ Total = (81 pulse correctly found + 53 pulse correctly thought absent)/ 206 = 65%

From American Heart Association/International Liaison Committee on Resuscitation (ILCOR). Guidelines 2000 for cardiopulmonary resuscitation and emergency cardiovascular care. An international consensus on science. _Circulation_ 2000;suppl:1-357:I-39.

techniques. This includes devices such as esophageal detectors, end-tidal CO_2 indicators, and capnometric devices. These are class IIa interventions in patients who are not in full arrest and IIb indications in patients in full arrest. In this situation, because of poor perfusion, they may misleadingly indicate esophageal intubation while the endotracheal tube is in the correct position within the trachea.

DEFIBRILLATION

Defibrillation has become a high-priority goal for all cardiac arrest victims both within and outside the hospital setting. In the last decade, public access to AEDs has made a significant contribution to reducing morbidity and mortality associated with cardiac arrest. A recent study by Jared Bunch and colleagues demonstrated comparable long-term outcomes for out-of hospital cardiac arrest patients who had successful early defibrillation, and survived to hospital discharge, compared to age-, sex-, and disease-matched controls. Early defibrillation is a class IIa intervention for health-care providers within the hospital and outpatient medical offices. Establishing programs within these institutions to facilitate early defibrillation should remain a high priority for resuscitation programs.

The importance of speed in defibrillation is illustrated in Figure 29-1, which shows how quickly the chance of successful resuscitation decreases with each minute that goes by prior to defibrillation. This fact alone has led to publications comparing resuscitation with an

AED and a manually applied and run defibrillator. Results of that study confirmed that the time to application of the AED, coupled with analysis and defibrillation by the automated device, was longer and therefore potentially

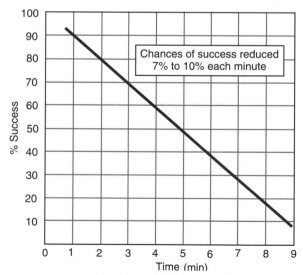

Figure 29-1   Composite data illustrating the relationship between probability of survival to hospital discharge (indicated as "success") after ventricular fibrillation cardiac arrest and interval between collapse and defibrillation. (From American Heart Association/International Liaison Committee on Resuscitation (ILCOR). Guidelines 2000 for cardiopulmonary resuscitation and emergency cardiovascular care. An international consensus on science. _Circulation_ 2000;suppl: I-61; data from Larsen MP, Eisenberg MS, Cummings RO, Hallstrom AP. Predicting survival from out-of-hospital cardiac arrest: a graphic model. _Ann Emerg Med_ 1993:22: 1652–1658.4)

detrimental to the patient compared to manual defibrillation, which would occur faster. However, this would only be true in a setting where both options were readily available – typically only in a hospital or clinic.

Defibrillators themselves are also undergoing significant transformation with the advent of biphasic defibrillators. Monophasic defibrillators have been used for over 30 years since the advent of direct current defibrillation. Two distinct waveforms have been utilized with equivalent efficacy: damped sinusoidal and truncated exponential. Recently, biphasic defibrillators have become available, which have been shown to be equally efficacious and safe in adults while using lower energy levels. Biphasic defibrillators deliver current in two directions between the electrodes, yielding positive and negative waveforms that have characteristic shapes depending upon the manufacturer. An example of these is shown in Figure 29-2. The ILCOR algorithms currently state that "equivalent biphasic energy" can be used for shocks applied during resuscitative efforts instead of the typical escalating doses of monophasic energy that have been in the algorithms for years.

It is likely that, as further research becomes available, more specific guidelines for biphasic defibrillator energies will be published.

ALGORITHMS FOR RESUSCITATION

Algorithms for resuscitation first appeared in the 1986 guidelines and have gradually become a major tool for critical decision making in emergency cardiac care for arrest victims. The algorithms promote recognition of clinical scenarios and guide decision-making steps for patient care. Many medications were trimmed from the 1992 guidelines and further modifications have taken place in the 2000 ILCOR guidelines for the administration of antiarrhythmics and drugs for circulatory support.

Algorithms are not intended to replace education and clinical judgment but may serve as a framework around which good clinical decisions can be made for patients needing resuscitation. The two major treatment algorithms shown in Figures 29-3 and 29-4 are an attempt to present these critical pathways in an organized, simplified way to promote greater retention by the student, quicker response time, and ultimately better care for patients.

In spite of the great efforts of the resuscitative councils to provide widespread education and training, many physicians, including anesthesiologists, continue to perform poorly during resuscitation simulation and classes. Certainly, full cardiac arrest is a rarity in the operating room, with a reported incidence below 1:10,000. This gives the average practitioner few opportunities to demonstrate these skills in a "live" environment and often little opportunity to practice. However, the onus is still on the practitioner to be fully trained and to maintain

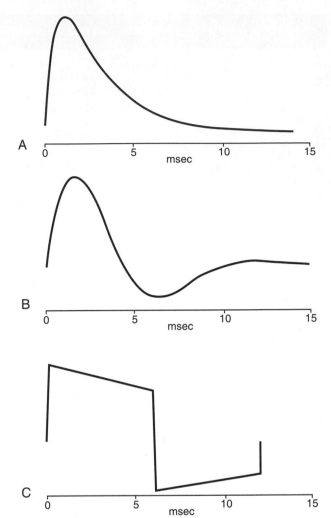

Figure 29-2   Relative efficacy of monophasic and biphasic waveforms for transthoracic defibrillation after short and long durations of ventricular fibrillation. (From Walcott GP, Melnick SB, Chapman FW, *et al*. Relative efficacy of monophasic and biphasic waveforms for transthoracic defibrillation after short and long durations of ventricular fibrillation. *Circulation* 1998; 98:2210–2215.)

and upgrade these skills on an annual or biannual basis to be prepared for the occurrence of cardiac arrest anywhere in the perioperative arena.

As mentioned, algorithms do not replace critical thinking and clinical awareness but should be used as a guideline or framework for patient care. Because of ongoing monitoring, the anesthesia care provider may commonly utilize fragments of these algorithms to prevent the patient from requiring "complete arrest" resuscitation.

Cardiac Rhythms

Primary algorithms

In Figure 29-3, the ILCOR Universal/International ACLS Algorithm, and Figure 29-4, the Comprehensive

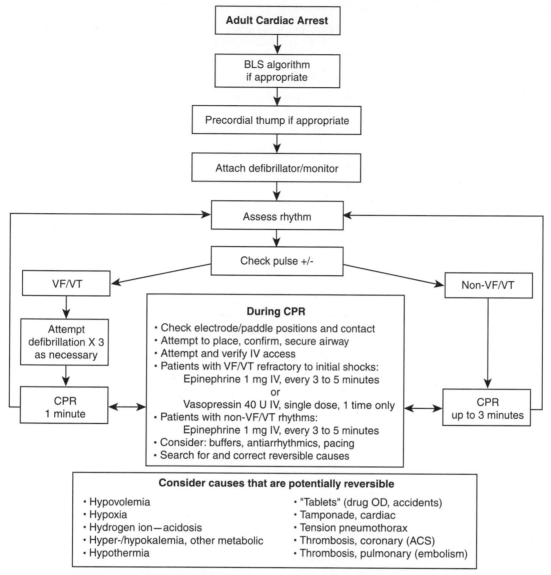

Figure 29-3   ILCOR universal/international Advanced Cardiothoracic Life Support algorithm. (From American Heart Association/International Liaison Committee on Resuscitation (ILCOR). Guidelines 2000 for cardiopulmonary resuscitation and emergency cardiovascular care. An international consensus on science. *Circulation* 2000;suppl:I-143.)

Emergency Cardiac Care (ECC) Algorithm, efforts were made to incorporate and integrate ACLS, defibrillation and BLS into two simple, easy to use algorithms. Both these algorithms categorize patients into two potential rhythm groups for treatment – ventricular fibrillation (VF) or ventricular tachycardia (VT) – and non-VF/VT. An essential element of these algorithms and others that will be discussed is prompt recognition of cardiac rhythm and assessment of circulation. In the operating room, postanesthesia care unit, and the intensive care unit, monitoring is already in place to detect and dis-

play significant changes in vital signs and cardiac rhythm.

Ventricular Fibrillation

Three significant changes appear in the algorithm for patients in VF (Figure 29-5). One of these changes is the incorporation of biphasic defibrillation. Rapid defibrillation is present on all algorithms and should certainly occur quickly in the operating room and perioperative area. It is a class I indication if it occurs within 3 minutes of cardiac arrest within the hospital. All algorithms that indicate defibrillation now state energy levels as either

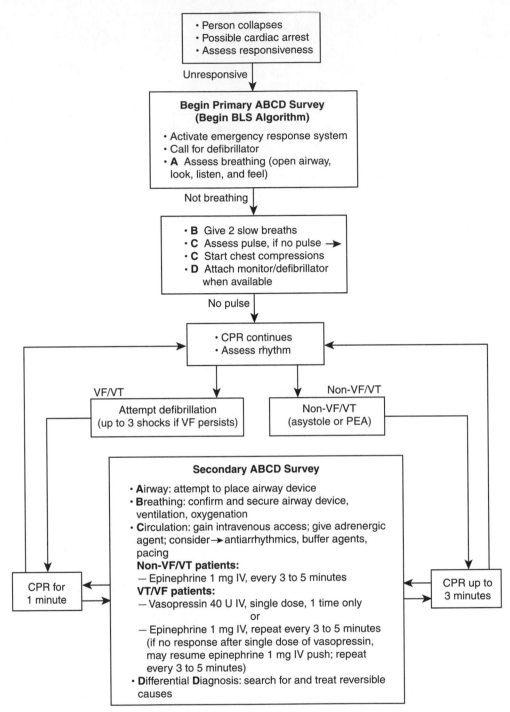

Figure 29-4   Comprehensive ECC algorithm. (From American Heart Association/International Liaison Committee on Resuscitation (ILCOR). Guidelines 2000 for cardiopulmonary resuscitation and emergency cardiovascular care. An international consensus on science. *Circulation* 2000;suppl:I-144.)

sequential monophasic defibrillators (200 J, 200–300 J, and 360 J) or equivalent biphasic energy. As discussed previously, energy levels for successful biphasic defibrillation have been shown to be consistently lower than monophasic defibrillators. The exact levels, however, have yet to be determined and future guidelines will probably give more specific recommendations for energy levels.

Other significant changes are in the recommended medications. The first change is the addition of vasopressin as an alternative to epinephrine as a first-line drug. Vasopressin becomes a potent vasoconstrictor

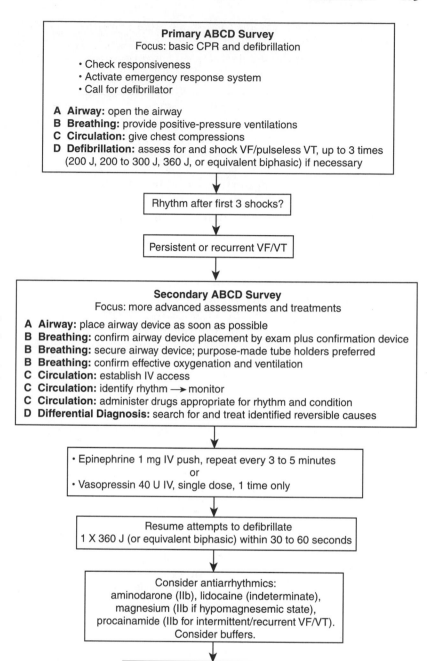

Figure 29-5   Ventricular fibrillation/pulseless VT algorithm. (From American Heart Association/ International Liaison Committee on Resuscitation (ILCOR). Guidelines 2000 for cardiopulmonary resuscitation and emergency cardiovascular care. An international consensus on science. *Circulation* 2000;suppl:I-147.)

in high doses, acting via direct stimulation of smooth muscle V_1 receptors. This may produce a variety of effects including pallor, intestinal cramps, nausea, and bronchial or uterine contractions. Its effects on V_1 receptors will cause significant vasoconstriction of skeletal muscles without increased myocardial oxygen consumption. Vasopressin has compared favorably with epinephrine in human and animal studies for resuscitation during cardiac arrest. It has done as well or better in studies on long-term arrest and has been shown in some

studies to maintain higher coronary perfusion pressures. At the time of the ILCOR guidelines, vasopressin was given as class IIb (acceptable, fair supporting evidence) for adult shock-refractory VF as an alternative to epinephrine. The half-life of vasopressin in animal models is 10–20 minutes, leading to the recommendations in the guidelines that it be given as a single one-time dose. Vasopressin is being studied for other dysrhythmias and may have a role in asystole and pulseless electrical activity in the future. It is also found a potential role in the intensive care unit for vasodilatory shock from sepsis as a continuous infusion. To date, there is no evidence to support repeating the administration of vasopressin after 10–20 minutes of unsuccessful resuscitation. If vasopressin is given as the first drug and there is no response, epinephrine may be given in doses of 1 mg IV and repeated every 3–5 minutes. High dose epinephrine (up to 0.2 mg/kg) is acceptable, but not recommended by ILCOR as there is growing evidence that this may be detrimental.

The last significant change in the algorithm concerns antiarrhythmic therapy. Lidocaine has been demoted to class Indeterminate status, based on the critical evaluation of the literature. Amiodarone, however, has been shown to improve early hospital survival and restore spontaneous circulation in patients with VF. It has moved to become the drug of choice in many of the algorithms including being given a class IIb recommendation for use in the VF/pulseless VT algorithm. Both magnesium and procainamide remain as potential choices depending upon the circumstances of the arrest, but bretylium has been removed from the algorithm.

Pulseless Electrical Activity

This group is defined by a rhythm other than VF or VT and the lack of a detectable pulse. It is often associated with specific reversible causes and a successful resuscitation usually implies treatment for one of these causes. The pulseless electrical activity algorithm in Figure 29-6 delineates the most frequent causes of this group of arrhythmias, which includes pseudo-EMD, idioventricular rhythms, ventricular escape rhythms, and bradyasystolic rhythms. The five Hs – hypovolemia, hypoxia, hyper- or hypokalemia, hypothermia, and acidosis (hydrogen ion) – as well as the five Ts – tablets (drug overdose, accidental), tamponade, tension pneumothorax, thrombosis (coronary), and thrombosis (pulmonary) – should be quickly investigated. Epinephrine remains on the algorithm as a class Indeterminate and, as mentioned, there has been insufficient evidence to include vasopressin to date. Sodium bicarbonate and atropine are included on the algorithm for specific circumstances. In patients with pre-existing hyperkalemia, bicarbonate-responsive acidosis, or drug overdose, sodium bicarbonate may be beneficial. When the rhythm of pulseless electrical activity is bradycardic, atropine may be given.

Asystole

Figure 29-7 illustrates the algorithm for asystole, which contains many of the same basic primary and secondary ABCD surveys that are common to many algorithms and prominent in the two basis ILCOR algorithms. These surveys are also more relevant to the out-of-hospital

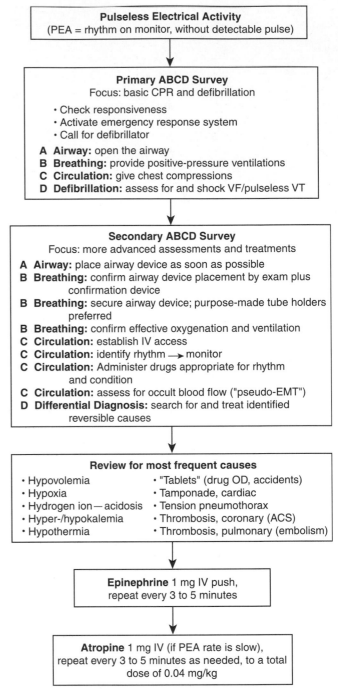

Figure 29-6 Pulseless electrical activity algorithm. (From American Heart Association/International Liaison Committee on Resuscitation (ILCOR). Guidelines 2000 for cardiopulmonary resuscitation and emergency cardiovascular care. An international consensus on science. *Circulation* 2000;suppl:p I-151.)

arrest or the in-hospital arrest on a regular medical ward. Transcutaneous pacing as an early intervention, epinephrine, and atropine remain on the algorithm for potential interventions. And, as with pulseless electrical activity, a rapid search should be conducted for any reversible causes.

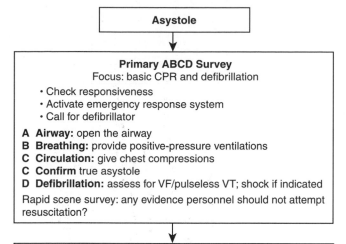

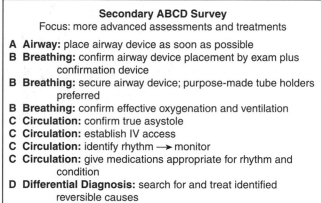

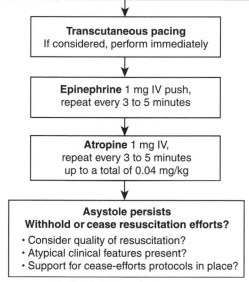

Figure 29-7   Asystole: the silent heart algorithm. (From American Heart Association/International Liaison Committee on Resuscitation (ILCOR). Guidelines 2000 for cardiopulmonary resuscitation and emergency cardiovascular care. An international consensus on science. *Circulation* 2000;suppl:I-153.)

Bradycardia

The bradycardia algorithm (Figure 29-8) requires, as do all the algorithms and the management of any patient with an unstable rhythm, constant patient surveillance

for signs or symptoms associated with the bradycardia. Possible complications of the rhythm could be hypotension, pulmonary congestion, chest pain, or shortness of breath. Careful attention should also be paid to any rhythm changes – i.e., is second- or third-degree heart block now present? If the patient is symptomatic, transcutaneous pacing is a class I intervention. Bradycardia is a relatively common occurrence during anesthesia and the vigilant practitioner is continually assessing the rhythm and looking for any serious associated signs. Atropine, dopamine, and epinephrine remain on the treatment algorithm as well as continued observation in the absence of any serious signs or symptoms associated with the bradycardia.

Tachycardia Algorithms

The tachycardia algorithms remain the most complex of all the algorithms because of the number of potential treatment arms available based upon rhythm determination. For the patient in no immediate need of cardioversion, the primary aim of the anesthesia care provider is to determine the specific rhythm and look for signs of impaired cardiac function. These two elements are critical to the application of antiarrhythmic therapy and are points of major emphasis in the 2000 guidelines. The tachycardia algorithms are also substantially more complex, which illustrates the diversity of the rhythms and the difficulty ILCOR had in attempting to simplify them. Simplification was a major theme for the guidelines overall but was untenable with the tachycardia algorithms.

The basic tenets of these algorithms are to first establish whether the patient is stable or not. If not – synchronized cardioversion is required with either monophasic or biphasic energy (Figure 29-9). If the patient is stable, the focus shifts to rhythm recognition and appropriate treatment is selected with one antiarrhythmic. At the same time, if unknown, some interpretation must be made of the suspected underlying cardiac function (if EF <40%, drug choices may be limited and/or dosage reduced).

There are four choices of rhythm type in the tachycardia algorithm:

- atrial fibrillation/flutter
- narrow complex tachycardias
- wide complex tachycardias of unknown type
- stable monomorphic/polymorphic tachycardia.

This decision tree is illustrated in Figure 29-10, with Figures 29-11 and 29-12 illustrating the specific algorithms for stable narrow-complex supraventricular tachycardia, and stable ventricular tachycardia. Note the emergence of amiodarone in both algorithms, particularly for the heart with decreased functional capacity.

The treatment of atrial fibrillation or atrial flutter is directed at rate control, assessment of need for anticoagulation, and conversion of rhythm via either

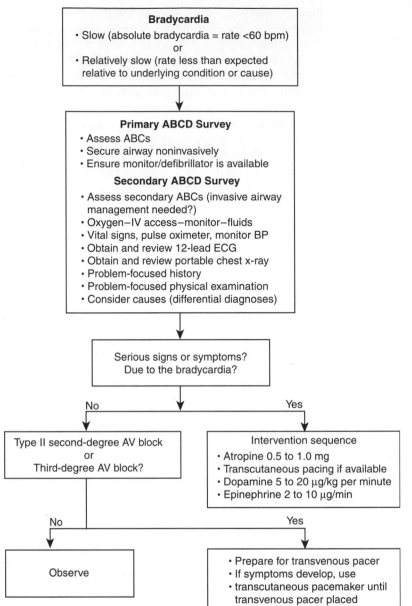

Figure 29-8 Bradycardia algorithm. (From American Heart Association/International Liaison Committee on Resuscitation (ILCOR). Guidelines 2000 for cardiopulmonary resuscitation and emergency cardiovascular care. An international consensus on science. *Circulation* 2000;suppl:I-156.)

medications or electrical cardioversion when urgent or necessary. In many institutions, including my own, cardiology services are often consulted for long-term management of stable atrial fibrillation or flutter.

Many antiarrhythmics may be used for rhythm control, including amiodarone, ibutilide, propafenone, flecainide, and procainamide (all class IIa in patients with normal cardiac function).

The key to the treatment of the other tachyarrhythmias is rapid determination of rhythm type, investigation for possible underlying causes, and continued assessment of the patient's stability.

Acute Coronary Syndromes

These algorithms are included here to underscore the need for vigilance in determining patients at risk for acute myocardial infarction or unstable angina and the current medical management that is applicable for the anesthesiologist in the operating room and perioperative setting. An ever-increasing percentage of patients presenting in operating rooms for surgery have known or suspected cardiac disease. It is imperative that the anesthesiologist has a good understanding of appropriate treatment in the different settings in

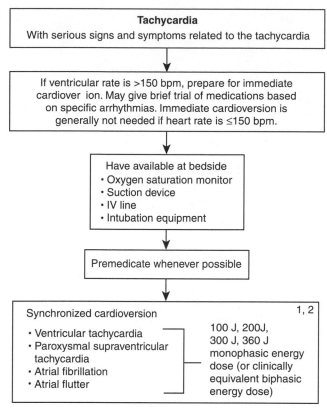

Tachycardia
With serious signs and symptoms related to the tachycardia

↓

If ventricular rate is >150 bpm, prepare for immediate cardiover ion. May give brief trial of medications based on specific arrhythmias. Immediate cardioversion is generally not needed if heart rate is ≤150 bpm.

↓

Have available at bedside
• Oxygen saturation monitor
• Suction device
• IV line
• Intubation equipment

↓

Premedicate whenever possible

↓

Synchronized cardioversion   1, 2
• Ventricular tachycardia
• Paroxysmal supraventricular tachycardia
• Atrial fibrillation
• Atrial flutter

100 J, 200J, 300 J, 360 J monophasic energy dose (or clinically equivalent biphasic energy dose)

Notes:
1. Treat polymorphic ventricular tachycardia (irregular form and rate) like ventricular fibrillation; see ventricular fibrillation/pulseless vetricular tachycardia algorithm.
2. Paroxysmal supraventricular tachycardia and atrial flutter often respond to lower energy levels (start with 50 J).

Figure 29-9 Synchronized cardioversion algorithm. (From American Heart Association/International Liaison Committee on Resuscitation (ILCOR). Guidelines 2000 for cardiopulmonary resuscitation and emergency cardiovascular care. An international consensus on science. *Circulation* 2000;suppl:I-164.)

which they may be asked to treat these patients. This includes the preoperative setting, the operating room, the postanesthesia care unit, and the intensive care unit if applicable.

Figures 29-13 and 29-14 illustrate the initial management for patients with chest pain suggestive of ischemia and electrocardiographic changes. Several of these interventions are applicable to patients in both preoperative and postoperative units, including oxygen, morphine, nitroglycerin, and aspirin (MONA). However, in postsurgical patients antithrombolytics and antiplatelet agents may be contraindicated because of the risk of bleeding, and the need for them will have to be balanced against the patient's clinical status.

FUTURE DIRECTIONS

Hypothermia in Reperfusion Injury

Moderate hypothermia (28–32 °C) has been used successfully for decades in cardiac surgery as a mechanism to protect the brain against ischemia. Its first use after cardiac arrest can be traced back to the middle of the 20th century but, because of problems and no well-defined benefit to the practice, its use was abandoned. In the 1990s several studies revived the interest in hypothermia in a cardiac arrest model after the return of spontaneous circulation.

Two prospective randomized trials were published in 2002, one from Europe and one from Australia, comparing mild hypothermia (range of 32–34 °C in one study and 33 °C in the other) with normothermia in survivors of out-of-hospital cardiac arrest. Patients were treated for 12 hours on one study and 24 hours in the other. Results showed improved outcomes for the treated group compared to the normothermic patients. Patients treated with hypothermia had increased neurologic outcome and fewer deaths at discharge and at 6 months. There were strict inclusion criteria for the study and there were more complications in the treatment groups, such as hyperglycemia, pneumonia, and sepsis.

How does hypothermia improve outcome? Possible mechanisms include a reduced cerebral metabolic rate and the suppression of reactions, such as free radical production and excitatory amino acid release, that may be associated with reperfusion injury. Because of these and other results, the Advanced Life Support Task Force of ILCOR has made recommendations for the use of therapeutic hypothermia, which are as follows:

• Unconscious adult patients with spontaneous circulation after out-of-hospital cardiac arrest should be cooled to 32–34 °C for 12–24 hours when the initial rhythm is ventricular fibrillation.
• Such cooling may also be beneficial for other rhythms or in-hospital cardiac arrest.

New Techniques for Cardiopulmonary Resuscitation

Although chest compressions have been part of modern CPR since its inception, controversy has existed over the ability of rescuers to provide meaningful consistent perfusion pressure, which remains the goal of chest compressions. There is also evidence that illustrates how quickly this pressure output drops off when compressions are stopped for either ventilation or defibrillation. Several alternative techniques have been developed recently in an attempt to improve perfusion pressure during CPR. For a complete review of these,

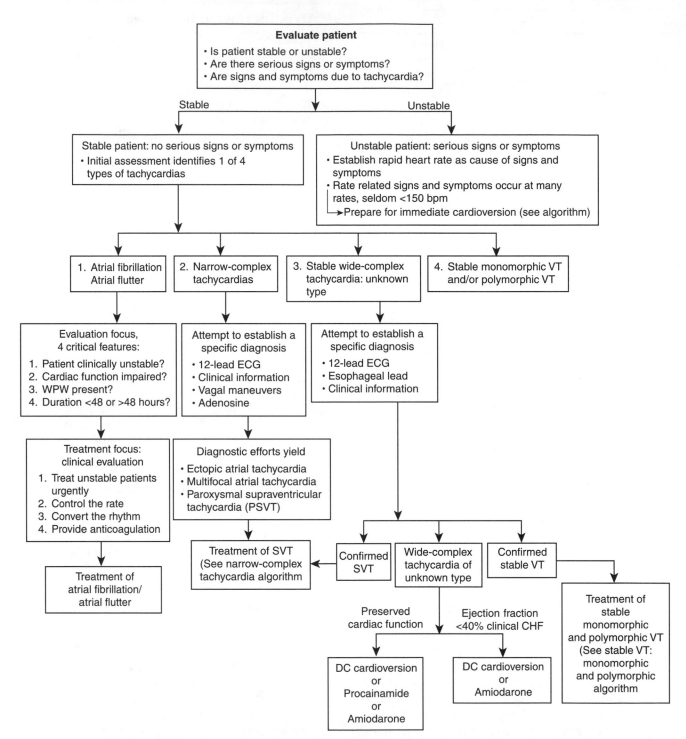

Figure 29-10   The tachycardia overview algorithm. (From American Heart Association/ International Liaison Committee on Resuscitation (ILCOR). Guidelines 2000 for cardiopulmonary resuscitation and emergency cardiovascular care. An international consensus on science. *Circulation* 2000;suppl:I-159.)

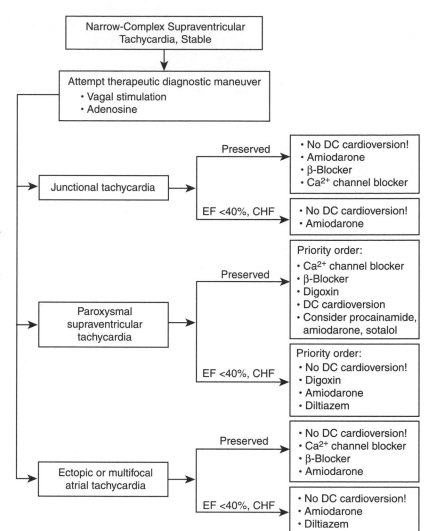

Figure 29-11 Narrow-complex supraventricular tachycardia algorithm. (From American Heart Association/International Liaison Committee on Resuscitation (ILCOR). Guidelines 2000 for cardio-pulmonary resuscitation and emergency cardio-vascular care. An international consensus on science. *Circulation* 2000;suppl:I-162.)

the reader is referred to Section 4, Part I of the ILCOR recommendations, and a recent review article by Tony Smith which is referenced at the end of this chapter.

Interposed Abdominal Compression Cardiopulmonary Resuscitation

Interposed abdominal compression (IAC)-CPR requires an extra rescuer be present to assist with compressions. The objective is to actively compress the abdomen in the midline between the xiphoid process and the umbilicus, alternating with the chest compressions. The goal of these alternating compressions is to increase blood return to the thorax and elevate aortic diastolic pressures. Randomized controlled trials have shown improved outcome for in-hospital trials but no improvement in survival for out-of-hospital arrest. ILCOR's guidelines have given IAC-CPR a class IIb indication as an alternative to standard CPR in the hospital, provided additional trained personnel are readily available.

Active Chest Decompression Cardiopulmonary Resuscitation

Another model to improve the efficiency of chest compressions has been the development of devices that allows an active chest decompression (ACD) phase to CPR. Active decompression by means of a suction cup device attached to the sternum may decrease intrathoracic pressure and increase venous return to the heart. This would increase available blood volume for the next compression (ejection) and increase perfusion pressures.

There have been concerns over a potentially higher incidence of rib fractures and difficulties with the application of the device. However, the technique has been studied both within and outside the hospital setting and results have been positive enough for ILCOR to recommend ACD-CPR as an alternative to standard CPR for in-hospital use, provided trained rescuers are available (class IIb).

Additional research has led to the development of devices that will perform interposed abdominal

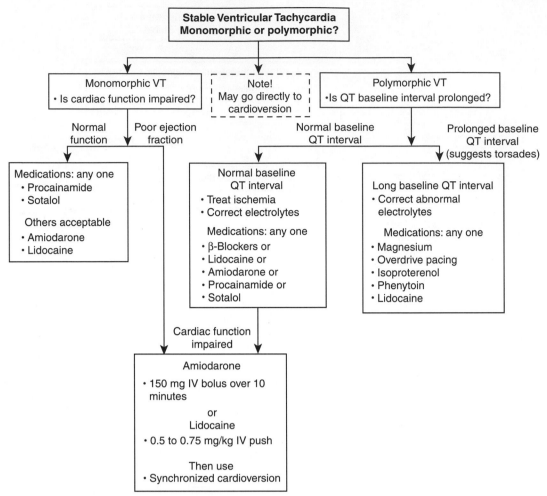

Figure 29-12   Stable ventricular tachycardia (monomorphic and polymorphic) algorithm. (From American Heart Association/International Liaison Committee on Resuscitation (ILCOR). Guidelines 2000 for cardiopulmonary resuscitation and emergency cardiovascular care. An international consensus on science. *Circulation* 2000;suppl:I-163.)

compression with chest compression/decompression or a combination of ACD-CPR and IAC-CPR. One such device, the LifeStick™ (Datascope, Fairfield, NJ) is currently under investigation.

Impedance Threshold Valve

This device has been tested in conjunction with ACD-CPR and given a class IIb recommendation as an adjunct to ACD-CPR. It works by preventing passive inspiration during the decompressive phase of ACD-CPR. This enhances the negative intrathoracic pressure being achieved by the decompressive phase and further augments venous return.

It must be used with an airway device in place such as an endotracheal tube and should be discontinued with the return of spontaneous respiration. It has the advantage of requiring little training and being simple and easy to use.

Open Cardiac Massage

There has been a resurgence of interest in internal cardiac massage and the development of a device to perform this task. Initial research has shown beneficial hemodynamics with open cardiac massage compared to external chest compressions. A device has been developed (MIDCM, TheraCardia, San Clemente, CA) that can be placed through a mini-thoracotomy incision. In a small trial with patients who had failed prolonged resuscitation attempts, the device helped to produce a return of spontaneous circulation in seven of 25 patients. None of these patients survived to hospital discharge.

Further research needs to be done on this technique, which will ultimately require specialized training and potentially expose the patient to increased risks during insertion of the device.

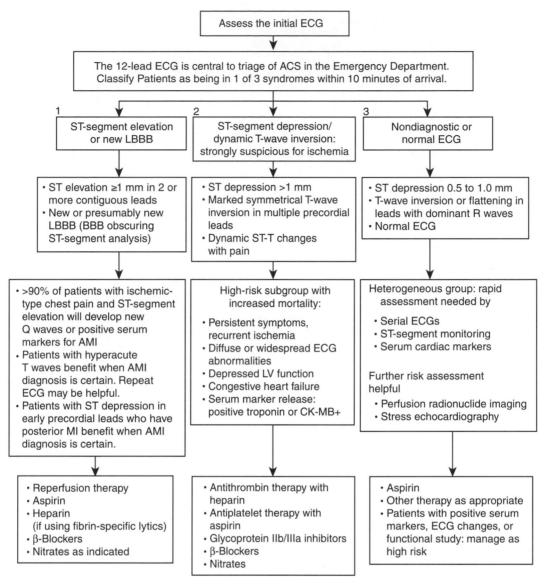

Figure 29-13   The acute coronary syndromes algorithm. (From American Heart Association/ International Liaison Committee on Resuscitation (ILCOR). Guidelines 2000 for cardiopulmonary resuscitation and emergency cardiovascular care. An international consensus on science. *Circulation* 2000;suppl:I-179.)

Vest Cardiopulmonary Resuscitation

Vest CPR typically uses a circumferential vest that is cyclically inflated and deflated to take advantage of the thoracic pump mechanism for blood flow. Historically, these devices have been difficult to install and operate, but experimental studies have shown improved peak aortic and coronary pressures as well as cerebral and blood flow.

ILCOR has designated this a class IIb intervention when there are trained personnel available.

Recently a newer, smaller, gas-driven, more easily transportable device has become available (LUCAS™)

that provides active mechanical compression/decompression. It is smaller and lighter (6.5 kg) than some of the previous devices and an initial study has shown superior pressures compared to manual CPR in an animal model. As with many of the adjuncts to traditional CPR, carrying, fitting, and operating the device safely adds to the complexity of its use. How effective they become at safely and efficiently improving patient outcomes will determine their ultimate inclusion in future algorithms and use by resuscitative personnel, including the anesthesiologist.

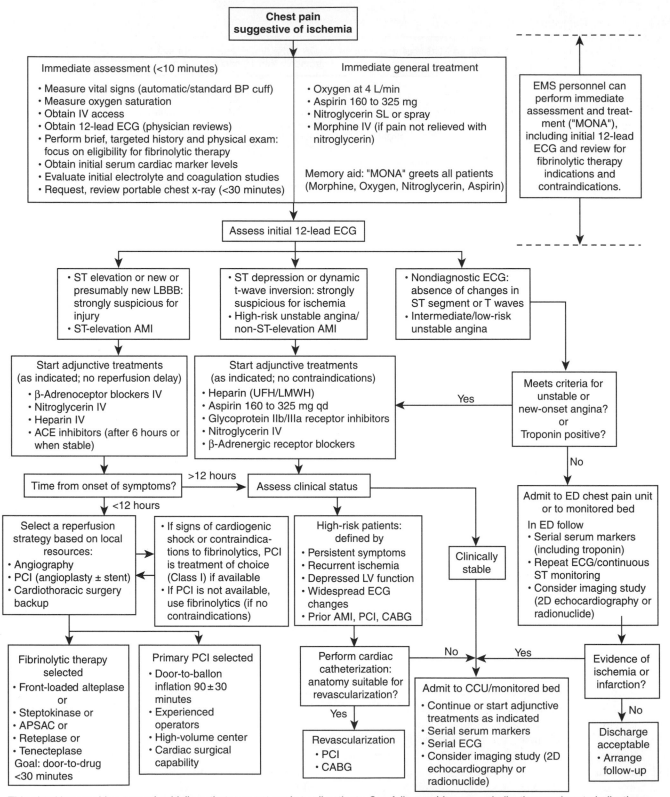

This algorithm provides general guidelines that may not apply to all patients. Carefully consider proper indications and contraindications.

Figure 29-14   Acute ischemia chest pain protocol. (From American Heart Association/ International Liaison Committee on Resuscitation (ILCOR). Guidelines 2000 for cardiopulmonary resuscitation and emergency cardiovascular care. An international consensus on science. *Circulation* 2000;suppl:I-178.)

SUGGESTED READING

ACC/AHA/ESC. Guidelines for the management of patients with supraventricular arrhythmias – executive summary: a report of the American College of Cardiology/American Heart Association Task Force on Practice Guidelines and the European Society of Cardiology Committee for Practice Guidelines (Writing Committee to Develop Guidelines for the Management of Patients With Supraventricular Arrhythmias). *Circulation* 2003;108:1871–1909.

American Heart Association/International Liaison Committee on Resuscitation (ILCOR). Guidelines 2000 for cardiopulmonary resuscitation and emergency cardiovascular care. An international consensus on science. *Circulation* 2000;suppl:1–357.

Nolan JP, Morley PT, Vanden Hoek TL, Hickey RW. Therapeutic hypothermia after cardiac arrest. An advisory statement by the Advanced Life Support Task Force of the International Liaison Committee on Resuscitation. *Resuscitation* 2003; 57:231–235.

Paiva EF, Kern KB, Hilwig RW, *et al*. Minimally invasive direct cardiac massage versus closed-chest cardiopulmonary resuscitation in a porcine model of prolonged ventricular fibrillation cardiac arrest. *Resuscitation* 2000;47:287–299.

Smith, T. Alternative cardiopulmonary resuscitation devices. *Curr Opin Crit Care* 2002;8:219–223.

Vincent R. Resuscitation. *Br Heart J* 2003;89:673–680.

Walcott GP, Melnick SB, Chapman FW, *et al*. Relative efficacy of monophasic and biphasic waveforms for transthoracic defibrillation after short and long durations of ventricular fibrillation. *Circulation* 1998;98:2210–2215.

White RD. Cardiopulmonary resuscitation: basic and advanced cardiac life support. In: Miller R, ed. *Anesthesia*, 5th ed. Philadelphia: Churchill Livingstone, 2000:2533–2559.

CHAPTER 30

Guidelines and Practice Parameters

JAMES S. HICKS

DANIEL J. COLE

INTRODUCTION

Anesthesiology is recognized as an early innovator and continuing leader in the development of various standards, guidelines, and other statements designed to provide guidance to the practitioner and improve patient care. These are described variously as practice standards, parameters, guidelines, advisories, and statements, depending on the source. These documents are generally derived from a consensus process involving a number of experts in the specific field, then subjected to review by the governing body prior to their publication. The body of material comprising the documents reviewed in this chapter is substantial. It is the intent here to present a distilled version suitable for brief review by the practicing anesthesiologist and identify the source for readers requiring a more detailed analysis.

Although there are a host of parameters with some relation to anesthesia practice (see http://www.guideline.gov), for purposes of this discussion we will focus primarily on those that are work products of the American Society of Anesthesiologists (ASA). In addition, relevant material from the American College of Cardiology/American Heart Association, the Brain Trauma Foundation/American Association of Neurological Surgeons, and the American Society for Regional Anesthesia and Pain Medicine will be discussed.

Each of these documents is a set of suggestions, commonly set forth as decision rules that reflect informed consensus on issues commonly presenting themselves to anesthesiologists. Some are specific to a given procedure (e.g., use of pulmonary artery catheters) while others are quite broad (standards for preanesthesia care). In general, they are generated as a means to assure the quality of care and, in some instances, contain costs. Anesthesiologists should critically assess all such instruments encountered for their relevancy to their clinical practice (Box 30-1).

Much of the material contained in this chapter is specifically identified at one of three levels of certainty in its intended effect on clinical practice: standards, guidelines, and advisories. Practice standards are authoritative statements for clinical practice, from which there should be little deviation except in an emergency or major extenuating circumstances. Practice guidelines are systematically developed recommendations for patient care that describe a range of basic management strategies. The content contained within them is often subcategorized by the strength of evidence supporting them and/or the strength of their applicability to clinical practice. They are supported by analysis of the current literature and by a

Box 30-1   Guide to Assessing a Practice Guideline

VALIDITY OF THE PROCESS

Who produced the guideline, and was their agenda congruent with your agenda?

Was the clinical question explicit and relevant?

What was the process used to identify, select, and analyze the evidence?

How contemporary is the guideline?

Has the guideline been subject to peer review?

RESULTS

How practical and clinically relevant are the recommendations?

What is the scientific validity of the recommendations?

What is the level of uncertainty regarding the recommendations?

CLINICAL APPLICATION

How can I integrate the guideline into patient care to improve quality?

Is the practice guideline a "cookbook" which requires rigid conformity, or does is leave room for discretion and professional judgment?

synthesis of expert opinion, open forum commentary, clinical feasibility data, and consensus surveys. Guidelines are not intended as standards or absolute requirements. They may be adopted, modified, or rejected according to the clinical situation. Practice advisories are similar to guidelines in their construct but usually represent the work of a less rigorous process than that used to develop guidelines.

Other statements and policies are work products of various task forces and committees within the ASA addressing issues that have arisen in the conduct of the practice of anesthesiology and for which the society has felt the need to make a written statement of policy; these statements and policies are not addressed within the scope of this chapter but are available from the ASA. Boxes 30-2 through 30-23 contain a synopsis of the various standards, guidelines, and advisories developed by the ASA.

In addition to the subjects addressed herein, the ASA publishes a number of additional statements of policy and position that address many aspects of anesthesiology practice but are neither standards nor clinical practice guidelines and have thus not been included here. These are all accessible through the ASA website, www.asahq.org.

Box 30-2   Standards for Basic Anesthetic Monitoring

Date published: 1998
Organization: American Society of Anesthesiologists
Purpose: To establish standards for intraoperative monitoring by anesthesiologists
Summary:

GENERAL CONDITIONS

- Standards apply to all anesthesia care, although appropriate life support measures take precedence
- Addresses only basic monitoring
- In rare or unusual circumstances, some may be clinically impractical and, even with their use, may not detect untoward clinical developments
- Brief interruptions in their use may be unavoidable
- The anesthesiologists may waive some (marked with asterisk) requirements and should explain such in the record
- Do not apply to the obstetrical patient in labor or the pain management patient
- Continual is defined as "repeated regularly and frequently in steady rapid succession;" continuous is defined as "prolonged without any interruption at any time"
- Standards with an asterisk (*) can be waived by the anesthesiologist but should be explained in the medical record

STANDARD I

Qualified anesthesia personnel shall be present in the room throughout the conduct of all general anesthetics, regional anesthetics, and monitored anesthesia care.
- If remote observation is necessary (e.g., magnetic resonance imaging), provision for monitoring the patient must be made
- If an emergency requires temporary absence of the anesthesiologist, the best judgment of the anesthesiologist should be used in selecting a person responsible for remaining with the patient, considering the patient's condition

Continued

Box 30-2   Standards for Basic Anesthetic Monitoring—cont'd

STANDARD II

During all anesthetics, patient oxygenation, ventilation, circulation and temperature shall be continually evaluated.

Oxygenation

- The concentration of oxygen in the breathing system shall be measured by an analyzer with a low oxygen limit alarm in use during general anesthesia with an anesthesia machine*
- During all anesthetics, a quantitative method of measuring patient blood oxygenation (such as pulse oximetry) shall be used*
- Adequate illumination and exposure of the patient are necessary to assess color*

Ventilation

- The adequacy of ventilation shall be continually evaluated
- Continual monitoring for end-tidal carbon dioxide ($ETCO_2$) shall be performed unless impractical or impossible
- Quantitative measurement of expired tidal volume is strongly encouraged*
- Endotracheal tube or laryngeal mask airway positioning must be verified by clinical assessment and $ETCO_2$ measurement, and continual $ETCO_2$ measurement shall be performed using capnography, capnometry, or mass spectroscopy*
- An audible breathing system disconnect alarm must be used when a mechanical ventilator is employed
- During regional anesthesia and monitored anesthesia care, ventilation shall be evaluated at minimum by continual observation of qualitative clinical signs

Circulation

- The electrocardiogram (ECG) must be continuously displayed from start to finish of anesthesia
- Blood pressure and pulse must be taken and recorded every 5 minutes
- Circulatory function must be continually monitored by one of the following: palpation of a pulse, auscultation of heart sounds, intra-arterial pressure, ultrasound, pulse plethysmography or oximetry

Body Temperature

- Shall be monitored when clinically significant changes in body temperature are intended, anticipated, or suspected.

Based on *Standards for basic anesthetic monitoring*, 1998, of the American Society of Anesthesiologists.

Box 30-3   Standards for Postanesthesia Care

Date published: 1994
Organization: American Society of Anesthesiologists
Purpose: To prescribe basic standards for anesthesiologists in the delivery of postanesthesia care
Summary:

GENERAL

- Standards apply to postanesthesia care in all locations
- May be exceeded at the judgment of the anesthesiologist

STANDARD I

All patients who have received anesthesia of any type shall receive appropriate postanesthesia care.

- A postanesthesia care unit (PACU) or equivalent area shall be available to receive patients
- All patients who receive anesthesia care shall be admitted to the PACU unless specifically ordered by the anesthesiologist
- Policies and procedures of the PACU shall govern care and be reviewed and approved by the Department of Anesthesiology
- Design, equipment, and staffing of the PACU shall meet all accrediting and licensing requirements in force

Continued

Box 30-3   Standards for Postanesthesia Care—cont'd

STANDARD II

Patients transported to the PACU shall be accompanied by a member of the anesthesia care team who knows the patient, shall be appropriately monitored, evaluated, and treated during transport.

STANDARD III

Upon PACU arrival, the patient shall be re-evaluated and a report given to the responsible PACU nurse by the transporting member of the team
- The patient's status on arrival in PACU shall be documented
- A review of the intraoperative course shall be provided to the PACU nurse
- The anesthesia care team member shall remain in the PACU until the PACU nurse accepts responsibility for the patient

STANDARD IV

The patient shall be evaluated continually in the PACU.
- Evaluation shall use methods appropriate to the patient's condition
- Particular attention should be given to oxygenation, ventilation, circulation, and temperature
- Oxygenation shall be assessed quantitatively during early recovery (does not apply to the labor patient post regional anesthesia)
- An accurate PACU report shall be maintained
- The use of a PACU scoring system is encouraged on admission, at appropriate intervals, and at discharge
- General medical supervision and coordination of patient care in the PACU shall be the responsibility of an anesthesiologist
- A policy should be in place to assure the presence in the facility of a physician capable of managing complications and provide cardiopulmonary resuscitation for patients in the PACU

STANDARD V

A physician is responsible for discharging the patient from the PACU.
- If discharge criteria are used, they must be approved by the Department of Anesthesiology and the medical staff
- Discharge criteria may vary based on the destination of the patient when leaving the PACU
- In the absence of the responsible physician, the PACU nurse may determine that the patient meets the discharge criteria, and record the name of the responsible physician on the record.

Based on *Standards for postanesthesia*, 1994, of the American Society of Anesthesiologists.

Box 30-4   Basic Standards for Preanesthesia Care

Date published: 1987
Organization: American Society of Anesthesiologists
Purpose: To establish standards of preanesthesia care for anesthesiologists
Summary:
- Standards apply to all patients who receive anesthesia or monitored anesthesia care
- If modified for circumstance, documentation should be made in anesthesia record

STANDARD I

An anesthesiologist shall be responsible for determining the medical status of the patient, developing a plan of anesthesia care, and acquainting the patient or the responsible adult with the proposed plan, which includes:
- Reviewing the medical record
- Interviewing the patient, discussing the medical history, previous anesthesia, and drug history
- Assessing the physical conditions of the patient that have an impact on care
- Obtaining or reviewing necessary tests
- Prescribing necessary preoperative medications
- Verifying that the above has been properly performed and documented

Based on *Basic standards for preanesthesia care*, 1987, of the American Society of Anesthesiologists.

Box 30-5 Practice Advisory for Preanesthesia Evaluation

Year published or revised: 2001

Organization: American Society of Anesthesiologists

Purpose: To survey current evidence, provide a standard reference, and stimulate research in preanesthesia evaluation

The following consensus findings were rendered by the task force preparing these guidelines:

- A preanesthesia review of the patient's history, patient interview, and pertinent physical examination is an essential component of good anesthetic practice.
- In general, patients with more severe disease and/or those having more complex procedures should be evaluated prior to the day of surgery
- A minimal preanesthetic physical examination should include an airway examination and an evaluation of the cardiovascular and pulmonary systems
- If a full examination in advance of the date of surgery is not practicable, the surgical scheduling system should at least make the anesthesiologist aware of the severity of patient illness and the invasiveness and complexity of the planned procedure.

Substantial attention continues to be given regarding the necessity for preoperative testing, and what conditions should trigger what specific tests. These guidelines support the following conclusions:

- **Electrocardiography (ECG)**: Recommended for patients with known cardiac risk factors. The validity of performing an ECG on all patients over a certain age was not supported in these guidelines
- Tests such as stress ECG, echocardiogram, radionuclide scanning, etc., are not supported for routine testing and should be reserved for patients with specific indications or specific procedures
- **Chest radiograph**: The guidelines support chest radiography for patients with pulmonary disease, but neither routine nor age-based testing was supported
- Such testing as spirometry or arterial blood gas determinations should be reserved for indicated patients and procedures
- **Hemoglobin/hematocrit determination**: Routine determination is not supported. Specific patient factors such as known anemia, coagulopathy, or hematologic disorders should trigger testing
- **Coagulation studies**: Known coagulopathy or disease of the blood and coagulation element forming organs should trigger coagulation studies. Routine coagulation studies were specifically not recommended for patients anticipating major regional/neuraxial blocks
- **Urinalysis**: Should be performed only with suspected disease or urinary tract symptoms
- **Pregnancy testing**: May be considered but is not considered necessary, for all females of childbearing age. Uncertain pregnancy history or a history of a current pregnancy should trigger testing
- **Timing**: Absent a material change in the patient's medical condition or history, values for laboratory and other testing obtained within the 6 months prior to surgery are probably sufficient.

Based on *Practice advisory for preanesthesia evaluation*, 2001, of the American Society of Anesthesiologists.

Box 30-6 Practice Guidelines on Acute Pain Management in the Perioperative Setting

Year published or revised: 1995

Organization: American Society of Anesthesiologists

Purpose: To facilitate efficient and safe pain management in the perioperative period and reduce the risk of adverse outcomes.

These guidelines encompass broad principles for the address of problems incident to the management of perioperative pain. They are divided into 12 sections, which address the following areas:

- The need for proactive planning
- The need for education and training of hospital personnel, patients, and families
- Proper assessment and documentation of perioperative pain management
- The use of standardized institutional policies and procedures for ordering, administering, discontinuing, and transferring responsibility for perioperative pain management
- Strong support for the use of patient controlled analgesia (PCA), epidural analgesia, and regional analgesia, and/or the use of a multimodal approach
- Interdisciplinary activities involving nurses, surgeons, and pharmacists
- Recognition of the special features of pediatric, geriatric, and ambulatory pain management.

Based on *Practice guidelines for acute pain management in the perioperative setting*, 1995, of the American Society of Anesthesiologists.

Box 30-7   Practice Guidelines for Chronic Pain Management

Year published or revised: 1997

Organization: American Society of Anesthesiologists

Purpose: To optimize pain control, enhance functional ability and physical and psychological wellbeing, and enhance the quality of life for patients with chronic pain while minimizing adverse outcomes and costs.

Recommendations:

The following fundamental issues should be assessed in a chronic pain patient:

- The patient's general medical condition and current medical and surgical diagnoses
- The presence of chronic pain syndromes
- The diagnosis and management of painful crises
- The diagnosis and management of emergencies and complications from the cause or treatment.

The following elements should be incorporated into a comprehensive evaluation and treatment plan:

- **History**: Characterization of the pain with respect to onset, quality, intensity, distribution, duration, course, affective components, exacerbating and relieving factors, previous tests and therapy, and current therapy
- **Physical examination**: Appropriate, directed neurologic and musculoskeletal evaluation and other systems as indicated, with attention to both causes and effects of the pain.
- **Psychosocial evaluation**: Presence of psychological symptoms, psychiatric disorders, personality, coping mechanisms, and the meaning of pain to the patient, involvement and expectation of family, work, or legal issues, involvement of outside agencies in payment and/or rehabilitation efforts
- **Impression and differential diagnosis**: Possible etiologies and effects of the pain
- **Treatment plan**: Should be formulated using the working diagnosis and involving the patient, other professionals, family, and/or significant others, and expected outcomes discussed with the patient.

The guidelines address use of the following general or specific diagnostic or therapeutic modalities:

- **Diagnostic evaluation**: Use of neural blockade, imaging, pharmacodiagnosis, electrodiagnosis, and laboratory studies
- **Counseling and coordination of care**: Appropriate counseling should be provided to the patient regarding the diagnosis, treatment, rehabilitation, and follow-up goals, with coordination of care
- **Monitoring and measurement of clinical outcomes**: Maintenance of complete records of therapy and results at appropriate intervals, and analysis of aggregate outcomes for quality improvement purposes
- The concept of multidisciplinary pain management is supported
- Multimodal pain management should be considered
- Use of adjuvant analgesics is supported
- Regional sympathetic blockade
- Corticosteroid injection
- **Neurostimulation therapy**: Transcutaneous electrical nerve stimulation and spinal cord stimulation at appropriate levels of difficulty in management
- **Opioid therapy**: Oral or neuraxial opioid therapy can be very effective, but can be fraught with difficulties; the use of a written agreement or evaluation from a second practitioner is to be considered
- **Neuroablative techniques**: Used as a last resort.

Based on *Practice guidelines for chronic pain management*, 1997, of the American Society of Anesthesiologists.

Box 30-8   Practice Guidelines for Cancer Pain Management

Year published or revised: 1996

Organization: American Society of Anesthesiologists

Purpose: To optimize cancer pain control and enhance function, well being, and quality of life while minimizing side effects, adverse outcomes and cost

Recommendations:

General requirements for the cancer pain practitioner

- Assess general medical condition and extent of disease
- Acquire a knowledge of common pain syndromes
- Acquire a knowledge of oncologic emergencies
- Acquire a knowledge of the management of painful crises

Continued

Box 30-8 Practice Guidelines for Cancer Pain Management—cont'd

Conduct a comprehensive evaluation and develop a treatment plan consisting of the following six features:
- A complete history including a careful characterization of the pain
- A psychological evaluation including pre-existing psychological or psychiatric disorders, mood, coping mechanisms and family function, support systems, and patient expectations
- A physical examination including general medical, neurologic, and focused examination of the pain area
- Impression and initial diagnosis
- Further diagnostic evaluations indicated
- Treatment plan, including expected outcome, contingencies, and reassessment

Conduct longitudinal monitoring of pain using three concepts:
- Patient self-report: the primary source of ongoing pain assessment
- Use of a rating scale
- Use of regular intervals for reporting pain and any changes. Frequency may need to be increased if new pain, change in pain or new interventions are done

Multidisciplinary management: Encouraged, should also involve patient's primary physician

Paradigm for cancer pain management: The continuum from indirect drug delivery to direct drug delivery. Use the World Health Organization analgesic ladder:
- Begin with oral systemic analgesia, first using acetaminophen, salicylates, or other nonsteroidal anti-inflammatory drugs (NSAIDs) for mild to early moderate pain
- Add oral opioids when pain is consistently moderate, maintaining awareness of acetaminophen and NSAID toxicity
- Use rectal and transdermal routes when oral is inappropriate
- Progress to subcutaneous and intravenous routes when previous are ineffective or impractical
- Use an individualized regimen, increasing dosage until effect occurs or adverse effects occur
- Give medications "around-the-clock" rather than prn, with additional doses for breakthrough pain
- When tolerance develops, consider substituting another opioid at a lower equianalgesic dose, since cross-tolerance is incomplete
- Use adjuvants as coanalgesics when indicated
- Consider progressing to direct delivery systems (neuraxial and neuroablative) when dose-limiting toxicity prevents effective therapy
- Neuraxial delivery is effective but requires cognizant patients and a logistical support system
- Neuroablative procedures are generally the last modality to use
- Use local anesthetic neural blockade as a diagnostic tool to predict neuroablative effectiveness.

Management of cancer-related symptoms and adverse effects
- Promptly identify, assess, and treat adverse effects (e.g., constipation, sedation, nausea/vomiting, myoclonus, pruritus, urinary retention, and respiratory depression
- Recognize, assess, and manage psychosocial factors of cancer pain
- Incorporate multidisciplinary management (e.g., hospice services) to facilitate home parenteral therapy and subsequent end-of-life care
- Recognize and give special attention to pediatric cancer pain management

Based on *Practice guidelines for cancer pain management*, 1996, of the American Society of Anesthesiologists.

Box 30-9 Practice Guidelines for Blood Component Therapy

Year published or revised: 1996

Organization: American Society of Anesthesiologists

Purpose: To provide evidence-based guidelines on the proper indications for administration of red blood cells (RBCs), platelets, fresh frozen plasma (FFP), and cryoprecipitate

Recommendations:

Transfusion of homologous red blood cells:
- Is rarely indicated for hemoglobin (Hg) concentrations greater than 10 g/dL, and almost always indicated for Hg of less than 6 g/dL
- In the interval between 6 and 10 g/dL Hg, transfusion is based on the patient's risk for complications of inadequate oxygenation

Continued

Box 30-9 Practice Guidelines for Blood Component Therapy—con'd

- Should not be based on a single "trigger" Hg concentration applicable to all patients
- Should be preceded by the use, whenever possible, of other measures such as preoperative autologous blood donation, intraoperative and postoperative blood recovery, acute normovolemic hemodilution, and measures to decrease blood loss (deliberate hypotension and pharmacologic agents)
- May have more stringent indications than those associated with autologous RBC transfusion, although autologous RBC transfusion is not without risk.

Transfusion of platelets:

- Is ineffective as a prophylactic measure and is rarely indicated when thrombocytopenia is due to increased platelet destruction
- May be indicated as a prophylactic measure or in surgical and obstetric patients with microvascular bleeding when the platelet count is less than 50,000/mm³, but is rarely indicated when the platelet count is greater than 100,000/mm³. Transfusion of platelets in the intermediate group (i.e., between 50,000 and 100,000/mm³) should be based on the risk of bleeding
- Vaginal deliveries or surgical procedures associated with insignificant blood loss may be undertaken in patients with platelet counts less than 50,000/mm³
- May be indicated despite adequate platelet numbers if there is known platelet dysfunction and microvascular bleeding.

Transfusion of FFP is recommended:

- For urgent reversal of warfarin therapy (usually requires 5–8 ml/kg of FFP)
- For correction of known coagulation factor deficiencies when specific factor concentrates are not available
- For correction of microvascular bleeding when the prothrombin time (PT) or partial thromboplastin time (PTT) is elevated greater than 1.5 times normal or when patients have been transfused more than one blood volume and PT/PTT is not available in a timely fashion
- To be given in doses to achieve at least 30% of normal plasma factor concentration (usually 10–15 ml/kg of FFP)
- For equivalence purposes, to 4–5 platelet concentrates, 1 unit of apheresis platelets, or 1 unit of whole blood (despite decreased but still hemostatic factor V and VIII in whole blood)
- Not for augmentation of plasma volume or albumin concentration.

Transfusion of cryoprecipitate is recommended:

- For prophylaxis in patients with congenital fibrinogen deficiencies or von Willebrand's disease unresponsive to 1-desamino-8-D-arginine vasopressin (DDAVP)
- For bleeding patients with von Willebrand's disease
- For correction of microvascular bleeding in massively transfused patients with fibrinogen concentrations less than 80–100 mg/dL or when fibrinogen assay is delayed.

Based on *Practice guidelines for blood component therapy*, 1996, of the American Society of Anesthesiologists.

Box 30-10 Practice Guidelines for Management of the Difficult Airway

Year published or revised: 2002
Organization: American Society of Anesthesiologists
Purpose: To facilitate management of the difficult airway and reduce adverse outcomes.
Recommendations:
Conduct an airway history; review of previous airway management is valuable
Conduct a multiple airway feature assessment (Box 30-11).
Conduct additional airway diagnostic testing if indicated
Prepare for encountering a difficult airway:

- Become familiar with the difficult airway algorithm (Figure 30-1)
- Inform the patient of risks and special procedures necessary
- Arrange for additional assistance during intubation
- Preoxygenate patient using 3 minutes of oxygen or four maximal breaths

---

Box 30-10   Practice Guidelines for Management of the Difficult Airway—cont'd

- Have a preplanned strategy for the management sequence, to include awareness of four basic problems that could occur:
  - Difficult ventilation
  - Difficult intubation
  - Difficulty with patient cooperation or consent
  - Difficult tracheostomy
- Consider relative merits of three basic strategies:
  - Whether to perform awake versus postinduction intubation
  - Whether to go directly to invasive techniques (surgical airway) or attempt a noninvasive airway
  - Whether to preserve spontaneous ventilation or use muscle relaxation
- Identify preferred methods of approach to:
  - Awake intubation
  - The patient who can be ventilated but not intubated
  - The patient who can neither be ventilated nor intubated
- Identify alternative methods of approach:
  - Management of the pediatric or uncooperative patient
  - Risk of use of regional or local techniques to attempt to obviate need for airway management
- Have available a means of end-tidal CO_2 measurement
- Formulate an extubation strategy for the patient who was difficult to intubate
  - Consider the merits of awake versus "deep" extubation
  - Enumerate factors affecting ventilatory drive or ability after extubation
  - Make provision for reintubation if necessary
  - Consider leaving some type of obturator in the trachea until the risk for reintubation has passed

Perform follow-up management:
- Describe airway management difficulties encountered
- Enumerate which devices were successful in maintaining ventilation or facilitating intubation
- Inform the patient and offer means of perpetuating this information (e.g., chart flags, Medic-Alert™ bracelet)
- Follow up patient clinically for complications related to difficult airway management

These guidelines further specify the suggested contents of a portable difficult airway management storage unit, enumerate the various useful ventilation and intubation devices and techniques, and summarize the existing literature supporting the use of many of these devices.

From *Practice guidelines for the management of the difficult airway*, 2002, of the American Society of Anesthesiologists. Anesthesiology 2003; 5:1269–1277.

Box 30-11   Airway Examination Component Nonreassuring Findings

Length of upper incisors: Relatively long
Relationship of maxilla and mandible: Prominent "overbite" (maxillary incisors during normal jaw closure – anterior to mandibular incisors)
Relationship of maxillary and mandibular incisors: Patient cannot bring incisors, during voluntary protrusion of mandibular incisors, anterior to maxillary incisors
Interincisor distance: Less than 3 cm
Visibility of uvula: Not visible when tongue is protruded with patient in sitting position (i.e., Mallampati class greater than II)
Shape of palate: Highly arched or very narrow
Compliance of mandibular space: Stiff, indurated, occupied by mass, or nonresilient
Thyromental distance: Less than 3 ordinary finger-breadths
Length of neck: Short
Thickness of neck: Thick
Range of motion of head and neck: Patient cannot touch tip of chin to chest, or cannot extend neck

From *Practice guidelines for the management of the difficult airway*, 2002, of the American Society of Anesthesiologists. *Anesthesiology* 2003;98:1273.

DIFFICULT AIRWAY ALGORITHM

1. Assess the likelihood and clinical impact of basic management problems:

    A. Difficult Ventilation
    B. Difficult Intubation
    C. Difficulty with Patient Cooperation or Consent
    D. Difficult Tracheostomy

2. Actively pursue opportunities to deliver supplemental oxygen throughout the process of difficult airway management.

3. Consider the relative merits and feasibility of basic management choices:

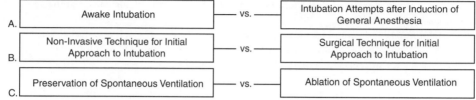

4. Develop primary and alternative strategies:

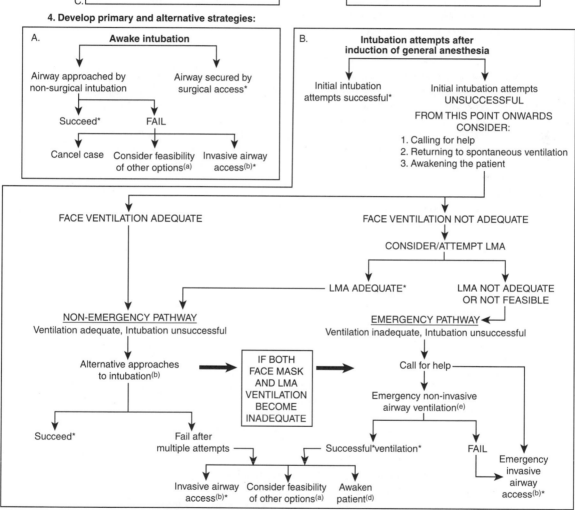

* Confirm tracheal intubation or LMA placement with exhaled CO_2

a. Other options include (but are not limited to): surgery utilizing face mask or LMA anesthesia, local anesthesia infiltration or regional nerve blockade. Pursuit of these options usually implies that mask ventilation will not be problematic. Therefore, these options may be of limited value if this step in the algorithm has been reached via the Emergency Pathway.

b. Invasive airway access includes surgical or percutaneous tracheostomy or cricothyrotomy

c. Alternative non-invasive approaches to difficult intubation include (but are not limited to): use of different laryngoscope blades, LMA as an intubation conduit (with or without fiberoptic guidance), fiberoptic intubation, intubating stylet or tube changer, light wand, retrograde intubation, and blind oral or nasal intubation

d. Consider re-preparation of the patient for awake intubation or canceling surgery.

e. Options for emergency non-invasive airway ventilation include (but are not limited to): rigid bronchoscope, esophageal-tracheal combitube ventilation, or transtracheal jet ventilation.

Figure 30-1   The difficult airway algorithm. LMA, laryngeal mask airway. (Redrawn from *Practice guidelines for the management of the difficult airway*, American Society of Anesthesiologists, 2002. Anesthesiology 2003; 98(5):1273.)

Box 30-12 Practice Guidelines for Obstetrical Anesthesia

Year published or revised: 1998
Organization: American Society of Anesthesiologists
Purpose: To enhance the quality of obstetric care, reduce anesthesia complications, and increase patient satisfaction

GENERAL RECOMMENDATIONS

- A focused history and physical examination should be performed, including an airway examination, and inspection of the back if neuraxial analgesia is planned
- Platelet count is recommend for patients with pregnancy-induced hypertension but not as a routine
- Type and screen or cross-match should be reserved for patients at increased risk of hemorrhage
- Fetal heart rate monitoring should precede and follow placement of a regional anesthetic/analgesic but may not always be continuously required
- Clear liquids may be allowed during labor for the uncomplicated patient but at-risk patients or those with nonreassuring fetal heart rate pattern may require restriction on a case-by-case basis
- Solid foods should be avoided in laboring patients

SPECIFIC RECOMMENDATIONS

- Although pain and a maternal request for pain relief constitute sufficient indication for pain relief, the specific technique is dependent on the status of the patient, progress of labor, and anesthesia resources
- A low concentration local anesthetic combined with an opioid and administered via a continuous infusion may provide improved analgesia and minimal motor block for a labor epidural anesthetic
- Spinal opioids, with or without local anesthetic, may be used for effective, although time-limited labor analgesia, or may be combined with epidural anesthesia administration using the combined spinal epidural technique
- Regional analgesia should be administered when desired and not based on cervical dilation
- Anesthesiologists should be willing to provide monitored/standby care for complicated vaginal delivery
- Regional, general, or sedation/analgesia may be appropriate for removal of a retained placenta, but general anesthesia may be preferable in the patient who has sustained significant hemorrhage
- Nitroglycerin is effective for use as a uterine dilator for removal of a retained placenta
- As compared to general anesthesia, regional anesthesia for cesarean delivery is:
  - Associated with fewer maternal and neonatal complications and increased maternal satisfaction
  - Associated with a longer induction to delivery time
  - Associated with fewer maternal deaths
  - Associated with higher Apgar scores at 1 and 5 minutes
  - Associated with occasional hypotension, nausea, vomiting, pruritus, and postdural puncture headache
- Choice of anesthesia for cesarean section should be individualized and based on obstetric indications and the mutual preferences of patient and anesthesiologist
  - With respect to postpartum tubal ligation (PPTL), the patient:
  - Should be re-evaluated post-partum for blood loss or other risks
  - Should be made NPO during labor if PPTL is planned within 8 hours of delivery
  - May have a higher risk of failure of the epidural catheter if longer delivery–PPTL times are employed
  - Should not be scheduled at a time that their surgery would compromise the delivery of obstetric care
  - May receive spinal, epidural, or general anesthesia based on individualized considerations, risk factors, and patient and anesthesiologist preference
- Institutions providing obstetric care should have resources to manage hemorrhage
- Labor and delivery units should have equipment and personnel available to manage airway emergencies, and difficult airway management equipment should be available in the obstetric operating area
- Performance of invasive hemodynamic monitoring (arterial, central venous, or pulmonary artery) should be based on clinical indications and may not be available in all obstetric units
- Regarding cardiopulmonary resuscitation:
  - Basic and advanced life support equipment and supplies should be available in obstetric areas
  - Standard resuscitative measures, but including left uterine displacement, should be employed in the case of cardiac arrest during labor
  - Several American Heart Association contributors suggest that the decision to perform a perimortem cesarean section should be made rapidly, with delivery accomplished within 4–5 minutes of the arrest

Based on *Practice guidelines for obstetrical anesthesia*, 1998, of the American Society of Anesthesiologists.

Box 30-13 Practice Guidelines for Perioperative Transesophageal Echocardiography

Year published or revised: 1996
Organization: American Society of Anesthesiologists
Purpose: To provide recommendations for the indications for use of perioperative transesophageal echocardiography (PTEE) and the proficiency necessary in the anesthesiologist performing PTEE
Recommendations:

Category I indications are supported by the strongest evidence or opinion (PTEE indicated); category II is supported by weaker evidence (PTEE useful); and category III by little scientific evidence or expert support.

CATEGORY I INDICATIONS

- Acute, life-threatening hemodynamic dysfunction and left ventricular function unresponsive to treatment
- Valve repair
- Most congenital heart surgery requiring cardiopulmonary bypass (CPB)
- Hypertrophic obstructive cardiomyopathy repair
- Emergency detection of thoracic aortic dissection or trauma in the unstable patient
- Patients undergoing pericardial window procedures to evaluate adequacy of treatment
- Diagnosis of unexplained hemodynamic disturbances, suspected valvular disease, or thromboembolic disease in critically ill patients

CATEGORY II INDICATIONS

- When there is an increased risk of myocardial ischemia or infarction
- When there is an increased risk for intraoperative hemodynamic problems for the patient or the procedure
- Assessing surgical repair of cardiac aneurysm
- Removal of cardiac masses
- Detection of foreign bodies
- Detection of air emboli during cardiotomy, heart transplant surgery, and upright neurosurgical procedures
- Use prior to CPB for intracardiac thrombectomy
- Diagnosis of cardiac trauma
- Evaluating potential anastomotic sites during heart–lung transplantation
- Detection of pericardial effusion or evaluation of the effectiveness of pericardiectomy
- Detection of suspected thoracic aortic aneurysm dissection, trauma, or atheromatous disease
- Monitoring the placement and function of cardiac assist devices

CATEGORY III INDICATIONS

- Use to evaluate perfusion, coronary artery anatomy, or graft patency
- Evaluation of cardiomyopathies other than hypertrophic obstructive cardiomyopathy
- Evaluation of endocarditis in patients undergoing noncardiac surgery
- Evaluation of pleuropulmonary diseases
- Monitoring the placement of balloon pumps, implantable cardiac defibrillators, or pulmonary artery catheters
- Monitoring the administration of cardioplegia solution

Procedures requiring an anesthesiologist with advanced TEE training to perform or confirm the findings of a basically trained TEE operator include:

- Detection of subtle changes in segmental wall motion or thickening
- Assessing valve function when surgery will be dictated by TEE
- Quantitative measurements of valve function when surgery will be dictated by TEE
- Interpretation of congenital heart lesions
- Interpretation of cardiac aneurysms when surgery will be dictated by TEE
- Interpretation of endocarditic disease when surgery will be dictated by TEE
- Detection of small or ill-defined cardiac masses
- Accurate detection of intracardiac foreign bodies
- Diagnosis of pulmonary emboli or monitoring of embolectomy or pulmonary thrombolysis
- Detection of traumatic cardiac injuries
- Diagnosis of thoracic aortic dissection or trauma

Continued

Box 30-13   Practice Guidelines for Perioperative Transesophageal Echocardiography—cont'd

- Detection of pericardial effusions, surgical guidance, and evaluation of the effectiveness of pericardiectomy
- Evaluation of the surgical results of heart transplant surgery
- Monitoring the placement and function of cardiac assist devices
- Use in nonoperative critical care situations
  Procedures that should be safely accomplished by the anesthesiologist with basic TEE training include:
- Recognition of clear changes in wall thickness and motion and distinction of them from artifact
- Ability to make qualitative assessments of hemodynamic status
- Ability to obtain multiple views of all valves, recognize gross valvular dysfunction, interpret Doppler findings, diagnose causes of hemodynamic disturbances, detect air emboli, and detect large pericardial effusions
- Recognition of large, unequivocal cardiac masses

Based on *Practice guidelines for perioperative transesophageal echocardiography (PTEE)*, 1996, of the American Society of Anesthesiologists.

Box 30-14   Practice Guidelines for Postanesthetic Care

Year published or revised: 2001
Organization: American Society of Anesthesiologists
Purpose: To improve postanesthetic care outcomes.
Recommendation:

MONITORING AND ASSESSMENT

- Periodic assessment of airway patency, respiratory rate, and oxygenation saturation
- Routine monitoring of pulse and blood pressure, with electrocardiographic monitoring immediately available
- Assessment of neuromuscular function and mental status during both emergence and recovery
- Periodic assessment of patient temperature, pain, nausea, and vomiting
- Assessment of postoperative fluid management and management according to surgical loss
- Case-by-case assessment of urine output and voiding ability for selected patients
- Assessment of drainage and bleeding

TREATMENT MODALITIES

- Antiemetic agents and metoclopramide or the combination should be used for the prevention or treatment of nausea and vomiting when indicated
- Oxygen should be administered during transportation to and in the postanesthetic area when the risk of hypoxia is present
- Normothermia should be a goal during emergence and recovery, and forced air warming is recommended for treatment of hypothermia
- Meperidine is indicated for shivering but other opioids or antagonists may be used
- Flumazenil and naloxone should be available, used when indicated but not routinely, and patients should be observed for a sufficient time following their use for secondary cardiorespiratory depression, maintaining awareness for the risks of acute complete antagonism of opioids
- Neuromuscular block antagonists should be administered when residual blockade is present
The guidelines recommend the following regarding discharge criteria:
- A requirement for voluntary voiding should not be a routine discharge criterion
- Drinking and retaining clear fluids should not be a routine discharge criterion
- Patients should be routinely required to have a responsible individual accompany them home
- Patients should be observed until they are no longer at risk for cardiorespiratory depression, but there should be no mandatory minimum postanesthesia stay

Based on *Practice guidelines for postanesthetic care*, 2001, of the American Society of Anesthesiologists.

Box 30-15 Practice Guidelines for Preoperative Fasting and the Use of Pharmacologic Agents to Reduce the Risk of Pulmonary Aspiration: Application to Healthy Patients Undergoing Elective Procedures

Year published or revised: 1999
Organization: American Society of Anesthesiologists
Purpose: To provide preoperative fasting recommendations and suggestions for administration of pharmacologic agents for modifying gastric volume and pH.
Recommendations:
(These guidelines do not address or apply to:
- Procedures where upper airway protective reflexes are not impaired
- Women in labor
- Patients with coexisting diseases or in whom airway management might be difficult)
Pertinent history and physical examination is important
- **2-hour fast**: Clear liquids (include waters, fruit juice without pulp, carbonated beverages, clear tea and black coffee; no alcohol)
- **4-hour fast**: Breast milk (neonates and infants)
- **6-hour fast**: Infant formula, nonhuman milk, light meal (i.e., toast and clear liquid)
- **8-hour fast**: Fried or fatty foods, meat
Although agents such as gastrointestinal stimulants, H_2-receptor antagonists, proton pump inhibitors, and antacids may decrease gastric pH and volume, none are recommended for *routine* use in the patient not at risk for aspiration
Anticholinergics are not recommended in any circumstance

Based on *Practice guidelines for preoperative fasting and the use of pharmacologic agents to reduce the risk of pulmonary aspiration: application to healthy patients undergoing elective procedures*, 1999, of the American Society of Anesthesiologists.

Box 30-16 Practice Guidelines for Pulmonary Artery Catheterization

Year published or revised: 2002
Organization: American Society of Anesthesiologists
Purpose: To establish appropriate indications for pulmonary artery catheterization (PAC)
Subjects addressed:
- **Effect on treatment decisions**: Although therapy is often changed, there is no association with mortality on patients whose therapy is altered based on information received from PAC
- **Preoperative catheterization**: No good data have shown that routine or selective preoperative PAC improves outcome
- **Perioperative catheterization**: Extensive reviews of numerous studies were conducted by the task group, who paid specific and separate attention to cardiac, vascular, neurosurgical, trauma, obstetric-gynecologic, and pediatric patient groups. Two separate meta-analyses, one of 16 trials and one of 4 trials, yielded conflicting results
- **Harm**: A section outlines the type and incidence of complications, which are often catastrophic. Attempts to quantify the rate of iatrogenic death from PAC have been difficult because of the underlying severe illness affecting most patients in whom they are used
Collective expert opinion:
- Monitoring of selected surgical and obstetric patients can reduce the incidence of perioperative complications, when this immediately accessed data is accurately interpreted and used to guide appropriate treatment, and subsequently reduce perioperative morbidity and mortality
- The quality of data available from PAC is superior to central venous catheter (CVC) data, and preplacement of PAC is often preferable to emergency placement in hastily prepared situations, which results in a doubling of catheter-related sepsis.
- Experience in catheter placement, catheter interpretation, and nursing management is an important factor in the usefulness of PAC
- Although the risk of severe morbidity or death from PAC is reported to be between 1% and 5%, the task force's opinion is that this risk is appropriate and necessary is properly selected surgical patients. The risk is related to the health of the patient, the risk associated with the specific surgical procedure, and the practice setting.
Nonclinical issues surrounding the placement and use of PAC:
- Cost and cost/benefit ratio
- Provider competency and training
- Reimbursement

Continued

Box 30-16 Practice Guidelines for Pulmonary Artery Catheterization—cont'd

- Utilization review
- Medicolegal liability

Recommendations (addressed with reference to three venues: patient, procedure, and practice setting):

- Patient conditions warranting consideration for PAC might include significant cardiovascular or pulmonary disease, hypoxia, renal insufficiency, or other hemodynamically unstable conditions. It emphasized that the assessment necessary to arrive at a decision must be based on a thorough analysis of the medical history and physical examinations findings rather than exclusive consideration of specific laboratory or other findings
- When a surgical procedure has a known increased risk of complications from hemodynamic changes, including potential damage to vital organs, patients may benefit from PAC. There are no specific procedures enumerated, however. Special circumstances may warrant exception
- The skill of both the inserting physician, ability to interpret data, and nursing and ancillary support capabilities should enter into the decision to employ PAC. Consideration should be given to the availability of specialists, facilities, and equipment that could manage complications detected by PAC. Multiple opinions are cited regarding the necessity for initial and recurring experience with PAC, with estimates of 25–50 catheterizations to obtain initial competency and 12–50 per year to maintain that competency

Based on *Practice guidelines for pulmonary artery catheterization (PAC)*, 2001, of the American Society of Anesthesiologists.

Box 30-17 Practice Guidelines for Sedation and Analgesia by Non-anesthesiologists

See Table 30-1 for definition of terms.
Year published or revised: 2001
Organization: American Society of Anesthesiologists
Purpose: To allow clinicians to safely provide their patients with the benefits of sedation and analgesia
Recommendations:

PATIENT EVALUATION AND PREPARATION

Includes:

- Major organ system abnormalities
- History of difficulty with anesthesia or sedation
- Pertinent allergies, medication, and potential drug interactions
- Recent oral intake
- Alcohol, tobacco, and recreational drug history
- Pertinent history and physical finding (vital signs, cardiopulmonary, and airway examinations)
- Patient counseling of risks, benefits, and alternatives improves satisfaction
- Preprocedure fasting improves safety

MONITORING OF LEVEL OF CONSCIOUSNESS, VITAL SIGNS, AND VENTILATION/OXYGENATION

- Response to spoken words, tactile, and painful stimuli is the best means of assessing consciousness
- Monitoring of ventilatory function by observation, auscultation, and qualitative capnography is useful
- Pulse oximetry is of major monitoring and predictive value in any patient receiving sedation/analgesia
- Regular monitoring of heart rate and blood pressure should be employed for moderate and deep sedation
- Electrocardiographic monitoring reduces risk in deep sedation

RECORDING OF MONITORED PARAMETERS

- Level of consciousness, ventilatory function, oxygenation and vital signs should be recorded
- Should be at least recorded preprocedure, after administration of agents, at regular intervals, during initial recovery, and just prior to discharge

INDIVIDUAL RESPONSIBLE FOR PATIENT MONITORING

- Should have an additional individual available for monitoring for moderate and deep sedative procedures
- During moderate sedation, this person may have other interruptible duties
- During deep sedation, this person should have no other duties

Continued

Box 30-17 Practice Guidelines for Sedation and Analgesia by Non-anesthesiologists—cont'd

- Monitoring individual should be trained in the recognition of sedation/analgesia complications
- Moderate sedation requires the immediate presence of a basic life support qualified person, and the immediate availability of an individual with advanced life support skills
- Deep sedation requires the constant attendance of a person with advanced life support skills

EQUIPMENT AND DRUGS

- All equipment required under "Monitoring"
- Defibrillator for moderate sedation of patients with cardiac disease and all deep sedation patients
- Pharmacologic reversal agents, advanced life support drugs, airway equipment and supplies
- Oxygen should be considered for moderate sedation and used for deep sedation

THERAPEUTIC REGIMENS FOR SEDATION/ANALGESIA

- Combination therapy is acceptable and preferable to fixed combinations
- Titration of intravenous agents is recommended over a single large bolus dose
- Use of anesthetic induction agents carries increased risk for inadvertent general anesthesia, does not allow for pharmacologic reversal, but may be associated with an increase in satisfactory deep sedation
- Patients receiving induction agents should be given care at the deep sedation level
- Continuous intravenous access until sedation/analgesia has abated increases satisfaction and safety
- Reversal agents should be reserved for specific indications
- Treatment of respiratory depression should be with stimulation, oxygen, and positive pressure ventilation

POSTPROCEDURE CARE

- Discharge criteria specific to the procedure and sedative regimen are likely to decrease complications
- Patients who have received sedation should be observed until their level of consciousness is near baseline

SPECIAL SITUATIONS

- Patients presenting special risks should be given special consideration, including consultation by a specialist appropriate to their disease or an anesthesiologist
- Consideration should be given to having an anesthesiologist present or available when performing moderate or – especially – deep sedation.

From *Practice guidelines for sedation and analgesia by non-anesthesiologists*, 2001, of the American Society of Anesthesiologists. *Anesthesiology* 2003; 96:1004–1017.

Table 30-1 Definition of General Anesthesia and Levels of Sedation/Analgesia

	Minimal Sedation (Anxiolysis)	Moderate Sedation/ Analgesia	Deep Sedation/ Analgesia	General Anesthesia
Responsiveness	Normal response to verbal stimulation	Purposeful response to verbal or tactile stimulation	Purposeful response following repeated or painful stimulation	Unarousable even with painful stimulus
Airway	Unaffected	No intervention required	Intervention may be required	Intervention often required
Spontaneous ventilation	Unaffected	Adequate	May be inadequate	Frequently inadequate
Cardiovascular function	Unaffected	Usually maintained	Usually maintained	May be impaired

Description of states:
Minimal sedation (anxiolysis): Normal response to verbal commands, no impairment of ventilatory and cardiovascular function
Moderate sedation/analgesia ("conscious sedation"): Depressed consciousness but purposeful response to verbal commands, with or without light tactile stimulation, no ventilatory impairment and cardiovascular function usually maintained
Deep sedation/analgesia: Patients not easily aroused but will respond purposefully to repeated or painful stimulation, possibly impaired spontaneous ventilation or ability to maintain patient airway, but cardiovascular function still usually maintained
General anesthesia: Loss of consciousness, no arousal to painful stimulation, frequent impairment of spontaneous ventilation or patent airway; may require positive pressure ventilation. Cardiovascular function may be impaired
Practitioners intending to produce a given level of sedation should have training, equipment, and equipment available to "rescue" patients whose level becomes greater than intended.

Box 30-18   Practice Advisory for the Prevention of Perioperative Peripheral Neuropathies

Year published or revised: 2000

Organization: American Society of Anesthesiologists

Purpose: This practice advisory provides suggested practices for positioning of the adult patient, use of protective padding, and avoidance of contact with hard surfaces or supports.

Recommendations:

- <90° abduction of the arms in supine patients (prone patients may tolerate >90°)
- Decreased pressure on the ulnar groove
- Neutral positioning of the tucked forearm, and
- Neutral or supine positioning of the abducted arm

Pressure on the spiral groove of the humerus should be avoided and it may be helpful to slightly flex the elbow to prevent stretching of the medial nerve

The lower extremity should be monitored for absence of stretch of the hamstrings (to avoid stretch on the sciatic nerve) and absence of pressure on the peroneal nerve at the head of the fibula

The hip may be positioned in flexion or extension without increased risk to the femoral nerve

The use of padded armboards, chest rolls for laterally positioned patients, and elbow and fibular head padding may decrease the risk of neuropathy

Caution should be exercised for properly functioning noninvasive blood pressure cuffs and in the use of shoulder braces for steep head-down positions. Simple postoperative assessment for extremity function is useful, and good documentation of positioning is important

Based on *Practice advisory for the prevention of perioperative peripheral neuropathy*, 2001, of the American Society of Anesthesiologists.

Box 30-19   ACC/AHA Guideline Update for Perioperative Cardiovascular Evaluation for Noncardiac Surgery – Executive Summary

Date published: 2002 (available online from http://www.acc.org/clinical/guidelines/perio/update/periupdate_index.htm)

Organizations: American College of Cardiology and American Heart Association

Purpose: To provide a consensus document outlining the appropriate indications and studies for patients with cardiac disease undergoing noncardiac surgery.

Recommendations: Strength of recommendations is divided into classes I, II, and III. Class I procedures/agents are considered to be useful and effective; class II exhibit conflicting evidence, and are divided into class IIa, in which the opinion is in favor and class IIb in which the usefulness or efficacy is less well established; and class III procedures are not useful or effective and may be harmful. Not all procedures/agents are so classified.

PREOPERATIVE EVALUATION

- History, physical examination and electrocardiogram (ECG)
- Identification of cardiac disorders: prior myocardial infarction, angina, heart failure, symptomatic arrhythmias, pacemaker or implantable cardioverter defibrillator, orthostatic intolerance, anemia
- Definition of disease severity, stability, and prior treatment
- Other factors including functional capacity, age, comorbidities (diabetes, peripheral vascular disease, renal dysfunction, chronic pulmonary disease), and type of surgical procedure
- Classification of major clinical predictors (Box 30-20)
- Evaluation of functional capacity in metabolic equivalents (METs) ranging from 1 MET for light activities to 4 METs for climbing a flight of stairs to 10 METs for strenuous exercise
- Evaluation of surgery specific risk (Figure 30-2)
- Cardiac risk stratification for noncardiac procedures (Box 30-21)

PREOPERATIVE MANAGEMENT OF SPECIFIC CARDIOVASCULAR CONDITIONS

Hypertension

- Control systolic and diastolic blood pressure <180 and <110 mmHg respectively.

Valvular Heart Disease

- Symptomatic stenotic lesions may require invasive intervention prior to noncardiac surgery
- Symptomatic regurgitant lesions better tolerated and may be medically stabilized preoperatively and repaired later
- Severe regurgitant lesions may require preoperative intervention

Continued

Box 30-19   ACC/AHA Guideline Update for Perioperative Cardiovascular Evaluation for Noncardiac Surgery – Executive Summary—cont'd

Myocardial Disease
- Dilated and hypertrophic cardiomyopathy associated with perioperative heart failure; preoperative hemodynamic status should be maximized with intensive postoperative medical therapy

Arrhythmias and Conduction Abnormalities
- Presence is reason for intense evaluation for etiology
- Therapy indicated for symptomatic or hemodynamically significant problems
- Antiarrhythmic therapy and cardiac pacing may be indicated
- Frequent premature ventricular contractions or asymptomatic nonsustained ventricular tachycardia not associated with increased risk of myocardial infarction or death in the perioperative period and aggressive therapy or monitoring not necessary

RECOMMENDATIONS FOR SUPPLEMENTAL PREOPERATIVE EVALUATIONS

Resting Left Ventricular Function
- Class I for poorly controlled heart failure
- Class IIa for prior heart failure and dyspnea of unknown origin
- Class III for routine evaluation

12-lead Electrocardiogram
- Class I for recent chest pain or ischemia in intermediate- or high-risk patients for intermediate- or high-risk operative procedures
- Class IIa for asymptomatic persons with diabetes mellitus
- Class IIb for patients with prior coronary artery bypass graft (CABG), asymptomatic males >45 years old or females >55 years old with two or more risk factors
- Class III for routine evaluations

Exercise or Pharmacological Stress Testing
- Class I for adults with intermediate pretest probability of coronary artery disease (CAD), prognostic assessment of suspected or proven CAD or significant change in clinical status, demonstration of proof of myocardial ischemia before CABG; evaluation of adequacy of medical therapy, or prognostic assessment after acute coronary syndrome
- Class IIa for evaluation of exercise capacity when subjective assessment unreliable
- Class IIb for diagnosis of CAD patients with high or low pretest probability (i.e., resting ST depression, 1 mm, digitalis therapy, or ECG criteria for left ventricular hypertrophy), detection or restenosis in high-risk asymptomatic patients after percutaneous coronary intervention (PCI)
- Class III for exercise stress testing of patients with resting ECG abnormalities that preclude adequate assessment, severe comorbidity likely to limit life expectancy or candidacy for CABG, routine screening, or investigation of isolated ectopy in young patients.

Coronary Angiography
- Class I for patients with suspected or known CAD
- Class IIa for multiple intermediate risk factors for vascular surgery, moderate or greater ischemia on noninvasive testing without high-risk features and low left ventricular ejection fraction, nondiagnostic noninvasive tests results in intermediate-risk patients undergoing high-risk surgery, urgent noncardiac surgery while convalescing from acute myocardial infarction
- Class IIb for perioperative myocardial infarction, stable class III or IV angina and planned low-risk or minor surgery
- Class III for low-risk surgery with known CAD and no high-risk results on noninvasive testing, asymptomatic post-CABG patients with 7 MET or greater tolerance, mild stable angina with good left ventricular function and no high-risk noninvasive test results, noncandidates for CABG secondary to medical illness, severe left ventricular dysfunction (e.g., left ventricular ejection fraction, <20%), or refusal to undergo CABG, or candidates for liver, lung or renal transplant, <40 years old unless other high-risk factors exist

CORONARY ARTERY BYPASS GRAFT OR PERCUTANEOUS CORONARY INTERVENTION PRIOR TO NONCARDIAC SURGERY

Coronary Artery Bypass Graft
- Indications for CABG are identical to those for CABG without impending noncardiac surgery
- Cardiac risk associated with noncardiac thoracic, abdominal, arterial, and head and neck surgery was reduced in patients with prior CABG
- Patients with prognostic high-risk coronary anatomy who would otherwise benefit from CABG should generally undergo CABG prior to noncardiac surgery of high or intermediate risk

Continued

Box 30-19   ACC/AHA Guideline Update for Perioperative Cardiovascular Evaluation for Noncardiac Surgery – Executive Summary—cont'd

Percutaneous Coronary Intervention
- No controlled trials comparing PCI with medical therapy prior to noncardiac surgery
- In general, indications for PCI prior to noncardiac surgery are the same as for PCI in the nonsurgical patient
- Delays of 1 week after balloon angioplasty or 2–4 weeks after coronary stenting seems appropriate to allow for vessel healing and re-endothelialization to occur

PERIOPERATIVE MEDICAL THERAPY
- Class I: Recent prior beta-blocker therapy to control angina, arrhythmias, or hypertension
  - Beta-blockers for patients at high cardiac risk from ischemia for vascular surgery
- Class IIa: Beta-blockers for hypertension, known CAD, or major risk factors for CAD
- Class IIb: Alpha-2-agonist for perioperative control of hypertension or known CAD or major risk factors for CAD
- Class III: Beta-blockers if contraindicated, alpha-2-agonists if contraindicated

ANESTHETIC CONSIDERATIONS AND INTRAOPERATIVE MANAGEMENT

Agents
- No one technique shown to be best for myocardial protection
- Consideration of all factors necessary in anesthesia choice

Perioperative Pain Management
- Patient controlled analgesia or epidural both effective
- Good pain management probably reduces catecholamine surges and hypercoagulability

Intraoperative Nitroglycerin
- Insufficient data to recommend prophylactic use
- Use as indicated in consideration of hemodynamic effects

Transesophageal Echocardiography
- Few data available
- Value for risk prediction is small
- ASA Guidelines explore in detail

Maintenance of Normothermia

PERIOPERATIVE SURVEILLANCE

Pulmonary Artery Catheters
- Three variables (disease severity, magnitude of surgery, and practice setting) have the greatest influence on the risk/benefit ratio of pulmonary artery catheterization
- Patients most likely to benefit are those with recent myocardial infarction with heart failure, significant CAD in procedures with increased hemodynamic stress, and those with systolic or diastolic left ventricular dysfunction, cardiomyopathy, and/or valvular disease undergoing high-risk procedures

Intraoperative and Postoperative ST-Segment Monitoring
- ST changes are strong predictors of perioperative myocardial infarction in patients at high risk having noncardiac surgery
- Postoperative ischemia is a good predictor of long-term risk of myocardial infarction and cardiac death
- ST depression in low-risk patients often not associated with wall motion abnormalities
- Intra-and postoperative ST segment analysis may improve detection of ischemia in properly selected patients

Surveillance for Perioperative Myocardial Infarction
- Optimum method not well studied
- Clinical symptoms, ECG changes, CK-MB, or troponin can be valuable
- Baseline, immediate postoperative, and 2-day postoperative ECG appears useful and cost-effective

POSTOPERATIVE AND LONG-TERM MANAGEMENT
- Despite best management, some patients will sustain perioperative myocardial infarction, which is associated with a 40–70% mortality
- Angioplasty should be considered
- Aspirin, beta-blockers, and angiotensin-converting enzyme inhibitors should be considered

From *ACC/AHA guideline update for perioperative cardiovascular evaluation for noncardiac surgery—executive summary*, 2002, American College of Cardiology and American Heart Association.

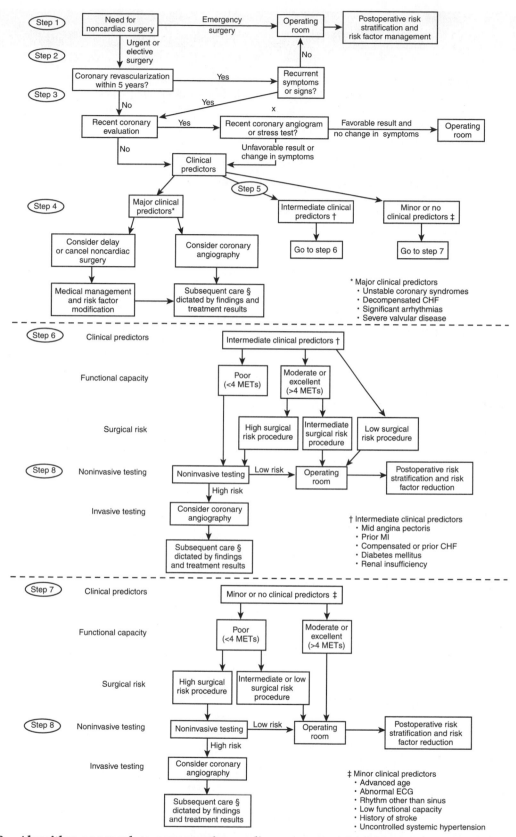

Figure 30-2   Algorithm approach to preoperative cardiac assessment. § Subsequent care may include cancellation or delay of surgery, coronary revascularization followed by noncardiac surgery, or intensified care. CHF, congestive heart failure; ECG, electrocardiogram; MET, metabolic equivalent; MI, myocardial infarction. (Redrawn from *ACC/AHA guideline update for perioperative cardiovascular evaluation for noncardiac surgery*. American Academy of Cardiology and American Heart Association, 2002.)

Box 30-20   Classification of Clinical Indicators for Perioperative Cardiovascular Risk

MAJOR

Unstable coronary syndromes
- Acute or recent myocardial infarction with evidence of important ischemic risk by clinical symptoms or noninvasive study
- Unstable or severe angina (Canadian class III or IV)
- Decompensated heart failure
- Significant arrhythmias
- High-grade atrioventricular block
- Symptomatic ventricular arrhythmias in the presence of underlying heart disease
- Supraventricular arrhythmias with uncontrolled ventricular rate
- Severe valvular disease

INTERMEDIATE
- Mild angina pectoris (Canadian class I or II)
- Previous myocardial infarction by history or pathological Q waves
- Compensated or prior heart failure
- Diabetes mellitus (particularly insulin-dependent)
- Renal insufficiency

MINOR
- Advanced age
- Abnormal electrocardiogram (left ventricular hypertrophy, left bundle branch block, ST–T abnormalities)
- Rhythm other than sinus (e.g., atrial fibrillation)
- Low functional capacity (e.g., inability to climb one flight of stairs with a bag of groceries)
- History of stroke
- Uncontrolled systemic hypertension

From *Practice guidelines for sedation and analgesia by non-anesthesiologists*, 1999, of the American Society of Anesthesiologists.

Box 30-21   Cardiac Risk Stratification for Noncardiac Procedures

HIGH

Reported cardiac risk often >5%
- Emergency major operations, particularly in the elderly
- Aortic and other major vascular surgery
- Peripheral vascular surgery
- Anticipated prolonged surgical procedures associated with large fluid shifts and/or blood loss

INTERMEDIATE

Reported cardiac risk generally <5%
- Carotid endarterectomy
- Head and neck surgery
- Intraperitoneal and intrathoracic surgery
- Orthopedic surgery

LOW

Reported cardiac risk generally <1%
- Endoscopic procedure
- Superficial procedure
- Cataract surgery
- Breast surgery

From *Practice guidelines for sedation and analgesia by non-anesthesiologists*, 1999, of the American Society of Anesthesiologists.

Box 30-22   Guidelines for the Management of Severe Traumatic Brain Injury

Date published: 2000
Organization: Brain Trauma Foundation and the American Association of Neurological Surgeons
Purpose: To provide consensus standards, guidelines, and options for all specialties managing traumatic brain injuries
The recommendations for the initial resuscitation are outlined in Figure 30-3.

SUMMARY OF MATERIAL OF INTEREST TO ANESTHESIOLOGISTS

Key: S, standard; G, guideline; O, option.
General
- All regions should have an organized trauma system (G)
- First priority is rapid physiologic resuscitation, aggressively treating hypotension and hypoxia, and treating for herniation or progressive neurologic deterioration with mannitol and hyperventilation only if present (O)
- Sedation and neuromuscular blockade are used as necessary at physician discretion, with awareness that both impair the ability to assess neurological function (O)
Specific
See Figure 30-4.
Blood Pressure and Oxygenation
- Closely monitor and correct systolic blood pressure <90 mmHg with fluid resuscitation (G)
- Closely monitor and correct arterial oxygen saturation (S_pO_2) <90% or arterial oxygen partial pressure (P_aO_2) <60 mmHg (G)
- Secure airway of patients with Glasgow Coma Scale (GCS) <9 if patient unable to maintain airway or remains hypoxemic despite oxygen therapy (O)
Intracranial Pressure and Cerebral Perfusion Pressure Monitoring and Treatment
- Intracranial pressure (ICP) monitoring is appropriate in severe head injury patients (GCS 3-8) with abnormal computed tomography scan (G)
- ICP also indicated if two of the following present: age >40 years, motor posturing, or systolic blood pressure <90 mmHg (G)
- ICP should be treated above 20-25 mmHg (G)
- Cerebral perfusion pressure should be maintained at a minimum of 70 mmHg (O)
- In the absence of increased ICP, chronic prolonged hyperventilation to P_aCO_2 ≤25 is not recommended (S)
- Prophylactic hyperventilation to P_aCO_2 ≤35 mmHg should be avoided during the first 24 hours after severe traumatic brain injury to avoid compromise of cerebral perfusion (G)
- Hyperventilation may be necessary for brief periods to treat acute neurologic deterioration or when other measures to decrease ICP fail (O)
- Use of S_jO_2, $A_{vd}O_2$, brain tissue oxygen and cerebral blood flow monitoring may help to identify cerebral ischemia when hyperventilation is necessary (O)
- Mannitol therapy (0.25-1.0 g/kg) is effective for control of increased ICP (G):
  - Indicated prior to ICP monitoring when signs of herniation or progressive neurological deterioration not otherwise explainable are present (O)
  - Should be accompanied by measurement and maintenance of serum osmolality below 320 mosmol/L for renal protection (O)
  - Should be accompanied by maintenance of euvolemia (O)
  - May be more effective as bolus versus infusion (O)
- High-dose barbiturate therapy may be considered if patient is hemodynamically stable, salvageable, and has ICP refractory to all other medical and surgical interventions (G)
- Steroids are not recommended in the treatment of increased ICP

From *Management and prognosis of severe traumatic brain injury (TBI), part I: Guidelines for the management of severe traumatic brain injury*, 2000. Brain Trauma Foundation and American Association of Neurological Surgeons.

Initial Management

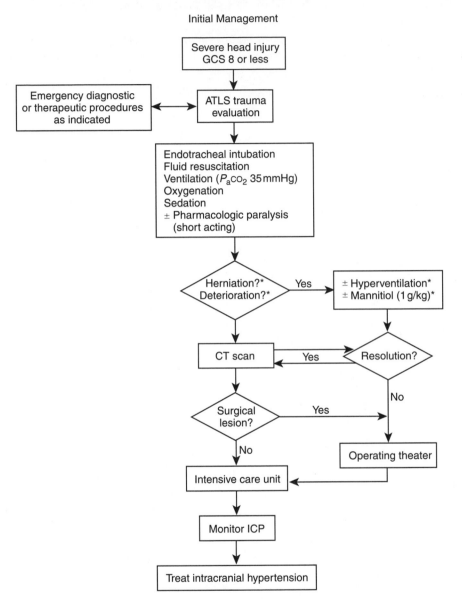

* Only in the presence of signs of herniation or progressive neurologic deterioration not attributable to extracranial factors.

Figure 30-3   Initial resuscitation of the severally head-injured patient. ATLS, Advanced Trauma Life Support; CT, computed tomography; GCS, Glasgow Coma Scale, ICP, intracranial pressure; Pt, patient. (Redrawn from *Management and prognosis of severe traumatic brain injury*. Brain Trauma Foundation, 2000.)

Critical pathway for treatment of intracranial hypertension

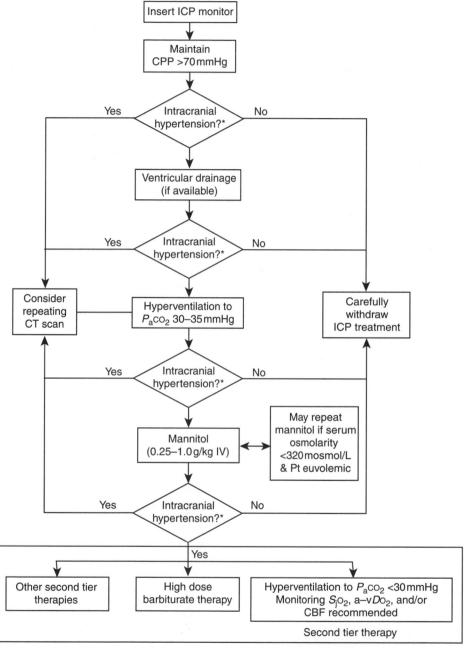

* Threshold of 20–25 mmHg may be used. Other variable may be substituted in individual conditions.

Figure 30-4   Critical pathway for treatment of intracranial hypertension. CT, computed tomography; CBF, coronary blood flow, CPP, cerebral perfusion pressure; ICP, intracranial pressure. (Redrawn from *Management and prognosis of severe traumatic brain injury*. Brain Trauma Foundation, 2000.)

Box 30-23   Guidelines on Regional Anesthesia in the Anticoagulated Patient

Date published: 2002 (available online from http://www.asra.com/items_of_interest/consensus_statements/index.iphtml
Organization: American Society of Regional Anesthesia and Pain Medicine
Purpose: To provide consensus recommendations for the use of neuraxial anesthesia in patients with various anticoagulant regimens in effect
Summary of recommendations:

PATIENTS RECEIVING THROMBOLYTIC THERAPY

- Should generally not receive neuraxial block during fibrinolytic or thrombolytic therapy, for probably 10 days thereafter
- Frequent (e.g., every 2 hr) neurological monitoring should be maintained for patients receiving thrombolytics with a neuraxial block, and local anesthetic agents should be adjusted to minimize sensory/motor blockade
- There are no specific recommendations for catheter removal during the period of thrombolytic effectiveness. Fibrinogen level may be helpful
- Concurrent heparin and thrombolytics place neuraxial block at an even higher risk, and antiplatelet therapy adds further risk

PATIENTS RECEIVING UNFRACTIONATED HEPARIN

- There are no contraindications to the use of subcutaneous or heparin. It may be helpful to administer heparin after block placement, and extended heparin therapy should warrant assessment of platelets
- Neuraxial anesthesia can be combined with intraoperative heparin under the following circumstances:
  - Do not use neuraxial anesthesia in patients with additional coagulopathies
  - Delay heparin until 1 hour after needle placement
  - Remove the catheter one hour prior to a heparin dose, or 2–4 hours after the last heparin dose
  - Monitor for unexpected motor blockade and use minimal local anesthetic concentrations
  - Bloody or difficult block is not necessarily a cause for case cancellation, but should be discussed with surgeons and monitored carefully postoperatively
- Insufficient data is available to assess the safety of neuraxial block after full anticoagulation
- Concurrent combination anticoagulant therapy may increase risk

PATIENTS RECEIVING LOW-MOLECULAR-WEIGHT HEPARIN

- Anti-Xa monitoring is not recommended
- Concomitant additional anticoagulant therapy may increase risk
- Bloody or difficult block should delay low-molecular-weight heparin (LMWH) therapy initiation for 24 hours
- Preoperative LMWH therapy may alter coagulation:
  - Single-dose spinal anesthesia may be safest, and should be delayed for 10–12 hours after the last LMWH dose
  - Higher doses of LMWH should have neuraxial anesthesia delayed for at least 24 hours
  - Avoid neuraxial anesthesia in patients receiving LMWH 2 hours preoperatively
- Postoperative LMWH therapy:
  - If using twice-daily dosing, there is increased risk of spinal hematoma, and indwelling catheters should be removed prior to LMWH, or the first dose of LMWH should be administered more than 2 hours after catheter removal
  - If using once-daily dosing, first dose given 6–8 hours postoperatively, and the second no sooner than 24 hours later. Indwelling catheters may be used safely, but should be removed no less than 10–12 hours after the last dose of LMWH, and subsequent LMWH dosing should occur no less than 2 hours after catheter removal

PATIENTS ON ORAL ANTICOAGULANTS (WARFARIN)

- Therapy should ideally be stopped 4–5 days prior to surgery
- Other anticoagulant/antiplatelet therapy may increase risk. The prothrombin time (PT)/international normalized ratio (INR) should be checked prior to neuraxial block if the first dose of warfarin was given more than 24 hours prior to block, or a second dose has been given. Patients on low-dose warfarin should have daily PT/INR monitoring, and should have PT/INR checked prior to catheter removal if initial warfarin therapy was started more than 36 hours preoperatively
- Catheters should be removed when INR is <1.5
- Routine neurologic testing should be done for patients with neuraxial catheters on warfarin therapy, and continued for 24 hours after catheter removal (longer if INR was >1.5 at the time of removal). As with other therapies, minimal concentrations of local anesthesia that produced satisfactory analgesia should be used
- If INR >3, warfarin should be held or reduced in the presence of a neuraxial catheter
- Decreased warfarin dosage should be used if patients have an enhanced response to warfarin

Continued

Box 30-23   Guidelines on Regional Anesthesia in the Anticoagulated Patient—cont'd

PATIENTS RECEIVING ANTIPLATELET MEDICATIONS

- No test is totally accepted for measuring antiplatelet activity. Clinical correlation is necessary.
- Nonsteroidal anti-inflammatory drugs do not appear to increase risk, and there are no concerns regarding timing or type of neuraxial block or the need for postoperative neurologic monitoring. The various specific antiplatelet agents (e.g., thienopyridine derivatives) and GP IIb/IIIa antagonists can increase risk, and each specific agent has a recommended time of discontinuation prior to placement of neuraxial block.
- There are no data indicating risk of combination of antiplatelet agents with other anticoagulation, but the consensus is that they may increase bleeding complications. COX-2 inhibitors appear to have a minimal effect on platelet function and should be considered.

PATIENTS RECEIVING HERBAL THERAPY

- Herbal medications do not appear to increase risk of bleeding with neuraxial blocks and there are no data to suggest that they should be discontinued prior to surgery or that surgery should be canceled for patients on herbal therapy
- Other anticoagulation therapy combined with herbal therapy may increase risk
- There is no well-accepted test for the adequacy of hemostasis in patients using herbal medications. Clinical correlation is indicated. The timing of neuraxial block is not a factor

NEWER ANTICOAGULANTS (FONDAPARINUX™)

- Extreme caution should be exercised in patients on this agent. Current clinical data are insufficient to make specific recommendations otherwise. Close monitoring of the surgical literature may be helpful

From *Guidelines on regional anesthesia in the anticoagulated patient*, 2002. American Society of Regional Anesthesia and Pain Medicine.

SUMMARY

Anesthesiology's lead in safety and quality management is directly attributable to the willingness of the specialty to provide extensive, authoritative, peer-reviewed information to the practitioners' setting, for the best methods of practice for a wide variety of clinical situations, and practice management. We have described in this chapter the important points contained in the guidelines prepared by the ASA and other formative bodies of interest to anesthesiologists. The reader can easily access the full text of these documents in publications available from the ASA, the other organizations, or the World Wide Web.

SELECTED READING

http://www.guideline.gov – a complete listing of the guidelines relevant to anesthetic practice.

http://www.anesthesiology.org – click on the link to ASA Practice Parameters to view all ASA Practice Parameters.

http://www.braintrauma.org – click on the guidelines link and then the link entitled "Management and Prognosis of Severe Traumatic Brain Injury" for a full copy of the 2000 Brain Trauma Foundation Guidelines.

http://www.acc.org/clinical/guidelines/perio/update/periupdate_index.htm – detail on the ACC/AHA Guideline Update for Perioperative Cardiovascular Evaluation for Noncardiac Surgery – Executive Summary.

http://www.asra.com/items_of_interest/consensus_statements/index.iphtml – detail on the Guidelines on Regional Anesthesia in the Anticoagulated Patient.

Index

Note: Page numbers followed by 'f' refer to figures; page numbers followed by 't' refer to tables.